W9-BQF-509

The Foundations of Chinese Medicine

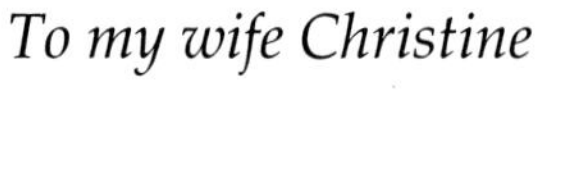

To my wife Christine

The Foundations of Chinese Medicine

A Comprehensive Text for Acupuncturists and Herbalists

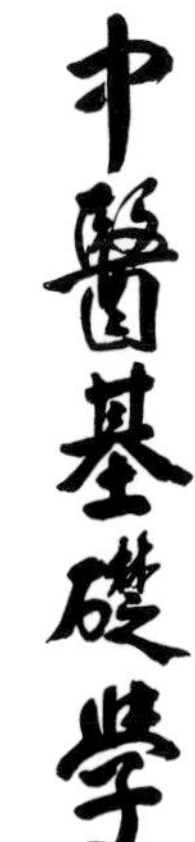

Giovanni Maciocia CAc (Nanjing)
Acupuncturist and Medical Herbalist, UK; Visiting Associate Professor at the Nanjing University of Traditional Chinese Medicine, Nanjing, People's Republic of China.

Foreword by

Dr Su Xin Ming
Associate Professor, Nanjing College of Traditional Chinese Medicine

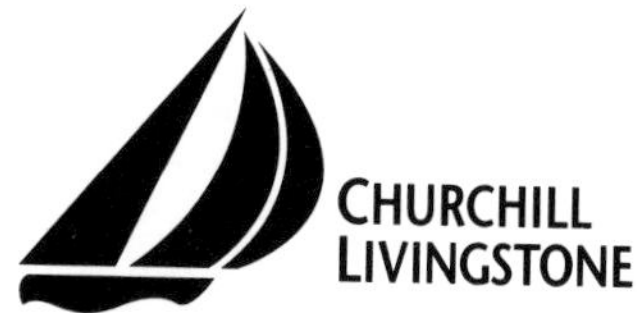

EDINBURGH LONDON NEW YORK OXFORD PHILADELPHIA ST LOUIS
SYDNEY TORONTO 1989

CHURCHILL LIVINGSTONE
An imprint of Elsevier Science Limited

First published 1989
Reprinted thirteen times between 1990 and 1998
Reprinted 2000, 2001, 2002, 2003

ISBN 0-443-03980-1

British Library Cataloguing in Publication Data
Maciocia, Giovanni
The foundations of Chinese medicine.
1. Chinese medicine
I. Title.
610'.951

Library of Congress Cataloging in Publication Data
Maciocia, Giovanni
The foundations of Chinese medicine.
Bibliography: p.
1. Medicine, Chinese-Philosophy. 2. Acupuncturists.
3. Herbalists. I. Title.
R601.M23 1989 610'.951 88-20339

Note
Medical knowledge is constantly changing. As new information becomes available, changes in treatment, procedures, equipment and the use of drugs become necessary. The editors, authors, contributors and the publishers have, as far as it is possible, taken care to ensure that the information given in this text is accurate and up to date. However, readers are strongly advised to confirm that the information, especially with regard to drug usage, complies with latest legislation and standards of practice.

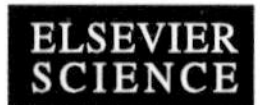

your source for books, journals and multimedia in the health sciences

www.elsevierhealth.com

The publisher's policy is to use **paper manufactured from sustainable forests**

Printed in China
C/19

Foreword

Acupuncture is an important part of Traditional Chinese Medicine. Over the past 2500 years medical scholars in every age have contributed to the development and refinement of the art of acupuncture in China.

During his three visits to China Giovanni Maciocia studied acupuncture conscientiously with Chinese doctors and teachers. He combined and adapted what he learned in China to Western conditions and successfully treated a large number of patients. He has also overcome language barriers to read Chinese medical classics. He spent many years studying and teaching Chinese Medicine in order to develop it for the benefit of patients and students. This spirit is highly appreciated by all those who know him.

His book "The Foundations of Chinese Medicine" is based on his many years of experience in practising and teaching Chinese Medicine. It is detailed in its contents, it adapts the theory of Chinese Medicine to a Western medical practice and is solidly based on the ancient Chinese classics. His book is unique in so far as it combines a rigorous scholarship with his wealth of clinical experience. It will be invaluable not only to students as a textbook, but also to acupuncturists and herbalists as a rich source of clinical information.

Nanjing 1989 Dr Su Xin Ming

Preface

Han dynasty, 154 BC, North China. A peasant works in the millet fields in springtime. A bitterly cold North wind is blowing. In the afternoon after work, she has an itchy throat, a runny nose, a cough and a severe stiff neck and headache. She visits the local acupuncturist who diagnoses an invasion of exterior Wind-Cold. The acupuncturist inserts a few needles in the peasant's hands and applies cupping to two points in the upper back, which produces a marked improvement after a few hours.

AD 1988, London, England. A fund manager from the City of London suffers from anxiety and insomnia. He works long hours and under considerable pressure as he is responsible for the management of several million-pound funds. A colleague at work had tried acupuncture to stop smoking and recommends him to his acupuncturist who diagnoses a case of Liver-Qi stagnation from the pressure of work. He inserts a few needles to remove the stagnation of Liver-Qi and calm the mind. After a few weekly treatments there is a considerable improvement.

Such is the awesome power of Chinese medicine that, even if it originated thousands of years ago and came to maturity a few hundred years before Christ, it can successfully diagnose and treat twentieth century health problems generated by a life-style which is light-years away from that of the ancient peasant society from which Chinese medicine originated.

Much is made of the cultural difference between the Chinese and Western societies. Of course, Chinese medicine arose out of China and therefore bears the cultural imprint of that society. Moreover, the way the theory of Chinese medicine is taught in modern China obviously reflects a materialistic approach. For example, the concept of *Shen* (the mental aspect of the Heart) is accepted, but not that of *Hun* or *Po* (the spiritual aspects of the Liver and Lungs). However, each society gives a particular imprint to the medicine they inherit. For example, Chinese herbal medicine during the Warring states period was mostly influenced by Daoist philosophy, whereas during the Han dynasty it was influenced by the Confucian and Legalist philosophies. During the Song dynasty, it was heavily influenced by the Neo-Confucian philosophy of the School of Principle (*Li*). Although the modern Chinese, with their materialistic philosophical orientation, have ignored or glossed over certain aspects of Chinese medicine, credit must be given to them for carrying out a useful and important sytematization of the theory of Chinese medicine. Moreover, we should not think that everything contained in the old classics is a pearl of wisdom. Even the greatest Chinese doctors such as Li Shi Zhen or Sun Si Miao clung to old superstitious beliefs and used some bizarre substances in their clinical practice. For example, Li Shi Zhen included the rope of a suicide victim as a medicinal "drug".[1] I feel we should be grateful for the work of modern Chinese doctors and teachers in sifting out such worthless aspects from the old classics.

Thus, although there are cultural differences between Chinese and Western societies, these should not be over-emphasized. One of the strongest points of Chinese medicine, and one which makes it truly universal, is its simplicity. For example, the causes of disease (climate, emotions, diet, and so on) are so basic that they can apply to any society and any time. Anger, sadness, grief, worry are such basic human feelings that they are certainly cross-cultural.

Of course, we do need to adapt Chinese medicine to Western culture and conditions, but this adaptation can only take place on the solid foundation of the theory of Traditional Chinese Medicine. One cannot adapt something if it is not mastered first. If the adaptation takes place without a true understanding of the theory and practice of Chinese medicine, it will result in spurious forms of "acupuncture" which are neither Chinese nor Western and which in the end will discredit Chinese medicine because of their poor therapeutic results.

When we talk about adapting Chinese medicine to Western conditions we must also remember that we cannot generalize about "Western culture". The cultural habits and beliefs of a Sicilian peasant are as far removed from those of a New York businessman as the latter's are from those of a Chinese peasant. In fact, the cultural beliefs of a Sicilian peasant are probably closer to those of a Chinese peasant than to those of a New York businessman.

One of the most important adaptations we need to make is semantic. The symptoms and signs found in Chinese medical books are those expressed by Chinese patients. Although Western patients will basically experience the same symptoms, they will be expressed in a different way. For example, "distending pain" (i.e. the typical sensation of distension and pain caused by Qi stagnation) is a commonly used term in China. An English person experiencing the same sensation will say that he or she feels "like bursting around the middle" or "bloated" Whenever possible, I have included some of these English expressions within the relevant patterns. On the other hand, sometimes Western patients can describe symptoms in a way that is remarkably similar to that of Chinese patients. For example, the following are three expressions used by English patients in my practice in the past month: "This rainy weather makes me damp", "I feel as if I have a stone in my throat" (a person presenting the pattern of "plum-stone in the throat") and "I have been sweaty on my chest and palms" (a person with Yin-deficient 5-palm sweating). It should be added that these patients were not acupuncture students.

Conversely, Western patients have a different life-style and a different cultural attitude to their emotional life than Chinese patients, and will tend to express their feelings much more. The following are examples of expressions used by English patients which are not found in Chinese medical books: "After treatment I felt more in touch with my grief", "I feel not grounded", "Lately I have been more withdrawn" and "I feel not properly in control". With experience, we can learn to interpret these feelings in the light of Chinese medical theory.

The aim of the present book is to give a detailed account of the theory of Chinese medicine and acupuncture. I have tried to present the theory of Chinese medicine based on a rigorous reference to ancient and modern Chinese books, as well as to explain its application in a Western practice. I am well aware that there are other perfectly valid acupuncture traditions, notably the Japanese and Korean ones, which differ considerably from the Chinese one. However, they differ more in their techniques than in their basic theoretical premises, which they share with Chinese acupuncture as presented in this book has proved its clinical validity all over the world in many different cultural situations for a wide variety of diseases. I believe it is a solid foundation from which one can build and branch out in many different directions.

This book presents the complete body of the theory of Chinese Medicine which is common to both acupuncture and Chinese herbalism. In addition, it discusses the use of the acupuncture points in detail and the principles of treatment. The location and indications of points as well as techniques of acupuncture have been left out, firstly because they can be found in other books and secondly because, had they been included, it would have made the book far too long and unwieldy. These subjects will be dealt with in a future book so that the two volumes will form a complete textbook of the theory of Chinese Medicine and the practice of acupuncture.

It is hoped that this book will help practitioners and students of Chinese Medicine in their practice and provide a solid foundation for the development of Chinese medicine in the world.

Amersham 1989 G.M.

NOTES

1 Unschuld P 1986 Medicine in China — A History of Pharmaceutics, University of California Press, Los Angeles, p. 151.

2 Wallis-Budge EA 1928 Divine Origin of the Herbalists, Society of Herbalists, p 51–52.

Acknowledgements

This book would not have been possible without the help of my teachers, friends and family.

Dr Su Xin Ming of the Nanjing College of Traditional Chinese Medicine first taught me the practical application of the principles of Chinese Medicine. During my three stays in China, he patiently shared with me his deep knowledge and skills.

I am indebted to Dr J H F Shen for communicating to me his great skills, particularly in pulse diagnosis.

My friend Michael McIntyre read the whole manuscript and provided immense help with the style. He also enhanced the book a great deal with his invaluable comments, suggestions and criticism.

My friend Linda Upton not only drew some of the drawings with neat skill, but also imaginatively and creatively expressed in her drawings the ideas I was trying to convey.

I am grateful to Dr Xiao Shao Qin of the Nanjing College of Traditional Chinese Medicine for painting the majority of the Chinese characters. I also wish to express my thanks to Miss Rose Li and Dr Huang Liu Xin for painting some of them.

I am also indebted to the director, teachers, interpreters and staff of the Nanjing College of Traditional Chinese Medicine for their constant support and encouragement with my book and for their help during my three stays there where I learned the theory and practice of Chinese Medicine.

Finally this book would not have come to reality without the help, support and inspiration of my wife Christine. To her I am deeply grateful.

Note on the Translation of Chinese Medicine Terms

Throughout the book I have adopted the principle of translating all Chinese Medicine terms, the only exception being *"Qi"*, *"Yin"*, *"Yang"*, the names of the acupuncture points and the abbreviations *"Du"* and *"Ren"* for the points of the Governing and Directing vessels.

The terms Qi, Yin and Yang are left untranslated since they are concepts which are so peculiar to Chinese Medicine as to be nearly impossible to translate. They are so well known that translation is not really necessary.

I have used the abbreviations *"Du"* and *"Ren"* for the points of the Governing and Directing vessels as, having introduced a new translation for the *Ren Mai* (Directing Vessel), an abbreviation such as "DV" (instead of the more usual "CV") might have been difficult to comprehend.

The English translation of the acupuncture point names is given in the chapter on the function of the points, but when a point is mentioned elsewhere in the text, both the Chinese name and the Western number is given. This was done because the Chinese name is still the only firm term of reference to identify a point, as the English translation may differ from text to text and so can the numbering system. The point numbering system used is the same as in the "Essentials of Chinese Acupuncture".[1] I have used abbreviations of the organ names to identify the points and a list of these abbreviations is given in the glossary. The only exception is, as explained above, in the use of *"Ren"* (as in Ren-12) for the Directing Vessel and *"Du"* (as in Du-14) for the Governing Vessel.

It is extremely difficult to translate Chinese medical terminology into English, and nearly every single Western acupuncture book uses different translations for the various Chinese terms. This is understandable as every writer tries to find as close an approximation as possible to the original Chinese meaning. The result is a very confusing variety of different translations for the same Chinese term. For example, *"Zong Qi"* (the Qi of the chest) is variously translated as "Essential Qi"[2], "Ancestral Qi"[3] and "Genetic Qi"[4].

I have reviewed afresh all Chinese medical terms and tried to tread a middle way between changing established translations whenever I thought it essential, and keeping certain others on account of established use. For example, one could not keep the term "sympathy" as a translation of the "emotion" corresponding to the Spleen in the 5-Element scheme of correspondences as it is obviously wrong (the term *"Si"* means "pensiveness" or "thought"). On the other hand, even though the term "Excess" is not quite right as a translation of the Chinese term *"Shi"*, I have kept it alongside the better translation of "Fullness" or "Full", as in some cases it provides a more fluent English style.

Being well aware of the reader's difficulties in encountering yet new translations of Chinese terms, I have tried to keep the changes to a minimum. The main instances where I have departed from established translations are:

— "Gathering Qi" for *Zong Qi* 宗气 (the Qi of the chest)

— "Back Transporting" points for *Bei Shu* 背俞 points, i.e. the points on the Bladder channel on the back.

— "Front Collecting" points for *Mu* 募 points , i.e. the so-called "alarm" points or "Front-Mu" points.

— "Gathering" points for *Hui* 会 points , i.e. the eight points corresponding to various tissues such as sinews, bones, blood vessels, etc.

— "Directing Vessel" for *Ren Mai*, usually translated as "Conception Vessel".

I have changed this last name because the term "Conception vessel" is obviously a mistranslation. The Chinese character for *Ren* 任 means "to direct", "to take up a job" or "to appoint". This fits in well with the function of this vessel as the director of all Yin channels (in the same way as the Governing Vessels governs all Yang channels). The translation of *Ren* as "conception" might have come from mistaking the character 任 with 妊 which does mean conception. It is easy to see how this could have been done as the Directing Vessel does influence conception, but this is only one of its many functions.

Most other terms are the same as in "The Essentials of Chinese Acupuncture", the "Web that has no Weaver", "Tongue Diagnosis in Chinese Medicine" [5] and "Acupuncture-A Comprehensive Text" [6].

As for the term " Elements", I have decided, after much consideration and pondering, to keep this translation not only because of a very strong established use, but also because it is actually semantically correct, and I explain this in the relevant chapter (see ch. 2). The term "5 Phases" is being increasingly used but is, in my opinion, not quite correct as the 5 Elements are much more than just "phases" of a cyclical movement.

I have translated Shen (of the Heart) as "Mind" rather than "Spirit". The reason for this is explained in the chapter on the Heart functions (p. 71) and, in this connection, I strongly recommend the reader to read also note 6) on page 75.

I have translated the terms "*Shi*" and "*Xu*" as either Fullness-Emptiness (or Full-Empty) or Excess-Deficiency according to the context and in order to provide a more readable style. Strictly speaking, "Excess" and "Deficiency" are not quite correct as they imply that they are two poles along the same axis, i.e. too much or too little of the same. In actual fact, they indicate two different terms of reference: "Excess" refers to excess of a pathogenic factor, whereas "Deficiency" refers to deficiency of the body's normal Qi. So while the term "Deficiency" is right, the term "Excess" does not adequately convey the Chinese idea. "*Shi*" means "solid", "full", and it indicates a condition characterized by "fullness" of a pathogenic factor, not an "excess" of normal body's Qi. Thus "Fullness" and "Emptiness" (or "Full" and "Empty") would, strictly speaking, be a better translation.

Whenever words indicate specific concepts and phenomena peculiar to Chinese Medicine, they are capitalized; when the same words refer to the common Western entities, they are not. For example, all the names of the internal organs are capitalized to indicate the concept of Internal Organ as understood in Chinese Medicine. Thus "Heart" refers to the Chinese medical concept of Heart, whereas "heart" indicates the actual anatomical organ in a Western medical sense.

Similarly, "Exterior" indicates the superficial energetic layers of the body in a Chinese Medicine sense. "Phlegm" denotes the Chinese concept of Phlegm as a pathogenic factor with very wide-ranging manifestations while "phlegm" indicates the mucus or sputum which is coughed up.

Finally, the translation of certain terms indicating Chinese medical disease entities should be explained. I use the term "Painful Obstruction Syndrome" for Bi syndrome (i.e. pain in the joints from external Dampness, Cold, Wind or Heat), "Atrophy Syndrome" for Wei syndrome (i.e. muscle weakness, flaccidity or atrophy), "Wind-stroke" for Zhong Feng (i.e. the sudden unconsciousness and paralysis caused by interior Wind) and "Difficult Urination Syndrome" for Lin syndrome (i.e. the symptoms of urinary difficulty and pain).

I have provided a full glossary with Chinese characters, pinyin transliteration and English translations (see p. 485).

NOTES

1 Nanjing-Beijing-Shanghai Colleges of Traditional Chinese Medicine and the Acupuncture Institute of the Academy of Traditional Chinese Medicine 1980 Essentials of Chinese Acupuncture, Beijing.
2 Essentials of Chinese Acupuncture.
3 Kaptchuk T 1983 The Web that has no Weaver-Understanding Chinese Medicine, Congdon & Weed, New York.
4 Porkert M., 1974 The theoretical Foundations of Chinese Medicine, Massachusetts Institute of Technology.
5 Maciocia G 1987, Tongue Diagnosis in Chinese Medicine, Eastland Press, Seattle.
6 O'Connor J, Bensky D 1981 Acupuncture — A Comprehensive Text. Eastland Press, Chicago.

Contents

Yin Yang 1 陰陽

The concept of Yin-Yang is probably the single most important and distinctive theory of Chinese Medicine. It could be said that all Chinese medical physiology, pathology and treatment can, eventually, be reduced to Yin-Yang. The concept of Yin-Yang is extremely simple, yet very profound. One can seemingly understand it on a rational level, and yet, continually find new expressions of it in clinical practice and, indeed, in life.

The concept of Yin-Yang, together with that of Qi, has permeated Chinese philosophy over the centuries and is radically different to any Western philosophical idea. In general, Western Logic is based upon the opposition of contraries which is the fundamental premise of Aristotelian logic. According to this Logic, contraries (such as "The table is square" and "The table is not square") cannot both be true. This has dominated Western thought for over 2,000 years. The Chinese concept of Yin-Yang is radically different to this system of thought: Yin and Yang represent opposite but complementary qualities. Each thing or phenomenon could be itself and its contrary. Moreover, Yin contains the seed of Yang and vice versa, so that, contrary to Aristotelian logic, A can also be *NON-A*.

HISTORICAL DEVELOPMENT

The earliest reference to Yin and Yang is probably the one in the "Book of Changes" (*Yi Jing*), dating back to about 700 BC. In this book Yin and Yang are represented by broken and unbroken lines (Fig. 1).

The combination of broken and unbroken lines in pairs forms four pairs of diagrams representing utmost Yin, utmost Yang and two intermediate stages (Fig. 2).

The addition of another line to these four diagrams forms, with varying combinations, the eight trigrams (Fig. 3).

Finally, the various combinations of the trigrams gives rise to the 64 hexagrams. These are supposed to symbolize all possible phenomena of the universe, and it therefore shows how all phenomena ultimately depend on the two poles of Yin and Yang.

The philosophical school that developed the theory of Yin Yang to its highest degree, is called the Yin -Yang School. Many schools of thought arose during the

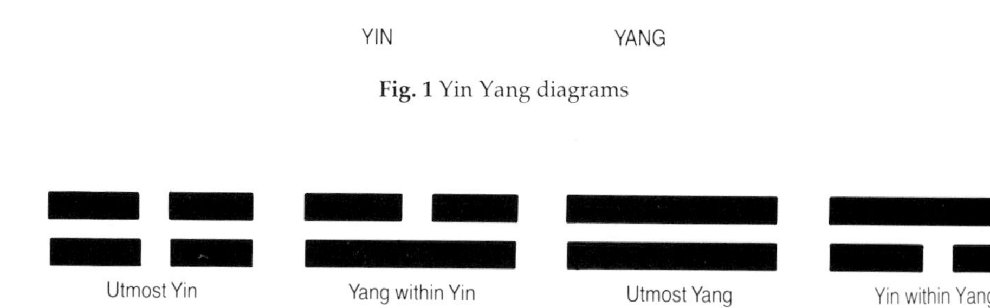

Fig. 1 Yin Yang diagrams

Fig. 2 Four stages of Yin Yang

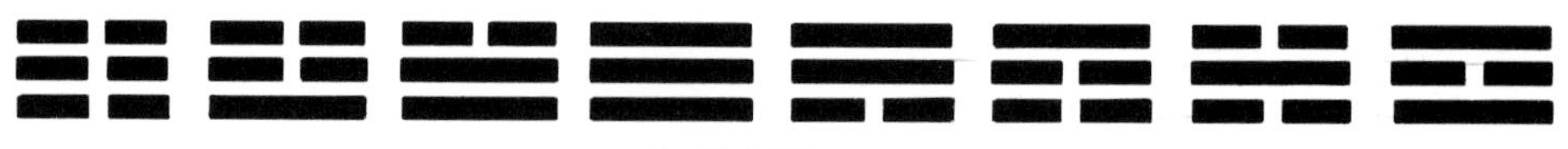

Fig. 3 The Eight Trigrams

Warring States period (476–221 BC), and the Yin-Yang school was one of them. It dedicated itself to the study of Yin-Yang and the 5 Elements and its main exponent was Zou Yan (c. 350–270 BC). This school is sometimes also called the Naturalist School as it set out to interpret Nature in a positive way and to use natural laws to man's advantage, not through attempting to control and subdue Nature (as in modern Western science), but by acting in harmony with its laws. This school represents a form of what we might call naturalist science today, and the theories of Yin-Yang and the 5 Elements served to interpret natural phenomena, including the human body, in health and disease.

The theories of Yin-Yang and the 5 Elements, systematically elaborated by the Naturalist school, later became the common heritage of subsequent schools of thought, particularly the Neo-Confucianist schools of the Song, Ming and Qing dynasty. These schools combined most of the elements from the previous schools of thought to form a coherent philosophy of Nature, Ethics, Social Order and Astrology.[1]

I will discuss Yin-Yang from a general philosophical point of view first, and then from a medical point of view.

NATURE OF YIN-YANG CONCEPT

The Chinese characters for "Yin" and "Yang" are related to the dark and sunny side of a hill. The characters are:

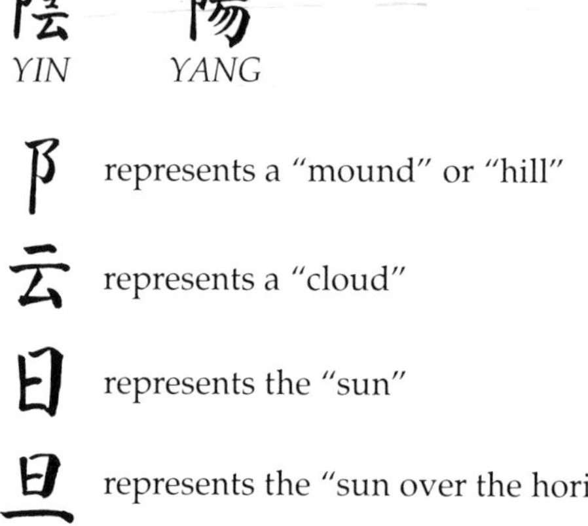

Thus the character for Yin indicates the shady side of a hill, whilst the character for Yang indicates the sunny side of a hill. By extension, they therefore also indicate "darkness" and "light" or "shady" and "bright".

YIN-YANG AS TWO PHASES OF A CYCLICAL MOVEMENT

The earliest origin of Yin-Yang phenomena must have derived from the peasants' observation of the cyclical alternation of day and night. Thus Day corresponds to Yang and Night to Yin, and, by extension, Activity to Yang and Rest to Yin. This led to the first observation of the continuous alternation of every phenomenon between two cyclical poles, one corresponding to Light, Sun, Brightness and Activity (Yang), the other corresponding to Darkness, Moon, Shade and Rest (Yin). From this point of view, Yin and Yang are two stages of a cyclical movement, one constantly changing into the other, such as the day giving way to night and vice versa.

Heaven (where the sun is) is therefore Yang and Earth is Yin. The ancient Chinese farmers conceived Heaven as a round vault, and the Earth as flat. Hence, Round is Yang and Square is Yin. The Heaven, containing the sun, moon and stars on which the Chinese farmers based their calendar therefore corresponds to Time; the Earth, which is parcelled out into fields corresponds to Space.

Because the sun rises in the East and sets in the West, the former is Yang and the latter Yin. If we face South, East will be on the left and West on the right. In Chinese cosmology, the compass directions were established assuming that one faced South. This was also reflected in imperial ceremonials when *"The Emperor faced South towards his subjects who faced North... The Emperor thus opened himself to receive the influence of Heaven, Yang and South. South is therefore like Heaven, at the top; North is therefore like Earth, at the bottom... By facing South, the Emperor indentifies his left with East and his right with West"*.[2]

Thus, Left corresponds to Yang and Right to Yin. The "Simple Questions" relates the correspondence Yang-Left and Yin-Right to physiology. It says: *"East represents Yang... West represents Yin... in the West and North there is a deficiency of Heaven, hence the left ear and eyes hear and see better than the right; in the East and South there is a deficiency of Earth, hence the right hand and foot are stronger than the left."* [3]

The characters for "left" and "right" clearly show their relation with Yin and Yang as that for left includes the symbol for work (activity = Yang), and that for right includes a mouth (which eats products of the Earth which is Yin).[4]

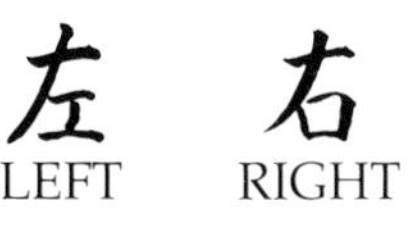

LEFT RIGHT

工 represents "work"

口 represents "mouth"

We therefore have the first correspondences:

Yang	*Yin*
Light	Darkness
Sun	Moon
Brightness	Shade
Activity	Rest
Heaven	Earth
Round	Flat
Time	Space
East	West
South	North
Left	Right

Thus, from this point of view, Yin and Yang are essentially an expression of a duality in time, an alternation of two opposite stages in time. Every phenomenon in the universe alternates through a cyclical movement of peaks and bases, and the alternation of Yin and Yang is the motive force of its change and development. Day changes into night, summer into winter, growth into decay and vice versa. Thus the development of all phenomena in the universe is the result of the interplay of two opposite stages, symbolized by Yin and Yang and every phenomenon contains within itself both aspects in different degrees of manifestation. The Day belongs to Yang but after reaching its peak at midday, the Yin within it gradually begins to unfold and manifest. Thus each phenomenon may belong to a Yang or Yin stage but always contains the seed of the opposite stage within itself. The daily cycle clearly illustrates this (Fig. 4):

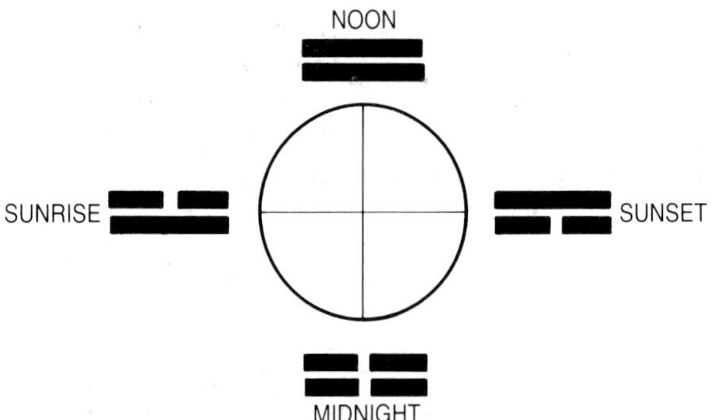

Fig. 4 Yin Yang in daily cycle

Exactly the same happens with the yearly cycle and we only need to substitute "Spring" for "dawn", "Summer" for "noon", Autumn" for "dusk" and "Winter" for "midnight".

Thus:

Spring	=	Yang within Yin
	=	growth of Yang
Summer	=	Yang within Yang
	=	maximum Yang
Autumn	=	Yin within Yang
	=	growth of Yin
Winter	=	Yin within Yin
	=	maximum Yin.

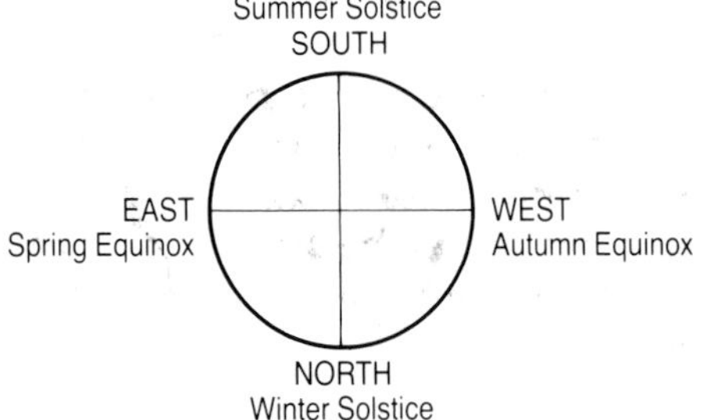

Fig. 5 Yin Yang in seasonal cycle

The two intermediate stages (dawn-Spring and dusk-Autumn) do not represent neutral stages in between Yin and Yang: they still pertain primarily to one or the other (i.e. dawn-Spring pertain to Yang and dusk-Autumn pertain to Yin), so that the cycle can always be narrowed down to a polarity of two stages.

YIN-YANG AS TWO STAGES OF TRANSFORMATION

From a different viewpoint, Yin and Yang stand for two stages in the process of change and transformation of all things in the universe. As we have seen above, everything goes through phases of a cycle, and in so doing, its form also changes. For example, the water in lakes and seas heats up during the day and is transformed into vapour. As the air cools down in the evening, vapour condenses into water again.

Form can be more or less dense material. From this point of view, Yang symbolizes the more immaterial, rarefied states of matter, whereas Yin symbolizes the more material, dense states of matter. To use the same example, water in its liquid state pertains to Yin, and the vapour resulting from heat pertains to Yang. This duality in the states of condensation of things was often symbolized in ancient China by the duality of "Heaven" and "Earth". "Heaven" symbolized all rarefied, immaterial, pure and gas-like states of things, whereas "Earth" symbolizes all dense, material, coarse and solid states of things. The "Simple Questions" in chapter 2 says: *"Heaven is an accumulation of Yang, Earth is an accumulation of Yin"*.[5]

The important thing to understand is that the two opposite states of condensation or aggregation of things are not independent of each other, but they change into each other. Yin and Yang also symbolize two opposite states of aggregation of things. Lie Zi, a Daoist philosopher (c. 300 BC) said: *"The purer and lighter [elements] tending upwards made the Heaven; the grosser and heavier, tending downwards, made the Earth"*.[6]

In its purest and most rarefied form, Yang is totally immaterial and corresponds to pure energy, and Yin, in its coarsest and densest form, is totally material and corresponds to matter. From this viewpoint, energy and matter are but two states of a continuum, with an infinite possible number of states of aggregation. The "Simple Questions" in chapter 2 says: *"Yin is quiet, Yang is active. Yang gives life, Yin makes it grow... Yang is transformed into Qi, Yin is transformed into material life"*.[7]

As Yang corresponds to creation and activity, it naturally also corresponds to expansion and it rises. As Yin corresponds to condensation and materialization, it naturally also corresponds to contraction and it descends. Thus we can add a few more qualities to the list of Yin-Yang correspondences:

Yang	*Yin*
Immaterial	Material
Produces energy	Produces form
Generates	Grows
Non-substantial	Substantial
Energy	Matter
Expansion	Contraction
Rising	Descending
Above	Below
Fire	Water

The relationship and interdependence of Yin-Yang can be represented in the famous symbol (Fig. 6). This symbol is called the "Supreme Ultimate" (*Tai Ji*) and it represents well the interdependence of Yin and Yang.

The main points of this interdependence are:

a) Although they are opposite stages, Yin-Yang form a unity and are complementary.

b) Yang contains the seed of Yin and vice versa. This is represented by the small black and white spots.

c) Nothing is totally Yin or totally Yang.

d) Yang changes into Yin and vice versa.

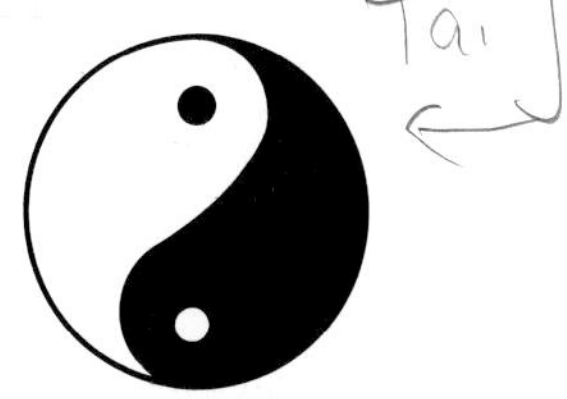

Fig. 6 Symbol of Yin and Yang

FOUR ASPECTS OF YIN-YANG RELATIONSHIP

The main aspects of the Yin-Yang relationship can be summarized into four.

1) The opposition of Yin and Yang

Yin and Yang are opposite stages either of a cycle or of states of aggregation as explained above. Nothing in the natural world escapes this opposition. It is this very inner contradiction that constitutes the motive force of all the changes, development and decay of things.

However, the opposition is relative, not absolute, in so far as nothing is totally Yin or totally Yang. Everything contains the seed of its opposite. Moreover, the opposition of Yin-Yang is relative as the Yin or Yang quality of something is not really intrinsic, but only relative to something else. Thus, strictly speaking, it is wrong to say that something "is Yang" or "is Yin". Everything only pertains to Yin or Yang in relation to something else. For example, hot pertains to Yang and cold pertains to Yin, so we might say that the climate in Naples is Yang in relation to that in Stockholm, but it is Yin in relation to that in Algiers.

Although everything contains Yin and Yang, these are never present in a static 50/50 proportion, but in a dynamic and constantly changing balance. For example, the human body's temperature is nearly constant within a very narrow range. This is not the result of a static situation, but of a dynamic balance of many opposing forces.

2) The interdependence of Yin and Yang

Although Yin and Yang are opposite, they are also interdependent: one cannot exist without the other. Everything contains opposite forces which are mutually exclusive, but, at the same time, they depend on each other. Day is opposite to night, there cannot be activity without rest, energy without matter or contraction without expansion.

3) Mutual consumption of Yin and Yang

Yin and Yang are in a constant state of dynamic balance, which is maintained by a continuous adjustment of the relative levels of Yin and Yang. When either Yin or Yang are out of balance, they necessarily affect each other and change their proportion and so achieve a new balance. Besides the normal state of balance of Yin and Yang, there are four possible states of imbalance:

Preponderance of Yin
Preponderance of Yang
Weakness of Yin
Weakness of Yang.

When Yin is preponderant, it induces a decrease of Yang, i.e. the excess of Yin consumes Yang. When Yang is preponderant, it induces a decrease of Yin, i.e. the excess of Yang consumes Yin.

When Yin is weak, Yang is in apparent excess, and when Yang is weak, Yin is in apparent excess. This is only apparent, as it is only in excess in relation to the deficient quality, not in absolute.

These four situations can be represented by the following diagrams (Fig. 7). These diagrams will be discussed again in detail when dealing with the application of Yin and Yang to Chinese Medicine. Although the diagram of a normal, balanced state of Yin and Yang shows equal proportion of the two qualities, this should not be interpreted literally: the balance is achieved with different dynamic proportions of Yin and Yang.

It is important to see the difference between Preponderance of Yin and Weakness of Yang: these may appear the same, but they are not. It is a question of what is primary and what is secondary. In case of Preponderance of Yin, this is primary and, as a consequence, the excess of Yin consumes the Yang. In case of Weakness of Yang, this is primary and, as a consequence, Yin is in apparent excess. It looks like it is in excess, but is only relative to the deficiency of Yang. The same applies to Preponderance of Yang and weakness of Yin.

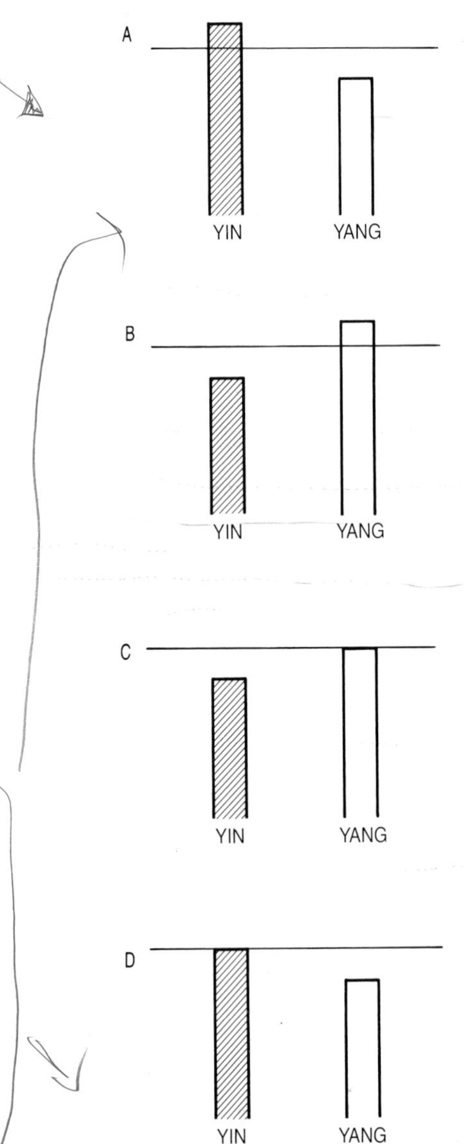

Fig. 7 Preponderance and weakness of Yin and Yang

4) The inter-transformation of Yin and Yang

Yin and Yang are not static, but they actually transform into each other: Yin can change into Yang and vice versa. This change does not happen at random, but only at a certain stage of development of something. Summer changes into Winter, day changes into night, life into death, happiness into unhappiness, heat into cold and vice versa. For example, the great euphoria of a drinking spree is quickly followed the next morning by the depression of a hang-over.

There are two conditions for the transformation of Yin into Yang or vice versa.

a) The first concerns internal conditions. Things can only change through internal causes primarily, and external causes secondarily. Change only takes place when the internal conditions are ripe. For example, an egg changes into a chick with the application of heat, only because the egg contains within itself the capacity of turning into a chick. Application of heat to a stone will not produce a chick.

b) The second condition is the time factor. Yin and Yang can only transform into each other at a certain stage of development, when conditions are ripe for the change. In the case of the egg, the chick will only hatch when the time is ripe.

APPLICATION OF YIN-YANG TO MEDICINE

It could be said that the whole of Chinese Medicine, its physiology, pathology, diagnosis and treatment, can all be reduced to the basic and fundamental theory of Yin and Yang. Every physiological process and every symptom or sign can be analysed in the light of the Yin-Yang theory. Ultimately, every treatment modality is aimed at one of these four strategies:

- To tonify Yang
- To tonify Yin
- To eliminate excess Yang
- To eliminate excess Yin.

Understanding the application of the theory of Yin-Yang to medicine, is therefore of supreme importance in practice: one can say that there is no Chinese Medicine without Yin-Yang.

YIN-YANG AND THE BODY STRUCTURE

Every part of the human body has a predominantly Yin or Yang character, and this is important in clinical practice. It must be emphasized, however, that this character is only relative. For example, the chest area is Yang in relation to the abdomen (because it is higher), but Yin in relation to the head.

As a general rule, the following are the characters of various body structures:

Yang	*Yin*
Superior	Inferior
Exterior	Interior
Posterior-lateral surface	Anterior-medial surface
Back	Front
Function	Structure

More specifically, the Yin-Yang characters of the body structures, organs and energies are:

Yang	*Yin*
Back	Front (chest-abdomen)
Head	Body
Exterior (skin-muscles)	Interior (organs)
Above the waist	Below the waist
Posterior-lateral surface of limbs	Interior-medial surface of limbs
Yang organs	Yin organs
Function of organs	Structure of organs
Qi	Blood-Body Fluids
Defensive Qi	Nutritive Qi

Each of these will need to be explained in detail.

Back-Front

The Back is the place where all the Yang channels flow. These carry Yang energy and have the function of protecting the body from exterior pathogenic factors. It is the nature of Yang to be on the Exterior and to protect. It is the nature of Yin to be in the Interior and to nourish. Thus the channels on the back belong to Yang and can be used both to strengthen Yang and therefore as resistance to exterior pathogenic factors, and to eliminate pathogenic factors after these have already invaded the body.

The Front (abdomen and chest) is the place where all the Yin channels flow. These carry Yin energy and have the function of nourishing the body. They are often used to tonify Yin.

Head-Body

The head is the place where all the Yang channels either end or begin: they therefore all meet and flow into each other on the head. The relation of the head to Yang energy is verified in different ways in practice. First of all, Yang energy tends to rise and in pathological situations, Heat or Fire will tend to rise. Since the head is the topmost area of the body, Yang energy (be it physiological or pathological) will tend to rise to the head. In pathological circumstances, this will cause red face and red eyes.

The head is also easily affected by Yang pathogenic factors such as Wind and Summer-Heat.

Finally, the head being the convergence place

of all the Yang channels, points in this area can be used to raise the Yang energy.

The rest of the body (chest and abdomen) pertains to Yin and is easily affected by Yin pathogenic factors such as Cold and Dampness.

Exterior-Interior

The Exterior of the body includes skin and muscles and pertains to Yang. It has the function of protecting the body from exterior pathogenic factors. The Interior of the body includes the internal organs and it has the function of nourishing the body.

Above-Below Waist

The area above the waist pertains to Yang and is easily affected by Yang pathogenic factors such as Wind, whereas the area below the waist pertains to Yin and is easily affected by Yin pathogenic factors such as Dampness.

Posterior-lateral and Anterior-medial surface of limbs

The Yang channels flow on the posterior-lateral surface of limbs, and the Yin channels on the anterior-medial one.

Yang and Yin organs

Some organs pertain to Yang and some to Yin. The Yang organs transform, digest and excrete "impure" products of food and fluids. The Yin organs store the "pure" essences resulting from the process of transformation carried out by the Yang organs. The "Simple Questions" in chapter 11 says: *"The 5 Yin organs store... and do not excrete... the 6 Yang organs transform and digest and do not store"*.[8]

Thus the Yang organs, in conformity with the correspondence of Yang to activity, are constantly filling and emptying, transforming separating and excreting the products of food in order to produce Qi. They are in contact with the exterior as most of the Yang organs (stomach, intestines, bladder) communicate with the exterior, via the mouth, anus or urethra.

The Yin organs, on the contrary, do not transform, digest or excrete, but store the pure essences extracted from food by the Yang organs. In particular they store the Vital Substances, i.e. Qi, Blood, Body Fluids and Essence.

Function-Structure of Organs

Yang corresponds to Function and Yin corresponds to Structure. We have just said that some organs "are" Yang and some "are" Yin. However, in accordance with the principle that nothing is totally Yang or Yin, each organ contains within itself a Yang and a Yin aspect. In particular, the structure of the organ itself and the Blood, Essence or Fluids contained within it, pertain to Yin; they are its Yin aspect.

The functional activity of the organ represents its Yang aspect. The two aspects are of course related and interdependent. For example, the Spleen function of transforming and transporting the essences extracted from food, represents its Yang aspect. The Qi extracted in this way from food, is then transformed into Blood which, being Yin, contributes to forming the structure of the Spleen itself. The "Simple Questions" in chapter 5 says: *"Yang transforms Qi, Yin forms the structure"*.[9] This would be represented with a diagram (Fig. 8).

Yang function of Spleen transforms and transports Food-Qi which goes to make...
...Blood which is Yin and represents the Yin part of the Spleen

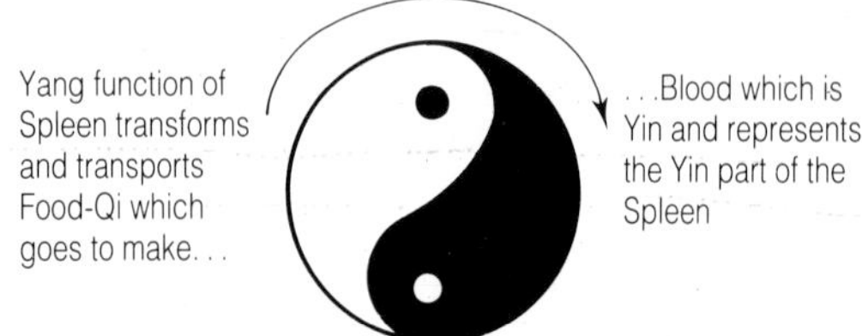

Fig. 8 Yin Yang in relation to function and structure

Qi-Blood

Qi is Yang in relation to Blood. Blood is also a form of Qi: it is a denser and more material form of Qi, and therefore more Yin.

Qi has the function of warming, protecting, tranforming and raising, all typically Yang functions. Blood has the function of nourishing and moistening, all typically Yin functions. The nature and functions of Qi and Blood will be dealt with in detail in chapter 3.

Defensive Qi-Nutritive Qi

Defensive Qi is Yang in relation to Nutritive Qi. Defensive Qi circulates in the skin and muscles (a Yang area) and has the function of protecting and warming the body (a Yang function). Nutritive Qi circulates in the internal organs (a Yin area) and has the function of nourishing the body (a Yin function). Again, the nature and functions of Defensive and Nutritive Qi will be dealt with in detail in chapter 3.

APPLICATION OF THE FOUR PRINCIPLES OF YIN-YANG TO MEDICINE

Let us now discuss in detail the application of the four principles of Yin-Yang interrelationship to Chinese Medicine.

Opposition of Yin-Yang

The opposition of Yin-Yang is reflected in medicine in the opposing Yin-Yang structures of the human body, the opposing Yin-Yang character of the organs and most of all, in the opposing symptomatology of Yin and Yang. No matter how complicated, all symptoms and signs in Chinese Medicine can be reduced to their elemental, basic character of Yin or Yang.

In order to interpret the character of the clinical manifestations in terms of Yin-Yang, we can refer to certain basic qualities which will guide us in clinical practice. These are:

Yang	*Yin*
Fire	Water
Hot	Cold
Restless	Quiet
Dry	Wet
Hard	Soft
Excitement	Inhibition
Rapidity	Slowness
Non-substantial	Substantial
Transformation, change	Conservation, storage sustainment

Fire-Water

This is one of the fundamental dualities of Yin-Yang in Chinese Medicine. Although these terms derive from the Five-Element theory, there is an interaction between that and the theory of Yin-Yang.

The balance between Fire and Water in the body is crucial. Fire is essential to all physiological processes: it represents the flame that keeps alive and stokes all metabolic processes. Fire, the physiological Fire, assists the Heart in its function of housing the Mind, it provides the warmth necessary to the Spleen to transform and transport, it stimulates the Small Intestine function of separation, it provides the heat necessary to the Bladder and Lower Burner to transform and excrete fluids and it provides the heat necessary for the Uterus to keep the Blood moving. If the physiological Fire declines, the Mind will suffer with depression, the Spleen cannot transform and transport, the Small Intestine cannot separate the fluids, the Bladder and Lower Burner cannot excrete the fluids and there will be oedema, the Uterus turns Cold and may cause infertility.

This physiological Fire is called the Fire of the Gate of Vitality (Ming Men) and derives from the Kidneys.

Water has the function of moistening and cooling during all the body's physiological functions, to balance the warming action of the physiological Fire. The origin of Water is also from the Kidneys. Thus, the balance between Fire and Water is fundamental to all physiological processes of the body. Fire and Water balance and keep a check on each other in every single physiological process. When Fire gets out of hand and becomes excessive, it has a tendency to flow upwards, hence the manifestations will show on the top part of the body and head, with headaches, red eyes, red face or thirst. When Water become excessive, it has a tendency to flow downwards causing oedema of the legs, excessive urination or incontinence.

Hot-Cold

Excess of Yang is manifested with Heat and Excess of Yin is manifested with Cold. For example, a person with Excess of Yang will feel hot, and one with Excess of Yin will tend to feel always cold. The hot and cold character can also be observed in certain signs themselves. For example, a large single boil that is red and hot to the touch indicates Heat. A lower back area very cold to the touch indicates Cold in the Kidneys.

Restless-Quiet

Restlessness, insomnia, fidgeting or tremors, indicate excess of Yang. Quiet behaviour, desire to be immobile or sleepiness, indicate excess of Yin.

Dry-Wet

Any symptom or sign of dryness such as dry eyes, dry throat, dry skin or dry stools, indicates excess of Yang (or deficiency of Yin). Any symptom or sign of excess wetness such as watery eyes, runny nose, damp pimples on skin or loose stools, indicates Excess of Yin (or deficiency of Yang).

Hard-Soft

Any lumps, swellings or masses that are hard are usually due to excess of Yang, whereas if they are soft they are due to excess of Yin.

Excitement-Inhibition

Whenever a function is in a state of hyperactivity, it indicates an excess of Yang; if it is in a state of hypoactivity, it indicates excess of Yin. For example, a rapid heart rate may indicate excess of Yang of the Heart, whereas a very slow heart rate may indicate excess of Yin of the Heart.

Rapidity-Slowness

This shows in two ways: in a person's movements and in the onset of the manifestations.

If a person's movements are rapid, and he or she walks and talks fast, it may indicate an excess of Yang. If a person's movements are slow, and he or she walks and talks slowly, it may indicate an excess of Yin.

If symptoms and signs appear suddenly and change rapidly, they indicate a Yang condition. If they appear gradually and change slowly, they indicate a Yin condition.

Substantial-Non-substantial

As explained above, Yang corresponds to a subtle state of aggregation, and Yin corresponds to a dense, coarse state of aggregation. If Yang is normal, things will be kept moving, Qi will flow normally and fluids will be transformed and excreted. If Yang is deficient, Qi stagnates, fluids are not transformed or excreted and therefore Yin will prevail. Thus, Yang keeps things moving and in a state of fluidity or "non-substantiality". When Yin prevails, the movement and transformation power of Yang fails, energy condenses into form and it becomes 'substantial". For example, if Qi moves normally in the abdomen, the intestines' function of separation and excretion of fluids will be normal. If Yang fails and Qi decreases, the Yang power of moving and transforming is impaired, fluids are not transformed, Blood is not moved, and in time, the stagnation of Qi gives rise to stasis of Blood and then to actual, physical masses or tumours.

Transformation/change-Conservation/storage:

Yin corresponds to conservation and storage: this is reflected in the function of the Yin organs, which store Blood, Body Fluids and Essence and guard them as precious essences. Yang corresponds to transformation and change: this is reflected in the function of the Yang organs which are constantly filled and emptied and constantly transform, transport and excrete.

The above are general guidelines, enabling us, through the theory of Yin-Yang, to interpret clinical manifestations. All symptoms and signs can be interpreted in the light of the above guidelines, because all clinical manifestations arise from a separation of Yin and Yang. In health, Yin and Yang are harmoniously blended in a dynamic balance. When Yin and Yang are so balanced, they cannot be identified as separate entities, hence symptoms and signs do not appear. For example, if Yin and Yang and Qi and Blood are balanced, the face will have a normal, pink, flourishing colour and will be neither too pale nor too red, nor too dark, etc. In other words, nothing can be observed. If Yin and Yang are out of balance, they become separated; there will be either too much of one or the other, and the face will be either too pale (excess of Yin) or too red (excess of Yang). Yin and Yang therefore show themselves as they are out of balance. One can visualize the Yin-Yang Supreme Ultimate symbol (see Fig. 6) spinning very fast: in this case the white and black colour will not be visible because they cannot be separated by the eye. Similarly, when Yin and Yang are balanced and moving harmoniously, they cannot be separated, they are not visible and symptoms and signs will not arise.

All symptoms and signs can be interpreted in this way, as a loss of balance of Yin and Yang. Another example: if Yin and Yang are balanced, urine will be of a normal pale-yellow colour and of normal amount. If Yin is in excess, it will be very pale nearly like water and profuse; if Yang is in excess, it will be rather dark and scanty.

Keeping in mind the general principles of the Yin and Yang character of symptoms and signs, we can list the main clinical manifestations as follows:

Yang	*Yin*
Acute disease	Chronic disease
Rapid onset	Gradual onset
Rapid pathological changes	Lingering disease
Heat	Cold
Restlessness, insomnia	Sleepiness, listlessness
Throws off bedclothes	Likes to be covered
Likes to lie stretched	Likes to curl up
Hot limbs and body	Cold limbs and body
Red face	Pale face
Likes cold drinks	Likes hot drinks
Loud voice, talks a lot	Weak voice, dislikes talking
Coarse breathing	Shallow, weak breathing
Thirst	No thirst
Scanty-dark urination	Profuse-pale urination
Constipation	Loose stools
Red tongue with yellow coating	Pale tongue
Full pulse	Empty pulse

Finally, having discussed the Yin and Yang character of symptoms and signs, it must be emphasized that, although the distinction of Yin and Yang in clinical manifestations is fundamental it is not detailed enough to be of much clinical use in practice. For example, if the face is too red, it indicates an excess of Yang. However, this conclusion is too general to give any indication as to what the appropriate treatment should be. In fact, the face could be red from Full-Heat or Empty-Heat (both of which can be classified as "excess of Yang"). If it was red from Full-Heat, one must further distinguish which organ is mostly involved: it could be red from Liver-Fire, Heart-Fire, Lung-Heat or Stomach-Heat. The treatment would be different in each case. The theory of Yin-Yang, although fundamental is thus too general to give concrete guidelines as to the treatment needed. As we will see later, it needs to be integrated with the 8-Principle and the Internal-Organ pattern theory to be applied to actual clinical situations. The theory of Yin-Yang is, nevertheless, the necessary foundation for an understanding of symptoms and signs.

The interdependence of Yin and Yang

Yin and Yang are opposite but are also mutually dependent on each other. Yin and Yang cannot exist in isolation, and this is very apparent when considering the body's physiology. All the physiological processes are a result of the opposition and interdependence of Yin and Yang. The functions of the internal organs in Chinese Medicine show the interdependence of Yin and Yang very clearly.

Yin and Yang Organs

The Yin and Yang organs are very different in their functions, but, at the same time, they depend on each other for the performance of their functions. The Yin organs depend on the Yang ones to produce Qi and Blood from the transformation of food. The Yang organs depend on the Yin ones for their nourishment deriving from Blood and Essence stored by the Yin organs.

Structure and function of the organs

Each organ has a structure represented by the

organ itself and the Blood and fluids within it. At the same time, each organ has a certain function which both affects and is affected by its structure. For example, the structure of the Liver is represented by the actual organ and the Blood stored within it. In particular, the Liver has the function of storing Blood. Another function of the Liver is that of ensuring the smooth flow of Qi all over the body. By ensuring the smooth flow of Qi, the Liver also keeps the Blood moving, therefore providing a correct storage of Blood within itself: this is an example of how the Liver function assists the Liver structure. On the other hand, in order to carry out its function, the Liver organ itself needs the nourishment of Blood: this is an example of how the Liver structure assists the Liver function

Without structure (Yin), the function (Yang) could not perform; without function, the structure would lack transformation and movement.

The "Simple Questions" in chapter 5 says: *"Yin is in the Interior and is the material foundation of Yang; Yang is on the Exterior and is the manifestation of Yin"*.[10]

The Mutual Consuming of Yin and Yang

Yin and Yang are in a constant state of change so that when one increases the other is consumed, to preserve the balance. This can easily be seen in the ebb and flow of night and day. As the day comes to an end Yang decreases and Yin increases. Exactly the same can be observed in the cycle of seasons. When Spring comes, Yin begins to decrease and Yang increases. Beyond, the mere preservation of their balance, Yin and Yang also mutually "consume" each other. When one increases, the other must decrease. For example, if the weather becomes unduly hot (Yang), the water (Yin) in the soil dries up. Thus:

If Yin is consumed, Yang increases
If Yang is consumed, Yin increases
If Yin increases, Yang is consumed
If Yang increases, Yin is consumed.

In the human body, the mutual consuming of Yin and Yang can be seen from a physiological and a pathological point of view.

From a physiological point of view, the mutual consuming of Yin and Yang is a normal process which keeps the balance of physiological functions. This process can be observed in all physiological processes, for example in the regulation of sweating, urination, temperature of the body, breathing, etc. For example in summertime the weather is hot (Yang) and we sweat (Yin) more; when the external temperature is very cold (Yin), the body starts trembling (Yang) in an attempt to produce some heat.

From a pathological point of view, Yin or Yang may increase beyond their normal range and lead to consumption of their opposite quality. For example, the temperature may rise (excess of Yang) during an infectious disease. This can lead to dryness and exhaustion of body fluids (consumption of Yin). Although some might still regard this as an attempt of the body to keep the balance between Yin and Yang (the body fluids and temperature), it is not a normal balance, but a pathological balance deriving from an excess of Yang. One might go further and say that the temperature itself was an attempt of the body to fight a pathogenic factor, but this does not change the fact that the rise in temperature represents an excess of Yang which leads to consumption of Yin.

From a pathological point of view, there can be four different situations of excess of Yin or excess of Yang leading to consumption of Yang or Yin respectively, or consumption of Yang or consumption of Yin leading to apparent excess of Yin or Yang respectively.

It is important to note that excess of Yang and consumption of Yin are not the same. In excess of Yang, the primary factor is the abnormal increase of Yang which leads to consumption of Yin. In consumption of Yin, the primary factor is the deficiency of Yin arising spontaneously and leading to an apparent excess of Yang.

Five diagrams will clarify this (Figs 9 to 13).

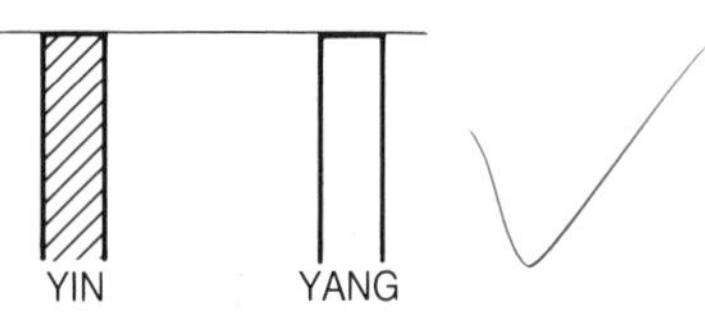

Fig. 9 Balance of Yin and Yang

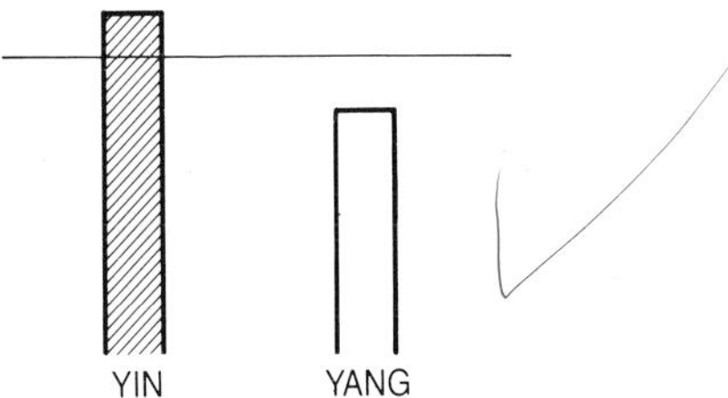

Fig. 10 Excess of Yin

Excess of Yin (Fig. 10)

An example of this is when excess Cold (interior or exterior) in the body consumes the Yang, especially Spleen-Yang. This is Full-Cold.

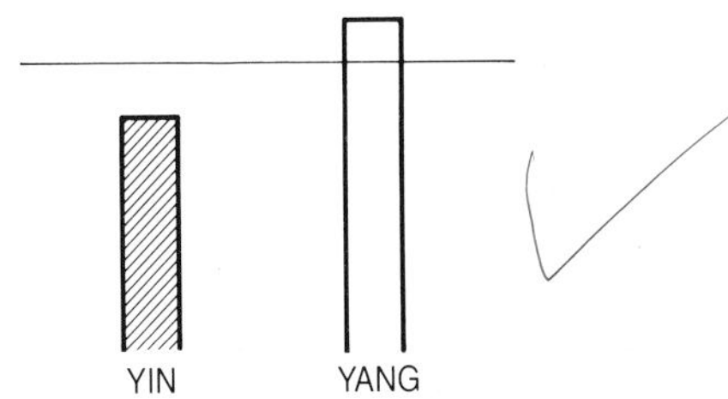

Fig. 11 Excess of Yang

Excess of Yang (Fig. 11)

An example of this is when excess Heat (which can be exterior or interior) consumes the body fluids (which pertain to Yin) and leads to dryness. This is Full-Heat.

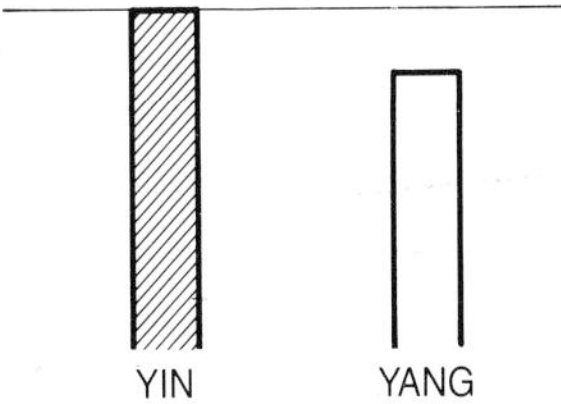

Fig. 12 Consumption of Yang

Consumption of Yang (Fig. 12)

This takes place when the body's Yang energy is spontaneously deficient. The decrease of Yang energy leads to cold, chilliness and other symptoms which, to a certain extent, are similar to those created by excess of Yin. The situation is, however, very different, as in excess of Yin, it is the excessive Yin which is the primary aspect and it causes consumption of Yang. In case of consumption of Yang, the decrease of Yang is the primary aspect and the Yin is only apparently in excess. This is called Empty-Cold.

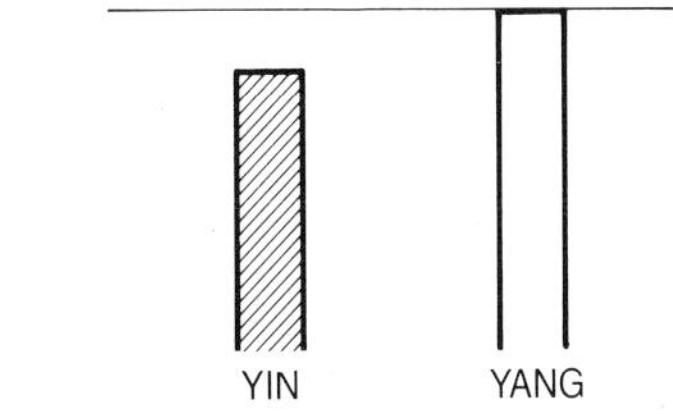

Fig. 13 Consumption of Yin

Consumption of Yin (Fig. 13)

This takes place when the body's Yin energies are depleted. The decrease of Yin may lead to symptoms of apparent excess of Yang, such as feeling of heat. Again, this situation is very different from that seen in excess of Yang. In excess of Yang, the excessive Yang is the primary aspect. In case of decrease of Yin, this is the primary aspect, and the Yang is only apparently in excess. This is called Empty-Heat.

The distinction between Empty-Cold and Full-Cold and between Empty-Heat and Full-Heat is all important in practice as, in case of Emptiness one needs to tonify, while in case of Fullness, one needs to sedate.

The Inter-Transformation of Yin and Yang

Although opposite, Yin and Yang can change into one another. This transformation does not take place at random, but is determined by the stage of development and by internal conditions.

First of all, the change takes place when conditions are ripe at a certain point in time. Day cannot turn into night at any time, but only when it has reached its point of exhaustion.

The second condition of change is determined by the internal qualities of any given thing or phenomenon. Wood can turn into coal, but a stone cannot.

The process of transformation of Yin and Yang into each other can be observed in many natural phenomena, such as in the alternation of day and night, the seasons, climate.

The principle of inter-transformation of Yin-Yang has many applications in clinical practice. An understanding of this transformation is important for the prevention of disease. If we are aware of how a thing can turn into its opposite, then we can prevent this and achieve a balance which is the essence of Chinese Medicine.

For example, excessive work (Yang) without rest induces extreme deficiency (Yin) of the body's energies. Excessive jogging (Yang) induces a very slow (Yin) pulse. Excessive consumption of alcohol creates a pleasant euphoria (Yang) which is quickly followed by a hang-over (Yin). Excessive worrying (Yang) depletes (Yin) the energy of the body. Thus, balance in our life, in diet, exercise, work, emotional life and sexual life, is the essence of prevention in Chinese Medicine, and an understanding of how Yang can turn into Yin and vice versa can help us to avoid the rapid swings from one to the other which are detrimental to our physical and emotional life. Of course, nothing would be more difficult to achieve in our modern Western societies, which seem to be geared to producing the maximum swing from one extreme to the other.

The transformation of Yin-Yang can also be observed in the pathological changes seen in clinical practice. For example, exterior Cold can invade the body and, after a time, it can easily change into Heat. An Excess condition can easily turn into a Deficiency one. For example, excessive Heat can damage the body fluids and lead to deficiency of fluids. A Deficiency condition can also turn into an Excess one. For example, a deficiency of Spleen-Yang can lead to Excess of Dampness. It is therefore extremely important to be able to discern the transformation of Yin-Yang in clinical practice in order to treat the condition properly.

Notes

1 A deeper discussion of the historical development of the theory of Yin-Yang over the centuries is beyond the scope of this book. The reader is referred to the following books:
Fung Yu-Lan 1966 A Short History of Chinese Philosophy. Macmillan, New York
Granet M 1968 La Pensee Chinoise. Albin Michel, Paris
Moore C A 1967 The Chinese Mind. University Press of Hawaii, Honolulu
Needham J 1956 Science and Civilization in China, vol 2. Cambridge University Press, Cambridge
Wing Tsit Chan 1969 A Source Book in Chinese Philosophy. Princeton University Press, Princeton.
2 Granet M 1968 La Pensee Chinoise. Albin Michel, p 367
3 1979 The Yellow Emperor's Classic of Internal Medicine—Simple Questions (*Huang Ti Nei Jing Su Wen* 黄帝内经素问) People's Health Publishing House, Beijing, p 44
4 It is interesting to compare this with the Western cultural attitude to left and right, according to which, left is somehow "bad" and right somehow "good". See, for example, certain words such as "sinister" etymologically related to "left", or "cack-handed" meaning both "left-handed" and "clumsy", or "dexterous" meaning both "right-handed" and "skilful".
5 Simple Questions, p 31.
6 Science and Civilization in China, vol 2, p 41.
7 Simple Questions, p 31.
8 Simple Questions, p 77–78.
9 Simple Questions, p 32.
10 Simple Questions, p 42–43.

The Five Elements 2

五行

Together with the theory of Yin-Yang, the theory of the 5 Elements constitutes the basis of Chinese medical theory. The term "5 Elements" has been used by most Western practitioners of Chinese Medicine for a long time. Some authors consider this to be a misunderstanding of the meaning of the Chinese term *"Wu Xing"*, perpetuated over the years. *"Wu"* means "five" and *"Xing"* means "movement", "process", "to go" or "conduct, behaviour". Most authors therefore think that the word *"Xing"* cannot indicate "element" as a basic constituent of Nature, as they were supposedly intended in ancient Greek philosophy.

This is, in my opinion, only partly true. First of all, the elements, as they were conceived by various Greek philosophers over the centuries, were not always considered basic constituents of Nature or "passive motionless fundamental substances".[1] Some Greek philosophers conceived the elements as dynamic qualities of Nature, in a way similar to Chinese philosophy.

Greek philosophers used different words to indicate the elements, which proves the lack of a uniform view of them. Empedocles called them "roots" (*rhizomata* ριζωματα), Plato called them "simple components" (*stoicheia* στοιχεια). Aristotle gave a definite dynamic interpretation to the four elements and called them "primary form" (*prota somata* πρωτα σωματα). He said: *"Earth and Fire are opposites also due to the opposition of the respective qualities with which they are revealed to our senses: Fire is hot, Earth is cold. Besides the fundamental opposition of hot and cold, there is another one, i.e. that of dry and wet: hence the four possible combinations of hot-dry* [*Fire*], *hot-wet* [*Air*], *cold-dry* [*Earth*] *and cold-wet* [*Water*] ... *the elements can mix with each other and can even transform into one another ... thus Earth, which is cold and dry, can generate Water if wetness replaces dryness"*.[2] To Aristotle, therefore, the four elements became the four basic qualities of natural phenomena, classified as combinations of four qualities, hot, cold, dry and wet. As is apparent from the above statement, the Aristotelian elements could even transform into one another and generate each other. This interpretation is very similar to the Chinese one, in which the elements are qualities of Nature.

Thus, it is not entirely true to say that the Greek elements were conceived only as the basic constituents of matter, the "building blocks" of Nature. Furthermore, the word "elements" does not necessarily imply that: it only does so in its modern chemical interpretation.

Finally, it is not entirely true either that the Chinese elements were not conceived as basic constituents of matter. Certainly, they are primarily basic qualities of natural phenomena, or movements; however, there are also statements which would seem to imply that the elements are that and basic constituents of Nature as well. For instance: "*When the Qi of the Elements settles, things acquire form.*"[3]

In conclusion, there is no real reason why the word "element" is not an acceptable translation of the Chinese word "*xing*". Moreover, considering the widespread and accepted use of this word in the world of Chinese Medicine, I find it unnecessary and confusing to change.

The five Elements, therefore, are not basic constituents of Nature, but five basic processes, qualities, phases of a cycle or inherent capabilities of change of phenomena.

The theory of the Five Elements was not applied to Chinese Medicine throughout its historical development but its popularity waxed and waned through the centuries. During the Warring States period it became immensely popular and was applied to medicine, astrology, the natural sciences, the calendar, music and even politics. Its popularity was such that most phenomena were classified in fives. However, voices of criticism were raised as early as the beginning of the 1st century. The great sceptical philosopher Wang Chong (AD 27–97) criticized the theory of the 5 Elements as being too rigid to interpret all natural phenomena correctly. He said: "*The rooster pertains to Metal and the hare to Wood: if Metal really conquers Wood, why is it that roosters do not devour hares?*"[4]

From the Han dynasty onwards, the influence of the theory of the 5 Elements in Chinese Medicine began to wane. For example, the great Chinese medical classic of the Han dynasty "Discussion of Cold-induced Diseases" by Zhang Zhong Jing makes no mention of the 5 Elements at all. It was not until the Song dynasty (960-1279) that the theory of the 5 Elements regained popularity and was systematically applied to diagnosis, symptomatology and treatment in Chinese Medicine.

From the Ming dynasty onwards, the influence of the theory of the 5 Elements again decreased as Chinese Medicine was dominated by the study of infectious diseases from exterior Heat for the diagnosis and treatment of which the Identification of Patterns according to the 4 Levels and 3 Burners was used.

For the best critical appraisal of the significance of the 5-Element theory in Chinese Medicine see "The Web that has no Weaver".[5]

THE FIVE ELEMENTS IN NATURE

The theory of Yin-Yang originated earlier than that of the 5 Elements. The first references to Yin-Yang date back to the Zhou dynasty (about 1000–770 BC), while the first recorded reference to the 5 Elements dates back to the Warring States Period (476–221 BC). [6]

Some of the earliest references to the Elements do not call them "elements" at all but either "seats of government" (*Fu* 府) or "ability, talent, material" (*cai* 材), and they were at one point considered to be six rather than five. They were in fact either called the "5 abilities" or the "6 seats of government". A book from the Warring States period says: "*Heaven send the Five Abilities and the people use them*".[7] And it also says :"*The 6 Seats of Government ... are Water, Fire, Metal, Wood, Earth and Grain*".[8] Thus "Grain" was considered to be the 6th "element".

A Western Han dynasty (206 BC–AD 24) book called the "Great Transmission of the Valued Book" says: "*Water and Fire provide food, Metal and Wood provide prosperity and the Earth makes provisions*".[9]

It could be said that the theory of the 5 Elements, and its application to medicine, marks the beginning of what one might call "scientific" medicine and a departure from Shamanism. No longer do healers look for a supernatural cause of disease: they now observe Nature and, with a combination of the inductive and deductive method, they set out to find patterns within it and, by extension, apply these in the interpretation of disease.

It is therefore not by chance that numbers and numeration are increasingly applied in the interpretation of Nature and the human body: 2 basic polarities (Yin-Yang), a three-tier cosmological "structure" (Heaven, Person, Earth), 4 seasons, 5 Elements, 6 climates in Nature, and 5 Yin and 6 Yang organs in the human body. The number 5 and the 5 Elements are associated with earthly phenomena, and the number 6 is associated with heavenly phenomena (the 6 climates). The classification of things in numbers is indicative of an increasingly searching and analytical mind. Interestingly, more or less the same process was taking place in Greece at roughly the same time, when the Greek theories of the Elements were developed. In his essay "On the sacred disease", Hippocrates launches in a in-depth criticism of the supernatural theory for the aetiology of epilepsy.[10]

The book "Shang Shu" written during the Western Zhou dynasty (1000–771 BC) said: *"The 5 Elements are Water, Fire, Wood, Metal and Earth. Water moistens downwards, Fire flares upwards, Wood can be bent and straightened, Metal can be moulded and can harden, Earth permits sowing, growing and reaping."*[11] We will return to this statement later as it contains many important concepts on the nature of the 5 Elements.

The theory of the 5 Elements was developed by the same philosophical school that developed the theory of Yin-Yang, i.e. the "Yin-Yang School", sometimes also called the "Naturalist School". The chief exponent of this school was Zou Yan (c. 350–270 BC). Initially, the theory of the 5 Elements had political implications as much as naturalistic ones. The philosophers of this school were highly esteemed, and perhaps somewhat feared, by the ancient Chinese rulers, as they purported to be able to interpret Nature in the light of Yin-Yang and 5 Elements and draw political conclusions from it. For example, a certain ruler was associated with a certain Element and every ceremonial had to conform to that particular Element colour, season, etc. Also, these philosophers claimed they could predict the succession of rulers by referring to the various cycles of the 5 Elements. Zou Yan said: *"Each of the 5 Elements is followed by one it cannot conquer. The dynasty of Shun ruled by the virtue of Earth, the Xia dynasty ruled by the virtue of Wood, the Shang dynasty ruled by the virtue of Metal, and the Zhou dynasty ruled by the virtue of Fire. When some new dynasty is going to arise, heaven exhibits auspicious signs to the people. During the rise of Huang Di [the Yellow Emperor] large earth-worms and large ants appeared. He said 'This indicates that the Element Earth is in the ascendant, so our colour must be yellow, and our affairs must be placed under the sign of Earth.' During the rise of Yu the Great, heaven produced plants and trees which did not wither in autumn and winter. He said 'This indicates that the Element Wood is in the ascendant, so our colour must be green, and our affairs must be placed under the signs of Wood' . . . "*.[12]

One could say that the philosophers of the Naturalist School developed a primitive natural science and occupied a respected social position comparable to that of modern scientists today.

Apart from its political connotation, the theory of the 5 Elements has many facets. The 5 Elements represent five different qualities of natural phenomena, five movements and five phases in the cycle of seasons.

THE FIVE ELEMENTS AS BASIC QUALITIES

It is worth repeating here and enlarging the passage from the "Shang Shu": *"The 5 Elements are Water, Fire, Wood, Metal and Earth. Water moistens downwards, Fire flares upwards, Wood can be bent and straightened, Metal can be moulded and can harden, Earth permits sowing, growing and reaping. That which soaks and descends [Water] is salty, that which blazes upwards [Fire] is bitter, that which can be bent and straightened [Wood] is sour, that which can be moulded and become hard [Metal] is pungent, that which permits sowing and reaping [Earth] is sweet"*.[13]

This statement clearly shows that the 5 Elements symbolize five different inherent qualities and states of natural phenomena. It also relates the tastes (or flavours) to the 5 Elements, and it is apparent that the tastes have more to do with an inherent quality of a thing (like its chemical composition in modern terms), rather than its actual flavour.

THE FIVE ELEMENTS AS MOVEMENTS

The 5 Elements also symbolize five different

directions of movement of natural phenomena. Wood represents expansive, outward movement in all directions, Metal represents contractive, inward movement, Water represents downward movement, Fire represents upward movement and Earth represents neutrality or stability.

THE FIVE ELEMENTS AS STAGES OF A SEASONAL CYCLE

Each of the 5 Elements represents a season in the yearly cycle. Wood corresponds to Spring and is associated with birth, Fire corresponds to Summer and is associated with growth, Metal corresponds to Autumn and is associated with harvest, Water corresponds to Winter and is associated with storage, Earth corresponds to the late season and is associated with transformation.

The position of Earth requires some explanation. Earth does not correspond to any season, as it is the centre, the neutral term of reference around which the seasons and the other elements spin. The "Classic of Categories" (1624) by Zhang Jie Bing says: "*The Spleen belongs to Earth which pertains to the Centre, its influence manifests for 18 days at the end of each of the four seasons and it does not pertain to any season on its own*".[14] The "Discussion of Prescriptions from the Golden Chest" (c. AD 220) by Zhang Zhong Jing says: "*During the last period of each season, the Spleen is strong enough to resist pathogenic factors*".[15] Thus, in the cycle of seasons, the Earth actually corresponds to the late stage of each season. In other words, towards the end of each season, the heavenly energies go back to the Earth for replenishment. In Western books, the Earth is often associated with "Late Summer" or "Indian Summer". It is true to say that Earth corresponds to Late Summer, but it also corresponds to "Late Winter", "Late Spring" and "Late Autumn".

This could be represented as in Figure 14.

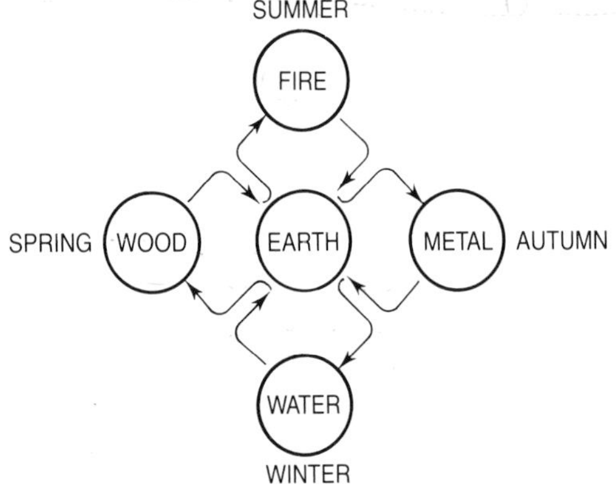

Fig. 14 The Five-Element seasonal cycle

THE FIVE-ELEMENT INTERRELATIONSHIPS

Essential to the very concept of the 5 Elements are the various interactions among them. Different philosophers stressed different relationships among the 5 Elements. For example, the main exponent of the Naturalist School, Zou Yan, only wrote about the "controlling" relationships among the Elements (see below). Thirty-six different arrangements of the 5 Elements are mathematically possible. The most common ones are five.

The Cosmological Sequence

As was mentioned above, the earliest reference to the 5 Elements, enumerates them as follows: "*As for the 5 Elements, the first is called Water, the second Fire, the third Wood, the fourth Metal and the fifth Earth*".[16]

The order in which the Elements are enumerated is not a chance one, and is closely related to their numerology. If we assign numbers to each of the Elements in the order in which they are listed, these would be:

1 Water
2 Fire
3 Wood
4 Metal
5 Earth

If we add 5 to each of these numbers, we get:

6 Water
7 Fire
8 Wood
9 Metal
10 (or 5) Earth.

These are the numbers usually associated with

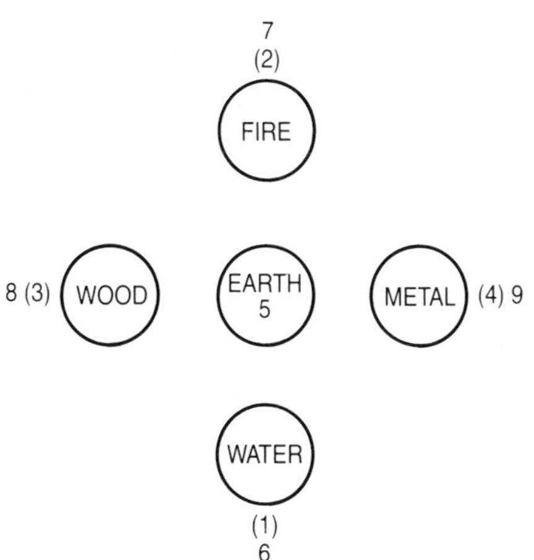

Fig. 15 The Five-Element numbers

the Elements in the list of correspondences (see below). If we arrange the Elements in the above order, they would look like Figure 15. In this arrangement Water assumes an important place, as it is the basis, the beginning of the sequence. Bearing in mind the correspondence of the Kidneys to Water, this reflects the important principle of the Kidneys being the foundation of all the other organs.

This sequence also bears out the importance of Earth being the Centre, the pivot of reference for all the other Elements. This has important implications in practice which will be discussed shortly.

The Generating Sequence

In this sequence each Element generates another and is generated by one. Thus, Wood generates Fire, Fire generates Earth, Earth generates Metal, Metal generates Water and Water generates Wood. Thus, for example, Wood is generated by Water, and it generates Fire. This is sometimes expressed as "Wood is the Child of Water and the Mother of Fire" (Fig. 16).

The Controlling Sequence

In this sequence each Element controls another and is controlled by one. Thus, Wood controls Earth, Earth controls Water, Water controls Fire, Fire controls Metal and Metal controls Wood. For example, Wood controls Earth, but is controlled by Metal (Fig. 17).

The controlling sequence ensures that a balance is maintained among the 5 Elements.

There is also an interrelationship between the Generating and the Controlling sequences. For example, Wood controls Earth, but Earth generates Metal which controls Wood. Furthermore, on the one hand Wood controls Earth, but on the other hand it generates Fire which, in turn, generates Earth. Thus a self-regulating balance is kept at all times.

The mutual generating and controlling relationships among the Elements is a fine model of the many self-regulating balancing processes to be seen in Nature and in the human body. Needham cites several interesting examples which clearly illustrate the above principles.[17]

The Over-acting Sequence

This follows the same sequence as the Controlling one, but in it, each Element "over-

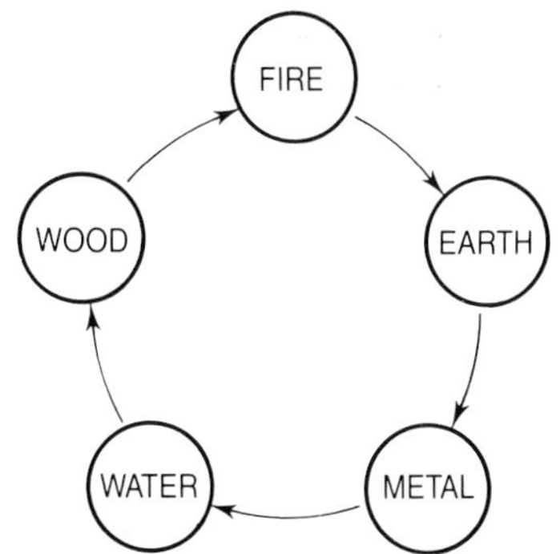

Fig. 16 The Generating Sequence

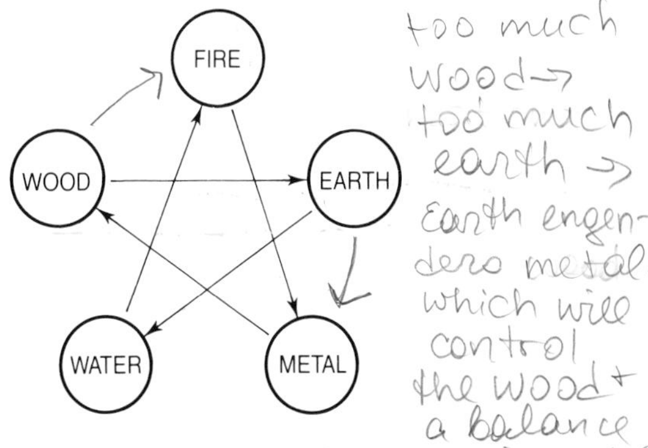

Fig. 17 The Controlling and Over-acting Sequence

controls" another, so that it causes it to decrease. This happens when the balance is broken and, under the circumstances, the quantitative relationship among the Elements breaks down, so that, at a particular time, one Element is excessive in relation to another (Fig. 17).

To return to a comparison with natural phenomena, the destructive actions of human beings towards Nature, especially in this century, provide numerous examples of this sequence.

The Insulting Sequence

This sequence is literally called "insulting" in Chinese. It takes place in the reverse order than the Controlling sequence. Thus, Wood insults Metal, Metal insults Fire, Fire insults Water, Water insults Earth and Earth insults Wood (Fig. 18). This also takes place when the balance is broken.

Thus, the first two sequences deal with the normal balance among the Elements, the second two (the Over-acting and the Insulting one) deal with the abnormal relationships among the Elements that take place when the balance is broken.

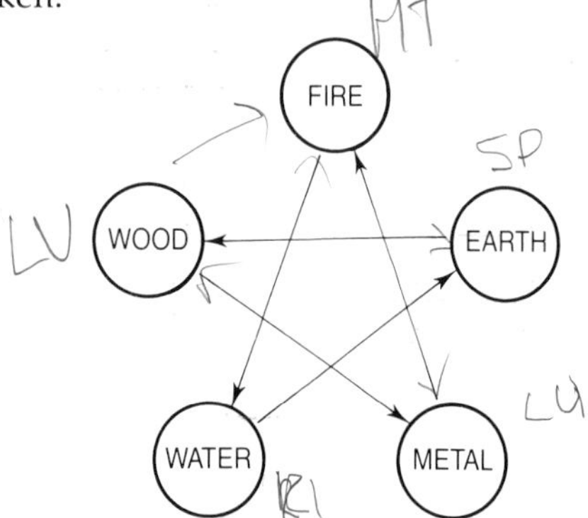

Fig. 18 The Insulting Sequence

THE FIVE-ELEMENT CORRESPONDENCES

The system of correspondences is an important part of the 5-Element theory. This system is typical of the ancient Chinese thought, linking many different phenomena and qualities within the microcosm and macrocosm under the aegis of a certain Element. The ancient Chinese philosophers saw the link among apparently unrelated phenomena as a kind of "resonance" among them. Various different phenomena would be unified by an indefinable common quality, much as two strings would vibrate in unison.

One of the most typical aspects of Chinese Medicine is the common resonance among phenomena in Nature and in the human body. Some of these correspondences are commonly verified and experienced all the time in clinical practice, some may seem far-fetched, but the feeling remains that there is a profound wisdom underlying all of them which is, at times unfathomable.

However they were determined, there are many sets of correspondences for each of the 5 Elements. The correlation between the Elements and seasons is a very immediate and obvious one, and so is that with the cardinal directions (Fig. 19).

The main correlations with regard to medicine are found in the "Simple Questions" chapters 4 and 5.[18]

Some of the main correspondences are as shown in Table 1.

These sets of correspondences, especially those related to the human body, show how the organs and their related phenomena form an inseparable and integrated whole. Thus, Wood corresponds to the Liver, eyes, sinews, shouting, green, anger, wheat, Spring and birth. All these phenomena are related and all pertain to the Element of Wood. Their application to Chinese Medicine will be explained shortly.

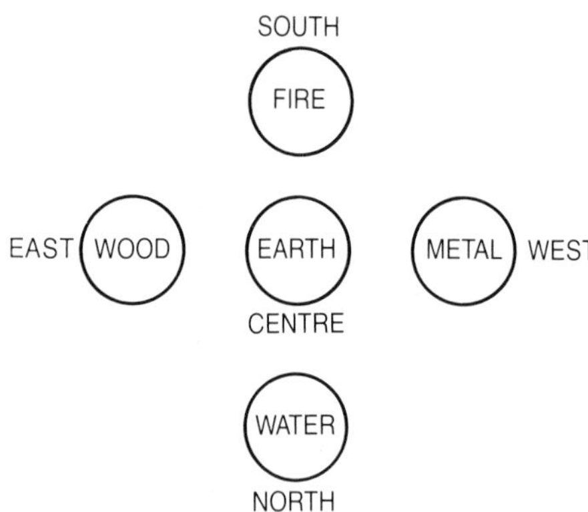

Fig. 19 The Five Elements and cardinal directions

Table 1 Some of the main correspondences of the 5 elements

	Wood	Fire	Earth	Metal	Water
Seasons	Spring	Summer	None[19]	Autumn	Winter
Directions	East	South	Centre	West	North
Colours	Green	Red	Yellow	White	Black
Tastes	Sour	Bitter	Sweet	Pungent	Salty
Climates	Wind	Heat	Dampness	Dryness	Cold
Stage of development	Birth	Growth	Transformation	Harvest	Storage
Numbers	8	7	5	9	6
Planets	Jupiter	Mars	Saturn	Venus	Mercury
Yin-Yang	Lesser Yang	Utmost Yang	Centre	Lesser Yin	Utmost Yin
Animals	Fish	Birds	Human	Mammals	Shell-covered
Domestic Animals	Sheep	Fowl	Ox	Dog	Pig
Grains	Wheat	Beans	Rice	Hemp	Millet
Yin organs	Liver	Heart	Spleen	Lungs	Kidneys
Yang organs	Gall-Bladder	Small Intestine	Stomach	Large Intestine	Bladder
Sense organs	Eyes	Tongue	Mouth	Nose	Ears
Tissues	Sinews	Vessels	Muscles	Skin	Bones
Emotions	Anger	Joy	Pensiveness	Sadness	Fear
Sounds	Shouting	Laughing	Singing	Crying	Groaning

THE FIVE ELEMENTS IN CHINESE MEDICINE

The applications of the theory of the 5 Elements to Chinese Medicine are numerous and very important. We shall explore them in five different areas:

Physiology
Pathology
Diagnosis
Treatment
Dietary and herbal therapy.

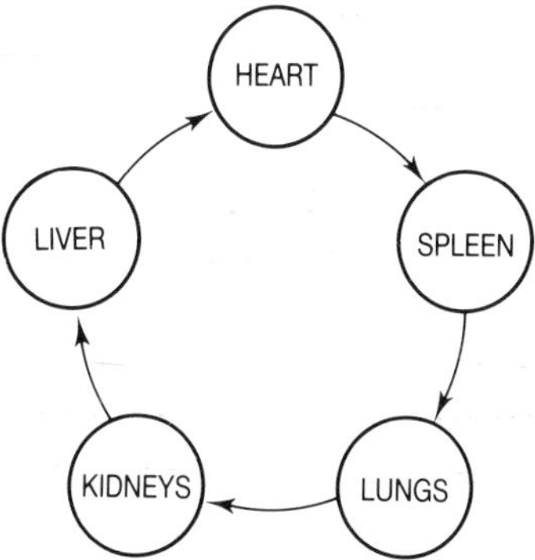

Fig. 20 The Organ Generating Sequence

THE FIVE ELEMENTS IN PHYSIOLOGY

The relationships among the 5 Elements are like a model of relationships among the internal organs and between them and the various tissues, sense organs, colours, smells, tastes and sounds.

The Generating and Controlling Sequences

These provide the basic model of physiological relationships among the internal organs. Just as "Wood generates Fire and is generated by Water", so we can say that the "Liver is the mother of the Heart and the child of the Kidneys". Thus, the Generating sequence among the organs is shown in Figure 20.

On the other hand, each organ is kept in check by another so that a proper balance among them is kept: this is the Controlling sequence (Fig. 21). This is as follows:

The Liver controls the Spleen
The Heart controls the Lungs

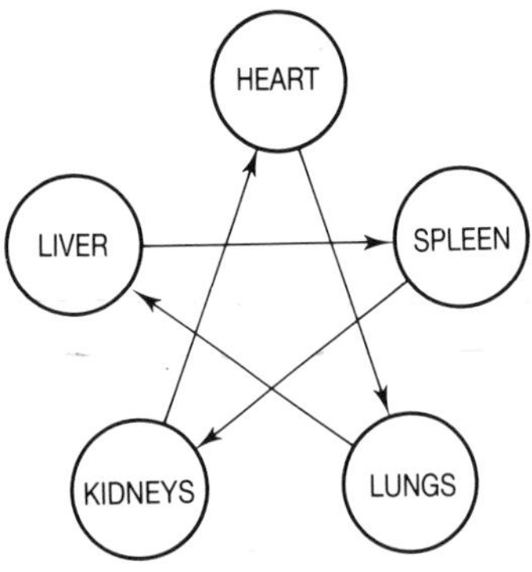

Fig. 21 The Organ Controlling and Over-acting Sequence

The Spleen controls the Kidneys
The Lungs control the Liver
The Kidneys control the Heart.

It is very important to remember in practice that the above sequences among the organs are only a 5-Element model of relationships and that, as such, it may suffer from inconsistencies, deficiencies and arbitrariness. Although this model can be extremely useful in clinical practice, one should not lose sight of the actual organ functions and how these interact with each other. In other words, we should not make the mistake of using the 5-Element model in practice in isolation from the actual organ functions which the model itself is trying to represent. There is the danger that one might use the symbols themselves (the 5 Elements), and not what they symbolize (the interaction of the internal organs' functions).

When properly used, however, the symbols can provide a quick and effective model to refer to in clinical practice and a guideline for diagnosis and treatment.

One could explain all the 5-Element relationships among the organs in terms of organ functions. The organ functions will be discussed in depth in chapter 5, but it is worth mentioning them at this stage to illustrate how the 5-Element interactions are a model of internal organs' functional relationships. It must be stressed, however, that not all the 5-Element relationships are equally meaningful as a model of organ-functions interactions. For example, the generating relationship between Kidneys and Liver has deep implications in practice, while that between Heart and Spleen less so. In fact, one should not lose sight of the fact that the Generating and Controlling sequences are only two of the possible models of relationships among the 5 Elements. Besides these two, I will discuss a third sequence, i.e. the Cosmological sequence, the relationships of which are different from those in the Generating sequence. For example, in the Generating sequence the Heart is the mother of the Spleen, but this relationship has no meaningful applications in practice. In the Cosmological sequence, on the contrary, the Spleen is a supporting organ for the Heart, and this has far more applications in practice as, for instance, the Spleen produces Blood which houses the Mind.

Let us look at some examples of Generating sequence relationships.

The Liver is the mother of the Heart: the Liver stores Blood and Blood houses the Mind. If Liver-Blood is weak, the Heart will suffer.

The Heart is the mother of the Spleen: Heart-Qi pushes the Blood and thus helps the Spleen function of transportation.

The Spleen is the mother of the Lungs: Spleen-Qi provides Food-Qi to the Lungs where it interacts with air to form the Gathering Qi.

The Lungs are the mother of the Kidneys: Lung-Qi descends to meet Kidney-Qi. The Lungs also send fluids down to the Kidneys.

The Kidneys are the mother of the Liver: Kidney-Yin nourishes Liver-Blood.

As for the Controlling sequence, "controlling" must not be taken literally, as the organs actually support rather than suppress each other's functions along the Controlling sequence. In fact, it will be seen that each organ actually helps the function of the organ it is supposed to "control". The following will be a few examples:

The Liver controls the Stomach and Spleen: the Liver actually helps the Stomach to rot and ripen food and the Spleen to transform and transport. It is only when the controlling function gets out of hand (in which case it is called "over-acting") that the Liver can actually interfere with and impair the Stomach and Spleen functions.

The Heart controls the Lungs: Heart and Lungs

are closely related as they are both situated in the Upper Burner. The Heart governs Blood and Lungs govern Qi: Qi and Blood mutually assist and nourish each other.

The Spleen controls the Kidneys: both Spleen and Kidneys transform Body Fluids. The Spleen activity in transforming and transporting fluids is essential to the Kidney transformation and excretion of fluids.

The Lungs control the Liver: in this case, unlike the others, there is a certain element of "control" of the Liver by the Lungs. The Lungs send Qi downwards, whereas the Liver spreads Qi upwards. If Lung-Qi is weak and cannot descend, Liver-Qi may tend to rise too much. This often happens in practice, when a deficiency of the Lungs leads to rising of Liver-Yang or stagnation of Liver-Qi

The Kidneys control the Heart: Kidneys and Heart actually assist and support each other. A proper communication and interaction between Kidneys and Heart is essential for health. This relationship will be discussed at length shortly, when dealing with the Cosmological sequence.

The Cosmological sequence

Western acupuncture books have surprisingly always left this sequence out. Yet, this is a very important and meaningful sequence in clinical practice, and in the philosophy of the 5 Elements in general.

As was mentioned above, the very first reference to the 5 Elements lists them in this order: Water, Fire, Wood, Metal and Earth (see note 11). Assigning them numbers, they would be 1 for Water, 2 for Fire, 3 for Wood, 4 for Metal and 5 for Earth. Adding 5 to each of these, we would get 6 for Water, 7 for Fire, 8 for Wood, 9 for Metal and 10 (or 5) for Earth. The number five is added, as 5 was associated with earthly phenomena in Chinese philosophy, whilst 6 was associated with heavenly phenomena. Since the 5-Element cosmology describes earthly phenomena, the number 5 is used. The climates, on the contrary, are heavenly phenomena, and they are classified in 6.

The Cosmological sequence can be represented as shown in Figure 22.

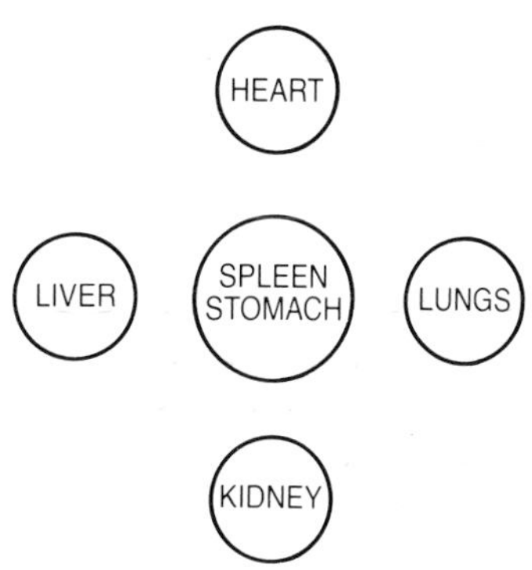

Fig. 22 The Organ Cosmological Sequence

This arrangement is significant in clinical practice in many ways:

Water as the foundation

In this sequence, Water is the beginning, the foundation of the other Elements. This corresponds well to the importance of the Kidneys as the foundation of Yin and Yang, the basis for the Yin and Yang of all the other organs. They pertain to Water and store Essence, but also store the Fire of the Gate of Vitality. They are therefore the source of Water and Fire, also called the Original Yin and Original Yang. From this point of view, Water can be considered the foundation of all the other Elements.

This principle is constantly applied in clinical practice as Kidney-Yin deficiency easily induces a deficiency of Liver-Yin and Heart-Yin, and Kidney-Yang deficiency easily induces a deficiency of Spleen-Yang and Lung-Qi.

Also, the Kidneys store the Essence which is the material foundation of Qi and Mind.

The relationship between Kidneys and Heart

Kidneys and Heart are related along the vertical axis. There is a direct communication between them, not an indirect one through Wood. This is a fundamental relationship between Water and Fire: it is probably the most important and basic balance of the body, as it reflects the basic balance between Yin and Yang.

The Kidneys govern Water and this has to flow upwards to nourish the Heart. The Heart governs Fire and this has to flow downwards to the Kidneys. Thus, far from being a relationship of control or over-action, the relationship between Kidneys and Heart is one of mutual nourishment and assistance.

This relationship also reflects that between Essence and Mind. The Essence is the material basis for the Mind: if Essence is weak, the Mind will necessarily suffer.

If Kidney-Yin is deficient, not enough Yin energy goes through to the Heart and Heart-Yin becomes deficient and Empty-Heat within the Heart will arise. This is a very common situation in clinical practice, particularly in women during the menopause.

The Stomach and Spleen as the Centre

From the Cosmological sequence the central role of Stomach and Spleen as a neutral pivot is very apparent. This is also fundamental in clinical practice. The Stomach and Spleen are the Root of the Post-Heaven Qi and the origin of Qi and Blood: they therefore nourish all the other organs and naturally occupy a central place in human physiology. Thus the Cosmological sequence accurately reflects the importance of the Pre-Heaven Qi (in so far as Water is the foundation), and of the Post-Heaven Qi (in so far as Earth is the Centre). The arrangement of the Elements in a circle along the Generating cycle does not highlight these two important concepts.

For this reason, tonifying Stomach and Spleen indirectly tonifies all the other organs.

The idea of the Stomach and Spleen being the centre and therefore the source of tonification of all the other organs appears throughout the classics, but the most famous and complete exponent of this idea was Li Dong Yuan who wrote the "Discussion on Stomach and Spleen" in 1249.

The Stomach and Spleen as support for the Heart

If we examine the Cosmological sequence diagram, we can see how the Earth is in between Water and Fire and is the support of Fire. Thus Stomach and Spleen are, in practice, the main support for the Heart. In all cases of chronic Heart-Qi or Heart-Blood deficiency, and particularly when the rhythm of the heart is irregular, it is essential to tonify the Stomach. The Spleen also produces Blood on which the Heart depends.

The role of Earth in the cycle of seasons

When the Earth is placed in the Centre, its role in relation to seasons is apparent. The Earth actually belongs to no season as it is the neutral pivot along which the seasonal cycle unfolds. On the other hand, the Earth does perform the role of replenishment at the end of each season (see Fig. 14).

Thus at the end of each season, the energy goes back to the Earth for regeneration. In the human body, this reaffirms the importance of the Stomach and Spleen as the Centre. Thus, the Stomach and Spleen could be tonified at the end of each season, particularly at the end of Winter, to regenerate the energy.

The vertical axis as symbol of Essence-Qi-Mind

The very important vertical axis of Water, Earth and Fire, can be seen as a symbol of Essence-Qi-Mind, which is the complex of physical and mental energies in human beings. The Essence belongs to the Kidneys, Qi is derived from Stomach and Spleen and the Mind is housed in the Heart.

The system of correspondences in 5-Element physiology

The system of 5-Element correspondences has wide applications in human physiology. According to this scheme, each Element encompasses numerous phenomena in the universe and the human body which are somehow "attributed" to that particular Element. Or it could be said that these phenomena "resonate" at a particular frequency and have particular qualities which respond to a certain Element.

As far as the internal organs are concerned, this theory has points of contact with the theory of the Internal Organs (see ch. 5), in so far as each organ is seen as a sphere of influence which encompasses many functions and phenomena beyond the organ itself. There are, however, some differences between the theory of 5-Element correspondences and that of the Internal Organs. First of all, the theory of 5-Element correspondences encompasses phenomena outside the human body, such as the 5 planets, the 5 grains, the 5 musical notes. Secondly, and most important, there are important discrepancies (or differences) between the two theories. For example, the Heart pertains to Fire from the 5-Element point of view, but from the Internal-Organ theory point of view, the Kidneys are the source of Fire in the body. Such discrepancies will be discussed in greater detail shortly. It will be seen that the two concepts are not mutually incompatible.

The system of 5-Element correspondences does, nevertheless, provide a comprehensive and clinically useful model of relationships between the organs and various tissues, sense organs, etc., and also between the organs and various external phenomena such as climates and seasons.

As a way of illustration, we can explore the system of correspondences related to Wood and how they apply in clinical practice.

Season: the season corresponding to Wood is Spring. In practice, it is very common for a Liver imbalance to be aggravated in Springtime. This is probably because the Liver energy flows upwards and is very active: in Springtime, Yang rises and the growing energy is bursting forward and can thus aggravate a Liver imbalance and cause Liver-Qi to rise excessively.

Direction: East winds easily affect the Liver. In practice, some patients suffering from chronic headaches or neck ache sometimes will remark that they get a headache whenever an East wind blows.

Colour: the face colour in Liver imbalances will often be greenish. This is applied in diagnosis.

Taste: a small amount of sour taste in the diet is beneficial to the Liver; and excess of it is detrimental. Also, an excess of sour taste can damage the Spleen and be beneficial to the Lungs. This will be discussed in greater detail when dealing with the application of 5-Element theory to diet and herbal therapy.

Climate: Wind very clearly affects those who suffer from an imbalance in the Liver, and often causes headaches and stiff neck.

Sense organ: the Liver moistens and nourishes the eyes.

Tissue: the Liver also moistens and nourishes sinews.

Emotion: anger is the emotion that is connected to Wood and the Liver. If the Liver energy stagnates or rebels upwards, the person may be prone to fits of anger.

Sound: related to the above, a person who suffers from a Liver disharmony will be prone to shouting (in anger).

The correspondences for the other Elements apply in the same way. However, it is important to realize that the system of 5-Element correspondences is only one of the theoretical models available, and by no means the only one. Chinese Medicine developed over thousands of years and, naturally, different theories arose at different times in its history. Thus, the model presented by the 5-Element system of correspondences may contradict, or complement, that available from other points of view, in exactly the same way that the Generating and Controlling sequences do not represent the only possible relationships among the 5 Elements.

Let us look at a few examples of discrepancies or differences between the 5-Element model and other theories of Chinese Medicine.

The Heart belongs to Emperor-Fire: in 5-Element theory, the Heart belongs to the so-called Emperor Fire and is the most important of all organs, sometimes called the Monarch. But from the point of view of Internal Organs physiology, the Heart has no such place, and the Kidneys are considered to be the foundation of all the other organs.

Fire pertains to the Heart: this may be true from the 5-Element point of view, but, again, from another point of view, the physiological Fire originates from the Kidney (Yang), and it is the Gate of Vitality that actually provides Fire to the Heart. This theory started from chapters 36 and 39 of the "Classic of Difficulties"[20] and later was taken up by many doctors, the most notable of them being Zhao Xian He of the Ming dynasty.

The eyes pertain to Wood (and Liver): although it is true and important in practice that the Liver moistens and nourishes the eyes, it is not the only organ that affects the eyes, and not every eye problem is related to the Liver. For example, Kidney-Yin also moistens the eyes and many chronic eye problems are related to the Kidneys. The Heart also reaches the eye via its Connecting channel. Some acute eye problems such as acute conjunctivitis are often related to no organ but simply due to exterior Wind-Heat. Many other channels are related to the eyes, such as the Lungs, Small Intestine, Gall Bladder and Triple Burner.

The tongue is related to Fire (Heart): this is true, but all the other organs are reflected on the tongue, and this forms the basis of tongue diagnosis.

The ears are related to Water (Kidneys): again, it is true that the Kidney-Essence nourishes the ears, but not every ear problem derives from the Kidneys. For example, acute ear problems, such as acute otitis media may be due to invasion of exterior Wind-Heat affecting the Gall Bladder channel.

The above are only a few examples of the limitations of the 5-Element model of correspondences. The basic limitation lies in the fact that the 5-Element model of correspondences became a rigid model of relationships between individual parts, and, in the process of fitting everything into a 5-fold classification, many assumptions and far-fetched correlations had to be made.

More important, the 5-Element model of correspondences sees one-to-one correlations between phenomena, for example Liver-eyes, Kidney-ears and Spleen-muscles. This may be useful in clinical practice, but the essence of Chinese Medicine is to see the whole disharmony and weave a pattern of various signs and symptoms. In this way, a one-to-one correlation is no longer valid, as one part could be related to a certain organ in the presence of a certain pattern, but to another organ in the presence of a different pattern. For example, if a woman suffers from blurred vision and, in addition, also has poor memory, scanty periods, numbness and dizziness, we can say that Liver-Blood is not nourishing the eyes: this therefore confirms the relationship between Liver and eye within the 5-Element theory. But if the same woman suffers from dry eyes and glaucoma and, in addition, has a lower back ache, vertigo, tinnitus and night sweating, we would say that Kidney-Yin is not moistening the eyes: this would therefore be outside the 5-Element model of correspondences.

THE FIVE ELEMENTS IN PATHOLOGY

The 5-Element model provides an important and clinically useful pattern of pathological relationships among the internal organs.

In the 5-Element relationships, two of the possible sequences only apply to pathological cases: these are the Over-acting and and Insulting sequences. The Generating sequence can also give rise to pathological conditions when it is out of balance.

The essence of the 5-Element relationships is balance: the Generating and Controlling sequences keep a dynamic balance among the Elements. When this balance is upset for a prolonged period of time, disease ensues.

The Over-acting Sequence

This occurs when the controlling relationship among the Elements gets out of control and becomes excessive. Similarly to the physiological relationships, the over-acting sequence relationships can be explained in terms of internal organs pathology.

The Liver over-acts on the Stomach and Spleen: if Liver-Qi stagnates, it "invades" the Stomach impairing its function of rotting and ripening, and the Spleen impairing its function of transforming and transporting. In particular, when Liver-Qi invades the Stomach, it prevents Stomach-Qi from descending causing nausea, and it prevents Spleen-Qi from ascending causing diarrhoea.

The Heart over-acts on the Lungs: Heart-Fire can

dry-up the Lung fluids and cause Lung-Yin deficiency.

The Spleen over-acts on the Kidneys: when the Spleen holds Dampness, this can obstruct the Kidney function of transformation and excretion of fluids.

The Lungs over-act on the Liver: this seldom happens in practice, as it is more a case of Lung deficiency triggering off stagnation of Liver-Qi.

The Kidneys over-act on the Heart: if Kidney-Yin is deficient, Empty-Heat forms and can be transmitted to the Heart.

The Insulting Sequence

These relationships along the Insulting sequence also occur in pathological conditions.

The Liver insults the Lungs: Liver-Qi can stagnate upwards and obstruct the chest and breathing.

The Heart insults the Kidneys: Heart-Fire can infuse downwards to the Kidneys and cause Kidney-Yin deficiency.

The Spleen insults the Liver: if the Spleen retains Dampness, this can overflow and impair the free flow of Liver-Qi.

The Lungs insult the Heart: if the Lungs are obstructed by Phlegm they can impair the circulation of Heart-Qi.

The Kidneys insult the Spleen: if the Kidneys fail to transform fluids, the Spleen will suffer and become obstructed by Dampness.

The Generating Sequence

The Generating sequence can also give rise to pathological states when out of balance. There are two possibilities:

a) The Mother-Element not nourishing the Child-Element.

b) The Child-Element taking too much from the Mother-Element.

The Liver (Mother) affecting the Heart (Child): this happens when the Liver fails to nourish the Heart. Specifically, when Liver-Blood is deficient, it often affects Heart-Blood which becomes deficient and palpitations and insomnia would ensue. There is another particular way in which Wood affects Fire, and that is in the way the Gall Bladder affects the Heart. This happens on a psychological level. The Gall Bladder controls the capacity of making decisions, not so much in the sense of being able to distinguish and evaluate what is right and what is wrong, but in the sense of having the courage to act on a decision. Thus, it is said in Chinese Medicine that a strong Gall Bladder makes one courageous.

This psychological trait of the Gall Bladder influences the Heart, as the Mind (housed in the Heart) needs the support of a strong drive and courage given by a strong Gall Bladder. In this way, a deficient Gall Bladder can affect the Mind (of the Heart) causing emotional weakness, timidity and lack of assertion.

The Heart (Child) affecting the Liver (Mother): if Heart-Blood is deficient, it can lead to general deficiency of Blood, which will affect the Liver storage of Blood. This would cause scanty periods or amenorrhoea.

The Heart (Mother) affecting the Spleen (Child): the Mind of the Heart needs to support the mental faculties and capacity of concentration which belong to the Spleen. Another aspect of this relationship is in Heart-Fire deficient being unable to warm Spleen-Yang and leading to cold feeling and diarrhoea. Ultimately, however, the physiological Fire of the Heart is itself derived from Kidney-Yang.

The Spleen (Child) affecting the Heart (Mother): the Spleen makes Qi and Blood and the Heart needs a strong supply of Blood. If the Spleen does not make enough Blood, the Heart will suffer and palpitations, insomnia, poor memory and slight depression will ensue.

The Spleen (Mother) affecting the Lungs (Child): if the Spleen function of transformation and transportation of fluids is impaired, Phlegm will be formed. Phlegm often settles in the Lungs and causes breathlessness and asthma.

The Lungs (Child) affecting the Spleen (Mother): the Lungs govern Qi and if Lung-Qi is deficient, Spleen-Qi will be affected, causing tiredness, no appetite and loose stools. In practice, Spleen-Qi and Lung-Qi deficiency often occur together.

The Lungs (Mother) affecting the Kidneys (Child): Lung-Qi normally descends towards the Kidneys which "hold" it down. Also, the Lungs send fluids down to the Kidneys. Thus, if Lung-

Qi is deficient, Qi and fluids cannot descend to the Kidneys, causing breathlessness (Kidney unable to receive Qi) and dryness of the Kidneys.

The Kidneys (Child) affecting the Lungs (Mother): if Kidney-Qi is deficient it will fail to hold Qi down, Qi will rebel upwards and obstruct the Lungs causing breathlessness.

The Kidneys (Mother) affecting the Liver (Child): Kidney-Yin nourishes Liver-Yin and Liver-Blood. If Kidney-Yin is deficient, Liver-Yin and/or Liver-Blood will become deficient and give rise to tinnitus, dizziness, headaches and irritability. This particular relationship is one of the most important and common in clinical practice.

The Liver (Child) affecting the Kidneys (Mother): Liver-Blood nourishes and replenishes the Kidney-Essence. If Liver-Blood is deficient over a long period of time, it can lead to deficiency of Kidney-Essence, causing dizziness, tinnitus, night sweating and sexual weakness.

In conclusion, each Element can be out of balance in four ways (Fig. 23):

a) it is in excess and over-acts on another along the over-acting sequence
b) it is deficient and is insulted by another along the insulting sequence
c) it is in excess and "draws" excessively from its Mother Element
d) it is deficient and fails to nourish its Child.

THE FIVE ELEMENTS IN DIAGNOSIS

The 5-Element model of correspondences is extensively used in diagnosis. This is based mostly on the correspondence between Elements and smell, colour, taste and sound. The "Classic of Difficulties" in chapter 61 says: *"By observation one can distinguish the five colours thus identifying the disease; by hearing one can distinguish the five sounds, thus identifying the disease; by interrogation one can distinguish the five tastes, thus identifying the disease."*[21]

Colours

Observation of the colours is the most important of all in the 5-Element scheme of diagnosis. The colour of the face is mostly observed and the

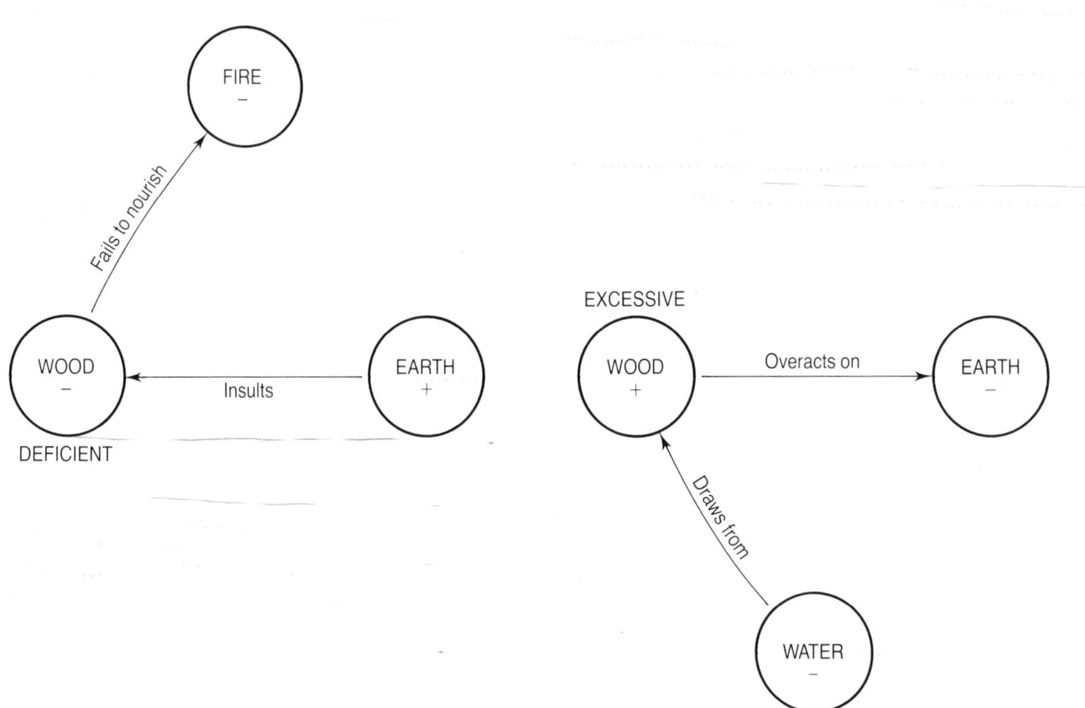

Fig. 23 Pathology of Generating, Over-acting and Insulting sequences

prevalence of one of the five colours indicates an imbalance in that particular Element, which could be either deficiency or excess.

Thus, a green colour of the face indicates an imbalance in Wood, which could be stagnation of Liver-Qi.

A red colour indicates an imbalance in Fire, which could be an excess of Heart-Fire.

A yellow, sallow complexion indicates an imbalance in Earth, which could be due to deficiency of Spleen-Qi.

A white colour indicates an imbalance in Metal, which could be deficiency of Lung-Qi.

A dark, purplish colour, sometimes grey, nearly black indicates an imbalance in Water, which could be due to Kidney-Yin deficiency.

Sometimes the complexion can show complex interactions between two Elements. For instance, a person may have a very pale-white face with red cheek-bones: this indicates Fire (red cheek-bones) over-acting on Metal (pale-white face). Or one might have a yellow complexion with a greenish tinge around the mouth: this would indicate Wood (green around mouth) over-acting on Earth (yellow complexion).

The face colour does not always accord with the clinical manifestations: in some situations, the face colour may contradict the pattern presented by the clinical manifestations. In these cases, the face colour usually shows the underlying cause of the imbalance. For example, if a person displays symptoms of Earth deficiency (tiredness, loose stools, no appetite, etc.) and has a greenish colour in the face, it may indicate that the Spleen is weak because the Liver is over-acting on it. Conversely, someone may display symptoms of Wood imbalance (such as gall stones, for instance) and have a yellow complexion. This may indicate that Earth is insulting Wood. If a person has symptoms of Fire imbalance (such as palpitations, bitter taste, mouth ulcers, insomnia, indicating Heart-Fire) and the complexion is dark, it may indicate that Water is over-acting on Fire. In the above cases then, the face colour shows the seat of the root imbalance and the clinical manifestations show the resulting pattern.

However, the 5-Element colour correspondences in diagnosis have to be used critically, and they should not be applied mechanically. In interpreting and making deductions from the face colour, one must be very careful to take into account not only the 5-Element theory, but also other aspects of Chinese Medicine. For example, a yellow complexion indicates an Earth problem from the 5-Element point of view, but it may also indicate retention of Dampness. A dark-black complexion indicates a Water problem according to the 5 Elements, but it may also indicate stasis of Blood. A white complexion indicates a Metal imbalance from the 5-Element point of view, but it also indicates a Cold condition (which could be of any organ) judged according to the 8 Principles (see page 179). According to the 5 Elements a green complexion indicates a Wood imbalance, but it also may indicate stasis of Blood or chronic pain. The 5-Element theory tells us that a red complexion indicates a Fire imbalance, but according to the 8 Principles, it may also indicate Heat, which could be in any organ.

As was pointed out before, in Chinese diagnosis it is not always possible to make a direct correlation between two phenomena on a one-to-one basis. What counts is the place of each phenomenon in the whole pattern. For example, a red face with bitter taste, insomnia, mouth ulcers and palpitations does indicate a problem in the Fire (Heart), but a red face with rapid breathing, yellow mucus and cough indicates a problem in the Lungs; a red face with irritability, bitter taste, headaches and dizziness indicates a problem in the Liver.

Sounds

Voice sounds and tone can also be used in diagnosis. If someone tends to shout a lot in anger, it indicates an imbalance in the Wood element. If someone laughs a lot without apparent reason (as it sometimes happens when a patient punctuates the interrogation with frequent laughs), it indicates an imbalance in the Fire element.

A singing tone of voice indicates an imbalance in the Earth element. Crying is related to Metal and it often indicates a deficiency of the Lungs (whose emotion is grief). A very thin and weak voice also indicates weakness of Lung-Qi. A groaning or husky tone of voice indicates an imbalance in Water.

Smells

Smells are also used in diagnosis according to the 5-Element model of correspondences. A rancid smell indicates an imbalance in Wood, often due to stagnation of Heat in the Liver. A burned smell indicates an imbalance in Fire, usually Heart-Fire.

A sweetish smell is often associated with Spleen deficiency or Dampness. A rank smell is often indicative of a Metal imbalance, usually due to chronic retention of Phlegm in the Lungs. A rotten or putrid smell is indicative of a Kidney or Bladder imbalance, usually retention of Damp-Heat.

In the same way that colours can be interpreted in other ways than those indicated by the 5-Element model, smells too sometimes do not correspond to this rather rigid system.

For example, a rotten or putrid smell is indicative of Heat of any organ. Also, other types of smells are sometimes described, such as leathery being indicative of Damp-Heat and fishy being indicative of Damp-Cold.

Emotions

The relationship between emotions and Elements is important in diagnosis. A person who is prone to outbursts of anger would manifest an imbalance in Wood (usually rising of Liver-Yang). The emotion may also be more subdued and less apparent when the anger is repressed.

Joy is the emotion related to Fire and the Heart. Obviously a state of joy is not a harmful emotion. What is meant by "joy" here, however, is rather a state of excessive or constant excitement which may be typical of some people in our society. An example of the negative effect of excess joy is the migraine attack that can sometimes be triggered not only by bad news, but also by sudden good news.

Pensiveness or over-concentration is the "emotion" related to Earth. Admittedly this is not an "emotion" in the way we conceive it, but it is nevertheless the mental activity related to the Spleen.[22]

An excessive use of our thinking faculties and study may lead to deficiency of the Spleen.

Grief and sorrow are the emotions related to Metal, and, in practice, there is a direct and common relationship between these emotions and the state of the Lungs. Lung-Qi is very much affected by grief or sadness (and also worry), and these emotions will cause a deficiency of Lung-Qi.

Fear is related to Water and, again, this emotion directly influences the Kidneys and Bladder. A deficiency of the Kidneys often causes anxiety and fears.

Tastes

The tastes related to the 5 Elements are a relatively minor aspect of Chinese diagnosis. The tastes are sour for Wood, bitter for Fire, sweet for Earth, pungent for Metal and salty for Water.

A sour taste often accompanies Liver disharmonies, a bitter taste is part of the pattern of Heart-Fire, a sweet taste is often indicative of Spleen deficiency, a pungent taste sometimes accompanies Lung disharmonies and a salty taste occasionally is associated with Kidney deficiency.

The taste correspondences also suffer from certain limitations, in the same way as for the colours. For example, a sour taste is more frequently present in Stomach disharmonies, a bitter taste is also more frequently indicative of Liver disharmonies such as Liver-Fire and a sweet taste can also indicate retention of Dampness.

Beside this, there are also other types of tastes often described by patients that do not fit into this scheme. For example, a "flat" taste indicates Spleen deficiency and a "sticky" taste indicates retention of Dampness.

Tissues

A pathological state of the tissues can be used in diagnosis as a pointer to disharmony of the relevant Elements. For example, if the tendons are tight and stiff, this indicates a Liver and Gall Bladder or Wood disharmony. A problem with blood vessels points to a Heart or Fire imbalance. A weakness or atrophy of the muscles indicates Spleen or Earth deficiency. The skin is related to Metal and the Lungs, and a Lung weakness is often manifested with spontaneous sweating (the pores being open).

The Kidneys are related to the bones, and bone degenerative diseases which occur in old age, such as osteoporosis, are often due to the decline of Kidney-Essence.

Sense orifices

Problems with the five senses can also reflect disharmonies in the relevant Elements. For example, blurred vision often reflects Liver-deficiency, a problem with the tongue can be related to the Heart, mouth and lips problems are often due to Spleen deficiency or Stomach Heat, dry nose or sneezing reflect Lung dryness or deficiency, a decrease in hearing of chronic tinnitus can be due to Kidney deficiency.

Again, this model of relationships is only partly applicable. For example, there are many eye disorders not related to Wood (as explained above), some tongue pathologies can also be due to Stomach or Kidneys, the lips also manifest the state of blood, mouth problems can also be due to a Kidney pathology and many ear problems are not due to a Kidney deficiency but to imbalances in other Elements, e.g. Wood Element.

Climates

A person's sensitivity to a particular climatic condition often reflects a disharmony in the relevant Element. Thus, a sensitivity to wind often reflects a disharmony in Wood. People with Heart disharmonies often feel much worse in the heat, dampness affects the Spleen, dryness injures the Lungs and Cold weakens the Kidneys.

However, this model has limitations too. For example, heat can aggravate a Heat condition of any organ, not just the Heart. Dampness can aggravate a Damp condition not only of the Spleen, but also Lungs, Kidneys, Gall Bladder and Bladder. Dryness injures the body fluids not only of the Lungs, but also Stomach and Kidneys. Cold affects virtually any organ (in particular Stomach, Spleen, Intestines, Lungs, Uterus and Bladder) and not just the Kidneys.

THE FIVE ELEMENTS IN TREATMENT

There are several ways in which the theory of the 5 Elements is applied in treatment. These could be summarized in two headings:

Treatment according to the various sequences

Treatment according to the 5 Transporting points.

These are not alternative ways of applying the 5-Element theory in treatment, but simply a convenient way to discuss their use, bearing in mind that they are often both used at the same time.

Treatment according to the various sequences

When considering a treatment of a certain Element, one should keep in mind the various relationships of that Element with the other along the Generating, Controlling, Over-acting, Insulting and Cosmological sequences.

Let us look for example at one Element, Wood; the other four Elements all follow the same general principle.

If there is a Wood disharmony, one must consider first of all if this disharmony may be affected by another Element, and, secondly, whether it is affecting another Element.

For example, if the Liver is deficient and the patient has several signs and symptoms of Liver-Blood deficiency, one should always consider and check whether the Mother Element (Water) is at fault, failing to nourish Wood. On the other hand, we must consider and check whether Wood is deficient from being over-acted upon by Metal, or because Fire (the Child) is drawing too much from Wood (the Mother), or even because it is being insulted by Earth. One should also consider and check whether the Liver deficiency is affecting the Child Element, i.e. the Heart (Fig. 24).

If the Liver is in excess and the patient for example, has symptoms and signs of Liver-Qi

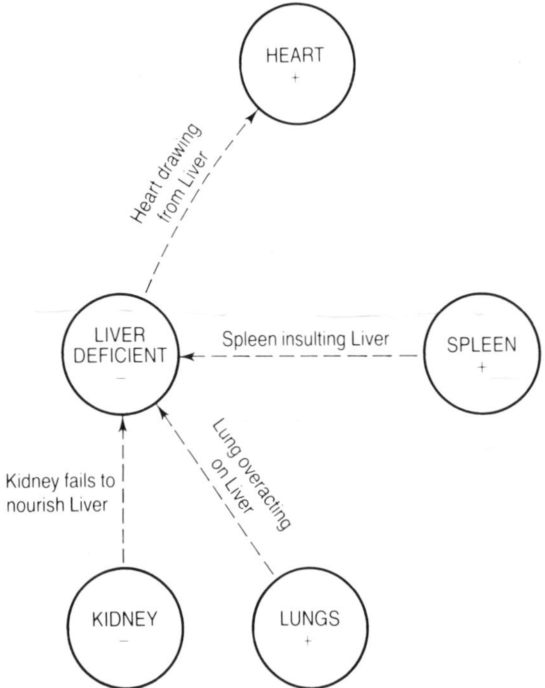

Fig. 24 Pathological influences between a deficient Liver and other organs

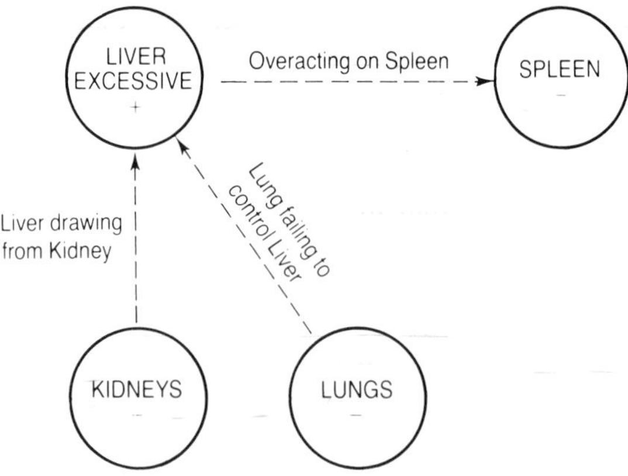

Fig. 25 Pathological influences between an excessive Liver and other organs

stagnation or Liver-Fire, one must check whether this excess is due to deficient Metal failing to control Wood. This often happens in chronic constitutional weakness of the Lungs.

On the other hand, one must check whether the excess in Wood has begun to affect other Elements. For example, when Wood is in excess, it can easily over-act on Earth. This is called "Wood invading Earth" and is very common in practice. If Wood is in excess, it could also make too much demand on the Mother Element, i.e. Water (Fig. 25). It is necessary to keep all these relationships in mind when determining the treatment.

Thus, if the Liver is deficient because it is not nourished by its Mother Element, Water, the Kidneys as well as the Liver must be tonified. If the Liver is deficient because it is being over-acted on by Metal, the correct course of action would be to sedate the Lungs (this is, however, a rather theoretical possibility as it hardly ever happens in practice). If the Liver is deficient because the Heart (Child) is drawing too much from it, one would have to sedate the Heart. If the Liver is deficient because it is being insulted by the Spleen, treatment demands sedation of the Spleen.

If the Liver deficiency is affecting its Child Element, one would tonify the Heart as well as the Liver.

If the Liver is in excess because Metal is not controlling it, one must tonify Metal (the Lungs), as well as sedating the Liver. If the Liver excess is affecting and depressing Earth, in this case the Spleen requires tonification. If the Liver is in excess and is drawing too much from the Mother Element, one must also tonify the Kidneys.

The "Classic of Difficulties" says in chapter 77: *"If the Liver is diseased, it can invade the Spleen, one must therefore tonify the Spleen first"*.[23]

Treatment according to the 5 Transporting points

This subject will be discussed in detail in chapter 37, and will therefore only be dealt with briefly here.

The 5 Transporting points are the points between the fingers and elbows and between the toes and knees: each of the 5 points is related to an Element, in the order of the Generating sequence, starting with Wood for the Yin channels and Metal for the Yang ones. This principle was established for the first time in the "Classic of Difficulties" in chapter 64.[24]

In chapter 69 it says: *"In case of Deficiency tonify the Mother, in case of Excess sedate the Child"*.[25]

This means that in case of deficiency of one organ one can choose the point on its channel related to its Mother Element. For example, in case of deficiency of the Liver channel, one can choose the point on the Liver channel related to its Mother Element, i.e. Water: this is Ququan LIV-8.

In case of excess of one organ one can choose the point on its channel related to its Child Element. For example, in case of excess of the Liver channel, one can choose the point on the Liver channel related to its Child Element, i.e Fire: this is Xingjian LIV-2.

Another way of using the 5-Element points in treatment is using them to expel pathogenic factors. Given that Wood corresponds to Wind, Fire to Heat, Earth to Dampness, Metal to Dryness and Water to Cold, one can use (usually sedate) the Element points to expel the relevant pathogenic factor. Thus one would use a Wood point to subdue Wind, a Fire point to clear Heat, an Earth point to resolve Dampness, etc.

THE FIVE ELEMENTS IN HERBAL AND DIET THERAPY

Diet therapy is a vast subject in Chinese Medicine and it will only be briefly mentioned here as it is partly based on the 5-Element model. The principles underlying diet therapy are largely the same as those in herbal therapy, and they will therefore be discussed together.

Each food or herb has a certain taste which is related to one of the Elements. The five tastes are: sour for Wood, bitter for Fire, sweet for Earth, pungent for Metal and salty for Water. Each food or herb is classified as having one of these tastes. The "taste" of a food or herb is not always related to its actual flavour: for instance, lamb is classified as "bitter", and so is apple. The "taste" of a food or herb is therefore more like its intrinsic quality, rather than its actual flavour, although in most cases the two will coincide.

Each of the tastes has a certain effect on the body: the sour taste generates fluids and Yin. It is astringent and can control perspiration and diarrhoea.

The bitter taste clears Heat, sedates and hardens. It clears Damp-Heat and it subdues rebellious Qi.

The sweet taste tonifies, balances and moderates. It is used to tonify deficiency and to stop pain.

The pungent taste scatters, and is used to expel pathogenic factors.

The salty taste flows downwards, softens hardness and is used to treat constipation and swelling.

Certain precautions should be used when choosing foods as these are consumed regularly over a long period of time and have therefore a deep and long-lasting effect on the body's functions. The same precautions apply if a certain herbal treatment is applied over a long period of time.

The sour taste goes to the nerves and can upset the Liver, so it should be used sparingly if a person suffers from chronic pain.

The bitter taste goes to the bones, and an excess of it should be avoided in bone diseases.

The sweet taste goes to the muscles and an excess of it can cause weakness of the muscles.

The pungent taste scatters Qi and should be avoided in Qi deficiency.

The salty taste can dry the Blood, and should be avoided in Blood deficiency.

The "Spiritual Axis" in chapter 56 deals with the effect of the five tastes. It says: *"The sour taste goes to the Liver, the bitter taste goes to the Heart, the sweet taste goes to the Spleen, the pungent taste goes to the Lungs, the salty taste goes to the Kidneys...if the Liver is diseased one should not eat pungent foods, if the Heart is diseased one should not eat salty foods, if the Spleen is diseased one should not eat sour foods, if the Kidney is diseased one should not eat sweet foods, if the Lung is diseased one should not eat bitter foods"*.[26]

Thus, if an organ is diseased one should avoid the taste related to the Element that controls that organ along the Controlling sequence.

NOTES

1 Science and Civilization in China, vol 2, p 244.
2 Lamanna E P 1967 *Storia della Filosofia* (History of Philosophy), vol 1.Le Monnier, Florence, p 220-221.
3 Science and Civilization in China, p 242.
4 Science and Civilization in China, p 266.
5 Kaptchuk T 1983 The Web that has no Weaver. Congdon & Weed, New York, p 343–354.
6 Science and Civilization in China, p 232, 242.
7 Gu He Dao 1979 History of Chinese Medicine (*Zhong Guo Yi Xue Shi Lue* 中国医学史略).Shanxi People's Publishing House, Taiyuan p 29.
8 History of Chinese Medicine, p 29.
9 Great Transmission of the Valued Book (*Shang Shu Da Chuan* 尚书大传), cited in History of Chinese Medicine, p 29.
10 Lloyd G, Chadwick J Mann W 1983 Hippocratic writings. Penguin Books, p 237.
11 *Shang Shu* (c. 659–627 BC), cited in 1975 Practical Chinese Medicine (*Shi Yong Zhong Yi Xue* 实用中医学). Beijing Publishing House, Beijing, p 32. The book *Shang Shu* is attributed by some to the early Zhou dynasty (hence c. 1000 BC), but the prevalent opinion is that it was written between 659 and 627 BC.
12 Science and Civilization in China, p 238.
13 Practical Chinese Medicine, p 32.
14 1982 Classic of Categories (*Lei Jing* 类经), People's Health Publishing House, Beijing, p 46 (first published 1624).
15 1981 Discussion of Prescriptions of the Golden Chest (*Jin Gui Yao Lue Fang Lun* 金匮要略方论). Zhejiang Scientific Publishing House, p 1 (first published c. AD 220).
16 See note 7 above.
17 Science and Civilization in China, vol 2, p 258–259.
18 Simple Questions, p 22–38.
19 As explained above, the Earth corresponds to a short period at the end of each season. In other words, at the end of each season the energy goes back to the Centre for replenishment. For this reason, the Earth does not correspond to any season in particular.
20 Nanjing College of Traditional Chinese Medicine 1979 A Revised Explanation of the Classic of Difficulties (*Nan Jing Jiao Shi* 难经校释). People's Publishing House, Beijing, p 90, 95.
21 Classic of Difficulties, p 134.
22 It is difficult to understand how the Chinese word "*Si*" 思 which is the "emotion" related to Earth and means "to think" or "pensiveness", could ever be translated as "sympathy" as it is in several Western acupuncture books.
23 Classic of Difficulties, p 163.
24 Classic of Difficulties, p 139.
25 Classic of Difficulties, p 151.
26 1981 Spiritual Axis, People's Health Publishing House, Beijing, p 104 (first compiled c. 200 BC).

The Vital Substances 3

氣血津液

Chinese Medicine sees the working of the body and mind as the result of the interaction of certain vital substances. These substances manifest in varying degrees of "substantiality", so that some of them are very rarefied and some totally non-material. All together, they constitute the ancient Chinese view of the body-mind. The body and mind are not seen as a mechanism (however complex) but as a vortex of energy and vital substances interacting with each other to form an organism. At the basis of all is Qi: all the other vital substances are but manifestations of Qi in varying degrees of materiality, ranging from the completely material, such as Body Fluids, to the totally immaterial, such as the Mind (*Shen*).

The Vital Substances are:

Qi
Blood
Essence (*Jing*)
Body Fluids.

THE CONCEPT OF QI IN CHINESE PHILOSOPHY

The concept of Qi has occupied Chinese philosophers of all times, right from the beginning of Chinese civilization to our modern times. The character for Qi indicates that it is something which is, at the same time, material and immaterial.

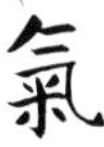

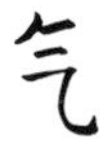 means "vapour", "steam", "gas"

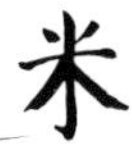 means (uncooked) "rice"

This clearly indicates that Qi can be as rarefied and immaterial as vapour, and as dense and material as rice. It also indicates that Qi is a subtle substance (steam, vapour) deriving from a coarse one (rice) just as steam is produced by cooking rice.

It is very difficult to translate the word "Qi" and many different ones have been proposed, none of which approximates the essence ot Qi exactly. It has variously been translated as "energy", "material force", "matter", "ether", "matter-energy", "vital force", "life force", "vital power", "moving power". The reason it is so difficult to translate the word "Qi" correctly, lies precisely in its fluid nature whereby Qi can assume different manifestations and be different things in different situations.

The way "Qi" is translated also depends on the particular view point taken. Most modern physicists would probably agree that "Qi" may be termed "energy" since Qi expresses the continuum of matter and energy as it is now understood by modern particle physics. The closeness of the concept of Qi and energy was highlighted by an article on the nature of Qi written by an eminent professor from the Institute of High Energy Physics of China.[1] According to Needham, "Qi" also conveys the idea of "aethereal waves" or "radioactive emanations", in a modern sense.[2]

Most sinologists generally agree that Qi corresponds to "matter", although not matter in a restrictive materialistic sense, as Qi can also assume very rarefied, dispersed, non-material forms. There is another term to indicate matter in its solid, hard and tangible state, and that is "JI". "Ji" is a form of Qi, but Qi is not always "Ji", as it can exist in tenuous and non-perceptible forms. Because of the difficulty in finding an appropriate translation for the term, I have chosen to leave it untranslated, together with "Yin" and "Yang".

Qi is at the basis of all phenomena in the universe and provides a continuity between coarse, material forms and tenuous, rarefied, non-material energies. It therefore completely sidesteps the dilemma that pervaded Western philosophy from the time of Plato down to the present day, i.e. the duality and contrast between materialism and idealism. Western philosophy either considered matter as independent of man's perception, or, at the other extreme, considered matter as a mere reflection of ideas. Needham puts this very well: "... *both* [*the macrocosm-microcosm doctrine and organic naturalism*] *were subject to what I call ... the characteristic European schizophrenia or split-personality. Europeans could only think in terms either of Democritean mechanical materialism or of Platonic theological spiritualism. A deus always had to be found for a machina. Animas, entelechiae, souls, archaei, dance processionally through the history of European thinking*".[3]

The infinite variety of phenomena in the universe is the result of the continuous coming together and dispersion of Qi to form phenomena of various degrees of materialization. This idea of aggregation and dispersion of Qi was discussed by many Chinese philosophers of all times.

Qi is the very basis of the universe's infinite manifestations of life, including minerals, vegetables and animals (including man). Xun Kuang (c. 313–238 BC) said: "*Water and Fire have Qi but not life; plants and trees have life, but not knowledge; birds and animals have knowledge, but no sense of what are rights.*"[4]

Lie Zi, a Daoist philosopher who lived around 300 BC said : "... *The purer and lighter* [*elements*], *tending upwards, made the heaven; the grosses and heavier* [*elements*], tending downwards, made the earth...".[5]

Thus "heaven" and "earth" are often used to symbolize two extreme states of utmost rarefaction and dispersion or utmost condensation and aggregation of Qi respectively.

Huai Nan Zi (c. 122 BC), a Daoist book, says: "*Dao orginated from Emptiness and Emptiness produced the universe. The universe produced Qi.... That which was clear and light drifted up to become heaven, and that which was heavy and turbid solidified to form earth.*".[6]

According to these ancient philosophers, life and death themselves are nothing but an aggregation and dispersal of Qi. Wang Chong (AD 27–97) said: "*Qi produces the human body just as water becomes ice. As water freezes into ice, so Qi coagulates to form the human body. When ice melts, it becomes water. When a person dies, he or she becomes spirit [shen] again. It is called spirit, just as melted ice changes its name to water.*"[7]

He also said: "*When it came to separation and differentiation, the pure* [elements] *formed heaven, and the turbid ones formed earth*"[8]

Zhang Zai (AD 1020–1077) further developed the concept of Qi. He proposed that the Great Void was not mere emptiness, but Qi in its state of continuity. He said the Great Void cannot but consist of Qi. He also further developed the idea of condensation and dissipation of Qi in giving rise to the myriad phenomena in the universe. He affirmed that extreme aggregation of Qi gives rise to actual form, "Xing", i.e. material substance. This concept has important applications in Chinese Medicine, as we shall see shortly. Zhang Zai said: *"The Great Void consists of Qi. Qi condenses to become the myriad things. Things of necessity disintegrate and return to the Great Void"*.[9] Also: *"If Qi condenses, its visibility becomes effective and physical form appears."*[10]

It is important to note that Zhang Zai clearly saw the indestructibility of matter-energy. He said: *"Qi in dispersion is substance, and so is it in condensation"*![11] Human life, too, is nothing but a condensation of Qi, and death is a dispersal of Qi. He said: *"Every birth is a condensation, every death a dispersal. Birth is not a gain, death not a loss...when condensed, Qi becomes a living being, when dispersed, it is the substratum of mutations"*![12]

Zhu Xi (1131–1200) also saw life as a condensation of Qi. He said: *"Qi, condensing, can form beings"*.[13]

Wang Fu Zhi (1619–1692) reaffirmed the concept of continuity of energy and matter and the condensation of formless Qi into physical shapes. He said: *"Life is not creation from nothing, and death is not complete dispersion and destruction"*![14] Also: "[*Despite the condensation and dispersion of Qi*] *its original substance can neither be added nor be lessened*"[15] Other quotations from his writings further clarify the nature of Qi: *"All that is void and empty is full of Qi which, in its state of condensation and thus visible, is called being, but in its state of dispersion and thus no longer visible, is called non-being"*.[16] *"When dispersing Qi makes the Great Void, only regaining its original misty feature but not perishing; when condensing, it becomes the origin of all beings"*.[17]

In conclusion, we can say that Qi is a continuous form of matter, resulting in physical shape ("*Xing*") when it condenses. *Xing* is a discontinuous form of matter, resulting in Qi when it disperses.

THE CONCEPT OF QI IN CHINESE MEDICINE

All that was said about Qi so far applies to Chinese Medicine. Chinese philosophers and doctors saw the interrelationship between the universe and human beings and considered the human being's Qi as a result of the interaction of the Qi of Heaven and Earth. The "Simple Questions" in chapter 25 says: *"A human being results from the Qi of Heaven and Earth...The union of the Qi of Heaven and Earth is called human being"*.[18] This stresses the interaction between the human being's Qi and natural forces. Chinese Medicine emphasizes the relationship between human beings and their environment and takes this into account in determining aetiology, diagnosis and treatment.

Just as Qi is the material substratum of the universe, it is also the material and spiritual substratum of human life. The "Classic of Difficulties" says: *"Qi is the root of a human being"*.[19]

In particular, two aspects of Qi are especially relevant to medicine:

a) Qi is an energy which manifests simultaneously on the physical and spiritual level;

b) Qi is in a constant state of flux and in varying states of aggregation. When Qi condenses, energy transforms and accumulates into physical shape.

According to the Chinese there are many different "types" of human Qi, ranging from the tenuous and rarefied, to the very dense and coarse. All the various types of Qi, however, are ultimately one Qi, merely manifesting in different forms.

It is important, therefore, to see the universality and particularity of Qi simultaneously. On the one hand, there is only one Qi energy that assumes different forms, but , on the other hand, in practice, it is also important to appreciate the different types of Qi.

Qi changes its form according to its locality and its function. Although Qi is fundamentally the same, it puts on "different hats" in different places assuming different functions. For example, Nutritive Qi exists in the Interior of the body. Its function is to nourish and it is denser than Defensive Qi, which is on the Exterior and protects the body. Derangement of either Defensive or Nutritive Qi will give rise to different clinical manifestations and will require different kinds of treatment. Ultimately, though, they are nothing but two different manifestations of the same Qi energy.

Poor circulation can result in excessive condensation of Qi which means that Qi becomes pathologically dense, forming lumps, masses or tumours.

In Chinese Medicine, "Qi" has two major aspects. Firstly, it indicates a refined essence produced by the internal organs, which has the function of nourishing the body and mind. This refined essence takes several forms depending on its location and function. Gathering Qi, for example, is in the chest and nourishes Heart and Lungs. Original Qi is in the Lower Burner and nourishes the Kidneys. Secondly, Qi indicates the functional activity of the internal organs. When used in this sense, it does *not* indicate a refined substance as above, but simply the complex of functional activities of any organ. For example, when we speak of Liver-Qi, it does not mean the portion of Qi residing in the Liver, but it indicates the complex of the Liver's functional activities, i.e. ensuring the smooth flow of Qi. In this sense, we can speak of Liver-Qi, Heart-Qi, Lung-Qi, Stomach-Qi, etc.

ESSENCE 精

"JING" is usually translated as "Essence". The Chinese character gives the idea of something derived from a process of refinement or distillation: it is a distilled, refined essence, extracted from some coarser basis. This process of extraction of a refined essence from a larger, coarser substance, implies that the Essence is a rather precious substance to be cherished and guarded.

The term "Essence" occurs in traditional Chinese medical books, used in three different contexts with slightly different meanings:

The "Pre-Heaven Essence"
The "Post-Heaven Essence"
The Essence (or Kidney-Essence).

Pre-Heaven Essence

Conception is a blending of the sexual energies of man and woman to form what the ancient Chinese called the "Pre-Heaven Essence" of the newly conceived human being. This Essence nourishes the embryo and fetus during pregnancy and is also dependent on nourishment derived from the mother's Kidneys. The Pre-Heaven Essence is the only kind of essence present in the fetus, as it does not have independent physiological activity.

This Pre-Heaven Essence is what determines each person's basic constitutional make-up, strength and vitality. It is what makes each individual unique.

Since it is inherited from the parents at conception, the Pre-Heaven Essence can be influenced only with difficulty in the course of adult life. Some say this Essence is "fixed" in quantity and quality. However, it can be positively affected, even if not quantitatively increased.[20]

The best way to affect positively one's Pre-Heaven Essence is by striving for balance in one's life activities: balance between work and rest, restraint in sexual activity and balanced diet. Any irregularity or excess in these spheres is bound to diminish the Pre-Heaven Essence. A direct way to positively influence one's Essence is through breathing exercises and such exercises as *Tai Ji Quan* and *Qi Gong*.

Post-Heaven Essence

This is the essence which is refined and extracted from food and fluids by the Stomach and Spleen after birth. After birth, the baby starts eating, drinking and breathing, its Lungs, Stomach and Spleen start functioning to produce Qi from food, drink and air. The "Golden Mirror of Medical Collection" says: *"The Pre-Heaven Essence originates from the parents, the Post-Heaven Essence originates from food"*.[21]

The complex of essences refined and extracted from food are collectively known as "Post-Heaven Essence". Because the Stomach and

Spleen are responsible for the digestion of food and the transformation and transportation of food essences ultimately leading to the production of Qi, the Post-Heaven Essence is closely related to Stomach and Spleen.

The Post-Heaven Essence is therefore not a specific type of essence, but simply a general term to indicate the essences produced by the Stomach and Spleen after birth, as opposed to the Pre-Heaven Essence which is formed before birth.

The Essence

Kidney-Essence is a more specific kind of vital substance which plays an extremely important role in human physiology. It derives from both the Pre-Heaven and Post-Heaven Essence. Like the Pre-Heaven Essence, it is a hereditary energy which determines the person's constitution. Unlike the Pre-Heaven Essence, though, the Kidney Essence interacts with the Post-Heaven Essence and is replenished by it. Kidney Essence therefore partakes of both the Pre-Heaven and Post-Heaven Essence.

This Essence is stored in the Kidneys, but having a fluid nature it also circulates all over the body, particularly in the 8 Extraordinary Vessels (see page 355).

Kidney Essence determines growth, reproduction, development, sexual maturation, conception and pregnancy.

There are many differences between Essence and Qi in the human body:

— Essence is mostly derived from the parents, whilst Qi is formed after birth.
— Essence is fluid-like, Qi is energy-like.
— Essence resides mostly in the Kidneys, Qi is everywhere.
— Essence is replenished only with difficulty, Qi can easily be replenished on a day-to-day basis.
—Essence follows very long cycles of 7 or 8 years, whereas Qi follows shorter cycles, some yearly, some circadian, some even shorter.
— Qi moves and changes quickly from moment to moment, whereas the Essence changes only slowly and gradually over long periods of time.

The functions of Essence are as follows:

1 Growth, reproduction and development

Essence is the organic substance which forms the basis for growth, reproduction and development. It controls the growth of bones in children, teeth, hair, normal brain development and sexual maturation. After puberty, it controls the reproductive function and fertility. It forms the basis for successful conception and pregnancy. The natural decline of the Essence during our lifetime, leads to the natural decline of sexual energy and fertility.

According to the first chapter of the "Simple Questions", men's Essence flows in 8-year cycles, and women's Essence in 7-year cycles.

"The Kidney energy of a girl becomes abundant at the age of 7, her baby teeth are replaced by permanent ones and the hair grows. At the age of 14 the dew of Heaven arrives [menstruation], the Directing Vessel begins to flow, the Penetrating Vessel is flourishing, the periods come regularly and she can conceive. At the age of 21 the Kidney Essence peaks, the wisdom teeth come out and growth is at its utmost. At the age of 28, tendons and bones become strong, the hair grows longest and the body is strong and flourishing. At the age of 35, the Bright Yang channels begin to weaken, the complexion starts to wither and the hair begins to fall. At the age of 42, the three Yang channels are weak, the face darkens and the hair begins to turn grey. At the age of 49, the Directing Vessel is empty, the Penetrating Vessel depleted, the dew of Heaven dries up, the Earth Passage [uterus] is not open, so weakness and infertility set in. In a man, at the age of 8 the boy's Kidney energy is abundant, his hair and teeth grow. At the age of 16 his Kidney energy is even more abundant, the dew of Heaven [sperm] arrives, the Essence is luxuriant and flowing, Yin and Yang are harmonized and he can produce a child. At the age of 24, the Kidney energy peaks, tendons and bones are strong, the wisdom teeth appear, and growth is at its peak. At the age of 32, tendons and bones are at their strongest, and the muscles are full and strong. At the age of 40, the Kidney is weakened, the hair begins to fall out and the teeth become loose. At the age of 48, Yang Qi is exhausted, the face becomes darker and the hair turns grey. At the age of 56, the Liver energy is weakened, the tendons cannot move, the dew of Heaven is dried up, the Kidney

becomes weak and the body begins to grow old. At the age of 64, hair and teeth are gone."[22]

2 The Essence as basis of Kidney-Qi

There is a close interaction among the various aspects of Kidney energy, i.e Kidney-Essence, Kidney-Yin, Kidney-Yang, Kidney-Qi.

Essence is fluid-like and naturally belongs to Yin; it can therefore be considered as an aspect of Kidney-Yin. In addition, it provides the material basis for Kidney-Yin to produce Kidney-Qi by the heating action of Kidney-Yang. In other words, the Kidneys can be compared to a large cauldron full of water. The fire under the cauldron is provided by Kidney-Yang and the Gate of Vitality (*Ming Men*, see page 98), the water inside the cauldron corresponds to the Kidney-Essence, and the resulting steam (i.e. Qi), corresponds to Kidney-Qi (Fig. 26).

Thus, Kidney-Essence is necessary for the transformation of Kidney-Yin into Kidney-Qi through the warming action of Kidney-Yang.

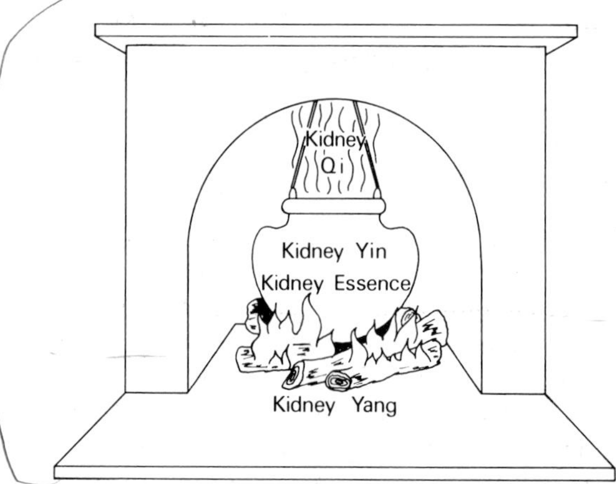

Fig. 26 Relationship among Kidney-Yin, Kidney-Essence, Kidney-Yang and Kidney-Qi

3 The Essence produces Marrow

The concept of Marrow in Chinese Medicine is different from that in Western medicine, and it does not correspond to bone marrow.

The Essence produces Marrow, which, in turn, produces bone marrow and fills the spinal cord and the brain. Thus, "Marrow" is a substance which is the common matrix of the bone marrow, brain and spinal cord: it has no equivalent in Western medicine.

Essence is therefore extremely important for healthy bone marrow, brain and spinal cord. The "Spiritual Axis"in chapter 33 says: *"The Brain is the Sea of Marrow"*.[23] Thus, if the Kidney-Essence is weak, the brain may lack nourishment and the person may lack concentration and memory and suffer from dizziness and a feeling of emptiness of the head.

4 The Essence as the basis of constitutional strength

Finally, the Essence determines our basic constitutional strength and resistance to exterior pathogenic factors. Although the Defensive Qi is mostly responsible for protection from exterior pathogenic factors, it also draws its strength and has its root in the Kidney-Essence. Thus the Kidney-Essence also plays a fundamental role in the protection against exterior pathogenic factors. The "Simple Questions" in chapter 4 says: *"If the Essence is properly stored [i.e. not dissipated], no exterior febrile diseases will be contracted in the Spring. . .if the Essence is not stored in Winter, exterior febrile diseases will be contracted in the Spring"*.[24]

From these four main functions of the Essence, one may deduce the kind of problems that may derive from a deficiency of Essence:

a) Growth, reproduction and development: stunted growth in children, poor bone development, infertility, habitual miscarriage, mental retardation in children, bone deterioration in adults, loose teeth and hair falling out or greying prematurely.

b) The Essence as basis for Kidney-Qi: poor sexual function, impotence, weakness of knees, nocturnal emissions, tinnitus and deafness.

c) The Essence as the basis of Marrow: poor concentration, poor memory, dizziness, tinnitus and a feeling of emptiness of the head.

d) The Essence as the basis of constitutional strength: being constantly prone to colds, influenza and other exterior diseases, chronic rhinitis and allergic rhinitis (hay fever).

Essence and Qi are also considered to be the material foundation of the Mind (*Shen*). Essence, Qi and Mind are the three fundamental physical and psychic substances of a human being. For this reason, they are called the "Three Treasures".

Essence, Qi and Mind also represent three different states of condensation of Qi, the Essence being the coarsest and densest, Qi being more rarefied, and the Mind being the most subtle and immaterial. According to Chinese Medicine, Essence and Qi are the essential foundation of the Mind. If Essence and Qi are healthy and flourishing, the Mind will be happy and this will lead to a healthy and happy life. If Essence and Qi are both depleted, then the Mind necessarily will suffer.

Thus a healthy Mind depends on the strength of the Essence, which is stored in the Kidneys, and Qi, which is produced by the Stomach and Spleen. In other words, the Mind is dependent on the Pre-Heaven and Post-Heaven Essence.

The triad of Essence, Qi and Mind is often expressed in Chinese Medicine as Heaven (the Mind), Person (Qi) and Earth (the Essence), corresponding to the three organs Heart, Stomach/Spleen and Kidneys respectively.

MIND	HEART	HEAVEN
QI	STOMACH-SPLEEN	PERSON
ESSENCE	KIDNEYS	EARTH

In practice, it is important to make a general assessment of the relative state of these three fundamental substances as the Essence gives an indication of the inherited constitution, Qi gives an indication of the state of Qi produced from day to day, and the Mind gives an indication of the state of the emotional and mental life.

The state of the Essence can to some degree be deduced from the patient's past: a history of serious childhood diseases would indicate a weak constitution. It can also be observed in the pulse: a pulse with a "Scattered" or "Leather" (see page 170) quality indicates poor and weakened Essence. The tongue can show a weakened Essence if its root has "no spirit" (see page 150).

The state of the Mind can be observed in the eyes. This can be deduced by observing the "glitter" of the eyes. Eyes with glitter, i.e. with a certain undefinable shine and vitality about them, show a healthy condition of the Mind. Eyes which look dull as if they had a curtain of mist in front of them, show that the Mind is disturbed. This can frequently be observed in those who have had serious emotional problems for a long period of time, or have had a serious shock, even if this occurred many years previously.

Some Chinese language expressions also show how these concepts are rooted in Chinese culture. "*Jing-shen*" (i.e. Essence-Mind) means "mind" or "consciousness", showing the interaction of body and mind. "*Jing-shen*" also means "vigour", "vitality", "drive", all qualities which are present when both the Essence and the Mind are healthy and strong. "*Jing-shen-bing*" means "mental illness".

QI 气

As we have discussed, Qi takes various forms in the body fulfilling a variety of functions. Let us now discuss the various forms of Qi.

Original Qi 原气

This type of Qi is closely related to Essence. Indeed, Original Qi is nothing but Essence in the form of Qi, rather than fluid. It can be described as Essence transformed into Qi. It is a dynamic and rarefied form of Essence having its origin in the Kidneys. Original Qi is also often said to include the "Original Yin" (*Yuan Yin*) and "Original Yang" (*Yuan Yang*): this means that Original Qi is the foundation of all the Yin and Yang energies of the body.

Original Qi, like Essence, relies on nourishment from the Post-Heaven Essence.

Original Qi has many functions:

1 *Motive force*

Original Qi can be seen as the dynamic motive force that arouses and moves the functional activity of all the organs. It does so because, like the Essence, it is the foundation of vitality and stamina. As a form of Qi, it circulates all over the body, in the channels. It could be said to be the link between Essence, which is more fluid-like and related to slow, long-term cycles and changes, and the day-to-day Qi, which is energy-like and is related to short-term cycles and changes.

2 Basis of Kidney-Qi

Original Qi is the basis for Kidney-Qi and is closely related to all the Kidneys functional activities. According to chapter 66 of the "Classic of Difficulties", Original Qi dwells between the two Kidneys below the umbilicus, at the Gate of Vitality.[25]

Thus, Original Qi is closely related to the Gate of Vitality and shares its role of providing the heat necessary to all the body's functional activities.

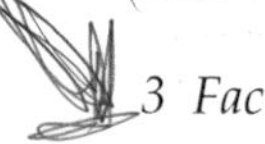

3 Facilitates the transformation of Qi

Original Qi acts as the agent of change in the transformation of Gathering Qi into True Qi (see below). This is one way in which the Kidneys (where the Original Qi arises from) participate in the production of Qi.

4 Facilitates the transformation of Blood

Original Qi also facilitates the transformation of Food-Qi (*Gu Qi*) into Blood in the Heart (see below). This is one way in which the Kidneys participate in the production of Blood.

5 Comes out at the Source points

From its origin in between the two Kidneys where the Gate of Vitality resides, Original Qi passes through the Triple Burner and spreads to the internal organs and channels. The places where the Original Qi stays are the Source points (Fig. 27).[25]

To sum up, Original Qi is like Essence in "Qi" form, it originates between the two Kidneys and is derived from the Pre-Heaven Essence. It is constantly replenished by the Post-Heaven Qi, it is related to the Gate of Vitality, it relies on the transporting function of the triple Burner to circulate all over the body and it circulates in the channels to emerge at the Source points.

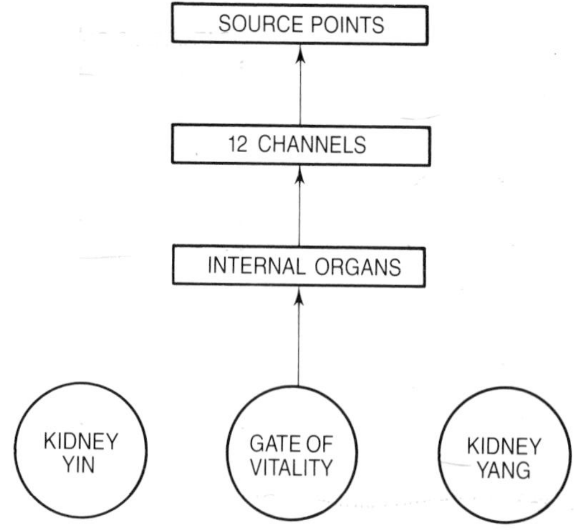

Fig. 27 Relationship among Gate of Vitality, Original Qi and Source points

How can the Original Qi be treated in acupuncture? There are three ways:

a) Needling the Source points (see page 345) on the twelve channels;

b) Needling and applying moxa to the points on the Directing Vessel below the navel, such as Yinjiao Ren-7, Qihai Ren-6, Shimen Ren-5 and Guangyuan Ren-4;

c) Needling and applying moxa to the point Mingmen Du-4, which corresponds to the place from which the Original Qi originates.

Food-Qi 谷

This is called "*Gu Qi*", meaning "Qi of grains" or "Qi of Food". This represents the first stage in the transformation of food into Qi.

Food entering the Stomach, is first "rotted and ripened", and then is transformed into Food-Qi by the Spleen. This Food-Qi is not yet in a useable form for the body.

From the Middle Burner, Food-Qi rises to the chest and goes to the Lungs where, combining with air, it forms Gathering Qi called in Chinese "*Zong Qi*" (Fig. 28).

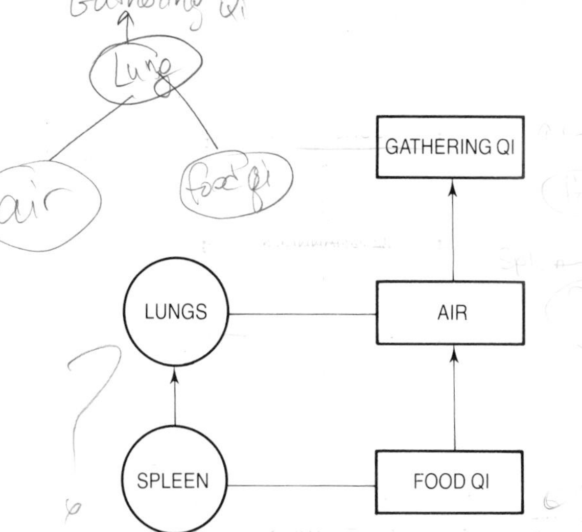

Fig. 28 Food-Qi and Gathering Qi

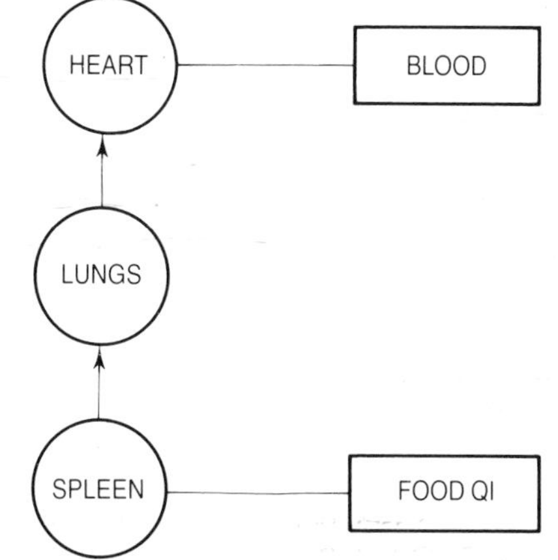

Fig. 29 Food-Qi and Blood

From the Middle Burner, Food-Qi also rises to the chest and goes first to the Lungs, and then to the Heart, where it is transformed into Blood. This transformation is helped by Kidney-Qi and Original Qi (Fig. 29).

Food-Qi is produced by the Spleen which has the very important function of transforming and transporting the various products extracted from food.

In so doing, the Spleen has to send the Food-Qi up to the chest: this is one reason why the Spleen is said to control the raising of Qi. Spleen-Qi normally flows up: if it flows down, the food is not transformed properly and there will be diarrhoea.

Although Food-Qi represents the crucial first stage in the transformation of food into Qi, it is still a coarse form of Qi that cannot be used by the body as it is: it therefore is the basis for the transformation into more refined forms of Qi.

Since Food-Qi is extracted from food and is the starting basis for the production of all Qi and Blood, it is easy to see what importance Chinese Medicine attributes to the quantity and quality of food eaten. The "Spiritual Axis" in chapter 56 says: *"If no food is eaten for half a day, Qi is weakened, if no food is eaten for a whole day, Qi is depleted".*[27] It is apparent from this statement that the ancient Chinese did not believe much in the therapeutic value of fasting!

Gathering Qi 宗气

This is called in Chinese *"Zong Qi"*. This is probably the type of Qi whose name has had the most translations. The character "Zong" 宗 usually means "ancestor", and for this reason, it is sometimes translated as "ancestral Qi" which is confusing as some authors call "ancestral Qi" either the Essence or the Original Qi. Some authors call it "genetic Qi", which is also confusing as, of all the types of Qi in the body, the Essence or the Original Qi would best qualify as being a "genetic" Qi. In the international acupuncture training courses run in China, it is usually called "Essential Qi".

I call it "Gathering Qi" as some authors think that the character "Zong" in this context means to "gather" or "collect together".[28] I am using this translation as I think it fits well the function of this type of Qi. The Gathering Qi is also sometimes called "Chest-Qi" (*Xiong Qi*) or "Big Qi" (*Da Qi*), or also "Big Qi of the Chest".

As mentioned before, the Gathering Qi derives from the interaction of Food-Qi with air. The Spleen sends Food-Qi up to the Lungs where, combining with air, it is transformed into Gathering Qi (Fig. 28).

Gathering Qi is a more subtle and refined form of Qi than Food-Qi, and it is usable by the body.

Its main functions are:

It nourishes Heart and Lungs

It enhances and promotes the Lung function

of controlling Qi and respiration, and the Heart function of governing Blood and blood vessels

It controls the speech and the strength of voice

It affects and promotes blood circulation to extremities.

Gathering Qi is closely related to the functions of Heart and Lungs. It assists the Lung and Heart in their functions of controlling Qi and respiration and Blood and blood vessels respectively. The "Simple Questions" in chapter 18 says: "*. . .the energy that comes out under the left breast and can be felt under the fingers, is the Gathering Qi*".[29]

This means that Gathering Qi assists the Heart and Lungs to push Qi and Blood to the limbs, especially hands. The "Spiritual Axis" in chapter 75 says: "*If the Gathering Qi does not descend, the blood will stagnate in the vessels*".[30] So if Gathering Qi is weak, the limbs and especially hands, will be cold.

Gathering Qi also gathers in the throat and influences speech (which is under the control of the Heart) and the strength of voice (which is under the control of the Lungs). Thus, if Gathering Qi is weak, the speech may be impeded, or the voice may be very weak and fine.

The "Spiritual Axis" in chapter 71 comments: "*The Gathering Qi accumulates in the chest, rises to the throat, enters the Heart channel and aids respiration*".[31]

In practice one can gauge the state of Gathering Qi from the health of the Heart and Lungs and from the circulation and voice. A weak voice shows weakness of Gathering Qi and so does poor circulation to the hands.

Gathering Qi being the energy of the chest, is also affected by emotional problems such as grief and sadness which weaken the Lungs and disperse the energy in the chest. In these cases, both Front positions of left and right (which correspond to Heart and Lungs) of the pulse are very weak or empty.

Finally, Gathering Qi and Original Qi assist each other. Gathering Qi flows downwards to aid the Kidneys, and Original Qi flows upwards to aid respiration. This is another aspect of the relationship of mutual assistance that exists between Lungs and Kidneys.

The chest area where Gathering Qi collects is also called the "Sea of Qi". This is one of the Four Seas discussed in chapter 33 of the "Spiritual Axis". The controlling point for the Sea of Qi (and the Gathering Qi) is Shanzhong Ren-17. Gathering Qi is also treated via the Heart and Lung channels, and, of course, by breathing exercises.

True Qi 真气

This is called in Chinese "*Zhen Qi*", which literally means "True Qi". This is the last stage of transformation of Qi. Gathering Qi is transformed into True Qi under the catalytic action of Original Qi. True Qi is the final stage in the process of refinement and transformation of Qi; it is the Qi that circulates in the channels and nourishes the organs (Fig. 30).

Like Gathering Qi, True Qi also originates from the Lungs, hence the Lung's function of controlling Qi in general.

True Qi assumes two different forms: Nutritive Qi (*Ying Qi*) and Defensive Qi (*Wei Qi*). We cannot therefore discuss the functions of the True Qi without referring to its two different forms.

Nutritive Qi 营气

This is called "*Ying Qi*" in Chinese. It literally means "Nutritive" or "Nourishing" Qi. As its name implies, this type of Qi has the function of nourishing the internal organs and the whole body.

Nutritive Qi is closely related to Blood and flows with it in the blood vessels, as well as, of course, in the channels.

The "Simple Questions" in chapter 43 says: "*Nutritive Qi is extracted from food and water, it regulates the 5 Yin organs, moistens the 6 Yang organs, it enters the blood vessels, it circulates in the channels above and below, is linked with the 5 Yin organs and connects with the 6 Yang organs*".

This is the Qi that is activated whenever a needle is inserted in an acupuncture point.

Defensive Qi 卫气

This is called "*Wei Qi*" in Chinese. "Wei" means "defend" or "protect".

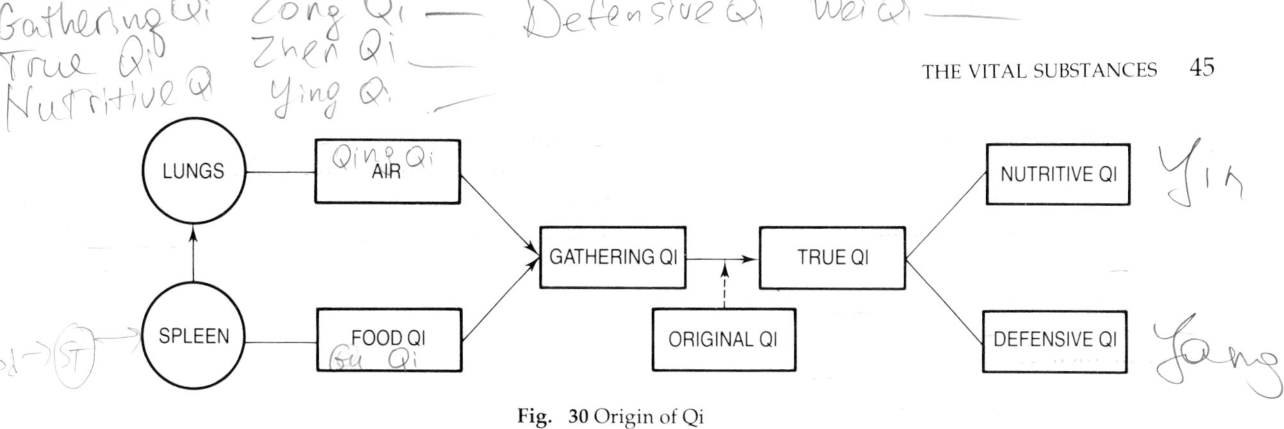

Fig. 30 Origin of Qi

This is another form assumed by True Qi: compared to the Nutritive Qi, it is a coarser form of Qi. It is Yang in relation to the Nutritive Qi as it flows on the outer layers of the body, whereas Nutritive Qi flows in the inner layers and the internal organs. The "Spiritual Axis" in chapter 18 says: *"The human being receives Qi from food: this enters the stomach, is transported to the Lungs [i.e. the Food-Qi]... it is transformed into Qi, the refined part becomes Nutritive Qi, the coarse part becomes Defensive Qi. Nutritive Qi flows in the blood vessels [and channels], Defensive Qi flows outside the channels"*.[33]

The "Simple Questions" in chapter 43 says: *"Defensive Qi is derived from the coarse part of food and water, it is slippery in nature, hence it cannot enter the channels. It therefore circulates under the skin, in between the muscles, it vapourizes in between membranes and diffuses over the chest and abdomen"*.[34]

To summarize: Nutritive Qi is in the Interior and nourishes, Defensive Qi is on the Exterior and protects.

The main function of Defensive Qi is to protect the body from attack of exterior pathogenic factors, such as Wind, Cold, Heat and Damp. In addition, it warms, moistens and partially nourishes skin and muscles, it adjusts the opening and closing of the pores (and therefore regulates sweating) and it regulates the body temperature (chiefly by regulating sweating).

The "Spiritual Axis" in chapter 47 says: *"Defensive Qi warms the muscles, fills up the skin, enters the space between skin and muscles, opens the pores"*.[35]

Being diffused under the skin, Defensive Qi comes under the control of the Lungs. The Lungs regulate the circulation of Defensive Qi to the skin and the opening and closing of the pores. Thus, a weakness of Lung-Qi may lead to a weakness of Defensive Qi. This can make someone prone to frequent colds.

Defensive Qi circulates outside the channels, in the skin and muscles: these are called the Exterior of the body, or also the "Lung-Defensive Qi Portion". The Lungs disperse body fluids to the skin and muscles. These fluids mix with Defensive Qi so that a deficiency of Defensive Qi may cause spontaneous daytime sweating, because if Defensive Qi is weak it fails to hold the fluids in.

This also explains the rationale in promoting sweating when the body is invaded by exterior Wind-Cold. In these cases invading Wind-Cold obstructs the circulation of Defensive Qi in the skin and muscles, blocking the pores and impairing the dispersing function of the Lungs. By restoring the Lung dispersing function and promoting sweating, the pores will be unblocked, the fluids come out as sweat and, mixed with them, the Wind-Cold is expelled. It is therefore said that the Defensive Qi spreads in the Upper Burner (see p. 119).

However, Defensive Qi also spreads in the Middle and Lower Burner. It spreads in the Middle Burner as it originates from the Food-Qi produced by Stomach and Spleen. On the other hand, the Essence and Original Qi stored in the Kidneys also play a role in the resistance to exterior pathogenic factors, as explained above. Thus, Defensive Qi originates also from the Essence and Original Qi and is transformed from Kidney-Yang. This is another reason why resistance to exterior pathogenic factors is determined not only by the strength of Lung-Qi, but also Kidney-Yang.

To summarize, Defensive Qi has its root in the Lower Burner (Kidneys), it is nourished by the Middle Burner (Stomach and Spleen), and it spreads outwards in the Upper Burner (Lungs).

A deficiency of Defensive Qi causes a weakening of the body's defences against exterior pathogenic factors, and the person will be prone to catching cold frequently. The person will always tend to feel easily cold, as the deficient Defensive Qi fails to warm the skin and muscles.

Defensive Qi circulates 50 times in 24 hours, 25 times in the day and 25 times at night. In the day it circulates in the Exterior of the body, and at night it circulates in the Yin organs.[36] In the daytime, it circulates on the Exterior in the Yang superficial channels from the Greater Yang to Lesser Yang to Bright Yang channels. According to the "Spiritual Axis", it is this very flow of Defensive Qi from the Interior towards the Exterior, emerging at the inner corner of the eye (meeting of Greater Yang Small Intestine and Bladder channels), that opens the eyes and wakes us up in the morning. At night, Defensive Qi flows into the Yin organs, first to the Kidneys, then to Heart, Lung, Liver, Spleen.[37]

Each twelve-hour period is divided into 25 periods. In the daytime, the Defensive Qi circulates first through Greater Yang, then Lesser Yang, Bright Yang, and then Yin, before repeating the circuit for 25 periods. At night it circulates in the above-mentioned order also for 25 periods (Fig. 31).

There are two other types of Qi to be discussed. One is the CENTRAL QI (*Zhong Qi*). "Zhong" means "middle" or "centre". In this case it indicates the Middle Burner. In fact, Central Qi is another way of defining the Qi of Stomach and Spleen, or the Post-Heaven Qi derived from food. It is also another term for the Spleen's function of transformation and transportation. In this sense we have already discussed Central Qi, but it does have one new feature in that the term Central Qi is usually also used in cases of deficiency of Spleen-Qi which give rise to prolapse of an organ. In these cases, the prolapse is often described as being due to "deficiency of Central Qi".

The other type of Qi to be described is the UPRIGHT QI (*Zheng Qi*). This too is not really another type of Qi, but simply a general term to indicate the various Qi having the function of protecting the body from invasion by exterior pathogenic factors. It is a term that is usually only used in relation and contrast to PATHOGENIC FACTOR (*Xie Qi*), and indicates the body's resistance to exterior diseases.

Functions of Qi

Before concluding the discussion of Qi, we need to summarize the basic functions of Qi as observed in clinical practice, irrespective of the various types of Qi.

The basic functions of Qi are:
— Transforming
— Transporting
— Holding

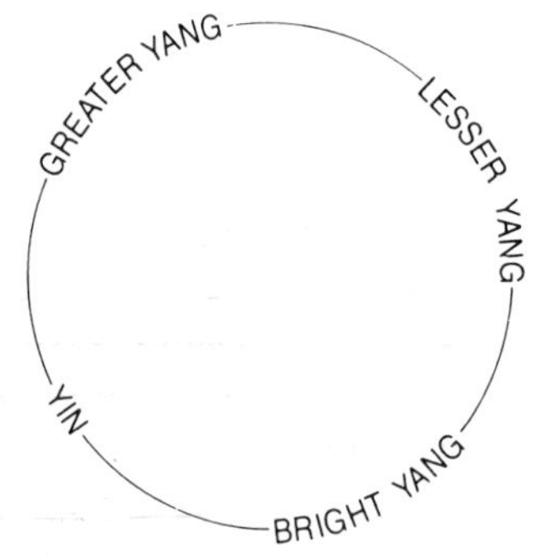

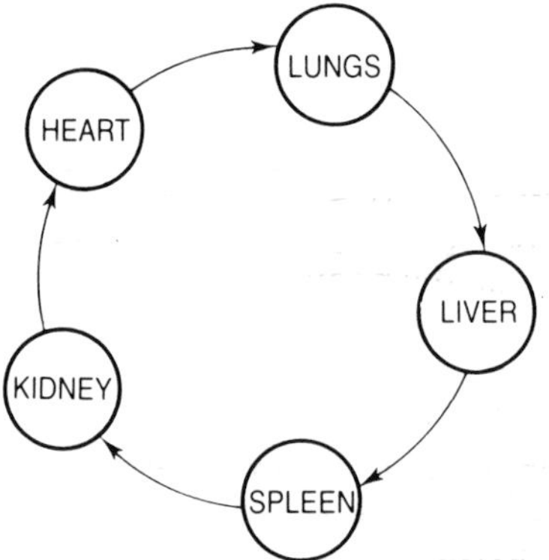

Fig. 31 Circulation of Defensive Qi

— Raising
— Protecting
— Warming.

It is worth giving some examples of these functions of Qi which will be clearer after reading chapter 5 on the function of the internal organs.

1 Transforming

Spleen-Qi transforms food into Food-Qi, Kidney-Qi transforms fluids, BL-Qi transforms urine, Heart-Qi transforms Food-Qi into Blood.

2 Transporting

Spleen-Qi transports Food-Qi, Lung-Qi transports fluids to the skin, Kidney-Qi transports Qi upwards, Liver-Qi transports Qi in all directions, Lung-Qi transports Qi downwards.

3 Holding

Spleen-Qi holds the Blood in the blood vessels and fluids, Kidney-Qi and Bladder-Qi hold urine, Lung-Qi holds sweat.

4 Raising

Spleen-Qi raises the organs, Kidney-Qi rises upwards.

5 Protecting

Lung-Qi protects the body from exterior pathogenic factors.

6 Warming

This is a function of Yang-Qi. Both Spleen-Yang and Kidney-Yang, especially the latter, have the function of warming the body.

Direction of Qi movement

The normal physiological functions of the internal organs and the various types of Qi rely on a complex balance not only among the internal organs and the Yin-Yang character of Qi, but also on the direction of movement of Qi.

There are various different types of Qi and twelve internal organs: each of these performs a specific function, usually in relation to a specific type of Qi, and in order to perform this function, the various types of Qi have to flow in the appropriate directions.

The complex of different directions of Qi is called "Ascending-descending and exiting-entering" in the Yellow Emperor's Classic. The "Simple Questions" in chapter 68 says: "*Without exiting-entering of Qi, there would be no birth, growth, maturity and ageing. Without ascending-descending, there would be no birth, growth, transformation, harvesting and storage. All organs rely on the ascending-descending and exiting-entering of Qi*".[38]

Let us look at some examples of the "ascending-descending and exiting-entering of Qi".

Lungs

The Lungs control respiration: clear Qi is inhaled and impure Qi is exhaled. In addition, the Lungs control the descending of Qi: they are the uppermost organ and are often compared to a "lid". They direct Qi downwards (to Kidneys and Bladder).

Liver

The Liver controls the smooth flow of Qi in all directions. In particular, Liver-Qi has to flow upwards. Thus, Lungs and Liver balance each other, in so far as Lung-Qi flows downwards and Liver-Qi flows upwards.

Kidneys

The Kidneys control the transformation of Water, so that the impure fluids flow downwards and the clear Qi flows upwards. Lungs and Kidneys also balance each other, as the Lung-Qi descends to the Kidneys, and Kidney-Qi ascends to the Lungs. Lungs send Qi down, Kidneys receive Qi, Lungs control exhalation, Kidneys control inhalation, one downwards one upwards, one's Qi exits, the other's Qi enters. Hence the "Classic of Difficulties" in chapter 4 says: *"Exhalation is controlled by Lungs and Heart, inhalation is controlled by Kidneys and Liver"*.[39]

The "Complete Book of [Zhang] Jing Yue" (1634) says: *"The Lungs govern Qi, and the Kidneys are the root of Qi"*.[40]

Spleen-Stomach

The Spleen sends Qi upwards (to Lungs and Heart) and the Stomach sends (impure) Qi downwards. The Spleen controls transformation, the Stomach controls receiving. Hence the ascending of clear Qi and descending of impure Qi depends on the ascending of Spleen-Qi and descending of Stomach-Qi. If Spleen-Qi descends, it causes diarrhoea; if Stomach-Qi ascends, it causes nausea, belching or vomiting.

Heart-Kidneys

Heart-Fire flows downwards to meet the Water of the Kidneys, and Kidney-Water rises to meet Heart-Fire.

Thus, the normal physiological functioning of the organs depends on the correct direction of Qi. A derangement of these different directions can cause various problems.

These arise when movement of Qi is impeded, or when the direction of movement is opposite to what it should be, and ascending-descending and exiting-entering are out of balance.

For example, Liver-Qi can stagnate (not flow smoothly in all directions) or it can ascend out of control. Stomach-Qi, as we have seen, can rise instead of descending, Spleen-Qi can descend instead of ascending, Lung-Qi could fail to descend, Kidney-Qi could fail to receive and ascend, Kidney and Heart could fail to communicate and respond to each other. All these are fairly common pathological occurrences.

Pathology of Qi

Qi pathology can manifest in four different ways:

1 Qi deficient

Qi can be deficient from various causes. This is so especially of the Qi of the Spleen, Lungs or Kidneys.

2 Qi sinking

If Qi is deficient it can sink, causing prolapse of the organs. This applies mostly to Spleen-Qi.

3 Qi stagnant

Qi can fail in its movement and stagnate. This applies mostly to Liver-Qi.

4 Qi rebellious

Qi can flow in the wrong direction: this is called "rebellious Qi". For example, Stomach-Qi failing to descend and flowing upwards, causing nausea or vomiting.

All these cases will be discussed in detail in chapter 9.

BLOOD 血

Blood in Chinese Medicine has a different meaning than in Western Medicine. In Chinese Medicine, Blood is itself a form of Qi, a very dense and material one, but Qi nevertheless. Moreover, Blood is inseparable from Qi itself, Qi infuses life into Blood; without Qi, Blood would be an inert fluid.

Source

Blood is derived mostly from the Food-Qi produced by the Spleen. The Spleen sends Food-Qi upwards to the Lungs, and through the pushing action of Lung-Qi, this is sent to the Heart, where it is transformed into Blood (Fig. 32). The "Spiritual Axis" says in chapter 18: *"The Stomach is in the Middle Burner, it opens onto the Upper Burner, it receives Qi, secretes the dregs, evaporates the fluids transforming them into a refined essence. This pours upwards towards the Lungs and is transformed into Blood."*[41]

The "Discussion on Blood" (by Tang Zong Hai, 1884) says: *"Water is transformed into Qi,*

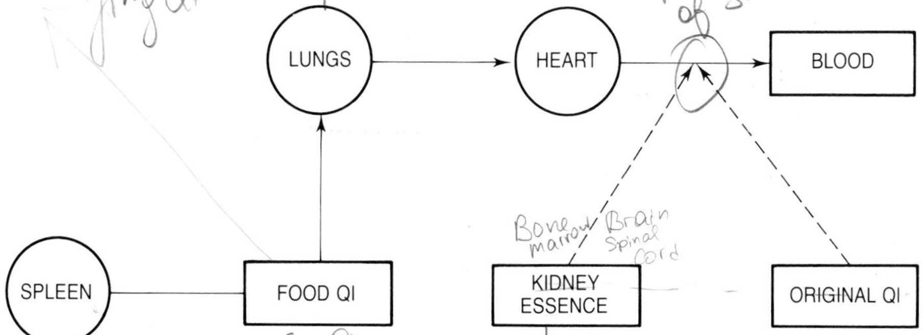

Fig. 32 Origin of Blood

Fire is transformed into Blood...How can we say that Fire is transformed into Blood? Blood and Fire are both red in colour, Fire resides in the Heart where it generates Blood, which moistens the whole body. Fire is Yang, and it generates Blood that is Yin." [42]

Figure 32 illustrates three aspects:

a) The Spleen and Stomach are the main source of Blood;

b) Lung-Qi plays an important role in pushing Food-Qi to the Heart: this is an example of the general principle that Qi makes Blood move;

c) Food-Qi is transformed into Blood in the Heart: this is one aspect of the principle that the Heart governs Blood.

According to Chinese Medicine there are two other important features in the manufacture of Blood.

One is that the transformation of Food-Qi into Blood is aided by the Original Qi. The other is that the Kidneys store Essence which produces Marrow: this, in turn, generates bone marrow which contributes to making Blood. A doctor of the Qing dynasty, Zhang Lu, in his book "Medical Transmission of the Zhang Family" (1695), says: *"If Qi is not exhausted, it returns essences to the Kidneys to be transformed into Essence; if the Essence is not depleted, it returns Essence to the Liver to be transformed into Blood"*.

From this it is evident that the Kidneys play an important role, as they store Essence and are the source of Original Qi. We can therefore say that Blood is generated by the interaction of the Post-Heaven Qi of the Stomach and Spleen (which are the source of Food-Qi) and the Pre-Heaven Qi (as the Kidneys play a role in its formation). This is illustrated in Figure 33. So to nourish Blood, we need to tonify the Spleen and Kidneys.

It seems remarkable that the Chinese account of the blood-forming function of bone marrow, so similar to that given by Western physiology was formulated during the Qing dynasty before the introduction of Western Medicine into China. Lin Pei Qin, a doctor of the Qing dynasty, formulated the theory that "Liver and Kidneys have the same source" and that Blood is transformed from the Kidney-Essence.[44]

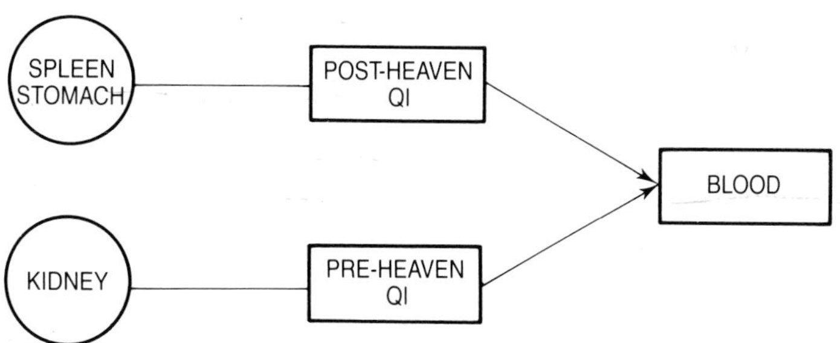

Fig. 33 Post-Heaven and Pre-Heaven sources of Blood

Function

The main function of Blood is that of nourishing the body. It complements the nourishing action of Qi. Blood is a dense form of Qi and it flows with it all over the body.

Besides providing nourishment, Blood also has a moistening function, which Qi does not have. The Blood ensures that body tissues do not dry out. For example, Liver-Blood moistens eyes and sinews, so that the eyes can see properly and the sinews are flexible and healthy. Liver-Blood also moistens the skin and the hair, ensuring that the skin is not too dry and the that the hair remains shiny and healthy. Heart-Blood moistens the tongue.

Blood is very important also in another way: it provides the material foundation for the Mind. Blood is part of Yin (as it is dense and fluid-like) and it houses and anchors the Mind. Blood embraces the Mind providing the harbour within which the Mind can flourish.

The "Simple Questions" says: *"Blood is the Mind of a person"*.[45] The "Spiritual Axis" says: *"When Blood is harmonized, the Mind has a residence"*.[46]

If the Blood is deficient, the Mind will lack its foundation and so become unhappy or uneasy. This is typically manifested by a "deficient restlessness" characterized by a vague anxiety, slight irritability, and a feeling of dissatisfaction. When we are asleep at night Blood naturally embraces the Mind, but if Blood is deficient the Mind "floats" and the person cannot sleep.

Relation with internal organs

Heart

The Heart governs the Blood and the blood vessels are responsible for its circulation. As we have seen, the Heart is also the place where the Blood is made through the agency of Heart-Fire. Fire is Yang and it transforms into Yin (Blood). Blood cools down the Fire preventing it from flaring up excessively. The "Discussion on Blood" written in 1884 by Tang Zong Hai says: *"Fire is Yang and generates Blood which is Yin. On the other hand, Blood nourishes Fire and makes sure that Fire does not flare up, whilst Blood moistens the lower Burner. It is stored in the Liver, it fills the Sea of Blood and the Penetrating, Directing and Girdle extraordinary vessels, and it warms and nourishes the whole body... When Blood moistens the Lower Burner and the Sea of Blood, and Heart-Fire follows it down to the umbilicus, then Blood is flourishing and Fire does not flare excessively, so that men are free of disease and women are fertile."*[47]

From this passage it is apparent that Heart-Fire is essential for the formation of Blood, and that it also has to flow downwards to the Lower Burner to interact with Blood.

Chinese pulse diagnosis confirms that the Heart corresponds to Blood and Lung to Qi. Since the Heart is felt on the left side and the Lung on the right, the left side can be taken to reflect the state of Blood, while the right pulse indicates the state of Qi.

Spleen

The Spleen is related to the Blood in two ways. First of all it is the origin of Blood as it produces Food-Qi which is the basis for the formation of Blood.

Secondly, Spleen-Qi makes sure that Blood remains in the blood vessels and does not extravasate. If Spleen-Qi is deficient, Qi cannot hold Blood, and haemorrhages may result. Such haemorrhages are of the deficient type, because they are due to deficient Qi not holding Blood.

Liver

When the Chinese say that the Liver stores Blood, they mean several things. Firstly, from a physiological point of view, when a person is erect and engaged in normal everyday movement, Blood flows to the muscles and sinews. When a person lies down, Blood flows back to the Liver. Wang Ping, a doctor from the Tang dynasty, said: *"When the person is active, Blood circulates in the vessels, when the person rests, Blood goes back to the Liver"*.[48]

When lying down, the Blood regenerates itself in the Liver, hence the importance of having adequate rest (especially lying down), in cases of deficient Liver-Blood.

As we have seen, Blood stored in the Liver has also the function of moistening the eyes and promoting good sight and moistening sinews promoting flexibility of joints. The "Simple Questions" says: "*Blood goes to the Liver during sleep, so that, when adequately supplied with Blood, the eyes can see, the hands can hold, the fingers can grasp, the feet can walk*".[49]

The "Spiritual Axis" says: "*When the Blood is harmonized ... the sinews are strong and the joints supple*".[50]

Another very important aspect of the Liver storage of Blood is in relation to the physiology and pathology of menstruation. The Blood of the Liver supplies the uterus with Blood and is closely related to the Penetrating extraordinary vessel. This vessel also supplies the uterus with Blood, but ultimately this also is dependent on the supply of Blood from the Liver. Thus Liver-Blood is extremely important for a regular and healthy menstrual function.

The importance of Liver-Blood in women's physiology is partly explained by the close connection existing between Kidneys and Liver. It is said in Chinese Medicine that "Kidneys and Liver have a common origin". The Kidneys store Essence and the Liver stores Blood. The Kidneys are the mother of the Liver according to the 5 Elements, and so Essence and Blood mutually influence each other. Essence can be transformed into Blood as mentioned above; on the other hand, Blood also nourishes and replenishes Essence. The Kidney-Essence controls the reproductive function and since it influences Blood, Blood also influences the reproductive function in women. The reason this is more relevant in women than men, is that women's physiology is more dependent on Blood than that of men. For these reasons, it is said that Kidney and Liver have a common origin, and the state of Liver-Blood is extremely important for women's menstrual function.

For example, if Liver-Blood is deficient, this can lead to amenorrhoea or scanty periods; stagnant Liver-Blood can be a cause of painful periods.

Lungs

The Lungs affect Blood in several ways. First of all they assist the Spleen in sending Food-Qi to the Heart where it is transformed into Blood.

Besides this, the Lungs control all the channels and blood vessels. This means that the Lungs infuse Qi into the blood vessels to assist the pushing action of the Heart. This is another aspect of the relationship between Qi and Blood, which will be discussed in detail.

Kidneys

As mentioned above, the Kidneys contribute to the production of Blood in two ways: Original Qi assists in the transformation of Food-Qi into Blood, and the Kidney-Essence can also be transformed into Blood.

The implication of this in clinical practice, is that, in order to nourish Blood, we need to tonify the Spleen and Kidneys.

Of all the above organs, however, the Heart, Spleen and Liver are the most important ones with relation to Blood. The Heart governs Blood, the Spleen holds Blood in, the Liver stores Blood.

Blood-Qi relationship

There is a very close relationship between Qi and Blood. Blood is also a form of Qi, albeit a very dense one. Qi is Yang compared to Blood (as it is more tenuous), Blood is Yin compared to Qi (as it is denser). Qi and Blood are inseparable: the Nutritive Qi circulates with Blood in the blood vessels. The close relationship between Blood and Qi can be observed in the clinical signs following a serious haemorrhage: often in these cases, after a massive loss of blood, the person develops signs of Qi deficiency, such as sweating, breathlessness and cold limbs. On the other hand, after prolonged and heavy sweating (which depletes Qi), one may develop signs of Blood deficiency, such as pallor, numbness, dizziness and palpitations.

There are four aspects to the Blood-Qi relationship.

Qi generates Blood

Qi generates Blood in so far as Food-Qi is the basis for Blood, and also Lung-Qi is essential for the production of Blood.

Thus, if Qi is deficient, Blood will eventually also be deficient. In practice, it is often necessary to tonify Qi in order to nourish Blood. This is particularly important in herbal practice, as the herbs to tonify Qi and nourish Blood are in different categories, whereas in acupuncture practice, the difference is not so clear-cut.

Qi moves Blood

Qi is the motive force for Blood. Without Qi, Blood would be an inert substance. Nutritive Qi is very closely related to Blood and flows with it in the blood vessels. Lung-Qi infuses the necessary Qi into the blood vessels.

This relationship between Qi and Blood is often expressed by a saying: "*When Qi moves, Blood follows*", and also "*If Qi stagnates, Blood congeals*".
If Qi is deficient or stagnant, it cannot push the Blood and this also stagnates.

Qi holds the Blood

Qi has also the function of holding Blood in the blood vessels, thus preventing haemorrhages. This function belongs primarily to the Spleen. If Spleen-Qi is deficient, Qi cannot hold Blood, and there may be haemorrhages.

The above three aspects of Qi-Blood relationship are often expressed in the saying: "*Qi is the commander of Blood*".

Blood nourishes Qi

While Blood relies on the generating, pushing and holding action of Qi, Qi, on the other hand, relies on the nutritive function of Blood.

Blood affects Qi in two ways. First of all, Qi relies on Blood for nourishment. Secondly, Blood provides a material and "dense" basis which prevents Qi from "floating" and giving rise to symptoms of Empty-Heat.

Both these aspects of Blood-Qi relationship are often expressed with the saying: "*Blood is the mother of Qi*".

Blood-Essence relationship

Blood and Essence mutually affect each other. Each of them can transform into the other.

As we have already seen, Essence plays an important role in the formation of Blood. On the other hand, Blood continually nourishes and replenishes the Essence.

Blood pathology

There are three basic cases of pathology of Blood:

1 Blood deficiency

Blood can be deficient when not enough is manufactured. This is mostly caused by Spleen Qi deficiency.

2 Blood Heat

Blood can be hot: this is mostly due to Liver-Heat.

3 Blood stasis

The Blood can fail to move properly and stagnate. This may be caused by stagnation of Qi (mostly of the Liver), by Heat, or by Cold.
All these cases will be discussed in detail in chapter 9.

BODY FLUIDS 津液

Body Fluids are called "*JIN-YE*" in Chinese. This word is composed of two characters, "*Jin*", meaning "moist" or "saliva", and "Ye", meaning "fluid". "*Jin*" indicates anything which is liquid, while "*Ye*" indicates fluids of living organisms (that found in fruit, for instance). Thus, "*Jin-Ye*" could be translated as "organic fluids". I will refer to them as "Body Fluids".

Source

Body Fluids originate from our food and drink. These are transformed and separated by the Spleen: a "clean" part goes up from the Spleen to the Lungs, which spreads part of them to the skin and sends part of them down to the Kidneys. A "dirty" part goes down to the Small Intestine where again it is separated into a pure and impure part. The pure part of this second separation goes to the Bladder and the impure part goes to the Large Intestine, where some water is re-absorbed. The Bladder further transforms and separates the fluids it receives into a pure and impure part. The pure part flows upwards and goes to the Exterior of the body where it forms sweat. The impure part flows downwards and is transformed into urine.

The Bladder effects this transformation and separation by the power of Qi, which it receives from Kidney-Yang: this function of the Bladder is called "function of Qi transformation".

The "Simple Questions" says: *"Fluids enter the Stomach and they are separated. A pure part flows upwards from the Spleen to the Lungs, which direct them to the Water Passages and then downwards to the Bladder."* [51]

The process of formation of Body Fluids is the result of an intricate series of purification processes, each stage further separating the fluids into a pure and impure part. For this reason the Chinese talk of a "pure within the impure" and "impure within the pure" part. The pure parts need to be transported upwards, the impure parts downwards. This correct movement of pure and impure parts of body fluids is essential to their proper transformation, and it is carried out principally by the Spleen. Hence the importance of the Spleen in the physiology and pathology of body fluids.

The pure fluids flow upwards to the Lungs which distribute some to the space under the skin, and some downwards to the Kidneys. For this reason, the Lungs are called the "Upper Source of Water". Impure fluids flow downwards to the Small Intestine and the Bladder which carries out its further separation and transformation as described above. The Bladder function of Qi transformation is controlled by Kidney-Yang, hence the Kidneys are called the "Lower Source of Water" (Fig. 34).

Relations with internal organs

Spleen

The Spleen is the most important organ in relation to the physiology and pathology of Body Fluids. It controls the initial transformation and separation into a pure and impure part, as described above. It also controls the crucial direction of pure and impure parts upwards and downwards respectively at all stages of body fluids production.

For this reason, the Spleen is always treated in any type of disorders of Body Fluids.

Lungs

The Lungs control the dispersion of the pure part of Body Fluids coming from the Spleen to the space under the skin. This is an aspect of the Lung dispersing function.

They also send part of the fluids down to the Kidneys and Bladder. This is an aspect of the Lung descending function.

Because of these two functions, the Lungs are said to regulate the "Water passages".

Kidneys

The Kidneys are extremely important in the physiology of Body Fluids. Firstly, they vaporize some of the fluids they receive and send them back up to the Lungs, to moisten the Lungs and prevent them from getting too dry.

Furthermore, the Kidneys, in particular Kidney-Yang, control many stages of the transformation of fluids.

a) They provide the heat necessary for the Spleen to transform Body Fluids. For this reason, a deficiency of Kidney-Yang nearly always results in deficiency of Spleen-Yang, with consequent accumulation of fluids.

b) They assist the Small Intestine in its function of separation of Body Fluids into a pure and impure part.

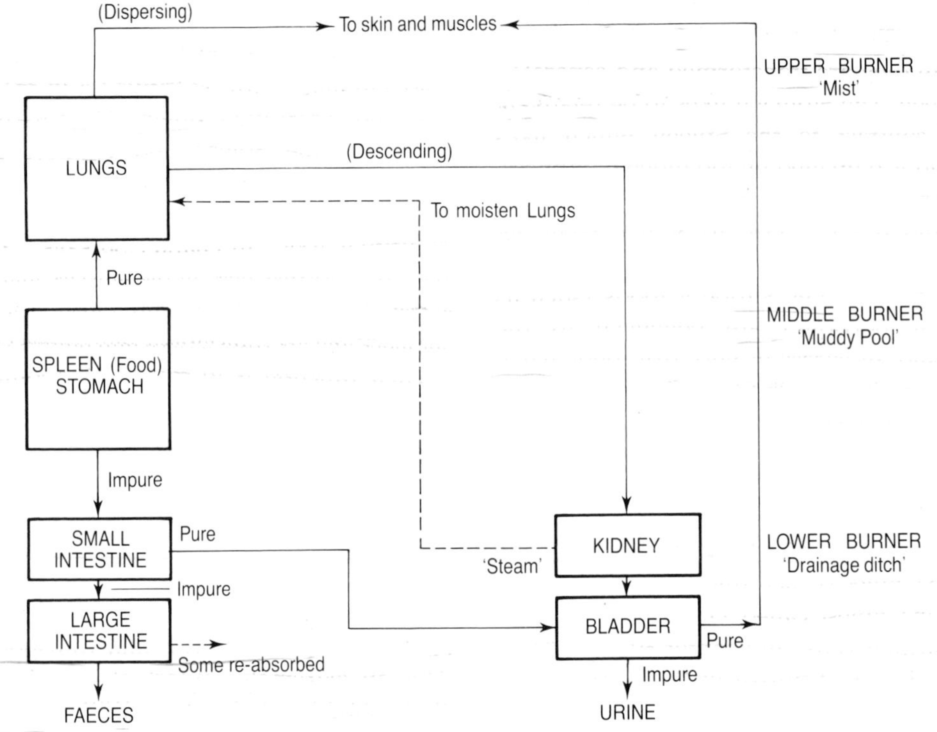

Fig. 34 Origin, transformation and excretion of Body Fluids

c) They provide Qi to the Bladder for its function of Qi transformation.

d) They assist the Triple Burner transformation and excretion of fluids.

For all these reasons, Kidney-Yang is extremely important for the transformation, separation and excretion of fluids.

Bladder

The Bladder separates the fluids it receives into a pure and impure part and it excretes urine by the power of Qi transformation.

Triple Burner

The Triple Burner assists the transformation, transportation and excretion of fluids at all stages. The "Simple Questions" in chapter 8 says: *"The Triple Burner is the official in charge of irrigation and it controls the water passages"*.[52]

The Upper Burner assists the Spleen in directing the pure fluids upwards, and the Lungs in dispersing them to the space under the skin. For this reason, the Upper Burner is compared to a "mist".

The Middle Burner assists the Stomach in its function of churning the fluids and directing the impure part downwards. For this reason, the Middle Burner is compared to a "muddy pool" (a reference to the Stomach function of rotting and ripening).

The Lower Burner assists the Small Intestine, Bladder and Kidneys in their functions of transforming, separating and excreting fluids. For this reason, the Lower Burner is compared to a "drainage ditch".

Stomach

Even though the Stomach does not appear to play an important role in the transformation of

Body Fluids, it nevertheless is the "source" of Body Fluids. The fluids first enter the Stomach from where they are transformed and separated by the Spleen. The Stomach likes to be relatively moist, in contrast to the Spleen which likes dryness and is damaged by too much dampness.

In fact, the Stomach easily suffers from excess dryness, and this can lead to Stomach-Yin deficiency.

For this reason, wet, slippery foods (such as rice or oat porridge) are beneficial to the Stomach, and an excess of very dry foods (such as foods roasted or broiled for a long time) may damage Stomach-Yin.

Types of Body Fluids

There are two types of body fluids:

Fluids in Chinese called *JIN*

Liquids in Chinese called *YE*.

The "Spiritual Axis" in chapter 30 says: *"The body fluids that are dispersed in the space between skin and muscles and come out as sweat are the fluids* [*Jin*]*...when food enters the body and Qi is abundant, fluids overflow to the bones, so that they can bend, the brain and marrow are irrigated and tonified, the skin is moistened, these are called liquids* [*Ye*]*."* [53]

Fluids (JIN)

These fluids are clear, light and thin-watery and they circulate with Defensive Qi on the Exterior (skin and muscles). They move relatively quickly. They are under the control of the Lungs, which spreads them to the skin all over the body, and of the Upper Burner, which controls their transformation and movement towards the skin.

Their function is to moisten and partially to nourish skin and muscles. These are the fluids that are exuded as sweat. They also manifest as tears, saliva and mucus.

Another important function of the fluids is to become a component of the fluid part of Blood. In other words, these fluids thin the Blood out and prevent its stasis. We discuss this further when dealing with the relation between Blood and fluids.

Liquids (YE)

These fluids are more turbid, heavy and dense. They circulate with Nutritive Qi in the Interior. They move relatively slowly. They are under the control of the Spleen and Kidneys for their transformation, and of the Middle and Lower Burner for their movement and excretion. The "Spiritual Axis" in chapter 36 says: *"The Qi of the Triple Burner goes to the muscles and skin and is transformed into fluids* [*Jin*]*. Other body fluids do not move and are transformed into liquids* [*Ye*]*"*.[54]

Their function is to moisten the joints, spine, brain and bone marrow. They also lubricate the orifices of the sense organs, i.e. eyes, ears, nose and mouth.

Relation between Qi and Body Fluids

Qi and Body Fluids are related in many ways. First of all Qi transforms and transports fluids. This an extremely important aspect of the Qi-Body Fluid relationship. Without the transforming and transporting power of Qi, Body Fluids would accumulate giving rise to disease.

Secondly, Qi also holds Body Fluids in, in the same way as it holds blood. If Qi is deficient, the fluids may leak out, and gives rise to urinary incontinence or enuresis (deficiency of Kidney-Qi), spontaneous sweating (deficiency of Lung-Qi) or chronic vaginal discharges (deficiency of Spleen-Qi).

Thirdly, while Qi produces Body Fluids, these, on the other hand, play a minor part in nourishing Qi. A deficiency of the Stomach and Spleen may, in the long run, cause deficiency of fluids (as the Stomach is the origin of fluids). Also, after a significant loss of fluids, such as it occurs in profuse sweating, Qi also becomes deficient, and the person may suffer from cold limbs, pallor, dislike of cold, i.e. symptoms of Yang deficiency.

This is because the fluids that form sweat in the space between skin and muscles are blended with Defensive Qi, and profuse sweating also causes a loss of Defensive Qi. Since Defensive Qi pertains to Yang, it is said in Chinese Medicine that "Profuse sweating injures Yang". Qi may also be consumed by excessive vomiting, hence the saying "Persistent vomiting certainly depletes Qi".

On the other hand, if Qi is deficient, fluids may leak out in the form of sweat, hence the saying "Qi deficiency causes sweating".

Relation between Blood and Body Fluids

There is a relation of mutual nourishment between fluids and Blood. On the one hand, Body Fluids constantly replenish Blood and make it thinner so that it does not coagulate or stagnate. The "Spiritual Axis" in chapter 71 says: *"Nutritive Qi secretes Body Fluids; these enter the blood vessels and are transformed into Blood"*.[55] And also in chapter 81: *"If Body Fluids are harmonized, they turn red and are transformed into Blood"*.[56]

On the other hand, Blood can also nourish and supplement Body Fluids. Both Blood and Body Fluids pertain to Yin and are somewhat interchangeable. For this reason, if there is a significant loss of Body Fluids over a long period of time, as in chronic spontaneous sweating (or excessive use of saunas), this can lead to deficiency of Blood. Vice versa, if there is a chronic loss of blood, as in menorrhagia, this can lead to deficiency of Body Fluids and dryness.

Because Blood and Body Fluids come from the same source and mutually nourish each other, sweating and bleeding treatment methods are contradictory in practice, and should never be used together. Also, if the patient is bleeding, one should not induce sweating while if the patient is sweating bleeding as a treatment is contraindicated. The "Spiritual Axis" says in chapter 18: *"If there is profuse bleeding, do not cause sweating; if there is profuse sweating, do not cause bleeding"*.[57] Also, the "Discussion on Cold-induced Diseases" says: *"In a patient with severe deficiency of Blood, do not cause sweating"*.[58]

Pathology of body fluids

The Body Fluids can be pathologically altered in two different ways:

a) Deficiency of Body Fluids;

b) Accumulation of Body Fluids in the form of oedema or Phlegm-Fluids.

These will be dealt with in detail in the chapter on the identification of Qi-Blood-Body Fluids patterns (ch. 19, p. 191).

NOTES

1 He Zuo Xiu 1968 The Materialistic Theory of Yuan Qi- One of the Brilliant Philosophical Ideas of the Legalist School, Institute of High Energy Physics, Academia Sinica. In: Scientia Sinica, vol. 18, no.6, Beijing.
2 Science and Civilization in China, p 472.
3 Science and Civilization in China p 302.
4 He Zuo Xiu 1968 The Materialistic Theory of Yuan Qi, p 697.
5 Science and Civilization in China, p 372.
6 Wing Tsit Chan 1969 A Source Book in Chinese Philosophy. Princeton University Press, Princeton, New Jersey, p 307.
7 A Source Book in Chinese Philsophy., p 300.
8 Science and Civilization in China, p 373.
9 A Source Book in Chinese Philosophy, p 501.
10 A Source Book in Chinese Philosophy, p 503
11 The Materialistic Theory of Yuan Qi, p 704.
12 Fung Yu Lan 1966 A Short History of Chinese Philosophy. Macmillan, New York, p 280.
13 Science and Civilization in China, p 480.
14 Science and Civilization in China, p 512.
15 The Materialistic Theory of Yuan Qi, p 704.
16 The Materialistic Theory of Yuan Qi, p 705.
17 The Materialistic Theory of Yuan Qi, p 705.
18 Simple Questions, p 158–159.
19 Classic of Difficulties, p 17.
20 The ability to enhance the Pre-Heaven Essence in the course of one's lifetime, can be compared to the process of adding peat to poor soil in order to "condition" it. Even though peat does not actually add fertilizing substances to the soil, it increases its fertility by improving the condition and structure of the soil and making the absorption of nutrients by the rootlet system of plants easier. Similarly, even though we cannot quantitatively increase one's Pre-Heaven Essence, we can improve the "soil" of all the body's energies, so that the Pre-Heaven Essence can issue forth and nourish the body more effectively.
21 Wu Qian 1742 The Golden Mirror of Medical Collection, cited in 1981 Syndromes and Treatment of the Internal Organs (Zang Fu Zheng Zhi 脏腑证治). Tianjin Scientific Publishing House, Tianjin, p 34.
22 Simple Questions, p 4–6.
23 Spiritual Axis, p 73.
24 Simple Questions, p 24.
25 Classic of Difficulties, p 144.
26 Classic of Difficulties, p 144.
27 Spiritual Axis, p 104.
28 Dr. Chen Jing Hua, personal communication, London 1986.
29 Simple Questions, p 111.
30 Spiritual Axis, p 137.

31 Spiritual Axis, p 126.
32 Simple Questions, p 245.
33 Spiritual Axis, p 51
34 Simple Questions, p 245.
35 Spiritual Axis, p 89
36 Ibid., ch 76, p 139.
37 Ibid., ch 76, p 140.
38 Simple Questions, p 400.
39 Classic of Difficulties, p 8.
40 Zhang Jing Yue 1634 Complete Book of [Zhang] Jing Yue (Jing Yue Quan Shu 景岳全书), cited in Syndromes and Treatment of the Internal Organs, p 24.
41 Cited in Syndromes and Treatment of the Internal Organs ch 8, p 52.
42 Tang Zong Hai 1884 Discussion on Blood (Xue Zheng Lun 血证论), edited by Pei Zheng Xue and Yin Xin Min, People's Health Publishing House, 1979, p 14 and 16.
43 Zhang Lu Medical Transmission of the Zhang Family (Zhang Shi Yi Tong 张氏医通), cited in Syndromes and Treatment of the Internal Organs, p 27.
44 Personal communication from Prof. Meng Jing Chun, Nanjing 1982. See also Academy of Traditional Chinese Medicine and Guangzhou College of Traditional Chinese Medicine, 1980 Concise Dictionary of Chinese Medicine (Jian Ming Zhong Yi Ci Dian 简明医辞票), People's Health Publishing House, Beijing, p 508.
45 Simple Questions, ch 26, p 168.
46 Spiritual Axis, ch 32, p 72.
47 Discussion on Blood, p 16.
48 Syndromes and Treatment of the Internal Organs, p 131.
49 Cited in Syndromes and Treatment of the Internal Organs, p 131.
50 Spiritual Axis, ch 47, p 89.
51 Simple Questions, ch 21, p 139–140.
52 Simple Questions, p 59.
53 Spiritual Axis, p 71.
54 Spiritual Axis, p 76–77.
55 Spiritual Axis, p 126.
56 Spiritual Axis, p 153.
57 Spiritual Axis, p 52.
58 Discussion on Cold-induced Diseases, cited in Syndromes and Treatment of the Internal Organs, p 41.

The Transformation of Qi

4

氣化

Human physiology is based on the transformation of Qi. As we have seen, Qi can assume different forms depending on its states of condensation or dispersal, and it is the motive force of all physiological processes. In the course of its work, Qi assumes many different forms: it is transformed, changed, transported, it enters, exits, rises, descends and disperses. All these functional activities of Qi are generally called "transformation of Qi", as constant transformation and transmutation is the essence of human Qi physiology.

Qi in condensation forms the material body and is Yin in nature, Qi in dispersal moves and is Yang in nature. The Yin and Yang aspects of Qi form the basis of human physiology. If Qi is transformed properly, movement, birth, growth and reproduction can take place.

If Qi is flourishing there is health, if it is weak there is disease, if it is balanced there is quiet, if it moves in the wrong direction there is disease. Thus the transformation and proper direction of movement of Qi is the basis for the movement of Blood, the transformation of the Essence, the movement of Body Fluids, the digestion of food, the absorption of nourishment, the excretion of waste, the moistening of sinews and bones, the moistening of skin and the resistance to exterior pathogenic factors.

In a broad sense transformation of Qi includes all the various physiological processes and movements of Qi; in a narrow sense, it indicates the transformation of Qi by the Triple Burner.

THE MOTIVE FORCE FOR THE TRANSFORMATION OF QI

The motive force for the transformation of Qi arises from between the Kidneys. The "Classic of Difficulties" says: *"The motive force between the Kidneys determines human life, it is the root of the 12 channels and is called Original Qi"*.[1]

Thus, the motive force between the Kidneys is related to the Original Qi but is also related to the fire of the Gate of Vitality. Zhang Jing Yue (1563–1640) said :*"The Fire of the Gate of Vitality is the Sea of Essence and Blood, the Stomach and Spleen are the Sea of Food and Water, the two together are the root of the 5 Yin and 6 Yang organs. The Gate of Vitality is the root of the Original Qi . . ."*.[2]

The "motive force between the Kidneys" is therefore the Fire of the Gate of Vitality. This is the root of Pre-Heaven Qi, the source of Post-Heaven Qi and the foundation for the Original Qi.

When we say that the "Kidney is the root of the Pre-Heaven" we mean two things:

1 The Kidneys store the Essence (including the Pre-Heaven and Post-Heaven Essence) which is the fundamental biological substance of life.

2 The Kidneys contain the Fire of the Gate of Vitality which is the motive force that transforms and sets things in motion.

The Essence and the Fire of Vitality are another example of Yin-Yang polarity and interdependence. The Fire of the Gate of Vitality relies on the Essence to provide the basic, fundamental biological substance for all life processes; the Essence relies on the Fire of the Gate of Vitality to provide the motive force and heat that transforms and moves the various physiological susbtances. Without the Fire of the Gate of Vitality, the Essence would be a cold, inert substance incapable of nurturing life.

The interrelationship between Essence and the Gate of Vitality is mirrored in the expressions *"Qi is transformed into Essence"* and *"Essence is transformed into Qi"*.[3]

The Fire of the Gate of Vitality is connected to the Gathering Qi of the chest: this has the function of assisting the Gate of Vitality by providing pure Qi from breathing. Gathering Qi has to flow down to the Gate of Vitality to provide Qi, and the Gate of Vitality has to flow up to the Lungs to provide heat.

THE DYNAMICS OF THE TRANSFORMATION OF QI

The direction of movement of the various types of Qi in various physiological processes is essential to the proper transformation of Qi. In certain physiological processes Qi needs to ascend, in others to descend. The ancient Chinese often expressed these two movements in relation to "Heaven" and "Earth". Heaven pertains to Yang and Yang descends; Earth pertains to Yin and Yin ascends. The "Simple Questions" in chapter 68 says: *"Descending pertains to Heaven; ascending pertains to Earth. The Qi of Heaven descends flowing to Earth; the Qi of Earth ascends mounting to Heaven"*.[4]

Most of the interrelationships between Yin and Yang and among the 5 Elements reflect the various ascending-descending and entering-exiting movements. For example, Yang floats (or exits), Yin sinks (or enters), Yang descends, Yin ascends, Water rises, Fire descends, Wood floats and Metal sinks.

The various ascending-descending and entering-exiting movements of Qi depend on the functions of the internal organs. Each organ has a particular effect on Qi with regard to its ascending or descending. For example, Spleen-Qi rises, Lung-Qi descends, Heart-Qi descends, Liver-Qi ascends and extends, Kidney-Qi descends, Stomach-Qi descends, and Bladder, Large and Small Intestine Qi all descend.

THE STOMACH AND SPLEEN AS THE CENTRAL AXIS

The movement of Qi of Stomach and Spleen is crucial for most physiological processes. Stomach and Spleen are the "centre" in more ways than one. They are the centre in a physiological sense, as they are the source of Qi and Blood and therefore all other organs depend on them for their nourishment. They are also anatomically the centre as they lie in the Middle Burner at the crossroads of many physiological activities and many different movements of Qi in all directions. The correct functioning of Stomach and Spleen in relation to the direction of movement of Qi is therefore crucial for a proper physiological activity.

Spleen and Stomach complement each other: the Spleen is Yin and its Qi rises: it transports and transforms which are Yang in nature. The Stomach is Yang and its Qi descends: its functions are to churn food and liquids and provide the source of Body Fluids, all activities which are Yin in nature.

Spleen-Qi ascends to send the essences extracted from food up to the Lungs and Heart where they are transformed into Qi and Blood. Stomach-Qi descends to send the impure part resulting from the transformation of food down to the Intestines.

Ye Tian Shi (1667–1746) said: "*After food has entered the Stomach, the Spleen transforms and moves it; if Spleen-Qi rises it is healthy. If Stomach-Qi descends there is harmony...Yang Qi [of the Spleen] moves...Yin Qi [of the Stomach] is quiet. The Spleen likes dryness, and the Stomach likes moisture*".[5]

Thus the ascending and descending of Spleen-Qi and Stomach-Qi is crucial for the production of Qi and Blood and for the harmonious crossing of Qi in the Middle Burner.

THE LIVER AND LUNGS AS THE OUTER WHEEL

The Liver is on the left and its Qi rises, the Lungs are on the right and its Qi descends. Being "on the left" or "on the right" should not be interpreted in a strict anatomical sense, but in relation to the 5-Element scheme which places Wood (Liver) on the left and Metal (Lungs) on the right.

Ye Tian Shi said: "*The human body mirrors the natural world* [so that]*, the Liver is on the left and its Qi ascends, the Lungs are on the right and their Qi descends. When their ascending and descending are harmonized, Qi can relax and develop...the Liver makes Qi ascend to the head and the upper orifices; the Lungs make Qi descend to the internal organs and sinews and bones. The two together permit Qi and Blood to flow and extend and the internal organs to be peaceful and balanced*".[6]

The Liver is in the Lower Burner (energetically, not anatomically) and sends Qi upwards, the Lungs are in the Upper Burner and send Qi downwards. The two together ensure the smooth flow of Qi between Upper and Lower Burner and among the internal organs.

THE HEART AND KIDNEYS AS THE ROOT

The Heart shelters the Mind and pertains to Fire; the Kidneys store Essence and pertain to Water. The polarity of Heart and Kidneys is the fundamental polarity between Fire and Water.

The Fire of the Heart[7] descends to the Kidneys to warm them; the Water of the Kidneys rises to the Heart to nourish its Yin aspect. The descending of the Fire of the Heart and ascending of the Water of the Kidneys keeps the fundamental balance between Fire and Water, Yang and Yin, Above and Below. There is a direct connection between Heart and Kidneys and the two have to communicate with each other and be harmonized.

The book "Wu's Collected Medical Works" (1792) says: "*The Heart pertains to Fire but there is Water within Fire; the Kidneys pertain to Water but there is Fire within Water. Fire governs Water and Heart-Qi descends. Water is the source of Fire and Kidney-Qi ascends. If Water does not ascend, disease ensues: this is due to Kidney-Yang deficient unable to raise Water upwards. If Fire does not descend, disease ensues: this is due to Heart Yin deficient unable to lower Fire downwards.*"[8]

We can now summarize these three relationships between Stomach and Spleen, Liver and Lungs and Heart and Kidneys by referring to the 5-Element cosmological sequence.

We can visualise the cosmological sequence as a three-dimensional model of the relationships of the internal organs and the movement of Qi in the various directions (Fig. 35).

The Heart and Kidney axis could be seen as an imaginary axis going through the centre of a horizontal wheel; the Stomach and Spleen could be seen as the hub of the wheel and the Liver and Lungs as the outer rim of the wheel. (Fig. 35A).

PATHOLOGY OF QI TRANSFORMATION

The correct direction of movement of the various types of Qi in different situations depends on the internal organs. Each of the internal organs moves its Qi in a particular direction to perform certain functions: thus, the direction of Qi is closely related to a particular internal organ's function. For this reason, any disruption of Qi transformation needs to be viewed in relation to the dysfunction of the internal organs.

Fig. 35 The Cosmological Sequence and the organ direction of Qi

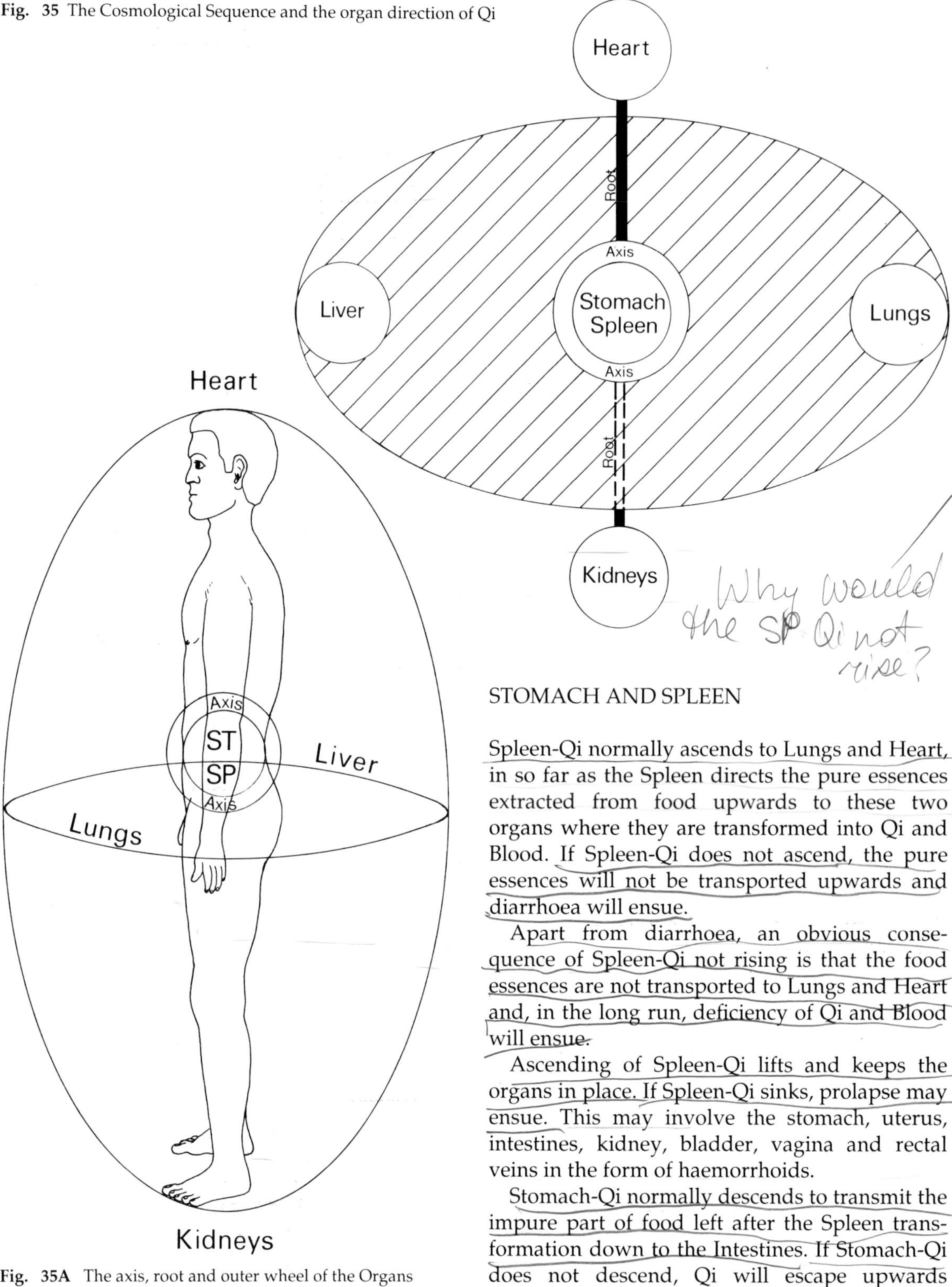

Fig. 35A The axis, root and outer wheel of the Organs

STOMACH AND SPLEEN

Spleen-Qi normally ascends to Lungs and Heart, in so far as the Spleen directs the pure essences extracted from food upwards to these two organs where they are transformed into Qi and Blood. If Spleen-Qi does not ascend, the pure essences will not be transported upwards and diarrhoea will ensue.

Apart from diarrhoea, an obvious consequence of Spleen-Qi not rising is that the food essences are not transported to Lungs and Heart and, in the long run, deficiency of Qi and Blood will ensue.

Ascending of Spleen-Qi lifts and keeps the organs in place. If Spleen-Qi sinks, prolapse may ensue. This may involve the stomach, uterus, intestines, kidney, bladder, vagina and rectal veins in the form of haemorrhoids.

Stomach-Qi normally descends to transmit the impure part of food left after the Spleen transformation down to the Intestines. If Stomach-Qi does not descend, Qi will escape upwards

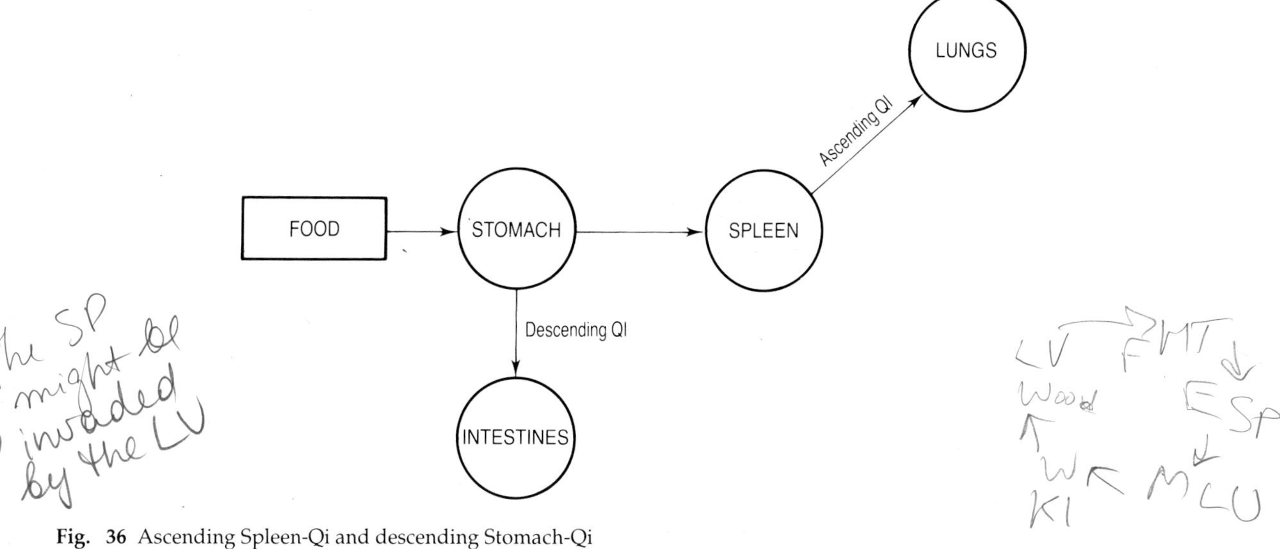

Fig. 36 Ascending Spleen-Qi and descending Stomach-Qi

causing nausea, hiccup, belching and vomiting (Fig. 36).

Both Spleen-Qi descending and Stomach-Qi ascending are called "rebellious" Qi, i.e. Qi flowing in the wrong direction. The former is a rebellious Qi of deficient nature, the latter a rebellious Qi of excess nature. Rebellious Qi is one of the possible pathologies of Qi, in addition to deficiency and stagnation.

LIVER AND LUNGS

Liver-Qi ascends and Lung-Qi descends: if the two are balanced, Qi flows freely and smoothly.

Liver-Qi can, however, fail to ascend and extend, and this becomes a major cause of stagnation of Qi. Stagnation of Liver-Qi can be manifested in many different areas of the body, such as the hypochondrium, epigastrium, abdomen, uterus, throat and head. When Liver-Qi stagnates, it can easily either invade the Stomach causing epigastric pain, nausea and vomiting or the Spleen causing diarrhoea.

Liver-Qi can stagnate in the throat causing a feeling of constriction of the throat. It can also infuse downwards to the Bladder causing a feeling of distension of the hypogastrium and slight retention of urine.

Ascending of Liver-Qi can also get out of hand and rise to the head causing headaches and irritability.

Excessive rising of Liver-Qi or its stagnation can affect the Lungs. In terms of 5 Elements this is called "Liver insulting the Lungs": this may cause cough and asthma. In such cases, the upward rush of Liver-Qi prevents Lung-Qi from descending which in turn causes cough and asthma.

Descending of Lung-Qi brings Qi and fluids down to the Kidneys and Bladder. If Lung-Qi fails to descend, it will stagnate in the chest and cause cough or asthma (Fig. 37).

If Lung-Qi fails to send down the fluids, this may cause urinary retention or oedema of the face.

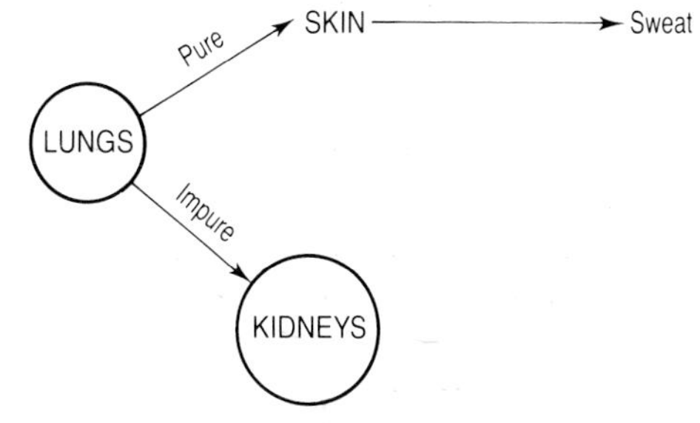

Fig. 37 Descending Lung-Qi

HEART AND KIDNEYS

In health, the Fire of the Heart goes downwards to communicate with the Water of the Kidneys: conversely, the Water of the Kidneys goes upwards to nourish Heart-Yin.

If the fire of the Heart does not descend to meet the Kidneys, Heart-Heat develops which can damage Kidney-Yin. If Water is deficient, it cannot rise to meet the Heart, Kidney-Yang is deficient and oedema develops.

This same situation is described by Zhang Jing Yue when he says: *"Fire is the root of Heat, if there is no Water within Fire the Heat becomes excessive and it depletes the Yin which causes the drying and withering of life. Water is the root of Cold, if there is no Fire within the Water, Cold becomes excessive and it injures the Yang which causes things to be lifeless and without Fire."*[9]

Wang Bing, author of the edition of the "Yellow Emperor's Classic of Internal Medicine" (AD 762) on which all modern versions are based, says: *"The Heart should not have excessive Heat but enough Yang; the Kidneys should not have excessive Cold but enough Yin."*[10]

The disharmony between Kidneys and Heart can also be manifested when the Water of the Kidneys, and in particular Kidney-Yin, fails to ascend to cool and nurture Heart-Yin: in this case the lack of nourishment from Kidney-Yin causes an uprising of pathological Fire in the Heart, with such symptoms as insomnia, mental restlessness and anxiety. These symptoms are caused by Empty-Heat of the Heart deriving from Yin deficiency.

Being the root for the ascending and descending of Qi, the axis of Heart and Kidneys affects many other organs. The Liver relies on the nourishment from Kidney-Yin: if Kidney-Yin does not nourish Liver-Yin, Liver-Qi may ascend too much causing headaches and irritability. The Heart, on the other hand, keeps the Lungs in check, and if Heart-Qi does not descend, Lung-Qi may fail to descend causing cough or asthma.

The function of Stomach and Spleen is also dependent on the ascending and descending of Heart and Kidney Qi, as these provide the Fire and the Water necessary for the function of digestion, transformation and transportation. He Bo Zhai (1694-?) said: *"The Internal Organs depend on the Stomach and Spleen for their nourishment. After food enters the Stomach, its essence is transported by the Spleen. The ability of the Spleen to transform food depends on the Qi of Fire and Water. If the Fire is in excess, the Stomach and Spleen are too dry; if Water is in excess the Stomach and Spleen are too damp: in both cases they will not be able to transform and disease will ensue"*.[11]

THE TRIPLE BURNER'S TRANSFORMATION OF QI

The Triple Burner is considered a Yang organ. The functions of the Triple Burner are expressed in the "Simple Questions" as "making things go through" and "letting out". In other words, the Triple Burner assists all the other organs in their functions and, in particular, it makes sure that all passages are open, that the various types of Qi flow smoothly and that wastes are excreted properly. This is therefore an essential function in relation to the movement of the various types of Qi and essences in any part of the body.

Each of the three Burners is in charge of particular functions and particular movements of Qi.

The Upper Burner (which comprises Lungs and Heart) is in charge of dispersing and scattering Qi to the skin and muscles. In particular, it controls the outward movement of Defensive Qi to the skin.

The Middle Burner (which comprises Stomach and Spleen) is in charge of digesting food, transforming it and transporting the Food-Qi upwards to Lungs and Heart. In particular, the Middle Burner controls the movement of Nutritive Qi and makes sure that Qi moves in the right directions, i.e. Spleen-Qi upwards and Stomach-Qi downwards.

The Lower Burner (which comprises Liver, Kidneys, Bladder and Intestines) is in charge of the transformation, transportation and excretion of fluids and wastes. Its Qi has a definite downward movement. In particular, the Lower Burner controls the downward movement of the Qi of the Intestines and Bladder.

To summarize, the Triple Burner is in charge of the correct direction of movement of all types of Qi in all parts of the body. If this function of the Triple Burner is impaired, Qi, Blood and Body Fluids will not flow smoothly, they will overflow, passages will be blocked and Qi will stagnate.

The "Classic of the Secret Transmission" by Hua Tuo (AD?-208) says: *"The Triple Burner ... assembles and directs the 5 Yin and 6 Yang organs, the Nutritive and Defensive Qi and the channels, [it harmonizes] the Qi of interior and exterior, left and right, upper and lower. If the Triple Burner is open, then the interior and exterior, left and right, upper and lower are also open; in this way it regulates and irrigates the body, it harmonizes interior and exterior, left and right, upper and lower."* [12]

NOTES

1 Classic of Difficulties, ch 66, p 144.
2 The Complete Book of Jing Yue, cited in Syndromes and Treatment of the Internal Organs, p 48.
3 Simple Questions, ch 5, p 33.
4 Simple Questions, p 398.
5 Cited in Syndromes and Treatment of the Internal Organs, p 51.
6 Simple Questions, p 51
7 What is described from now on as "the fire of the Heart" should not be confused with what is later described as "Heart-Fire". The "Fire of the Heart" indicates Fire in a 5-Element sense, the normal, physiological Fire to which the Heart pertains. "Heart-Fire" indicates a pathological conditions of the Heart characterized by excess Heat.
8 1792 Wu's Collected Medical Works, cited in Syndromes and Treatment of the Internal Organs, p 52.
9 The Complete Book of Jing Yue, cited in Syndromes and Treatment of the Internal Organs, p 52.
10 Wang Ping, cited in Syndromes and Treatment of the Internal Organs, p 56.
11 He Bo Zhai, cited in Syndromes and Treatment of the Internal Organs, p 56.
12 Hua Tuo (c. AD 180) The Classic of the Secret Transmission (Zhong Cang Jing 中藏经), Jiangsu Scientific Publishing House, 1985, p 39.

5 The Functions of the Internal Organs 脏腑

The theory of the Internal Organs is often described as the core of Chinese medical theory, because it best represents the Chinese Medicine view of the body as an intergrated whole. At core, this theory represents a landscape of functional relationships which provide total integration of bodily functions, emotions, mental activities, tissues, sense organs and environmental influences.

When studying the Chinese theory of the Internal Organs, it is best to rid oneself of the Western concept of internal organs entirely. Western Medicine sees each organ only in its material-anatomical aspect, whereas Chinese Medicine sees each organ as a complex system encompassing its anatomical entity and its corresponding emotion, tissue, sense organ, mental faculty, colour, climate and more. Throughout this book, organs are described in this way and not in the Western anatomical sense. However, it is often said that Chinese Medicine disregards anatomy entirely and only considers the functional relationships: this is not entirely true. While Chinese Medicine excels in its acute and detailed observation of complex functional relationships, it does not entirely disregard the study of anatomy. There are many chapters of the "Yellow Emperor's Classic" and the "Classic of Difficulties" that describe the anatomy of the internal organs, muscles and bones.[1]

The Internal Organs are functionally related to various vital substances , emotions, tissues, senses: the following are the main aspects of these interrelationships.

THE INTERNAL ORGANS AND THE VITAL SUBSTANCES

One of the main functions of the Internal Organs is to ensure the production, maintenance, replenishment, transformation and movement of the Vital Substances. Each of the Vital Substances, Qi, Blood, Essence, and Body Fluids is related to one or more of the organs. Thus:

The Heart governs Blood
The Liver stores Blood
The Lungs govern Qi and influence Body Fluids
The Spleen governs Food-Qi, holds Blood and influences Body Fluids
The Kidneys store Essence and influence Body Fluids.

THE INTERNAL ORGANS AND THE TISSUES

Each organ influences one of the tissues of the body: this means that there is a functional relationship between certain tissues and each organ, so that the state of the organ can be deduced by observation of the tissue related to it. Thus, the Heart controls the blood vessels and manifests in the complexion, the Liver controls the sinews and manifests in the nails, the Lungs control the skin and manifest in the body hair, the Spleen controls the muscles and manifests in the lips, the Kidneys control the bones and manifest in the hair.

THE INTERNAL ORGANS AND THE SENSE ORGANS

Each organ is functionally related to one of the sense organs. This means that the health and acuity of a particular sense organ relies on the nourishment of an internal organ. Thus, the Heart controls the tongue and taste, the Liver controls the eyes and sight, the Lungs control the nose and smell, the Spleen controls the mouth and taste, the Kidneys control the ears and hearing.

THE INTERNAL ORGANS AND THE EMOTIONS

This extremely important aspect of the Chinese theory of the Internal Organs illustrates the unity of body and mind in Chinese Medicine. The same Qi that is the basis for all the physiological processes, is also the basis for emotional and mental processes, since Qi, as we have seen, exists in many different states of refinement. Whereas in Western physiology emotional and mental processes are attributed to the brain, in Chinese Medicine they are part of the sphere of action of the internal organs. The relation between each organ and a particular emotion is mutual: the state of the organ will affect the emotions, and emotions will affect the state of the organ. Thus: the Heart relates to joy, the Liver to anger, the Lungs to sadness and worry, the Spleen to thinking and the Kidneys to fear. These emotions usually only become a cause of imbalance when they are excessive and prolonged. By treating a specific organ, we can influence the particular emotion related to that organ and help a person to achieve a more balanced emotional state.

THE INTERNAL ORGANS AND CLIMATES

Chinese Medicine considers that differing climatic conditions influence specific organs. Heat influences the Heart, wind influences the Liver, dryness influences the Lung, dampness influences the Spleen and cold influences the Kidneys. An excess of these climatic conditions for a prolonged period may adversely affect the relevant organ.

There are two types of Internal Organs: Yin (called *"Zang"*) and Yang (called *"Fu"*) organs. The Chinese name for Internal Organs is simply *"Zangfu"*.

Both *"Zang"* and *"Fu"* mean "organ", but an analysis of the Chinese characters can clarify the difference between the two.

ZANG 臟 (simplified: 脏) means organ, viscus.

月 this part indicates "flesh"

藏 this part indicates "to store".

This indicates that the Yin organs are in charge of storing the vital substances.

FU 腑 also means organ

月 this part indicates "flesh"

府 this part indicates "seat of government"

This indicates that the Yang organs are in charge of transforming food and drink to produce Qi and Blood, just as the government in ancient China was considered to be in charge of food distribution.

The "Simple Questions" in chapter 11 says: *"The 5 Yin organs store Essence and Qi and do not excrete: they can be full but not in excess. The 6 Yang organs transform and digest and do not store: they can be in excess but not full. In fact, after food enters the mouth, the stomach is full and the intestines empty; when the food goes down, the intestines are full and the stomach empty."* [2]

Thus the Yin organs store the Vital Substances, i.e. Qi, Blood, Essence and Body Fluids. They only store pure, refined substances which they receive from the Yang organs after transformation from food.

The Yang organs, on the contrary, do not store but are constantly filled and emptied. They transform and refine food and drink to extract the pure essences which are then stored by the Yin organs. As well as carrying out this process of transformation, the Yang organs also excrete waste products. The essence of the Yang organs is therefore to "receive", "move", "transform", digest" and "excrete". The functions of the Yang organs are often summarized by the two words *"chuan"* and *"xing"* meaning "to transmit" and "to move" because they are constantly receiving, transmitting, moving and excreting substances. Perhaps because of this constant moving in and out of substances, the Yang organs are also compared to a government office with a constant coming and going of people, as their name "Fu" implies. The "Simple Questions" in chapter 9 says: *"The Stomach, Small and Large Intestine, Triple Burner and Bladder are the roots of food storage, they are the residence of Nutritive Qi, they are called containers, they transform waste substances and transmit the incoming and outgoing flavours"*. [3]

There is a close interrelationship between Yin and Yang organs: the two groups of organs are different in function but their difference is only relative.

The relationship between Yin and Yang organs is a structural-functional relationship. The Yin organs correspond to structure and store the Vital Substances, while the Yang organs correspond to function. Structure and function are interdependent and we can view each Yang organ as the functional aspect of its corresponding Yin organ. For example, one can view the Gall Bladder as the functional aspect of the Liver. Although one Yang and one Yin, the two organs can be seen as a unit, the Liver being the structure and the Gall Bladder its functional expression. This view of the Yin-Yang relationship of the organs is particularly useful in pulse diagnosis where it may be more meaningful to see each pulse position at the superficial level as the function aspect of the relevant Yin organ, rather than considering each of the 12 pulse positions individually and in isolation.

In the Chinese theory of the organs, the Yin organs are the core: they are more important than the Yang organs both in terms of physiology and pathology. The Yin organs are more important because they store all the Vital Substances, while the Yang organs are their functional aspect. For this reason, in what follows, the main focus of attention is on the Yin organs. However, it should be stressed that the priority of the Yin over the Yang organs is not reflected in the theory of the channels: from an acupuncturist's (as opposed to a herbalist's) perspective, all the 14 channels are equally important.

There are 12 organs, 6 Yin and 6 Yang:

Yin organs	*Yang organs*
Heart	Small Intestine
Liver	Gall Bladder
Lungs	Large Intestine
Spleen	Stomach
Kidneys	Bladder
Pericardium	Triple Burner

For each organ the following aspects will be discussed in detail:

Its main function or functions

The tissue it controls

The sense organ into which it "opens" and the part of the body on which it "manifests".

Any other function peculiar to each organ.

In addition to the above, a few sayings for each organ will be given to illustrate certain other aspects of the organ functions not normally included in the itemized functions.

NOTES

1 See Spiritual Axis, ch 10, 13, 14, 31, and Classic of Difficulties, ch 41, 42.

2 Simple Questions, p 77.

3 Simple Questions, p 67.

The Functions of the Heart

Xin

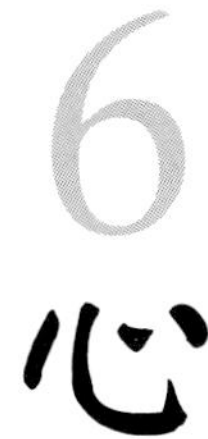

The Heart is considered to be the most important of all the internal organs, sometimes described as the "ruler" or "monarch" of the internal organs. The "Simple Questions" in chapter 8 says: *"The Heart is like the Monarch and it governs the Mind . . ."*[1]. The "Spiritual Axis" in chapter 71 says: *"The Heart is the Monarch of the 5 Yin organs and the 6 Yang organs and it is the residence of the Mind . . ."*[2]

The Heart's main functions are to govern Blood and blood vessels and to house the Mind.

The functions of the Heart are:

It governs Blood
It controls the blood vessels
It manifests in the complexion
It houses the Mind
It opens into the tongue
It controls sweat.

1 GOVERNS BLOOD

The Heart governs Blood in two ways:

a) The transformation of Food-Qi into Blood takes place in the Heart.

b) The Heart is responsible for the circulation of Blood just the same as in Western Medicine (although in Chinese Medicine, other organs, notably the Lungs, Spleen and Liver, also play a role in the circulation of Blood).

A healthy Heart is essential for a proper supply of blood to all the body tissues. When its function is impaired, i.e. Heart-Blood is deficient, the circulation of Blood is slack and the hands may be cold.

The relation between Heart and Blood is important in another way as it determines the strength of constitution of an individual.

Although our constitution is primarily related to the Essence and the Kidney, it is also partly determined by the relative constitutional strength of the Heart and Blood. If the Heart is strong, Blood in ample supply and its circulation good, a person will be full of vigour and have a good constitution. If the Heart is constitutionally weak and Blood deficient, a person will have a poor constitution and lack strength. A constitutional weakness of the Heart is sometimes manifested with a shallow long crack in the midline of the tongue and a weak pulse on both the Heart and Kidney positions (see p. 151).

The "Simple Questions" in chapter 10 says: *"Blood pertains to the Heart"*.[3]

2 CONTROLS THE BLOOD VESSELS

The state of the Heart's energy is reflected in the state of the blood vessels. Blood vessels depend on the Heart's Qi and Blood. If Heart Qi is strong, the blood vessels will be in a good state and the pulse will be full and regular. If Heart Qi is weak, the pulse may be feeble and irregular. The "Simple Questions" in chapter 44 says: *"The Heart governs the blood vessels . . ."*.[4]

3 MANIFESTS IN THE COMPLEXION

The Heart governs Blood and blood vessels and distributes Blood all over the body. The state of the Heart and Blood can therefore be reflected in the complexion. If Blood is abundant and the Heart strong, the complexion will be rosy and lustrous. If Blood is deficient, the complexion will be pale or bright-white. If Blood is stagnant, the complexion will be bluish-purple, and if the Heart has Heat, the complexion will be too red. The "Simple Questions" in chapter 10 says; *"The Heart . . . manifests in the complexion . . ."*.[5]

4 HOUSES THE MIND[6]

Chinese Medicine holds that the Heart is the residence of the Mind (*Shen*). The word *Shen* can have many different meanings and, in Chinese Medicine, it is used in at least two different contexts.

Firstly, *Shen* indicates the complex of mental faculties which are said to "reside" in the Heart. In this sense, the *Shen* corresponds to the Mind and is specifically related to the Heart.

Secondly, *Shen* is used to indicate the whole sphere of emotional, mental and spiritual aspects of a human being. In this sense, it is related not only to the Heart, but it encompasses the emotional, mental and spiritual phenomena of all the other organs, notably the Yin organs.

Let us now discuss the nature and functions of the Mind in the first sense outlined above.

According to Chinese Medicine, mental activity and consciousness "reside" in the Heart. This means that the state of the Heart (and Blood) will affect the mental activities including the emotional state. In particular, five functions are affected by the state of the Heart:

Mental activity (including emotions)
Consciousness
Memory
Thinking
Sleep.

If the Heart is strong and Blood abundant, there will be a normal mental activity, a balanced emotional life, a clear consciousness, a good memory, keen thinking and good sleep. If the Heart is weak and Blood deficient there may be mental problems (such as depression), poor memory, dull thinking, insomnia or somnolence and in extreme cases, unconsciousness. The "Simple Questions" in chapter 9 says: *"The Heart . . . is in control of the Mind..."*[7]. The "Spiritual Axis" in chapter 71 says: *"The Heart...is the residence on the Mind"*.[8]

Thus, some of the Heart functions in relation to the Mind (such as memory and intelligence) correspond to the brain's mental activities from a modern medical viewpoint. For example, the intellectual power of slow-to-learn children can, to a certain extent, be stimulated by tonifying the Heart.

The Heart's function of housing the Mind depends on an adequate nourishment from the Blood and conversely, the Heart's job of governing Blood depends on the Mind. Thus there is a relation of mutual dependence between the function of controlling Blood and that of housing the Mind. The Blood is the root of the Mind. This concept is important in practice as Heart-Blood roots the Mind, it embraces it and anchors it, so that the Mind will be peaceful and happy. If Heart-Blood is deficient and does not root the Mind, this will result in mental restlessness, depression, anxiety and insomnia. Conversely, mental restlessness, emotional problems and sadness can induce a deficiency of Blood of the Heart causing palpitations, a pale complexion and a weak or irregular pulse.

Apart from the mental activity aspect, the Mind also affects the emotional state. If the Heart is strong, the Mind will also be strong and the person will be happy. If the Heart is weak, the Mind lacks vitality and the person will be sad or depressed or in low spirits. If the Heart is in an excess condition, the Mind will be affected and the person may display symptoms of mental illness, such as manic depression. Of course, this is an oversimplification, as a person's emotional state is related to all the other organs too.

On an emotional level, the state of the Heart determines a person's capacity to form meaningful relationships. A healthy Heart and Mind will positively influence our ability to relate to other people, and conversely, emotional problems due to difficult relationships can weaken the Heart and the Mind.

Chinese Medicine sees the Mind closely linked to the body. Essence and Qi form the physical basis for the Mind. If the Essence is flourishing and Qi vital, then the Mind will be happy and peaceful. Conversely, if the Essence is weak and Qi deficient, the Mind will suffer. For this reason, the glitter of the eyes shows both the state of Essence and the Mind. Essence, Qi and Mind are called the "Three Treasures" (see also p. 41).

We can now discuss the nature of *Shen* in its second sense, i.e. not as the Mind residing in the Heart, but as the whole complex of emotional, mental and spiritual aspects of a human being. In this sense, it is related not only to the Heart, but it also encompasses mental and spiritual aspects related to other organs, and particularly the Yin organs. For this reason, it would be wrong to identify our mental and spiritual life simply with the Heart. All 5 Yin organs influence emotions, Mind and Spirit in different ways.

Each of the 5 Yin organs is related to a certain mental aspect. These are:

— the Mind (*Shen*) for the Heart
— the Ethereal Soul (*Hun*) for the Liver
— the Corporeal Soul (*Po*) for the Lungs
— the Will Power (*Zhi*) for the Kidneys
— Thought (*Yi*) for the Spleen.

The "Simple Questions" in chapter 23 says: *"The Heart houses the Mind (Shen), the Lungs house the Corporeal Soul (Po), the Liver houses the Ethereal Soul (Hun), the Spleen houses Thought (Yi) and the Kidneys house Will Power (Zhi)".*[9] The commentary, based also on passages from the "Spiritual Axis" adds: *"The Mind is a transformation of Essence and Qi: both Essences* [i.e. the Pre-Heaven and Post-Heaven Essences] *contribute to forming the Mind. The Corporeal Soul is the assistant of Essence and Qi: it is close to Essence but it moves in and out. The Ethereal Soul complements the Mind and Qi: it is close to the Mind but it comes and goes. Thought corresponds to memory: it is the memory which depends on the Heart. The Will Power is like a purposeful and focused mind: the Kidneys store Essence . . . and through the Will Power they can fulfil our destiny".*[10]

The complex of these five mental and spiritual phenomena represents the Chinese medical view of body and mind. Each of these will be discussed in more detail with the functions of their relevant organ.

The Ethereal Soul (*Hun*) pertaining to the Liver broadly corresponds to our Western concept of "Soul" or "Spirit". According to ancient Chinese beliefs it enters the body shortly after birth. It is ethereal in nature, as opposed to the Corporeal Soul which is more physical, and after death it survives the body. The Ethereal Soul can be described as *"that part of the Soul* [*as opposed to the Corporeal Soul*] *which at death leaves the body, carrying with it an appearance of physical form".*[11] This corresponds closely to the ancient Greek views on "spirit" as being πγευμα (which means "breath") or "soul" as being φυκη (which means "wind or vital breath").

The Corporeal Soul (*Po*) can be defined as *"that part of the Soul* [*as opposed to the Ethereal Soul*] *which is indissolubly attached to the body and goes down to Earth with it at death".*[12] The Corporeal Soul is closely linked to the body and it could be described as the somatic expression of the Soul. As the "Simple Questions" says in the passage mentioned above, the Corporeal Soul is close to Essence and Qi. The "Classic of Categories" (1624) says: *"The Corporeal Soul moves and accomplishes things and* [when it is active] *pain and itching can be felt".*[13] This passage illustrates just how physical the Corporeal Soul is. It gives us the capacity of sensation, feeling, hearing and sight.

The Will Power (*Zhi*) resides in the Kidneys and is the mental drive that gives us determination and single-mindedness in the pursuit of our goals.

Thought (*Yi*) resides in the Spleen and corresponds to our capacity for applied thinking, studying, concentrating and memorizing. Although Thought is said to reside in the Spleen, the Heart also affects thinking and memory, as shown by the passage from the "Simple Questions" (chapter 23) mentioned above.

Thus, while the *Shen* which resides in the Heart corresponds to the Mind, the *Shen* which indicates the complex of mental and spiritual aspects of a human being more appropriately corresponds to "Spirit".

In some cases, the word *Shen* is used in Chinese medical classics to indicate the outward appearance of something. For example, the *shen* of a face indicates an appearance of vitality. A tongue is said to have "spirit" (*Shen*) when it looks vital, bright and flourishing.

Before concluding this section on the relation between the Heart and the Mind, mention should be made of a different viewpoint which emerged during the historical development of Chinese Medicine.

Ever since the Ming dynasty (1368–1644), a few doctors attributed the functions of intelligence and memory to the brain, not the Heart as is traditional in Chinese Medicine. Li Shi Zhen (1518–1593), the famous herbalist of the Ming dynasty said: *"The brain is the residence of the Original Mind"*.[14]

Wang Qing Ren, of the early Qing dynasty (1644–1911), dealt at length with the role of the brain in relation to intelligence and memory. He believed that intelligence and memory are functions which depend on the brain rather than the Heart. He said: *"Intelligence and memory reside in the brain. Food generates Qi and Blood ... the clear Essence is transformed into marrow which ascends along the spine to the brain and is called Brain Marrow, or Sea of Marrow"*.[15]

From this it is obvious that, from the Ming dynasty onwards, a new medical theory developed in parallel with the traditional one, whereby the intellectual functions were attributed to the brain rather than the Heart. Significantly, these new theories emerged before the introduction of Western Medicine into China.

5 OPENS INTO THE TONGUE

The tongue is considered to be the "offshoot" of the Heart. The Heart controls the colour, form and appearance of the tongue, it is in particular related to the tip of the tongue. It also controls the sense of taste. If the Heart is normal, the tongue will have a normal pale-red colour and the sense of taste will be normal.

If the Heart has Heat, the tongue may be dry and dark red, the tip may be redder and swollen and there may be a bitter taste. If the Heat is severe the tongue may have ulcers which are red and painful. If the Heart is weak and the Blood deficient, the tongue may be pale and thin. The "Spiritual Axis" in chapter 17 says: *"Heart-Qi communicates with the tongue, if the Heart is normal the tongue can distinguish the five tastes"*.[16]

The condition of the Heart also affects speech and abnormalities may cause stuttering or aphasia. Apart from speech difficulties themselves, the Heart also influences talking and laughing. Often a disharmony of the Heart (whether excess or deficiency) can cause a person to talk incessantly or laugh inappropriately.

6 CONTROLS SWEAT

Blood and Body Fluids have a common origin. Sweat is one of the Body Fluids which comes from the space between skin and muscles. As we have seen, Blood and Body Fluids mutually interchange. When Blood is too thick, Body Fluids enter the blood vessels and thin it down. The "Classic of the Jade Letter of the Golden Shrine" says: *"Body fluids enter the blood vessels and change into Blood"*.[17]

Because of the relationship of interchange between Body Fluids and Blood, a patient who is haemorrhaging should not be subjected to sweating, and a patient who is sweating profusely should not have drying herbs, nor should a bleeding technique in acupuncture be used. The

"Spiritual Axis" in chapter 18 says: "*Big bleeding, do not cause sweat; big sweat, do not cause bleeding*".[18]

Since the Heart governs Blood and this has a relation of mutual interchange with Body Fluids, of which sweat is part, the Heart is related to sweat. A deficiency of Heart-Qi may often cause spontaneous sweating, while a deficiency of Heart-Yin may often cause night sweating and the treatment should be aimed at tonifying Heart-Yang in the former case and Heart-Yin in the latter.

Furthermore any profuse and continuous sweating in a patient with Heart deficiency should be treated without delay, as a loss of sweat implies loss of Body Fluids which, in turn, will lead to a deficiency of Blood because of the continuous interchange between Blood and Body Fluids.

DREAMS

Since the Heart stores the Mind, it is very closely related to sleep. The Mind should reside in the Heart and if the Heart (particularly Heart-Blood) is strong, a person will fall asleep easily and the sleep will be sound. If the Heart is weak, the Mind has no residence and it will "float" at night causing inability to fall asleep, disturbed sleep or excessive dreaming. All dreams therefore are, in a way, related to the Heart. Certain dreams, however, are more directly indicative of a Heart disharmony.

The "Simple Questions" in chapter 80 says: "*When the Heart is weak, one dreams of fires; if the dream takes place in summertime, one dreams of volcanic eruptions*".[19] The "Spiritual Axis" in chapter 43 says:"*When the Heart is in excess, one dreams of laughing. . .when the Heart is deficient, one dreams of mountains, fire and smoke*".[20]

"THE HEART LOATHES HEAT"

Of all the exterior pathogenic factors, Heat is the most pernicious to the Heart. Strictly speaking, Chinese Medicine holds that the Heart cannot be invaded by exterior Heat. The Pericardium is closely related to the Heart and can be invaded by exterior Heat which clouds the "Heart orifices". As the Heart houses the Mind, clouding of the Heart orifices can cause coma, delirium or aphasia.

"THE HEART CONTROLS SPEECH"

The Heart influences speech and this relationship is manifested in different ways. A condition of Heart-Fire (see p. 208) will cause a person to talk a lot. On the other hand, invasion of the Pericardium by Heat can result in aphasia. Stuttering can be due to a Heart disharmony, as explained above.

NOTES

1 Simple Questions, p 58.
2 Spiritual Axis, p 128.
3 Simple Questions, p 72.
4 Simple Questions, p 246.
5 Simple Questions, p 70.
6 I translate the word *Shen* as "Mind" as its functions, as described in the Chinese medical classics, closely correspond to the mental activities (including emotions) attributed to the "Mind" in Western psychology. The word *Shen* has many different meanings. In order to obtain a clearer idea of the meaning of this word it is useful to consult pre-1949 dictionaries which are not influenced by a Marxist-materialistic philosophical outlook. The 1912 "Chinese-English Dictionary" by H Giles (Kelly and Walsh Ltd, Shanghai, p 1194) gives the following possible translations for the word *Shen*: "Spirits; gods (used by some Protestant sects for "God"); divine; supernatural; mysterious; spiritual (as opposed to material); the soul; the mind; the animal spirits; inspiration; genius; force (as language); expression". Thus, as it is apparent from the above passage, the translation of *Shen* simply as "Spirit" (as opposed to the material body) was influenced by Western Christian missionaries in China during the second half of the 19th century. A Christian philosophical outlook would use the word *Shen* indicating the "Spirit" (or even "God") as opposed to the "body", reflecting a typical Western dualistic attitude to Matter and Spirit which is totally alien to Chinese philosophy. Although the word Shen can have the meaning of "spiritual", in Chinese medical classics it was always used to indicate the mental faculties attributed to the Heart, i.e. the Mind. Indeed, the word *Xin* itself (meaning "Heart") is often used as synonymous with "Mind" in Chinese medical classics. The problem is not simply semantic as it has

repercussions in diagnosis and treatment. Western acupuncture has concentrated entirely on the role of the Heart in mental and spiritual phenomena, based on the idea that "the Heart houses the Spirit". This approach is rather partial as, on the one hand, it ignores the role of the Heart for mental faculties, thinking and memory and, on the other hand, it ignores the role of the other Yin organs in the mental-spiritual sphere.

7 Simple Questions, p 67.
8 Spiritual Axis, p 128.
9 Simple Questions, p 153.
10 Simple Questions, p 153.
11 Giles H 1912 Chinese-English Dictionary, Kelly & Walsh, Shanghai, p 650.
12 Chinese-English Dictionary, p 1144
13 Concise Dictionary of Chinese Medicine, p 953.
14 Cited in Wang Xin Hua 1983 Selected Historical Theories in Chinese Medicine (*Zhong Yi Li Dai Yi Lun Xuan* 中医历代医论选), Jiangsu Scientific Publishing House, Jiangsu, p 31.
15 Correction of the Mistakes of the Medical Forest (*Yi Lin Gai Cuo* 医林改错) by Wang Qing Ren, 1830, cited in Selected Historical Theories in Chinese Medicine, p 30.
16 Spiritual Axis, p 50.
17 The Classic of the Jade Letter of the Golden Shrine (*Jin Gui Yu Han Jing* 金匮玉函经), Song Dynasty, cited in 1978 Fundamentals of Chinese Medicine (*Zhong Yi Ji Chu Xue* 中医基础学) Shandong Scientific Publishing House, Jinan, p 35.
18 Spiritual Axis, p 52.
19 Simple Questions, p 569.
20 Spiritual Axis, p 84–85.

7 The Functions of the Liver

肝

The Liver has many important functions among which are those of storing Blood and ensuring the smooth movement of Qi throughout the body. It is also responsible for our capacity for recovering energy and it contributes to the body's resistance to exterior pathogenic factors.

The Liver is often compared to an army general because it is responsible for overall planning of the body's functions by ensuring the smooth flow and proper direction of Qi (see below). Because of this quality, the Liver is also said to be the origin of courage and resoluteness, if the organ is in a good state of health.[1]

The "Simple Questions" in chapter 8 says: *"The Liver is like an army's general from whom the strategy is derived"*.[2] Owing to this quality, the Liver is also said to influence our capacity of planning our life.

The functions of the Liver are:

It stores Blood
It ensures the smooth flow of Qi
It controls the sinews
It manifests in the nails
It opens into the eyes
It houses the Ethereal Soul.

1 STORES BLOOD

The Liver is the most important organ for storing Blood and by so doing, it regulates the volume of Blood in the whole body at any one time. The Liver function of storing of Blood has two aspects:

It regulates the Blood volume according to physical activity
It regulates menstruation.

a) The Liver regulates the volume of Blood in the body according to physical activity. When the body is at rest Blood flows back to the Liver, when the body is active, Blood flows to the muscles. This is a self-regulating process, co-ordinated with physical activity.

The "Simple Questions" in chapter 62 says: *"The Liver stores Blood"*.[3] In chapter 10 it says: *"When a person lies down Blood returns to the Liver"*.[4] Wang Ping (Tang dynasty) says: *"The Liver stores Blood ... when a person moves, Blood goes to the channels, when at rest it goes to the Liver"*.[5]

When Blood returns to the Liver with the body at rest, it contributes to restoring the persons's energy; when it flows to the muscles during exercise, it nourishes and moistens the muscles to enable them to perform during exercise.

The Liver's job of regulating Blood volume throughout the body has an important influence on a person's level of energy. When the Blood flows to the appropriate places in the body at the appropriate times, it will nourish the necessary tissues, and therefore give us energy. If this regulatory function is impaired, there will be lack of Blood and therefore nourishment where and when it is needed, and the person will become easily tired. The "Simple Questions" in chapter 10 says: *"When the Liver has enough Blood...the feet can walk, the hands can hold and the fingers can grasp"*.[6]

Finally, the Liver function of storing and regulating Blood volume also indirectly influences our resistance to external pathogenic factors. If this Liver function is normal, the skin and muscles will be well nourished by Blood and be able to resist attacks of exterior pathogenic factors. If this function is impaired, the skin and muscles will not be irrigated and nourished by Blood at the appropriate times (during exercise), and the body will therefore be more liable to attack by exterior pathogenic factors. There are other more important factors involved in determining the resistance to exterior pathogenic factors, notably the strength of the Defensive Qi and Lung-Qi. However, it is necessary not to overlook the importance of this Liver function in this respect.

b) The Liver function of storing Blood has a marked influence on menstruation and is of great relevance in clinical practice. If the Liver stores Blood normally, menstruation will be normal. If the Blood of the Liver is deficient, there will be amenorrhoea or oligomenorrhoea. If the Blood of the Liver is in excess or hot, there may be menorrhagia or metrorrhagia.

The Liver function of storing Blood is extremely important in women's physiology and pathology. Many gynaecological problems are due to malfunction of Liver Qi or Blood. If Liver-Qi is stagnant, this may lead to stagnation of Blood of the Liver causing painful periods with premenstrual tension and the menstrual blood will have dark clots. The Liver storage of Blood also influences the Directing (*Ren Mai*) and Penetrating Vessels (*Chong Mai*), the two extraordinary vessels which are closely related to the uterus. Any malfunction of the Liver will induce an imbalance in these two vessels affecting menstruation.

The Blood of the Liver also moistens eyes and tendons. If Liver-Blood is deficient, there will be blurred vision, muscle cramps and contraction of the tendons.

Finally, there is a relationship of reciprocal influence between Blood and Liver: if Blood is abnormal (deficient or hot), it may affect the Liver function. If, on the other hand, the Liver function is abnormal, it may affect the quality of the Blood, causing certain kinds of skin diseases, such as eczema or psoriasis. This last concept has been advanced by Dr J. Shen, who holds that, just as an improper storing medium can spoil food (for instance a dirty container encouraging the growth of bacteria), similarly, an improper Liver function (the storing medium for Blood) can "spoil" Blood, giving rise to skin diseases.[7]

2 ENSURES THE SMOOTH FLOW OF QI

This is the most important of all the Liver functions and it is central to nearly all Liver disharmonies. The impairment of this function is one of the most common patterns seen in practice. What does it mean that the Liver ensures the "smooth flow of Qi"? The Chinese words for this function literally mean "to flow" and "to let out". When Chinese books explain this function they use such terms as "disperse", "extend", "loosen", "relax", "circulate", "make smooth and free" and "stop extremes". Thus the Liver ensures the smooth flow of Qi throughout the body, in all organs and in all directions.

This last point is important. As we have seen, every organ's Qi has a normal direction of flow: some organs's Qi flows downward (such as that of the Lungs and Stomach), other's flows upwards (such as that of the Spleen). The normal direction of movement of Liver-Qi is upwards and outwards in all directions to ensure the smooth and unimpeded flow of Qi everywhere. This explains the importance of this function, as it involves all parts of the body and can affect all organs. This movement of Liver-Qi can be related to the character of Wood in terms of the 5 Elements, with its expansive movement in all directions.

There are three aspects to this function:

In relation to the emotional state

In relation to digestion

In relation to the secretion of bile.

a) The Liver function of ensuring the smooth flow of Qi has a deep influence on the emotional state. If this function is normal, Qi flows normally and the emotional life is happy. If this function is impaired, the circulation of Qi is obstructed, Qi becomes restrained giving rise to emotional frustration, depression or repressed anger, accompanied by such physical symptoms as hypochondriac pain, sensation of oppression in the chest, a feeling of "lump" in the throat or abdominal distension. In women, it may give rise to pre-menstrual tension including depression, irritability and distension of the breasts. This is a reciprocal relationship: a restrained Liver function will lead to emotional tension and frustration, and a tense emotional life characterized by frustration or repressed anger will impair the Liver function and lead to a breakdown of the smooth flow of Qi.

The "Simple Questions" in chapter 3 says: *"Anger makes Qi rise and Blood stagnate in the chest"*.[8]

b) In health, the Liver function of ensuring the smooth flow of Qi assists the Stomach and Spleen digestive function. If Liver-Qi flows smoothly, the Stomach can ripen and rot food and the Spleen can extract Food-Qi. In disease, if Liver-Qi becomes stagnant it may "invade" the Stomach preventing the downward movement of Stomach-Qi resulting in belching, sour regurgitation, nausea or vomiting. If it invades the Spleen, it obstructs the transformation and transportation of food and prevents Spleen-Qi from flowing up-wards resulting in diarrhoea. In 5-Element terms this corresponds to "Wood overacting on Earth".

This is a pathological aspect of what is normally a physiological function of Liver-Qi in aiding Stomach and Spleen. The smooth flow of Liver-Qi is all important in ensuring a harmonious movement of Qi in the Middle Burner. Since Stomach-Qi should go down and Spleen-Qi should go up, the Middle Burner is a crossing place of Qi moving in different directions and the Liver makes sure that the Qi of the Stomach and Spleen flow smoothly in the proper directions.

c) Finally, the Liver function of ensuring a smooth flow of Qi affects the flow of bile. If Liver-Qi is stagnant, the flow of bile may be obstructed resulting in bitter taste, belching or jaundice.

3 CONTROLS THE SINEWS

The state of the sinews (including tendons) affects our capacity for movement and physical activity. The contraction and relaxation of sinews ensures the movement of joints. The sinews' capacity for contraction and relaxation depends on the nourishment and moistening of the Blood from the Liver. The "Simple Questions" in chapter 21 says: *"The Qi of food enters the Stomach, the refined essence extracted from food goes to the Liver and the excess Qi from the Liver overflows into the sinews"*.[9]

If Liver-Blood is abundant, the sinews will be moistened and nourished, ensuring smooth movement of joints and good muscle action. If Liver-Blood is deficient, the sinews will lack moistening and nourishment which may cause contractions and spasms or impaired extension / flexion, numbness of limbs, muscle cramps, tremors, tetany or lack of strength of the limbs. This is why the "Simple Questions" in chapter 1 says: *"When Liver-Qi declines, the sinews cannot move"*.[10]

The Liver influence on the sinews has also another meaning, corresponding to certain neurological conditions from a Western medical perspective. For example, if a child contracts an infectious disease such as meningitis manifesting with a high temperature eventually causing convulsions, in Chinese terms this is due to Heat stirring Liver-Wind. The interior Wind of the Liver causes a contraction and tremor of the sinews which leads to convulsions.

Finally, mention should be made of the fact that most Western books on acupuncture list the "muscles" as being controlled by the Liver and "flesh" by the Spleen. This is a mistranslation as the Liver controls the sinews, and the Spleen the muscles.

4 MANIFESTS IN THE NAILS

The nails are considered in Chinese Medicine as a "by- product" of the sinews, and, as such, they are under the influence of Liver-Blood. If Liver-Blood is abundant the nails will be moist and healthy, if Liver-Blood is deficient, the nails will lack nourishment and become dark, indented, dry and cracked. The "Simple Questions" in chapter 10 says: *"The Liver controls the sinews and its flourishing condition manifests on the nails"*.[11] In chapter 9 it says:*"The Liver is a regulatory organ, it is the residence of the ethereal Soul, it manifests in the nails, controls the sinews . . ."*[12]

5 OPENS INTO THE EYE

The eye is the sense organ connected to the Liver. It is the nourishment and moistening of Liver-Blood that gives the eyes the capacity to see. If Liver-Blood is abundant, the eyes will be normally moist and the vision will be good. If Liver-Blood is deficient, there may be blurred vision, myopia, "floaters" in eyes, colour blindness or the eyes may feel dry and gritty. The "Simple Questions" in chapter 10 says: *"When the Liver receives Blood the eyes can see . . ."*[13] The "Spiritual Axis" in chapter 17 says: *"Liver-Qi extends to the eyes, when the Liver is healthy the eyes can distinguish the five colours"*.[14]

The "Spiritual Axis" in chapter 37 says: *"The eye is the sense organ pertaining to the Liver"*.[15] The "Simple Questions" in chapter 4 says: *"The Liver corresponds to the direction East and the green colour, and it opens into the eye"*.[16]

If the Liver has Heat, the eyes may be bloodshot, and feel painful or burning. If the Liver has internal Wind, the eyeball may turn upwards and move involuntarily (nystagmus).

Aside from the Liver, many other Yin and Yang organs affect the eye, in particular the Heart, Kidney, Lungs, Gall-Bladder, Bladder and Small Intestine. The "Spiritual Axis" in chapter 80 says: *"The Essence from the 5 Yin and 6 Yang organs flows upwards to irrigate the eyes"*.[17]

In particular, the Essence of the Kidneys nourishes the eyes, so that many chronic eye diseases are related to the decline of Kidney-Essence. The Heart is also closely related to the eye. The "Spiritual Axis" in chapter 80 says: *"The eyes mirror the state of the Heart, which houses the Mind"*.[18]

The "Simple Questions" in chapter 81 says: *"The Heart concentrates the Essence of the 5 Yin organs and this manifests in the eye"*.[19]

Thus the eyes also reflect the state of the Mind and the Heart. In conclusion, the Kidney and Heart are the two other Yin organs besides the Liver which are most closely related to the eyes. Heart-Fire can cause pain and redness of the eye and Kidney-Yin deficiency can cause failing eyesight and dryness of the eyes.

6 HOUSES THE ETHEREAL SOUL

The Ethereal Soul, called Hun in Chinese, is the mental-spiritual aspect of the Liver. The "Simple Questions" in Chapter 9 says: *"The Liver is the residence of the Ethereal Soul"*.[20] The concept of Ethereal Soul is closely linked to the ancient Chinese belief in "spirits" and "demons". According to these beliefs spirits and demons are spirit-like creatures who preserve a physical appearance and wander in the world of spirit. Some are good and some are evil. In the times prior to the Warring States Period (476–221 BC), such spirits were considered to be the main cause of disease. Since the Warring State Period, naturalistic causes of disease (such as the weather) replaced this belief, which, however, has never really disappeared even to the present day. The character for *Hun* contains the radical *Gui* which means "spirit" in the above sense, and the radical *Yun* for "cloud". The combination of these two characters conveys the idea of the nature of the Ethereal Soul: it is like a "spirit" but it is Yang and ethereal in nature and essentially harmless, i.e. it is not one of the evil spirits (hence the presence of the "cloud" radical).

The Ethereal Soul is thus Yang in nature (as

opposed to the Corporeal Soul) and at death survives the body to flow back to a world of subtle, non-material energies.

A discussion of the nature of the Ethereal Soul is not complete without discussing the Corporeal Soul as the two are but two poles of the same phenomenon. The Corporeal Soul represents a very physical aspect of the Soul, the part of the Soul which is indissolubly linked to the body. At death, it goes back to the Earth. The Chinese concept of "soul" therefore includes both the Ethereal and Corporeal Souls.

The Ethereal Soul has not a great relevance in Chinese Medicine compared to the other four spiritual aspects (Corporeal Soul, Mind, Will Power and Thought).

The Ethereal Soul is said to influence the capacity of planning our life and find a sense of direction in life. A lack of direction in life and mental confusion could be compared to the wandering of the Ethereal Soul alone in space and time. Thus, if the Liver (in particular Liver-Blood) is flourishing, the Ethereal Soul is firmly rooted and can help us to plan our life with wisdom and vision. If Liver-Blood is weak, the Ethereal Soul is not rooted and cannot give us a sense of direction in life. If Liver-Blood or Liver-Yin is very weak, at times the Ethereal Soul may even leave the body temporarily at night during sleep or just before going to sleep. Those who suffer from severe deficiency of Yin may experience a sensation as if they were floating in the few moments just before falling asleep: this is said to be due to the "floating" of the Ethereal Soul not rooted in Blood and Yin.

The Ethereal Soul is also related to resoluteness and a vague feeling of fear at night before falling asleep is also said to be due to a lack of rooting of the Ethereal Soul.

The "Discussion on Blood Diseases" says: *"If Liver-Blood is deficient Fire agitates the Ethereal Soul resulting in nocturnal emissions with dreams"*.[21] This confirms that the Ethereal Soul can become unrooted at night when Blood or Yin are deficient.

DREAMS

The "Simple Questions" in chapter 17 says: *"When the Liver is in excess, one dreams of being angry"*.[22]

And in chapter 80 it says: *"When the Liver is deficient, one dreams of very fragrant mushrooms. If the dream takes place in Spring, one dreams of lying under a tree without being able to get up"*.[23]

The "Spiritual Axis" in chapter 43 says: *"When the Liver is deficient one dreams of forests in the mountains"*.[24]

"THE LIVER IS A RESOLUTE ORGAN"

Just as in disease Liver-Qi easily becomes stagnant and excessive and Liver Yang easily flares upwards causing irritability and anger, in health the same type of energy deriving from the Liver can give a person great creative drive and resoluteness.

For this reason, it is said in Chinese Medicine that a healthy Liver function can confer on a person resoluteness, an indomitable spirit and drive.

"THE LIVER INFLUENCES RISING AND GROWTH"

In health, Liver-Qi rises upwards and spreads in all directions to promote the smooth flow of Qi in all parts of the body. "Growth" here should be intended in a symbolical sense as the Liver pertains to Wood and this particular quality is compared to the rising of sap promoting growth in a tree.

In disease, the rising movement of Liver-Qi can get out of control, resulting in a separation of Yin and Yang and the excessive rising of Liver-Yang or Liver-Fire. This causes irritability, outbursts of anger, a red face, dizziness, tinnitus and headaches.

"THE LIVER CONTROLS PLANNING"

This idea is derived from chapter 8 of the "Simple Questions" already mentioned. The Liver is said to impart to us the capacity to plan our life smoothly and wisely. In disease, a Liver disharmony can manifest with an inability to plan our life and a lack of direction.

"THE LIVER IS A REGULATING AND HARMONIZING ORGAN"

This is a loose translation of a difficult expression that literally means "The Liver is the Root of stopping extremes". This expression was first used in chapter 9 of the "Simple Questions" where it says: *"The Liver has a regulating function [lit. is the Root of stopping extremes], it houses the Ethereal Soul, manifests in the nails . . ."*[25]

This means that the Liver has an important regulating activity which is mostly derived from its function of storing Blood.

As was mentioned, the Liver regulates the volume of Blood needed by the body according to physical activity. During movement and exercise the Blood flows to the muscles and sinews and at rest, it flows back to the Liver. By flowing back to the Liver during rest, the Blood helps us to recover energy. Conversely, if the Blood of the Liver is deficient a person will find it difficult to recover energy by resting.

"THE LIVER LOATHES WIND"

Windy weather often affects the Liver. Thus the relationship between Liver and "Wind" concerns not only interior but also exterior Wind. It is not infrequent to hear patients who suffer from a Liver disharmony complaining about headaches and stiffness of the neck appearing after a period of windy weather.

"THE LIVER CAN CAUSE CONVULSIONS"

Convulsions are a manifestation of interior Wind which is always related to the Liver.

"THE LIVER ARISES FROM THE LEFT SIDE"

Although anatomically situated on the right side, the Liver is related to the left side of the body in various ways.

Headaches on the left side of the head are said to be related to the Liver, and in particular deficiency of Liver-Blood, while those on the right are said to be related to the Gall Bladder. Of course, this is not always so in practice.

The left side of the tongue reflects more the state of the Liver, while the right side reflects the state of the Gall Bladder.

In pulse diagnosis, of course, the energy of the Liver is felt on the left side.

NOTES

1 Practical Chinese Medicine, p 53
2 Simple Questions, p 58
3 Simple Questions, p 334
4 Simple Questions, p 73
5 Syndromes and treatment of the Internal Organs, p 131.
6 Simple Questions, p 73
7 Personal communication from Dr J H F Shen.
8 Simple Questions, p 17.
9 Simple Questions, p 139.
10 Simple Questions, p 5.
11 Simple Questions, p 70.
12 Simple Questions, p 68.
13 Simple Questions, p 73.
14 Spiritual Axis, p 50.
15 Spiritual Axis, p 78
16 Simple Questions, p 25
17 Spiritual Axis, p 151.
18 Spiritual Axis, p 151.
19 Simple Questions, p 572.
20 Simple Questions, p 67
21 Discussion on Blood Diseases, p 29.
22 Simple Questions, p 102.
23 Simple Questions, p 569.
24 Spiritual Axis, p 85.
25 Simple Questions, p 68.

The Functions of the Lungs

8 肺

The Lungs govern Qi and respiration and in particular are in charge of inhaling air. For this reason, and also because they influence the skin, they are the intermediary organ between the organism and the environment.

They control the blood vessels in that the Qi of the Lungs assists the Heart in controlling blood circulation. They are also said to control the "Water passages". This means that they play a vital role in the movement of Body Fluids.

"The Simple Questions" in chapter 8 says that *"The Lungs are like a Minister from whom policies are issued"*.[1] This statement refers to the part that the Lung plays in aiding the Heart (which is the Monarch) to circulate the Blood.

The functions of the Lungs are:

They govern Qi and respiration
They control channels and blood vessels
They control dispersing and descending
They regulate Water passages
They control skin and hair
They open into the nose
They house the Corporeal Soul.

1 GOVERN QI AND RESPIRATION

This is the most important Lung function since, from the air, the Lungs extract "clean Qi" for the body which then combines with Food-Qi coming from the Spleen.

Let us look at the two aspects of this vital work:

a) When we say that the Lungs govern respiration we mean that they inhale "pure Qi" (air) and exhale "dirty Qi". The constant exchange and renewal of Qi performed by the Lungs ensures the proper functioning of all the body's physiological processes which take Qi as their basis. The "Simple Questions" in chapter 5 says: *"Heavenly Qi goes to the Lung"*.[2] "Heavenly Qi" here indicates air.

b) The second way in which Lungs govern Qi is in the actual process of formation of Qi. As we saw in the chapter on Qi (see p. 42), Food-Qi is extracted from food by the Spleen. This is directed to the Lungs where it combines with the inhaled air to form what is called Gathering Qi (*Zong Qi*). Because this process takes place in the chest, the chest is also called "Sea of Qi" or "Upper Sea of Qi" (as opposed to the Lower Sea of Qi below the navel). The Gathering Qi is sometimes also called "Big Qi of the chest".

After its formation, the Lung spreads Qi all over the body to nourish all tissues and promote all physiological processes.

The "Spiritual Axis" in chapter 56 says: *"Big Qi gathers together without moving to accumulate in the chest; it is called the Sea of Qi which comes out of the Lungs, goes to the throat and facilitates inhalation and exhalation"*. Gathering Qi (or Big Qi) resides in the chest and aids the Lung and Heart functions, promoting good circulation to the limbs and controlling the strength of voice. Weak Lung-Qi can therefore cause tiredness, weak voice and breathlessness.

Because of their role in extracting Qi from air, the Lungs are the most external of the Yin organs; they are the connection between the body and the outside world. For this reason, the Lungs are easily attacked by exterior pathogenic factors and are sometimes referred to as the "tender" organ, i.e. delicate and vulnerable to invasion by climatic factors.

2 CONTROL CHANNELS AND BLOOD VESSELS

As we have seen, the Lungs govern Qi and Qi is essential to aid the Heart to circulate Blood. For this reason, although the Heart controls the blood vessels, the Lungs also play an important part in maintaining the health of blood vessels. In this respect, their scope is somewhat wider than that of the Heart since the Lungs not only control circulation in the blood vessels themselves, but also in all channels. As we have seen in the chapter on Qi, Nutritive Qi is closely related to Blood and the two flow together both in blood vessels and channels. Since the Lungs govern Qi, they control the circulation of Qi in both blood vessels and channels.

If Lung-Qi is strong, the circulation of Qi and Blood will be good and the limbs will be warm. If Lung Qi is weak, Qi will not be able to push the Blood, and the limbs, particularly the hands, will be cold.

3 CONTROL DISPERSING AND DESCENDING

These two functions are extremely important and essential to grasp in order to understand the Lung pathology.

DISPERSING FUNCTION

The Lungs have the function of dispersing or spreading Defensive Qi and body fluids all over the body to the space between skin and muscles. This is one way in which the Lungs are physiologically related to the skin. This function ensures that Defensive Qi is equally distributed all over the body under the skin performing its function of warming the skin and muscles and protecting the body from exterior pathogenic factors. If Lung-Qi is weak and its dispersing function is impaired, Defensive Qi will not reach the skin and the body will be easily invaded by exterior pathogenic factors. One can have a good idea of what the dispersing function really is by observing what happens when this function is impaired. When a person contracts a cold, most of the symptoms and signs are a manifestation of the impairment of the Lung dispersing function. The exterior Wind-Cold obstructs the skin, prevents the spreading of Defensive Qi and therefore interferes with the Lung dispersing function. Qi cannot be dispersed and everything feels "blocked". That is precisely how one may feel during a heavy cold, with a headache, stuffed nose, sneezing, etc.

The "Spiritual Axis" in chapter 30 says: *"The Qi of the Upper Burner is in communication with the outside and spreads out, it disseminates the essences of food, it warms the skin, it fills the body and it moistens the hair like irrigation by fog and dew"*.[3]

Besides Qi, the Lungs also spread Body Fluids to the skin in the form of a fine "mist". This is one reason why the Upper Burner is compared to "Mist". The fine mist of Body Fluids moistens the skin and regulates the opening and closing of pores and sweating. When this function is normal, the pores open and close normally, and there is a normal, physiological, amount of sweating. When this function is impaired, and the condition is one of Excess, the pores become blocked and there is no sweating (this happens in invasion of Wind-Cold with the prevalence of Cold). If the condition is one of Deficiency, the pores are over-relaxed and remain open so that there is spontaneous sweating (this happens in invasion of exterior Wind-Cold with prevalence of Wind, or in interior conditions of Yang deficiency). If the Lung function of dispersing body fluids is impaired, fluids may accumulate under the skin causing oedema (usually of the face).

DESCENDING FUNCTION

Because the Lungs are the uppermost organ in the body, Chinese medical texts often referred to them as the "lid", or "imperial carriage roof".[4] Because they are the uppermost organ in the body, their Qi must descend. This is what is meant by descending function. As we have seen, Lung-Qi must descend to communicate with the Kidneys and these respond by "holding" Qi. The descending function applies not only to Qi but also to body fluids, because the Lungs also direct fluids down to the Kidneys and Bladder. If this descending movement of Qi is impaired, Lung-Qi does not flow down and Qi will accumulate in the chest causing cough, breathlessness and oppression of the chest. In some cases, it may affect the function of the Large Intestine. If the Large Intestine does not receive Qi from the Lungs, it will not have the power necessary for defecation (this happens particularly to old people). In certain cases, the impairment of the Lung descending function may also cause retention of urine (again, particularly in old people).

The role of the Lung dispersing and descending functions can be summarized as follows:

a) They ensure the "entering and exiting" of Qi (see p. 61), ensure the free movement of Qi and regulate breathing and the exchange of Qi between the body and the environment.

b) They ensure that all organs receive the necessary nourishment of Qi, Blood and Body Fluids and prevent the fluids from accumulating and stagnating.

c) They prevent the scattering and exhaustion of Lung-Qi.

4 REGULATE WATER PASSAGES

After receiving the refined fluids from the Spleen, the Lungs reduce them to a fine mist and "spray" them throughout the area under the skin. This process is part of the dispersing function of the Lungs. In health, the fluids are evenly spread all over the body and the opening and closing of the pores is normal. If this function is impaired, the fluids may accumulate and give rise to oedema.

The Lungs also direct fluids down to the Kidneys and Bladder. The Kidneys receive the fluids and vaporize part of these before sending them back up to the Lungs to keep them moist. The Lung's job of directing fluids downwards has also an influence on the Bladder function. If this Lung function is normal, urination will be normal, but if it is impaired, there may be urinary retention, especially in old people. For this reason, the Lungs are sometimes called the "Upper Source of Water". The "Simple Questions" in chapter 21 says: *"Fluids enter the Stomach, the refined part is transmitted upward to the Spleen. Spleen-Qi, in turn, spreads it upwards to the Lungs who, regulating the Water passages, send it down to the Bladder"*.[5]

Through its dispersing and descending functions, the Lungs are therefore responsible for the excretion of Body Fluids through sweat or urine.

5 CONTROL SKIN AND HAIR

This function is closely related to the previous two functions. The Lungs receive fluids from the Spleen and spread them to the skin all over the body. This gives the skin and hair nourishment and moisture. If the Lung function of dispersing fluids is normal, the skin will have lustre, the hair will be glossy, the opening and closing of the pores and sweating will be normal. If this function is impaired, the skin and hair will be deprived of nourishment and moisture, and the skin may be rough and dry, and the hair have a withered and dry quality.

The Lungs influence Defensive Qi which flows under the skin. If Lung Qi is strong, Defensive Qi will be strong and the person will have a good resistance to attack by exterior pathogenic factors. If Lung Qi is weak, the Defensive Qi will also be weak and because the pores will be open, there may be spontaneous sweating. The person will also be prone to attack by exterior pathogenic factors. When this kind of sweating occurs, a certain amount of Defensive Qi is lost with the sweat. For this reason, the "Simple Questions" in chapter 3 calls the pores *"doors of Qi"*[6] Conversely, if an exterior pathogenic factor does invade the exterior portions of the body, i.e. skin and muscles (which can happen even if the Defensive Qi is relatively good), it will obstruct the skin and therefore the circulation of Defensive Qi, which, in turn, will impair the Lung dispersing function causing sneezing, cough, etc.

The "Simple Questions" in chapter 10 says: *"The Lungs control the skin and manifest on the hair"*.[7] In chapter 9 it says: *"The Lungs are the root of Qi, the residence of the Corporeal Soul (Po), they manifest in the hair, they fill up the skin, they represent Yin within the Yang and pertain to Autumn"*.[8]

6 OPEN INTO THE NOSE

The nose is the opening of the Lungs, and through it respiration occurs. If Lung-Qi is strong, the nose will be open, respiration will be easy and the sense of smell will be normal. If Lung-Qi is weak, or if the Lungs are invaded by an exterior pathogenic factor, the nose will be blocked, there may be loss of the sense of smell and sneezing. If the Lungs have Heat, there may be bleeding from the nose, loss of the sense of smell and the alae nasi will flap rapidly (as in pneumonia). The "Spiritual Axis" in chapter 17 says: *"The Lungs open into the nose, if the Lung is harmonious, the nose can smell"*.[9]

Finally, it must be remembered that there are also other organs which affect the sense of smell apart from the Lungs, notably the Spleen.

7 HOUSE THE CORPOREAL SOUL

The Lungs are said to be the residence of the Corporeal Soul (*Po*), which forms the Yin or physical counterpart of the Ethereal Soul (*Hun*). Similarly to *Hun* the Chinese character for *Po* also contains the radical *Gui*, which means "spirit" or "demon".

The Corporeal Soul is the most physical and material part of a human being's soul. It could be said to be the somatic manifestation of the soul. The "Classic of Categories" (1624) by Zhang Jie Bing says: *"The Corporeal Soul moves and does, . . . through it pain and itching can be felt"*.[10]

The Corporeal Soul is closely related to Essence and it could be said to be a manifestation of the Essence in the sphere of sensations and feelings. Essence is the foundation for a healthy body and the Corporeal Soul makes for sharp and clear sensations and movements.

Being related to the Lungs, the Corporeal Soul is also closely linked to breathing. The ancient Greeks called the soul αγεμοϭ which means "wind or vital breath" and the spirit πγευμα which also means "breath". The Corporeal Soul, residing in the Lungs, is a direct manifestation of the breath of life.

On an emotional level, the Corporeal Soul is directly affected by emotions of sadness or grief which constrain its feelings and obstruct its movement. Since the Corporeal Soul resides in the Lungs, such emotions have a powerful and direct effect on breathing which could be seen as the pulsating of the Corporeal Soul. Sadness and grief constrict the Corporeal Soul, dissolve Lung-Qi and suspend our breathing. The shallow and short breathing of a person who is sad and depressed is an example of this. Similarly, the rapid and shallow breathing taking place at the very top of the chest only, almost in the neck, is an expression of the constraint of the Corporeal Soul and Lung-Qi. For this reason, treatment of the Lungs is often very important in emotional problems deriving from depression, sadness, grief, anxiety or bereavement. Lieque LU-7 has a powerful releasing effect on constrained emotions, while Pohu BL-42 tonifies Lung-Qi and firms the Corporeal Soul (see chapter on the Function of the Points). Thus, the implication of the Corporeal Soul in clinical practice is greater than that of the Ethereal Soul.

DREAMS

The "Simple Questions" says in chapter 17: *"When the Lungs are in excess, one dreams of weeping"*.[11] In chapter 80 it says: that *"If the Lungs are deficient, one will dream of white objects or about bloody killings. If the dream takes place in the Autumn, one will dream of battles and war"*.[12]

The "Spiritual Axis" in chapter 43 says: *"When the Lungs are in excess, one will have dreams of worry and fear, or crying and flying ... if the Lungs are deficient one will dream of flying and seeing strange objects made of gold or iron"*.[13]

"THE LUNGS GOVERN THE 100 VESSELS"

The Lungs govern Qi, which is closely related to Blood and flows in the blood vessels together with Blood. Thus the Lungs have an influence on all the blood vessels in the way already mentioned above. Since Lung-Qi affects the blood vessels, the pulse at the radial artery, situated on the Lung channel, reflects the state of all the organs.

"THE LUNGS LOATHE COLD"

The Lungs influence the skin and the Defensive Qi and are easily invaded by exterior pathogenic factors, particularly Cold.

"THE LUNGS GOVERN THE VOICE"

The strength, tone and clarity of voice are all dependent on the Lungs. When the Lungs are healthy they are compared to a bell, giving off a clear ringing sound, which is the voice. If the Lungs are weak, the voice may be low, while if the Lungs are obstructed by Phlegm, the voice tone may be muffled.

NOTES

1 Simple Questions, p 58.
2 Ibid., p 45.
3 Spiritual Axis, p 71.
4 Zhao Xian Ke 1687 Medicine Treasure (*Yi Guan* 医贯) cited in Selected Historical Theories in Chinese Medicine, p 1.
5 Simple Questions, p 139.
6 Simple Questions, p 19.
7 Simple Questions, p 70.
8 Simple Questions, p 67.
9 Spiritual Axis, p 50.
10 Cited in Concise Dictionary of Chinese Medicine, p 953.
11 Simple Questions, p. 102.
12 Simple Questions, p 569.
13 Spiritual Axis, p 85.

9 The Functions of the Spleen 脾

The Spleen's main function is to assist the Stomach digestion by transporting and transforming food essences, absorbing the nourishment from food and separating the usable from the unusable part of food. The Spleen is the central organ in the production of Qi: from the food and drink ingested, it extracts Food-Qi (*Gu Qi*), which is the basis for the formation of Qi and Blood. In fact, Food-Qi produced by the Spleen combines with air in the Lungs to form the Gathering Qi (see p. 43) which itself is the basis for the formation of True Qi (*Zhen Qi*). Food-Qi of the Spleen is also the basis for the formation of Blood which takes place in the Heart. Because the Food-Qi extracted by the Spleen is the material basis for the production of Qi and Blood, the Spleen (together with the Stomach) is often called the Root of Post-Heaven Qi.

Since the Spleen is the central organ in the digestive process, it is often referred to as the *"Granary official from whom the five tastes are derived"*.[1]

The functions of the Spleen are:

It governs transformation and transportation
It controls the Blood
It controls the muscles and the four limbs
It opens into the mouth and manifests in the lips
It controls the "raising Qi"
It houses Thought.

1 GOVERNS TRANSFORMATION AND TRANSPORTATION

The Spleen transforms the ingested food and drink to extract Qi from it: this is called Food-Qi and is the basis for the production of Qi and Blood. Once Food-Qi is formed, the Spleen transports this and some other refined parts of food, called "food essences", to the various organs and parts of the body.

The "Simple Questions" in chapter 21 says: *"Food enters the Stomach, the refined part goes to the Liver, the excess goes to the sinews. Food enters the Stomach, the unrefined part goes to the Heart, the excess goes to the blood vessels ... fluids enter the Stomach ... the upper part go to the Spleen, the Spleen transports the refined essence upwards to the Lungs"*.[2] This passage describes the Spleen's role of separating the usable from unusable part of food and directing Food-Qi upwards to the Lungs to combine with air to form Gathering Qi and to the Heart to form Blood. The various transformations and movements described, "the refined part to the Liver", "the unrefined to the Heart" "the refined upwards to the Lungs", are all under the control of the Spleen. For this reason the Spleen function of transforming and transporting is crucial to the process of digestion and production of Qi and Blood. If this function is normal, the digestion will be good, with good appetite, normal absorption and regular bowel movements. If this function is impaired, there may be poor appetite, bad digestion, abdominal distension and loose stools.

Apart from governing the movement of the various food essences the Spleen also controls the transformation, separation and movement of fluids. The Spleen separates an usable from unusable part from the fluids ingested; the "clear" part goes upwards to the Lungs to be distributed to the skin and the "dirty" part goes downward to the Intestines where it is further separated. If this Spleen function is normal, the transformation and movement of fluids will be normal. If this function is impaired, the fluids will not be transformed or transported properly and may accumulate to form Dampness or Phlegm or cause oedema. The implication here is that the Spleen must always be treated when there is Dampness, Phlegm or oedema. Moreover, the Spleen is also easily affected by external Dampness which may impair its function of transformation and transportation.

In connection with the transformation of food and digestion, it is said that the Spleen "likes dryness": this means that the Spleen's activity of transformation and transportation can be easily impaired by the excessive consumption of cold liquids or icy drinks (so common in many Western countries). In contrast, the Stomach "likes wetness", i.e. foods which are moist and not drying.

2 CONTROLS BLOOD

The Spleen is said to keep the Blood in the vessels. The "Classic of Difficulties" in chapter 42 says that the *"the Spleen is in charge of holding the Blood together"*.[3] While it is Qi in general that holds the blood in the vessels, it is Spleen-Qi in particular that performs this function.

If Spleen-Qi is healthy, Blood will circulate normally and stay in the vessels. If Spleen-Qi is deficient, Blood may spill out of the vessels resulting in haemorrhages.

Besides controlling the Blood and preventing haemorrhages, the Spleen also plays an important role in making Blood. In fact, the Spleen extracts Food-Qi from food and this forms Blood in the Heart with the assistance of the Original Qi from the Kidneys. The Spleen is therefore the central, essential organ for the production of both Qi and Blood. This is another reason why it is called the "Root of Post-Heaven Qi". If we wish to tonify the Blood, therefore, we must always tonify the Spleen.

Li Dong Yuan (1180–1251), author of the famous "Discussion on Stomach and Spleen", says: *"The Original Qi can only be strong if the Spleen and Stomach are not weakened and can nourish it. If the Stomach is weak and food is not transformed, the Stomach and Spleen are weakened, they cannot nourish the Original Qi which becomes empty and disease results."*[4]

3 CONTROLS THE MUSCLES AND THE FOUR LIMBS

The Spleen extracts Food-Qi from food so as to nourish all tissues in the body. This refined Qi is transported throughout the body by the Spleen. If the Spleen is strong, refined Qi is directed to the muscles, particularly those of the limbs. If Spleen-Qi is weak, the refined Qi cannot be transported to the muscles and the person will feel weary, the muscles will be weak and, in severe cases, may atrophy. The state of the Spleen is one of the most important factors determining the amount of physical energy a person has. Tiredness is a common complaint and in these cases the Spleen must always be tonified.

The "Simple Questions" in chapter 44 says: *"The Spleen governs the muscles . . . if the Spleen has Heat, there will be thirst, the muscles will be weak and atrophied"*.[5] In chapter 29 it says: *"The four limbs depend on the Stomach for Qi, but Stomach-*

Qi can only reach the channels through the transmission of the Spleen. If the Spleen is diseased it cannot transport the fluids of the Stomach, with the result that the four limbs cannot receive the Qi of Food".[6]

4 OPENS INTO THE MOUTH AND MANIFESTS IN THE LIPS

The action of chewing prepares food for the Spleen to transform and transport its food essences. For this reason the mouth has a functional relationship with the Spleen. When Spleen-Qi is normal, the sense of taste is good and the lips are moist and rosy. If Spleen-Qi is abnormal, there may be impairment of the sense of taste or the presence of an abnormal taste ("flat" or "sticky"), lack of appetite and the lips may be pale and dry. In particular, if the Spleen has Heat, the lips will tend to be dry and the patient may complain of a sweet taste; if Spleen-Qi is deficient, the lips may be pale. The "Simple Questions" says in chapter 10 that the *"Spleen controls the muscles and manifests in the lips"*.[7] The "Spiritual Axis" in chapter 17 says: *"Spleen-Qi connects with the mouth, if the Spleen is healthy, the mouth can taste the five grains"*.[8]

5 CONTROLS THE RAISING OF QI

The Spleen produces a "lifting" effect along the midline of the body. It is this force that makes sure that the internal organs are in their proper place.

If Spleen-Qi is deficient and its "raising Qi" function weak, there may be prolapse of various organs such as uterus, stomach, kidney, bladder or anus.

The Spleen action of raising of Qi is another expression of its function of extracting the refined Food-Qi and sending it upwards to the Lungs and Heart. Ye Tian Shi (1667–1746), the celebrated specialist in Warm Diseases, said: *"Spleen-Qi goes up, Stomach-Qi goes down"*.[9]

Li Dong Yuan said: *"Food enters the Stomach and the Spleen directs the clear essence of food up to the Lungs ... to nourish the whole body"*.[10] The upward movement of Spleen-Qi is coordinated with the downward movement of Stomach-Qi. The two together are essential for a proper movement of Qi in the body during digestion, so that the clear Qi is directed upwards by the Spleen and the dirty Qi downwards by the Stomach. Qi connects upwards with the Lungs and Heart and downwards with the Liver and Kidneys. Only if these ascending and descending movements of Qi are coordinated, can the clear Yang ascend to the upper (sense) orifices and the dirty Yin descend to the two lower orifices. If the descending and ascending movements are impaired, the clear Yang does not ascend, refined Qi extracted from food cannot be stored and dirty Qi cannot be excreted.

6 HOUSES THOUGHT

The Spleen is said to be the "residence" of Thought. This means that the Spleen influences our capacity for thinking, studying, concentrating, focusing and memorizing.

If Spleen-Qi is flourishing, we will think clearly and be able to concentrate and memorize easily. If Spleen-Qi is weak, thinking will be dull, concentration will be slack and memory will be poor. Conversely, excessive studying, mental work and concentration for sustained periods can weaken the Spleen.

The Spleen, Heart and Kidneys, all have an influence on thinking and memory in different ways. The Spleen influences our capacity for thinking in the sense of studying, concentrating and memorizing work or school-work subjects. The Heart houses the Mind and influences thinking in the sense of being able to think clearly when faced with life problems and it affects long-term memory of past events. The Kidneys nourish the brain and influence short-term memory in everyday life. For example, in old age there is a decline of Kidney-Essence which fails to nourish the brain. For this reason, many old people often forget recent events (which is due to a Kidney weakness), and yet may be able to remember long-past events (which is dependent on the Heart). Similarly, some people may have an extraordinary memory in their work or study field (which is dependent on the Spleen) and yet be very forgetful in every-day life (which is dependent on the Kidneys).

DREAMS

The "Simple Questions" in chapter 80 says: *"If the Spleen is deficient, one dreams of being hungry; if the dream takes place in late summer, one dreams of building a house"*.[11]

The "Spiritual Axis" in chapter 43 says: *"If the Spleen is in excess one dreams of singing and being very heavy. . .if the Spleen is deficient one dreams of abysses in mountains and of marshes"*.[12]

"THE SPLEEN GOVERNS THE FOUR LIMBS"

The Spleen distributes food essences to all parts of the body and in particular to the limbs. For this reason, when the Spleen is deficient, the food essences cannot reach the limbs which will feel cold and weak.

"THE SPLEEN TRANSFORMS FLUIDS FOR THE STOMACH"

The Stomach is the origin of fluids in the body and the Spleen transforms and transports them. The Stomach fluids are part of Stomach-Yin, while the activity of fluid transformation and transportation is part of Spleen-Yang.

"THE SPLEEN IS THE ROOT OF POST-HEAVEN QI"

The Spleen is the origin of Qi and Blood in the body. For this reason, it is called the Root of Post-Heaven Qi, i.e. the Qi and Blood produced after birth, as opposed to the Pre-Heaven Qi which nourishes a fetus before birth.

"THE SPLEEN IS THE ORIGIN OF BIRTH AND DEVELOPMENT"

This refers to the central role played by the Spleen in nourishing the body and promoting development.

"THE SPLEEN RAISES THE CLEAR (YANG) UPWARDS"

Spleen-Qi flows upwards to raise the clear Yang energies towards the head. If Dampness obstructs the Spleen, the clear Yang cannot rise to the head resulting in a feeling of heaviness and muzziness of the head.

"THE SPLEEN LOATHES DAMPNESS"

Dampness easily obstructs the Spleen causing a dysfunction of its activity of transformation and transportation. This can cause abdominal distension, urinary problems or vaginal discharges.

NOTE

Chinese medical books never mention the pancreas and it is often said that, functionally, the pancreas is included with the "Spleen". It would seem that many of the Spleen functions affecting digestion could be correlated with the pancreas secretion of digestive enzymes.

One of the few mentions of the pancreas is in chapter 42 of the "Classic of Difficulties" where it says: *"The spleen weighs 2 pounds and 3 ounces, it is 3 inches wide, 5 inches long and has ½ pound of fatty tissues surrounding it"*.[13] It would appear that the *"½ pound of fatty tissue surrounding it"* is the pancreas.

NOTES

1 Simple Questions, p 58.
2 Simple Questions, p 139.
3 A Revised Explanation of the Classic of Difficulties, p 99.
4 Syndromes and Treatment of the Internal Organs, p 168.
5 Simple Questions, p 246.
6 Simple Questions, p 180.
7 Simple Questions, p.70.
8 Spiritual Axis, p 50.
9 Syndromes and Treatment of the Internal Organs, p 170.
10 Syndromes and Treatment of the Internal Organs, p 170.
11 Simple Questions, p 569.
12 Spiritual Axis, p 85.
13 Classic of Difficulties, p 99.

10 The Functions of the Kidneys 肾

The Kidneys are often referred to as the "Root of Life" or the "Root of the Pre-Heaven Qi". This is because they store the Essence which is partly derived from the parents and established at conception.

Like every other Yin organ, the Kidneys have a Yin and a Yang aspect. However, these two aspects acquire a different meaning for the Kidneys because they are the foundation of the Yin and Yang for all the other organs. For this reason, Kidney-Yin and Kidney-Yang are also called "Primary Yin" and "Primary Yang" respectively. We could look upon Kidney-Yin as the foundation of all the Yin energies of the body, in particular that of the Liver, Heart and Lungs, and Kidney-Yang as the foundation of all the Yang energies of the body, in particular that of the Spleen, Lungs and Heart.

Kidney-Yin is the fundamental substance for birth, growth and reproduction while Kidney-Yang is the motive force of all physiological processes. Kidney-Yin is the material foundation for Kidney-Yang, and Kidney-Yang is the exterior manifestation of Kidney-Yin. In health, these two poles form a unified whole. In disease, however, a separation of Kidney Yin and Yang occurs.

Kidney-Yin and Kidney-Yang have the same root and they rely on each other for their existence. Kidney-Yin provides the material substratum for Kidney-Yang, and Kidney-Yang provides the Heat necessary to all the Kidney functions. Because they are fundamentally one, deficiency of one necessarily implies deficiency of the other. Kidney-Yin and Kidney-Yang could be likened to an oil lamp, the oil representing Kidney-Yin and the flame representing Kidney-Yang. If the oil decreases, the flame will also decrease and vice versa. It follows that, in treating Kidney disharmonies, one usually needs to tonify both Kidney-Yin and Kidney-Yang to prevent the exhaustion of one of them. In fact, if the flame (Kidney-Yang) is increased without increasing the oil, this will only lead to a decrease of the oil (Kidney-Yin). On the other hand, if the oil is increased too much without increasing the flame, the excess oil may only smother the flame. A good example of this principle can be seen in the composition of two classic herbal prescriptions to tonify Kidney-Yin and Kidney-Yang. The classic prescription to tonify Kidney-Yin is the "Six-Taste Rehmannia Decoction", while the classic prescription to tonify Kidney-Yang, the "Golden Chest Kidney-Qi Decoction", is nothing but the "Six-Taste Rehmannia Decoction" with the addition of two very hot herbs, i.e. aconite and cinnamon. This shows very clearly that in order to tonify Kidney-Yang, one must also, to a certain extent, tonify Kidney-Yin.

The Kidneys are different from other Yin organs because they are the foundation for all the Yin and Yang energies of the body, and also because they are the origin of Water and Fire in the body. Although according to the 5 Elements the Kidneys belong to Water, they are also the source of Fire in the body which is called the "Fire of the Gate of Vitality" (see below).

The functions of the Kidneys are:

They store Essence and govern birth, growth, reproduction and development

They produce Marrow, fill up the brain and control bones

They govern Water

They control the reception of Qi

They open into the ears

They manifest in the hair

They control the two lower orifices

They house Will Power.

1 STORE ESSENCE AND GOVERN BIRTH, GROWTH, REPRODUCTION AND DEVELOPMENT

As we discussed in chapter 3, the Essence of the Kidneys is a precious substance which is inherited from the parents and also partly replenished by the Qi extracted from food. The Kidneys function of storing Essence has two aspects:

a) They store Pre-Heaven Essence, i.e. the inherited Essence which before birth nourishes the fetus and after birth controls growth, sexual maturation, fertility and development. This Essence determines our basic constitution, strength and vitality. It is also the basis of sexual life, and the material foundation for the manufacture of sperm in men and ova in women. Insufficient Essence may be a cause of infertility, impotence, underdevelopment in children (physical or mental), retarded growth and premature senility.

b) They store Post-Heaven Essence, i.e. the refined essence extracted from food through the transforming power of the internal organs.

The Essence of the Kidneys also controls the various stages of change in life, i.e. birth, puberty, menopause and death. Ageing itself is due to a physiological decline of Essence during life. The first chapter of the "Simple Questions" describes the various stages of life in cycles of 7 years for women and 8 years for men.

Kidney-Essence provides the material basis for both Kidney-Yin and Kidney-Yang, even though in disease a deficiency of Kidney-Essence is part of the pattern of Kidney-Yin deficiency. To put it differently, Kidney-Essence is the organic basis for the transformation of Kidney-Yin into Kidney-Qi by the warming and evaporating action of Kidney-Yang (see p. 40).

The state of the Essence determines the state of the Kidneys. If Essence is flourishing and abundant, the Kidneys are strong and there will be great vitality, sexual power and fertility. If Essence is weak, the Kidneys are weak and there will be lack of vitality, infertility or sexual weakness.

2 PRODUCE MARROW, FILL UP THE BRAIN, CONTROL BONES

This function of the Kidney is also derived from the Essence. Essence is the organic foundation for the production of Marrow. "Marrow" does not correspond to bone marrow of Western Medicine. "Marrow" in Chinese Medicine is a substance which is the common matrix of bones, bone marrow, brain and spinal cord. Thus the Kidney-Essence produces Marrow which generates the spinal cord and "fills up" the brain. For this reason, in Chinese Medicine the brain has a physiological relationship with the Kidneys. If Kidney-Essence is strong, it will nourish the brain and memory and concentration, thinking and sight will all be keen. Chinese Medicine holds that "the Kidneys are the origin of skill and intelligence". If the brain is not adequately nourished by the Essence, there may be poor memory and concentration, dizziness, dull thinking and poor sight. Brain and spinal cord are also referred to as "Sea of Marrow".

The Marrow is also the basis for the formation of bone marrow which nourishes the bones. Thus the Kidneys also govern the bone marrow and bones. If the Kidney-Essence is strong, the bones will be strong, and the teeth will be firm.

If the Kidney-Essence is weak, the bones will be brittle and the teeth loose. A weak Kidney-Essence in children will cause poor bone development, pigeon-chest, etc. The "Simple Questions" in chapter 44 says: *"Kidneys control the bone marrow ... if the Kidneys have Heat, the spine will not be straight, the bones will wither, the marrow will decrease"*.[1]

The Kidney-Essence has also an important influence on vitality and mental vigour. The "Simple Questions" says in chapter 8: *"The Kidneys are the strong official from whom ingenuity is derived"*.[2] This means that the Kidneys determine both the physical and mental strength of an individual. They also determine our will power as will be explained shortly.

3 GOVERN WATER

As we have seen, according to the 5 Elements, the Kidneys belong to Water and they govern the transformation and transportation of Body Fluids in many different ways:

a) The Kidneys are like a gate that opens and closes in order to control the flow of Body Fluids in the Lower Burner. Under normal physiological conditions there will be a correct balance between Kidney-Yin and Kidney-Yang resulting in the correct regulation of the opening and closing of the "gate". Urination will therefore be normal in quantity and colour. In disease, there is an imbalance between Kidney-Yin and Kidney-Yang resulting in a malfunctioning of the "gate" in opening and closing: it will either be too open (deficiency of Kidney-Yang) causing profuse and pale urination, or too closed (deficiency of Kidney-Yin) causing scanty and dark urination.

b) The Kidneys belong to the Lower Burner, which is sometimes compared to a "drainage ditch". The organs of the Lower Burner are particularly concerned with the excretion of impure Body Fluids. The Kidneys have the function of providing Qi for the Bladder to store and transform urine.

c) The Small Intestine and Large Intestine, also in the Lower Burner, play a part in separating clean from dirty fluids. This intestinal function of separating fluids is also under the control of the Kidneys, in particular Kidney-Yang.

d) The Kidneys receive fluids from the Lungs, some of which are excreted and some of which are vaporized in which form they return to the Lungs to keep them moist.

e) The Spleen plays a very important role in the transformation and transportation of Body Fluids. Kidney-Yang provides the Spleen with the heat it needs to carry out its function of transforming and transporting fluids.

4 CONTROL THE RECEPTION OF QI

To make use of the clear Qi of the air, the Lungs and Kidneys work together. The Lungs have a descending action on Qi, directing it down to the Kidneys. The Kidneys respond by "holding" this Qi down. If the Kidneys cannot hold Qi down it "rebels" upward creating congestion in the chest resulting in breathlessness and asthma. This is a very frequent cause of chronic asthma.

5 OPEN INTO THE EARS

The ears rely on the nourishment of the Essence for their proper functioning, and are therefore physiologically related to the Kidneys. The "Spiritual Axis" in chapter 17 says: *"The Kidneys open into the ears, if the Kidneys are healthy the ears can hear the five sounds"*.[3]

If the Kidneys are weak, hearing may be impaired and there may be tinnitus.

6 MANIFEST ON THE HAIR

The hair also relies on the nourishment of the Kidney-Essence to grow. If the Kidney-Essence is abundant, the hair will grow well and will be healthy and glossy. If the Kidney-Essence is weak or is declining, the hair will become thin, brittle, dull-looking and may fall out altogether. The first chapter of the "Simple Questions" says: *"If the Kidneys are strong, the teeth will be firm and the hair grow well ... if the Kidneys are declining in energy, the hair will fall out and the teeth become loose."*[4]

The quality and colour of the hair are also related to the state of the Kidney-Essence. If the Kidney-Essence is strong, the hair will be thick and of a good colour.

If the Kidney-Essence is weak, the hair will be thin and become grey. The "Simple Questions" in chapter 10 says: *"The Kidneys control the bones and manifest in the hair"*.[5]

7 CONTROL THE TWO LOWER ORIFICES

The two lower orifices are the front and the rear lower orifices. The front orifice includes urethra and spermatic duct in men, the rear orifice is the anus. These orifices are functionally related to the Kidneys. The urethra is obviously related to the Kidneys since the Bladder derives the Qi necessary for the transformation of urine from the Kidneys. If the Kidney energy is weak, urine may leak out causing incontinence or enuresis. The spermatic duct is related to the Kidney as sperm is the outer manifestation of the Kidney-Essence. A deficiency of Kidney-Qi or Kidney-Essence may cause spermatorrhoea or nocturnal emissions. Finally, the anus, although anatomically related to the Large Intestine, is also functionally related to the Kidneys. If Kidney-Qi is weak, there may be diarrhoea or prolapse of the anus.

In conclusion, Kidney-Qi is essential for the normal functioning of all the lower orifices and a deficiency of Kidney-Qi will induce a "leaking" of each orifice, i.e. urinary incontinence, spermatorrhoea and diarrhoea.

8 HOUSE WILL POWER

It is said in Chinese Medicine that the Kidneys are the "residence" of Will Power (Zhi). The Simple Questions" says in chapter 23: "*... The Kidneys house Will Power ...*".[6] This means that the Kidneys determine our will power. If the Kidneys are strong, the Will Power will be strong, the Mind will be focused on goals that it sets itself and it will pursue them in a single-minded way. Conversely, if the Kidneys are weak, Will Power will be lacking and the Mind will be easily discouraged and swayed from its aims.

Lack of will power and motivation are often important aspects of mental depression and tonification of the Kidneys will often give very good results.

THE GATE OF VITALITY ("MING MEN")

A discussion of the Kidney functions would not be complete without reference to the Gate of Vitality (*Ming Men*). The first discussion of the Gate of Vitality can be found in the "Classic of Difficulties", especially in chapters 36 and 39. Chapter 36 says: *"The Kidneys are not really two, as the left Kidney is a Kidney proper and the right Kidney is the Gate of Vitality. The Gate of Vitality is the residence of the Mind and is related to the Original Qi: in men it stores Essence, in women it is connected to the uterus. That is why there is only one Kidney"*.[7]

Chapter 39 says: *"Why does the classic say that there are 5 Yang and 6 Yin organs? The reason is that the Yin organs count as 6 since there are two Kidneys. The left Kidney is the Kidney proper, the right Kidney is the Gate of Vitality. ... the reason that there are 6 Yang organs is that each of the 5 Yin organs has a corresponding Yang organ, plus an extra one being the Triple Burner"*.[8]

These two passages clearly show that according to the "Classic of Difficulties" the Gate of Vitality corresponds to the right Kidney, and is therefore functionally inseparable from the Kidneys. The "Pulse Classic" written by Wang Shu He in the Han dynasty confirms this in assigning the Kidney and Gate of Vitality to the right Rear (proximal) position on the pulse. Chen Wu Ze of the Song dynasty wrote: "*The ancients considered the left Kidney as Kidney proper, related to the Bladder, and the right Kidney as the Gate of Vitality related to the Triple Burner*".[9] However, for several centuries, up to the Ming dynasty, medical writers seldom discussed the Gate of Vitality as something separate from the Kidney, and simply referred to "Kidney-Qi".

With the beginning of the Ming dynasty, the concept of Gate of Vitality was greatly developed, and ideas on it differed from the "Classic of Difficulties". During the Ming dynasty, Chinese physicians no longer considered the Gate of Vitality as part of the right Kidney, but as occupying the place between the two Kidneys. Zhang Jie Bin (1563-1640) said: *"There are two Kidneys . . . the Gate of Vitality is in between them. . . . The Gate of Vitality is the organ of Water and Fire, it is the residence of Yin and Yang, the Sea of Essence and it determines life and death"*.[10] Li Shi Zhen also said that the Gate of Vitality is in between the two Kidneys. Zhao Xian He was a doctor who discussed the Gate of Vitality in greatest depth in his book "Medicine Treasure" (*Yi Gui*) published in 1687. Most of this book deals with physiological and pathological aspects of the Gate of Vitality. Zhao Xian He also regarded the Gate of Vitality as being between the two Kidneys. He wrote that it is the motive force of all functional activities of the body, being the physiological Fire which is essential to life. This Fire is also called "True Fire" or "Minister Fire" (in the same sense that is sometimes attributed to the Pericardium). The importance of the Fire nature of the Gate of Vitality is that it provides heat for all our bodily functions and for the Kidney-Essence itself. The Kidneys are unlike any other organ in so far as they are the origin of Water and Fire of the body, the Primary Yin and Primary Yang. The Gate of Vitality is the embodiment of the Fire within the Kidneys.

In this respect the Gate of Vitality theory is at variance with the 5-Element theory according to which Fire is derived from the Heart, not from the Gate of Vitality, i.e. the Kidneys. These theories simply spring from two different perspectives and are both valid. However, in clinical practice, the theory that attributes the origin of Fire to the Gate of Vitality and hence the Kidneys is more significant and more widely used.

The main functions of the Gate of Vitality can be summarized as follows.

A) IT IS THE ROOT OF THE ORIGINAL QI

Both Gate of Vitality and Original Qi are related to the Kidneys, and are interdependent. Original Qi is a form of dynamically activated Essence which has many functions, among which that of assisting in the making of Blood. Original Qi relies on heat for its performance and this heat is provided by the Gate of Vitality. If the Fire of the Gate of Vitality is deficient, Original Qi will suffer, and will inevitably lead to a general deficiency of Qi and Blood.

B) IT IS THE SOURCE OF FIRE FOR ALL THE INTERNAL ORGANS

If the Fire of the Gate of Vitality declines, the functional activity of all organs will be impaired, leading to tiredness, mental depression, lack of vitality, negativity and a feeling of cold.

C) IT WARMS THE LOWER BURNER AND BLADDER

The Lower Burner transforms and excretes fluids, with the assistance of the Bladder. The Heat of the Gate of Vitality is essential to transform fluids in the Lower Burner. If the Gate of Vitality Fire is weak, the Lower Burner and Bladder will lack the Heat necessary to transform fluids: these will therefore accumulate giving rise to Dampness or oedema.

D) IT WARMS THE STOMACH AND SPLEEN TO AID DIGESTION

Heat is essential to the Spleen for its functions of transportation, separation and transformation. All this requires heat supplied by the Gate of Vitality. If the Fire of the Gate of Vitality is deficient the Spleen cannot transform and the Stomach cannot digest the food leading to diarrhoea, tiredness, feeling of cold and cold limbs.

E) IT HARMONIZES THE SEXUAL FUNCTION AND WARMS THE ESSENCE AND UTERUS

The Fire of the Gate of Vitality is essential for a healthy sexual function and to warm the Essence and the uterus. Sexual performance, fertility, puberty and menstruation, all depend on the Fire of the Gate of Vitality. If the Fire of the Gate of Vitality declines, the Essence in men and the uterus in women will turn cold causing impotence and infertility in men and leucorrhoea and infertility in women.

F) IT ASSISTS THE KIDNEY FUNCTION OF RECEPTION OF QI

The function of reception of Qi depends on Kidney-Yang which requires the Fire of the Gate of Vitality for its performance. For Kidney-Yang to function normally, there must be communication between the Gathering Qi of the chest and the Original Qi of the lower abdomen, which itself relies on the heat from the Gate of Vitality for its activity. If the Fire of the Gate of Vitality is deficient, the Kidney ability to receive Qi will be impaired causing breathlessness, asthma, stuffiness of the chest and cold hands.

G) IT ASSISTS THE HEART FUNCTION OF HOUSING THE MIND

The Fire of the Gate of Vitality has to ascend from the Kidney and communicate with the Heart, to provide it with the Heat necessary for its functions. Because of this, the Fire of the Gate of Vitality assists the Heart in housing the Mind. This means that the Fire of the Gate of Vitality has a strong influence on the mental state and happiness. If the Fire of the Gate of Vitality is deficient, the Heart cannot house the Mind, and the person will be depressed, unhappy and lack vitality.

DREAMS

The "Simple Questions" in chapter 80 says: *"When the Kidneys are weak, one dreams of swimming after a shipwreck; if the dream takes place in winter, one dreams of plunging in water and being scared"*.[11]

The "Spiritual Axis" in chapter 43 says: *"When the Kidneys are in excess one dreams that the spine is detached from the body ... when they are weak, one dreams of being immersed in water"*.[12]

"THE KIDNEYS CONTROL OPENING AND CLOSING"

The Kidneys function like a "gate" in relation to urination. As was mentioned before, if Kidney-Yang is deficient (i.e. the gate is open) urine will be abundant and clear. If Kidney-Yin is deficient (i.e. the gate is closed), urine will be scanty and dark.

Besides controlling urination, the Kidneys also influence the anus and defecation and if Kidney-Yang is deficient there may be diarrhoea. For this reason, the Kidneys influence the "opening and closing" of both lower Yin orifices, i.e anus and urethra.

"THE KIDNEYS CONTROL STRENGTH AND SKILL"

The Kidneys control our capacity for hard work. If the Kidneys are strong, a person can work hard and purposefully for long periods of time. If the Kidneys are weak, a person will lack the strength necessary for long periods of hard work. Conversely, a Kidney disharmony can sometimes drive a person to overwork beyond measure becoming a "workaholic".

Besides strength, the Kidneys also influence our capacity for skilled and delicate activities.

"THE KIDNEYS ARE THE ROOT OF PRE-HEAVEN QI"

Just as the Spleen is the Root of Post-Heaven Qi, being the origin of Qi and Blood produced after birth, the Kidneys are the Root of Pre-Heaven Qi because they store the Essence which is inherited from our parents.

"THE KIDNEYS LOATHE DRYNESS"

Dry weather or internal Dryness can injure

Kidney-Yin. Interior Dryness can be produced by a Stomach deficiency, by profuse and continued loss of fluids (such as occurs in sweating or diarrhoea) or by smoking. According to Chinese Medicine, tobacco dries Blood and Essence and it can injure Kidney-Yin. Although the Kidneys dislike dryness and the Lungs dislike cold, some doctors also say that the Kidneys dislike cold and the Lungs dryness. This view is also valid.

"THE KIDNEYS ARE THE GATE OF THE STOMACH"

The Stomach is the origin of fluids and the Kidneys transform and excrete fluids. If the Kidneys cannot excrete fluids properly, these will stagnate and affect the Stomach. Conversely, a lack of Stomach fluids can lead to Kidney-Yin deficiency.

NOTES

1 Simple Questions, p 247
2 Simple Questions, p 58.
3 Spiritual Axis, p 50.
4 Simple Questions, p 4.
5 Simple Questions, p 70.
6 Simple Questions, p 153
7 A Revised Explanation of the Classic of Difficulties, p 90.
8 A Revised Explanation of the Classic of Difficulties, p 95
9 1979 Patterns and treatment of Kidney diseases (*Shen Yu Shen Bing de Zheng Zhi* 肾与肾病的证治) Hebei People's Publishing House, Hebei, p 2.
10 Patterns and treatment of Kidney diseases, p 3
11 Simple Questions, p 569
12 Spiritual Axis, p 85.

11 The Functions of the Pericardium 心包

The Pericardium is closely related to the Heart. The traditional view of the Pericardium is that it functions as an external covering of the Heart, protecting it from attacks by exterior pathogenic factors. The "Spiritual Axis" in chapter 71 says: *"The Heart is the Ruler of the 5 Yin organs and 6 Yang organs, it is the residence of the Mind and it is so tough that no pathogenic factor can take hold in it. If the Heart is attacked by a pathogenic factor, the Mind suffers, which can lead to death. If a pathogenic factor does attack the Heart, it will be deviated to attack the Pericardium instead. For this reason, the Heart channel has no Stream Transporting point"*.[1]

The "Simple Questions" in chapter 8 says: *"The Pericardium is the ambassador and from it joy and happiness derive"*.[2]

The Pericardium is thus of secondary importance to the Heart and it displays many of the same functions. In herbal medicine, the Pericardium is usually only referred to in the context of infectious diseases caused by exterior Heat. Such diseases correspond to the Upper Burner stage in the model of Identification of Patterns according to the Three Burners characterized by delirium, mental confusion, aphasia and very high temperature, all symptoms of invasion of the Pericardium by extreme Heat. In terms of acupuncture, however, the Pericardium channel has as much importance as the Heart or any other channel.

The Yellow Emperor's Classic normally only mentions 11 organs: the book constantly refers to 5 Yin and 6 Yang organs, the Pericardium being a mere appendage of the Heart. In fact, the "Spiritual Axis" in chapter 1 says that the Stream and Source point of the Heart is Daling, i.e. Pericardium-7.[3]

According to the theory of the internal organs, the functions of the Pericardium are more or less identical with those of the Heart: it governs Blood, and it houses the Mind. In fact, many Pericardium channel points have a powerful influence on the mental and emotional state.

From the point of view of channels, the Pericardium channel is quite distinct from the Heart channel and has a different sphere of action, influencing the area at the centre of the thorax. The "Yellow Emperor's Classic" often refers to the Pericardium as the "centre of the thorax", hence the important action of Neiguan P-6 on the chest.

Like the Heart, the Pericardium also influences a person's relations with other people, and the points on its channel are often used to treat emotional problems caused by relationship difficulties.

Before concluding this section on the Pericardium, mention should be made of the question of the so-called "Ministerial Fire". The prevailing view in the history of Chinese Medicine has been that the so-called "Ministerial Fire" is the Fire of the Gate of Vitality (*Ming Men*). As we have seen in the chapter on the Kidneys this Fire is essential to the health functioning of the body.

Although many doctors such as Zhu Zhen Heng (1281–1358) identified "Ministerial Fire" with the Fire of the Gate of Vitality,[4] others, such as Zhang Jie Bin (1563–1640), identified the "Ministerial Fire" with such internal organs as the Kidney, Liver, Triple Burner, Gall Bladder and Pericardium.[5]

For this reason, it is incorrect to identify "Ministerial Fire" merely with the Pericardium.

NOTES

1 Spiritual Axis, p 128.
2 Simple Questions, p 58.
3 Spiritual Axis, p 3.
4 Selected Historical Theories in Chinese Medicine, p 195.
5 Selected Historical Theories in Chinese Medicine, p 195.

12 Yin Organ Interrelationships

脏与脏之间的生理

Interrelationship is the essence of Chinese Medicine since the body is regarded as an integrated whole. Because of this it is not enough to consider the Yin organs merely on an individual basis. To understand them properly we must consider how they interrelate since a person's health depends on a proper balance being maintained among the internal organs.

HEART AND LUNGS

The Heart governs Blood and the Lungs govern Qi: the relationship between Heart and Lungs is thus essentially the relationship between Qi and Blood (Fig. 38). Qi and Blood are mutually dependent on each other: Qi pushes Blood, if Qi stagnates Blood congeals. On the other hand, Blood nourishes Qi. Blood needs the power of Qi in order to circulate in the blood vessels and Qi can only circulate throughout the body by "concentrating" in the blood vessels. That is why it is said in Chinese Medicine that "Qi controls warmth" (here "warmth" means warm nourishment), and that "Blood controls immersion" ("immersion" here means the fluids which transport this nourishment).[1]

Although it is the Heart that drives the Blood through the blood vessels, it relies on the Lungs to provide the Qi for this job. On the other hand, the Lungs rely on Blood from the Heart for nourishment.

Because of this, if Lung-Qi is deficient, it can lead to stagnation of Qi of the Heart, which in turn, causes stagnation of Blood of the Heart. This manifests with palpitations, pain in the chest and blue lips. Excessive Heart-Fire dries up the Lung fluids causing a dry cough, dry nose and thirst.

In practice it is common for both Heart and Lung Qi to be deficient at the same time as they are so closely related and they are both situated in the chest. Furthermore, Gathering Qi which collects in the chest influences both Heart and Lung functions and the circulation of both Qi and Blood. If Gathering Qi is weak, the voice will be weak and the hands will be cold, as Qi and Blood of Lung and Heart will be diminished.

Sadness often depletes both Lung and Heart Qi and is manifested with a pulse that is Weak in the Front position of both left and right side.

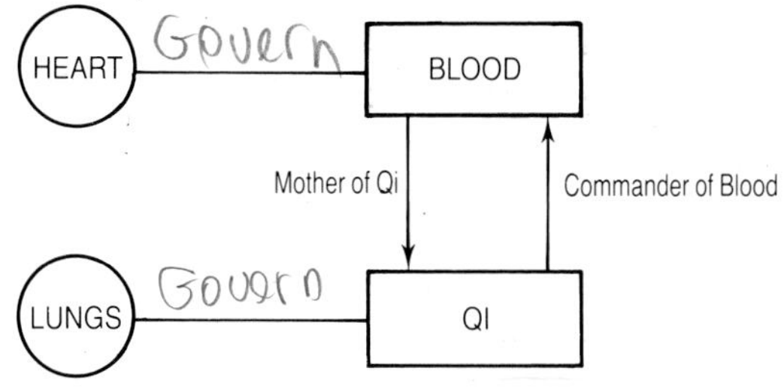

Fig. 38 Heart and Lung interrelationship

HEART AND LIVER

The interrelationship between Heart and Liver hinges on their roles in respect of Blood. The Heart governs Blood while the Liver stores Blood and regulates its volume: these two activities must be coordinated and harmonized. If Heart-Blood is deficient, this may disrupt the Liver's ability to regulate the Blood and gives rise to dizziness and excessive dreaming. More commonly, a deficiency of Liver-Blood causes a deficiency of Heart-Blood as not enough Blood is stored by the Liver to nourish the Heart, causing palpitations and insomnia. In 5-Element terms this situation would be described as the "Mother not nourishing the Child".

On a mental level, the Heart stores the Mind and vitality, while the Liver is responsible for a "smooth flow" of the emotions. The Mind and the emotions mutually support one another. A weak Heart and a low Mind, may lead to depression and anxiety, while constrained emotions and unhappiness due to stagnation of Liver-Qi may lead to a weakening of the Mind and a lowering of vitality (Fig. 39).

HEART AND KIDNEYS

The interrelationship of Heart and Kidneys is very important in clinical practice. This relationship has two aspects:

- the mutual assistance of Fire and Water
- the common root of Mind and Essence.

1 THE MUTUAL ASSISTANCE OF FIRE AND WATER

Heart belongs to Fire and is in the Upper Burner: Fire is Yang in nature and corresponds to movement.

Kidneys belong to Water and are in the Lower Burner: Water is Yin in nature and corresponds to stillness. Heart and Kidneys must be in balance as they represent two fundamental poles of Yang and Yin, Fire and Water. Heart-Yang descends to warm Kidney-Yin; Kidney-Yin ascends to nourish Heart-Yang. The energy of the Heart and Kidneys is in constant interchange above and below. Chinese Medicine refers to this as the "mutual support of Fire and Water", or the "mutual support of Heart and Kidneys".

If Kidney-Yang is deficient, the Kidneys cannot transform the fluids which can overflow towards the top causing the pattern called "Water insulting the Heart". If Kidney-Yin is deficient, it cannot rise to nourish Heart-Yin which leads to hyperactivity of Heart-Fire causing mental restlessness, insomnia, red flushed cheek-bones, night sweats, and a Red-Peeled tongue with a crack in the centre. These two situations are characterized by a loss of contact between Heart and Kidneys. It should be noted that the rela-

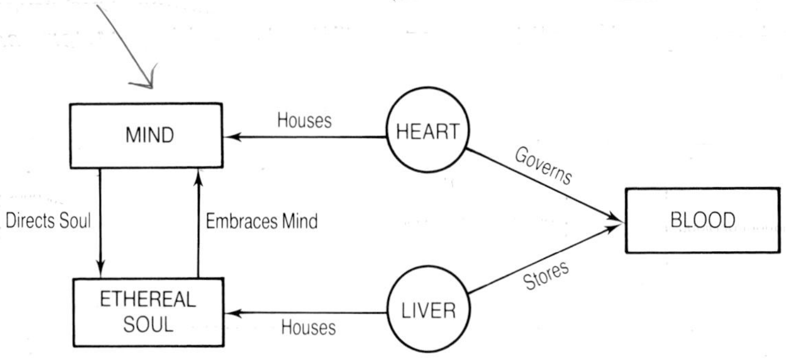

Fig. 39 Heart and Liver interrelationship

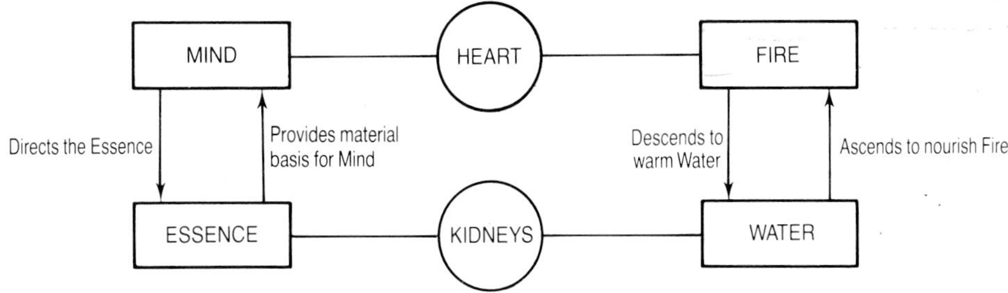

Fig. 40 Heart and Kidney interrelationship

tionship between Heart and Kidneys just described is different from that postulated by the 5-Element model in which the Heart and Kidney have a relationship of mutual control.

2 THE COMMON ROOT OF MIND AND ESSENCE

The Heart houses the Mind, the Kidneys store Essence. Mind and Essence have a common root. Essence is the fundamental substance from which the Mind is derived. In other words, the Mind is the external manifestation of the Essence. The Pre-Heaven Essence is the foundation of the Mind, while the Post-Heaven Essence provides nourishment for the Mind. An ample supply of Essence is the pre-condition for a normal activity of the Mind and a vigorous Mind is the pre-condition for a productive Essence. The relationship between Essence and Mind highlights the Chinese view of the body and mind as an integrated whole, one influencing the other with both body and mind having a common root in Qi.

If Essence is weak, the Mind will suffer and the person will lack vitality, self-confidence and will power. If the Mind is perturbed by emotional problems, the Essence will not be directed by the Mind and the person will feel permanently tired and lack motivation (Fig. 40).

LIVER AND LUNGS

The relationship between Lungs and Liver reflects the relationship between Qi and Blood. Lungs governs Qi, the Liver regulates and stores Blood, and the two rely on each other to perform their respective functions. The Liver relies on Lung-Qi to regulate Blood, and the Lungs rely on Liver-Qi for a smooth movement of Qi.

Deficient Lung-Qi can affect the Liver function of smooth flow of Qi. In such cases, a person will experience listlessness (from deficiency of Qi), depression (from stagnation of Liver-Qi), cough and hypochondriac pain. This situation corresponds to "Metal not controlling Wood" from the 5-Element point of view.

If Liver-Qi stagnates in the chest, it can obstruct the flow of Lung-Qi, impairing its descending function and causing cough, breathlessness or asthma. This situation corresponds to "Wood insulting Metal" according to the 5

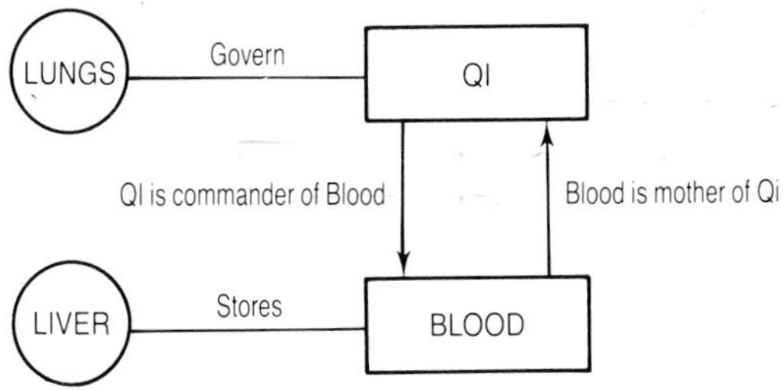

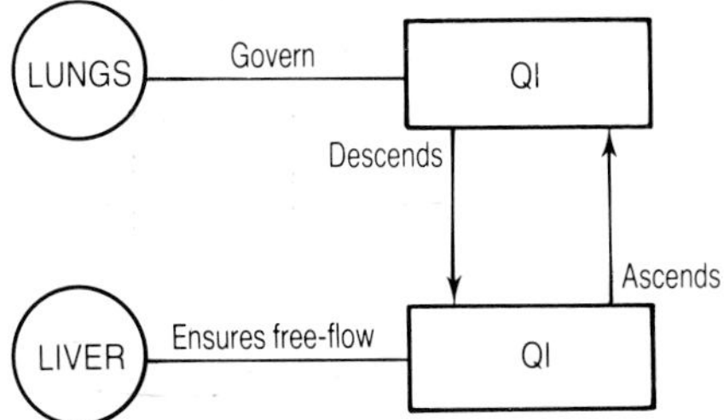

Fig .41 Liver and Lung interrelationship

Elements. Furthermore, stagnation of Liver-Qi can lead to Liver-Fire rising upwards to injure Lung-Yin causing hypochondriac pain, coughing of blood and pain on breathing. This is called "Fire of Liver insulting Metal" (Fig. 41).

LIVER AND SPLEEN

Liver and Spleen have a very close relationship, disturbances of which frequently occur in clinical practice. Under normal circumstances, Liver-Qi aids the Spleen function of transformation, separation and transportation. Furthermore, Liver-Qi also ensures the smooth flow of bile, which also helps digestion. If Liver-Qi is normal, digestion will be good and the Spleen will be aided in the performance of its function. By ensuring the smooth flow of Qi all over the body and in all directions, the Liver ensures that Spleen-Qi flows upwards, the normal direction of Spleen-Qi.

Stagnant Liver-Qi disrupts the Spleen ability to transform and transport food and fluids and in particular, the upward flow of Spleen-Qi. This manifests as abdominal distension, hypochondriac pain and diarrhoea. This situation corresponds to "Wood overacting on Earth" according to the theory of the 5 Elements, and is a common clinical finding.

As usual there is a reciprocal relationship, and the Spleen also aids the Liver function of smooth flow of Qi. If Spleen-Qi is deficient and its transformation and transportation function impaired, the food will not be digested properly and will be retained in the Middle Burner. This in turn may affect the circulation of Liver-Qi and impair the smooth flow of Qi in the Middle Burner, causing abdominal distension, hypochondriac pain and irritability. This situation corresponds to "Earth insulting Wood" according to the theory of the 5 Elements (Fig. 42).

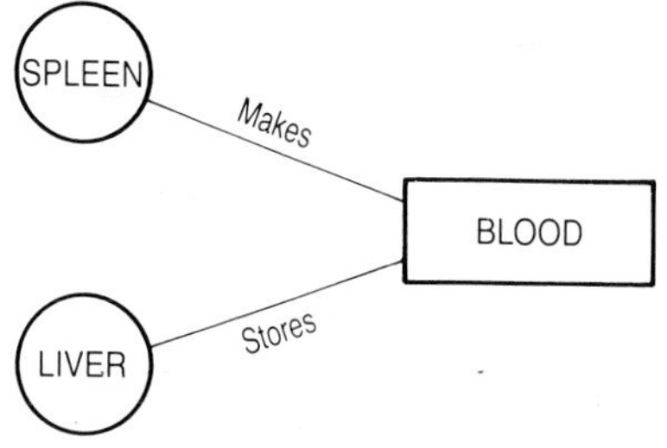

Fig. 42 Liver and Spleen interrelationship

LIVER AND KIDNEYS

The relationship between Liver and Kidneys, of considerable clinical significance, is based on the mutual exchange between Blood and Essence. Liver-Blood nourishes and replenishes Kidney-Essence, and this in turn contributes to the making of Blood (because the Essence produces bone marrow which makes Blood). This is why it is said that "Liver and Kidneys have a common origin" and "Essence and Blood have a common source". Moreover, Kidney-Yin nourishes Liver-Yin (which includes Liver-Blood), in agreement with the 5-Element theory which states that "Water nourishes Wood".

Deficient Kidney-Essence may in turn lead to deficiency of Blood, with symptoms of dizziness, blurred vision and tinnitus. If Kidney-Yin is deficient it fails to nourish Liver-Yin. Deficient Liver-Yin leads to hyperactivity and rising of Liver-Yang causing blurred vision, tinnitus, dizziness, irritability, and headaches.

Deficient Liver-Blood may cause weakness of Kidney-Essence, since this will lack the nourishment of Liver-Blood: the result will be deafness, tinnitus and nocturnal emissions (Fig. 43).

SPLEEN AND LUNGS

The Spleen and Lungs also mutually assist each other in their functions. The Spleen extracts the

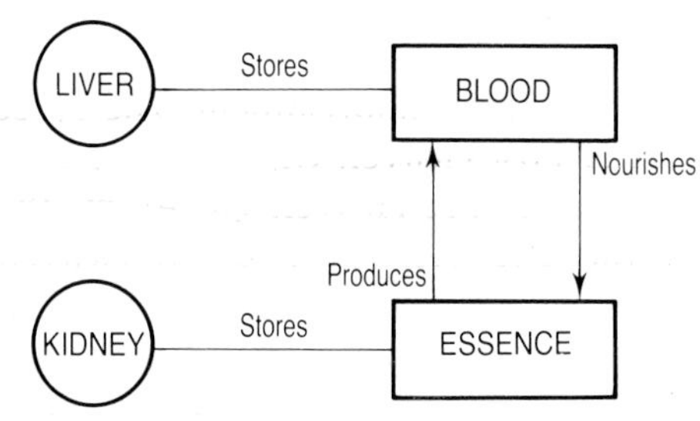

Fig. 43 Liver and Kidney interrelationship

refined Essence of Food and sends it up to the Lungs where it combines with air to form Gathering Qi. In this way, Spleen-Qi benefits Lung-Qi, as it provides Food-Qi from which Qi is formed. In its turn, the Spleen relies on the Lung descending function to help in the transformation and transportation of food and body fluids. This Lung-Qi has an influence on Spleen-Qi. Hence the saying: "The Spleen is the origin of Qi and the Lungs are the axis of Qi".

If Spleen-Qi is deficient Food-Qi will be deficient and the production of Qi, particularly that of the Lungs, will be impaired. This will result in tiredness, weak limbs, breathlessness and a weak voice. The theory of the 5 Elements describes this as "Earth not producing Metal".

Another important consequence of Spleen deficiency is that the fluids will not be transformed and may accumulate to form Phlegm which usually settles in the Lungs impairing the Lung functions. Hence the saying "The Spleen is the origin of Phlegm and the Lungs store it".

If Lung-Qi is weak and its descending function impaired, the Spleen cannot transform and transport the fluids causing oedema (Fig. 44).

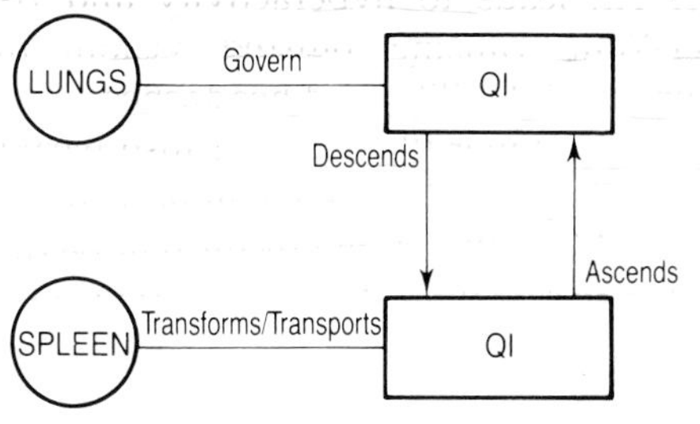

Fig. 44 Spleen and Lung interrelationship

SPLEEN AND KIDNEYS

The relationship between Spleen and Kidneys is also one of mutual nourishment. The Spleen is the Root of Post-Heaven Qi, while the Kidneys are the Root of Pre-Heaven Qi. As mentioned before, the Post-Heaven and Pre-Heaven Qi mutually support one another. The Post-Heaven Qi continually replenishes the Pre-Heaven Qi with the Qi produced from food, and the Pre-Heaven Qi assists in the production of Qi by providing the Heat necessary for digestion and transformation (through the Fire of the Gate of Vitality).

If Spleen-Qi is deficient, not enough Qi will be produced to replenish Kidney-Essence; this may cause tiredness, lack of appetite, tinnitus, dizziness and lower back ache.

If Kidney-Yang is deficient, the Fire of the Gate of Vitality cannot warm the Spleen in its activity of transformation and transportation causing diarrhoea and chilliness. This is termed by the 5-Element theory "Fire not producing Earth".

The Spleen and Kidney also assist each other in the transformation and transportation of body fluids. If Spleen-Qi cannot transform and transport the fluids, these may accumulate to form Dampness which can impair the Kidney function of governing Water, further aggravating the Dampness. On the other hand, if Kidney-Yang is deficient, the Gate of Vitality cannot provide the Heat necessary for the Spleen to transform the fluids and this can cause Dampness or oedema, diarrhoea and chilliness (Fig. 45).

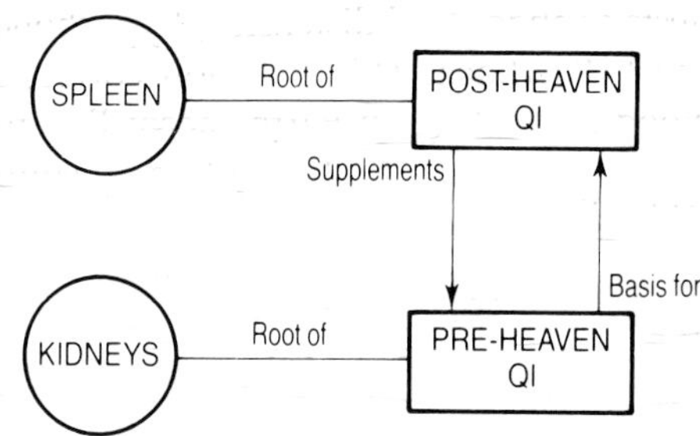

Fig. 45 Spleen and Kidney interrelationship

LUNGS AND KIDNEYS

The Lungs and Kidneys are related in many ways. First of all, the Lungs send Qi and fluids down to the Kidneys, and the Kidneys respond by holding the Qi down and evaporationg some of the fluids and sending the resulting vapour back up to the Lungs to keep them moist. The relationship between Lungs and Kidneys can therefore be analysed in terms of Qi or fluids:

1) In terms of Qi, the Lungs govern Qi and

respiration and send Qi down to the Kidneys. The Kidneys respond by holding Qi down. Thus, Lungs and Kidneys must communicate with and respond to each other. This relationship is also mirrored in the relationship between Gathering Qi in the lower abdomen (which belongs to the Kidneys). Gathering Qi has to flow down to obtain nourishment from the Original Qi while this has to flow up to the chest to assist in the production of Qi and Blood. Thus, the Lung function of governing Qi and respiration is dependent on the Kidney function of reception of Qi and viceversa.

If the Kidneys are weak and their function of reception of Qi is impaired, the Kidneys will fail to hold Qi down and Qi will flow back up to the chest obstructing the Lung descending function and causing breathlessness (more on inhalation), cough and asthma.

In terms of fluids, the Lungs control the Water passages and send fluids down to the Kidneys; the Kidneys respond by evaporating some of the fluids and sending them back up to the Lungs to keep them moist. This is why it is said in Chinese Medicine that the "Kidneys govern Water and the Lungs are the Upper Source of Water".

If Lung-Qi is deficient, it cannot send fluids downwards and the Lungs cannot communicate with the Kidneys and Bladder, causing incontinence or retention of urine. If Kidney-Yang is deficient and cannot transform and excrete the fluids in the Lower Burner, they may accumulate to cause oedema which will impair the Lung descending and dispersing function. Deficiency of Kidney-Yin results in deficiency of fluids in the Lower Burner. The consequence of this is that fluids fail to rise to keep the Lungs moist, thus causing deficiency of Lung-Yin. The symptoms of this are a dry throat at night, a dry cough, night sweating and a feeling of heat in the palms and soles of feet (Fig. 46).

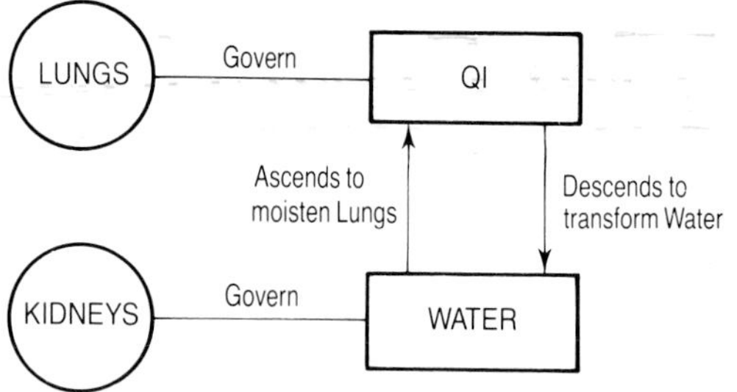

Fig. 46 Lungs and Kidney interrelationship

SPLEEN AND HEART

Spleen and Heart are interrelated because of their connection with Blood. The Spleen makes Blood (because it provides the Essence of Food which is the basis for Blood) and it is therefore of paramount importance to the Heart which governs Blood. If Spleen-Qi is deficient and cannot make enough Blood, this will inevitably lead to deficiency of Heart-Blood, with symptoms of dizziness, poor memory, insomnia and palpitations.

Moreover, Heart-Yang pushes Blood in the vessels and Heart-Blood nourishes the Spleen. If Heart-Yang is deficient it will fail to push the Blood in the vessels and the Spleen will suffer as it makes and controls Blood (Fig. 47).

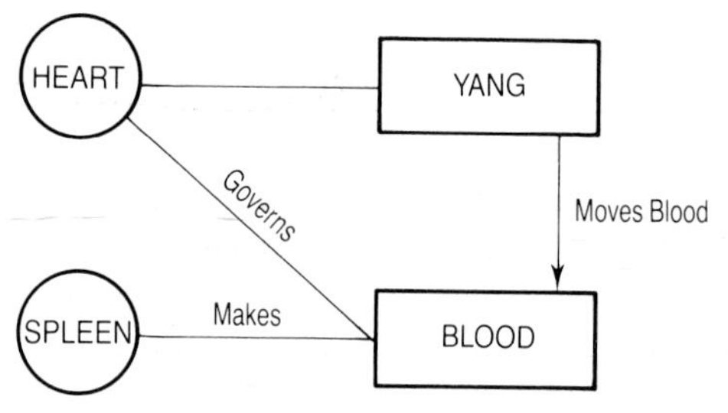

Fig. 47 Heart and Spleen interrelationship

NOTES

1 Practical Chinese Medicine, p 51.

The Functions of the Yang Organs 13 腑

THE FUNCTIONS OF THE STOMACH 胃

The Stomach is the most important of all the Yang organs. Together with the Spleen, it is known as the "Root of Post-Heaven Qi" because it is the origin of all Qi and Blood produced after birth (as opposed to the Pre-Heaven Qi which is formed at conception). The "Simple Questions" says in chapter 8: *"The Spleen and Stomach are the officials in charge of food storage and from whom the 5 flavours are derived"*.[1]

In chapter 11 it says: *"The Stomach is the Sea of water and grains and the great Source of nourishment for the 6 Yang organs. The 5 flavours enter the mouth to be stored in the Stomach for nourishing the 5 Yin organs ... and thus the flavours of the 5 Yin and 6 Yang organs are all derived from the Stomach ..."*.[2]

The functions of the Stomach are:

It controls the "rotting and ripening" of food

It controls the transportation of food essences

It controls the descending of Qi.

It is the origin of fluids.

1 CONTROLS THE "ROTTING AND RIPENING" OF FOOD

The Stomach transforms ingested food and drink by a process of fermentation described as "rotting and ripening". The "Classic of Difficulties" in chapter 31 says: *"The Middle Burner is in the Stomach ... and controls the rotting and ripening of food and drink"*.[3] This activity of the Stomach prepares the ground for the Spleen to separate and extract the refined essence from food. Because of the Stomach function of rotting and ripening, the Middle Burner is often compared to a bubbling cauldron. After transformation in the Stomach, food is passed down to the Small Intestine for further separation and absorption.

The Stomach role in transforming food means that the Stomach, together with the Spleen, is the origin of Qi in the body, and for this reason it is called the "Root of Post-Heaven Qi".

The "Simple Questions" in chapter 19 says: *"The 5 Yin organs all derive Qi from the Stomach, and thus the Stomach is the root of the 5 Yin organs."*[4]

Throughout the development of traditional Chinese medical theory, the Stomach was taken to be the origin of the Qi of the body. No matter how serious the disease, if Stomach-Qi is still strong, the prognosis will be good. Hence the saying *"If there is Stomach-Qi there is life, if there is no Stomach-Qi there is death"*. Yu Jia Yan (1585–1664) said: *"If Stomach-Qi is strong the 5 Yin organs are healthy, if Stomach-Qi is weak they* ***will decline"***.[5] **Zhang Jie Bin said:** ***"Stomach-Qi is the nourishment of life itself, if the Stomach is*** *strong life will be healthy, if the Stomach is weak, life will be unhealthy"*.[6] He also said: *"The doctor who wants to nourish life has to tonify Stomach and Spleen"*.[7]

A school of thought developed which stressed the importance of "Preserving Stomach-Qi" as the most important treatment method. The most famous exponent of this school was Li Dong Yuan (1180–1251), author of the celebrated "Discussion on Stomach and Spleen".

2 CONTROLS THE TRANSPORTATION OF FOOD ESSENCES

The Stomach, together with the Spleen, is responsible for the transportation of food essences to the whole body, in particular the limbs. From this point of view, the Spleen and Stomach roles are inseparable.

If the Stomach is strong and has enough Qi to extract and transport food essences throughout the body, a person will feel strong and full of energy. If the Stomach is deficient, food essences will be weak too and the Stomach will lack Qi to transport them to the whole body so that the person will feel tired and suffer from weakness of the muscles.

The Stomach function of transporting food essences also has an influence on the pulse. The "Simple Questions" in chapter 19 says: *"The Qi of the organs relies on Stomach-Qi to reach the Lung channel"*.[8]

This means that, by transporting food essences to all the organs, Stomach-Qi also ensures that the Qi of the organs reaches the pulse (which, of course, is on the Lung channel). There are certain qualities of a normal pulse that are associated with a good Stomach-Qi. A pulse with good Stomach Qi is said to be neither weak nor strong, with Yin and Yang perfectly harmonized, having a regular and rather slow beat. Strong Stomach-Qi is also said to make the pulse "soft and gentle": if a pulse feels too rough or hard, it indicates that it lacks Stomach-Qi.

Finally, in relation to the Stomach function of transporting food essences, the Stomach is very closely related to the tongue coating. This is formed by the "dirty dampness" that is generated as a by-product of the Stomach activity of rotting and ripening: this dirty dampness subsequently rises up to the tongue to form the coating. A thin white coating therefore indicates that the Stomach is functioning properly. The absence of coating indicates that the Stomach function of digestion is impaired and Stomach-Qi is severely weakened. The colour of the coating also closely reflects Stomach pathology: a thick white coating indicates Cold in the Stomach, while a thick yellow coating indicates Heat.

3 CONTROLS THE DESCENDING OF QI

The Stomach sends transformed food downwards to the Small Intestine: for this reason in health, Stomach-Qi has a downward movement. If Stomach-Qi descends, digestion will be good and trouble-free. If Stomach-Qi fails to descend, food will stagnate in the stomach leading to a feeling of fullness and distention, sour regurgitation, belching, hiccup, nausea and vomiting. Under normal conditions, Liver-Qi contributes to the descending of Stomach-Qi and so helps digestion. If Liver-Qi stagnates in the Middle Burner, it can interfere with the descending of Stomach-Qi giving rise to the above-mentioned symptoms.

4 IS THE ORIGIN OF FLUIDS

To rot and ripen food the Stomach needs an abundance of fluids, just as sufficient fluids are needed to extract the vital principles from a herbal decoction. Furthermore, fluids themselves are derived from the food and drink ingested. The Stomach ensures that the part of food and drink which does not go to make essences of food, condenses to form body fluids.

The Stomach is thus an important source of fluids in the body, and for this reason it is said that the Stomach "likes wetness and dislikes dryness".

If Stomach fluids are abundant, digestion will be good and the sense of taste normal. If Stomach fluids are deficient, a person will be thirsty, the tongue will be dry and cracked and digestion will be poor. One of the main reasons for deficiency of Stomach fluids is eating large meals late at night.

The Stomach function as origin of fluids is closely related to the Kidneys. The Kidneys are sometimes called the "Gate of the Stomach", because they transform fluids in the Lower Burner. If this Kidney function is impaired, fluids will stagnate in the Lower Burner and overflow upwards to the Stomach, impairing the digestion.

Furthermore, a long-standing deficiency of Stomach-fluids will often lead to a deficiency of Kidney-Yin, so that in very chronic cases, deficiency of Stomach-Yin is nearly always associated with deficiency of Kidney-Yin.

The Stomach's role as origin of fluids points to a rather strange anomaly in the theory of the Internal Organs. Although the Spleen is a Yin and the Stomach a Yang organ, in many ways the situation is reversed, the Stomach having many Yin functions and the Spleen many Yang functions:

a) The Stomach is the origin of fluids which are Yin
b) The Spleen has the function of transporting and moving, which is Yang in nature
c) Spleen-Qi ascends (Yang ascends) and Stomach-Qi descends (Yin descends)
d) The Spleen is Yin but likes dryness, the Stomach is Yang but likes wetness.
e) The Stomach channel is the only Yang channel in the anterior aspect of the body.
f) The Stomach often suffers from Yin deficiency, whilst the Spleen seldom suffers from Yin deficiency, but very often from Yang deficiency instead.

MENTAL ASPECT

Mention should be made here of the Stomach influence on the mental state. The Stomach easily suffers from Excess patterns, such as Fire, or Phlegm-Fire. Fire easily agitates the Mind and causes mental symptoms. On a mental level, a condition of Excess of the Stomach can manifest as shutting oneself in the house, closing all doors and windows, wanting to be by oneself, uncontrolled talking or laughing or singing, violent behaviour and taking off of one's clothes. These symptoms described in the ancient classics correspond to what we would today call manic behaviour.

In less serious cases, Stomach-Fire or Stomach Phlegm-Fire can cause mental confusion, severe anxiety, hypomania and hyperactivity.

DREAMS

The "Spiritual Axis" in chapter 43 says: "*When the Stomach is deficient one dreams of having a large meal*".[9]

RELATIONSHIP WITH THE SPLEEN

According to the 5 Elements Stomach and Spleen belong to the Earth Element, one Yang and the other Yin. The relationship between these two organs is very close indeed, so much so that they could be considered as two aspects of the same organ-system. In fact, the Stomach function of rotting and ripening is closely coordinated with the Spleen function of separating and moving essences of food. The Spleen function of transporting Food-Qi to the whole body is closely dependant on Stomach-Qi. The Stomach is the origin of fluids and must rely on the Spleen function of transforming and separating the body fluids. The coordination between Stomach and Spleen may be summarized as follows:

a) The Stomach is Yang, the Spleen is Yin.
b) Stomach-Qi descends, Spleen-Qi ascends.
c) The Stomach likes wetness and dislikes dryness, the Spleen likes dryness and dislikes wetness.

d) If the Stomach is too dry, Stomach-Qi cannot descend and food cannot be moved down to the Small Intestine. If the Spleen is too damp, Spleen-Qi cannot ascend and fluids and food cannot be transformed.
e) The Stomach easily suffers from Excess, the Spleen easily suffers from Deficiency.
f) The Stomach is prone to Heat, the Spleen prone to Cold.
g) The Stomach tends to suffer from deficiency of Yin, the Spleen from deficieny of Yang.

THE FUNCTIONS OF THE SMALL INTESTINE

小腸

The Small Intestine receives food and drink after digestion by the Stomach and Spleen. This it transforms further by separating a "clean" from a "dirty" part. The "Simple Questions" says in chapter 8: *"The Small Intestine is the official in charge of receiving, being filled and transforming"*.[10]

From a psychological point of view, the Small Intestine has an influence on mental clarity and judgement. It also has an influence on our capacity to take decisions, but in a different way from the Gall Bladder. Whereas the Gall Bladder has an influence on the capacity and courage to take decisions, the Small Intestine gives us the power of discernment, that is the ability to distinguish relevant issues with clarity before we make a decision.

The functions of the Small Intestine are:
It controls receiving and transforming
It separates fluids.

1 CONTROLS RECEIVING AND TRANSFORMING

As we have seen, the Small Intestine receives food and drink from the Stomach to carry out its job of separating a "clean" (i.e. re-usable) part from a "dirty" part. The clean part is then transported by the Spleen to all parts of the body to nourish the tissues. The "dirty" part is transmitted to the Large Intestine for excretion as stools, and to the Bladder for excretion as urine. From this it can be seen that the Small Intestine has a direct functional relation with the Bladder and it influences the urinary function.

2 SEPARATES FLUIDS

The Small Intestine plays an important role in the movement and transformation of fluids. This process is similar to the one outlined above in relation to food. After the "dirty" fluids are passed down from the Stomach, they are further separated by the Small Intestine into a "clean" part which goes to the Large Intestine for re-absorption, and a "dirty" part which goes to the Bladder for excretion as urine.

The Small Intestine function of separating fluids is controlled by the action of Kidney-Yang which provides the Qi and the heat necessary for this separation to take place. If the Small Intestine's function is impaired, there may be excessive or scanty urination, depending on whether the organ is Cold or Hot.

DREAMS

The "Simple Questions" in chapter 17 says: *"When one has small intestinal parasites, one will dream of crowds; when one has long intestinal parasites, one will dream of fights and mutual destruction"*.[11]

The "Spiritual Axis" in chapter 43 says: *"When the Small Intestine is deficient, one dreams of large cities"*.[12]

RELATIONSHIP WITH THE HEART

The relationships between Yin and Yang organs within the 5 Elements are not all equally close. For example, the relationship between Stomach and Spleen is very close indeed, as is that between the Liver and Gall Bladder. The relationship between Small Intestine and Heart, on the other hand, is rather tenuous. Chinese books normally say that Heart-Qi helps the Small Intestine function of separating, but it is not clear how this is achieved.

The closest link between Heart and Small Intestine can probably be found on the psychological level. The Heart houses the Mind and governs our mental life as a whole. Our mental activities all rely on our capacity of clear judgement and decisions, which in turn are dependent on the Small Intestine. Conversely, the capacity of clear judgement must rely on our mental capacity as a whole, which is dependent on the Heart.

There is a certain similarity between the Gall Bladder's role in helping us to make decisions and the Small Intestine's influence on judgement. However, there are some differences: the Gall Bladder gives us the courage to make decisions, while from the Small Intestine we derive the clarity of mind necessary to distinguish right from wrong in order to make a choice in life.

When the Gall Bladder is deficient, the person will lack the courage and initiative to take decisions, whereas when the Small Intestine is deficient, the person cannot make a decision because he or she cannot distinguish the various options and make the right choices. The Gall Bladder and Small Intestine in this respect, depend on each other since it is not enough to have the vision to see what is the right option, if we then lack the courage to act on it. The best points to affect these mental influences are Qiuxu G.B.-40 for the Gall Bladder and Yanggu S.I.-5 for the Small Intestine.

The relationship between Heart and Small Intestine can sometimes be observed in certain pathological situations when Heart-Fire can be transmitted to the Small Intestine, with such manifestations as thirst, bitter taste, tongue ulcers and blood in the urine.

THE FUNCTIONS OF THE LARGE INTESTINE

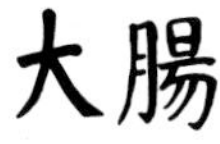

The main function of the Large Intestine is to receive food and drink from the Small Intestine. Having re-absorbed some of the fluids, it excretes the stools.

Chinese medical theory is usually extremely brief with regard to the Large Intestine functions. This is not because its functions are unimportant, but because many of the functions attributed to the Large Intestine in Western Medicine, are attributed to the Spleen from a Chinese medical perspective. The Spleen controls the transformation and transportation of food and fluids throughout the digestive system, including the Small and Large Intestine. For this reason, in disease, symptoms and signs such as diarrhoea, abdominal distension and pain are usually attributed to a Spleen disharmony.

RELATIONSHIP WITH THE LUNGS

The Lungs and Large Intestine are interiorly-exteriorly related. This relationship is important for the execution of common bodily functions, such as when descending Lung-Qi lends the Large Intestine the necessary Qi for the effort of defecation.

If Lung-Qi is deficient, it does not give enough Qi to the Large Intestine for the act of defecation, resulting in constipation. This is particularly common in old people with declining Lung-Qi.

Conversely, the Lung's ability to send Qi downwards depends on the Large Intestine's role in excreting waste food material. If this function is impaired and there is constipation, the stagnation of food in the Large Intestine may impair the Lung descending function giving rise to breathlessness.

DREAMS

The "Spiritual Axis" in chapter 43 says: "*When the Large Intestine is deficient, one dreams of open fields*".[13]

THE FUNCTIONS OF THE GALL BLADDER

胆

The Gall Bladder occupies a special place among the Yang organs because it is the only one that does not deal with food, drink and their waste products, but stores bile which is a refined product. Furthermore, it neither communicates with the exterior directly as all the other Yang organs do (via the mouth, rectum or urethra) nor does it receive food or transport nourishment, as do the other Yang organs. In fact, because it stores a refined substance, the Gall Bladder resembles a Yin organ.

On a psychological level, the Gall Bladder is said to influence the capacity of making decisions. The "Simple Questions" in chapter 8 says: *"The Gall Bladder is the upright official that takes decisions"*.[14]

The functions of the Gall Bladder are:

It stores and excretes bile
It controls judgement
It controls sinews.

1 STORES AND EXCRETES BILE

The Gall Bladder receives bile from the Liver which it stores ready to excrete when needed during digestion. From this point of view, the function of the Gall Bladder is identical with that of Western Medicine.

The Gall Bladder is the only Yang organ that stores a "clean" fluid such as bile, instead of "dirty" substances such as food, drink and their wastes.

Excretion of bile by the Gall Bladder is an expression of the Liver's role in ensuring the smooth flow of Qi since the Liver provides the necessary Qi for bile secretion.

Under normal circumstances, the smooth flow of bile aids the Stomach and Spleen function of digestion. In disease, when Liver-Qi is stagnant and the bile does not flow smoothly, both Stomach and Spleen functions may be impaired. In particular, the Stomach ability to direct Qi downwards will be impaired giving rise to nausea and belching.

2 CONTROLS JUDGEMENT

While the Liver is said to control the ability of planning one's life, the Gall Bladder controls the capacity to make decisions. The two functions have to be harmonized so that we can plan and act accordingly.

Besides controlling decision-making, the Gall Bladder is also said to give an individual courage and initiative. For this reason, in Chinese, there are several expressions such as "big gall bladder" meaning "courageous" and "small gall bladder" meaning "timid or fearful".

This is an important function of the Gall Bladder on a psychological level. It controls the spirit of initiative, the "drive" and the courage to take decisions and make changes. Although as we have seen, the Kidneys also control the "drive" and vitality, the Gall Bladder gives us the capacity to turn this drive and vitality into positive and decisive action. Thus a deficient Gall Bladder will cause indecision, timidity and the affected person will be easily discouraged at the slightest adversity.

The Gall Bladder provides the courage for the Mind, governed by the Heart, to carry out decisions. This reflects the Mother-Child relationship existing between Gall Bladder and Heart according to the 5 Elements. In cases of weak Mind from Heart deficiency, it is often necessary to tonify the Gall Bladder to support the Heart.

3 CONTROLS THE SINEWS

This function is almost identical to the Liver function of controlling sinews. The only slight difference is that in so far as the Liver nourishes the sinews with its Blood, the Gall Bladder provides Qi to the sinews to ensure their proper movement and agility. This explains why the gathering point for sinews, Yanglingquan G.B.-34, is on the Gall Bladder channel.

DREAMS

The Gall Bladder has an influence on the quality and length of sleep, and if it is deficient, a person will wake early in the morning and be unable to fall asleep again. The "Spiritual Axis" in chapter 43 says: *"When the Gall Bladder is deficient one dreams of fights, trials and suicide"*.[15]

RELATION WITH LIVER

The Liver and Gall Bladder depend on each other to perform their respective functions. The Gall Bladder function of storing and excreting bile depends on the Liver function of smooth flow of Qi. Conversely, the Liver relies on Gall Bladder-Qi to aid its function of smooth flow of Qi.

On a psychological level, the Liver's influence on the planning of our life is dependent on the Gall Bladder capacity to help us make decisions.

THE FUNCTIONS OF THE BLADDER

膀胱

The Bladder has a wider sphere of activity in Chinese Medicine than in Western Medicine. It stores and excretes urine, but also participates in the transformation of fluids necessary for the production of urine. The "Simple Questions" in chapter 8 says: *"The Bladder is like a district official, it stores the fluids so that they can be excreted by its action of Qi transformation"*.[16]

On a mental level, an imbalance in the Bladder can provoke negative emotions such as jealousy, suspicion and the holding of long-standing grudges.

The function of the Bladder is:

It removes water by Qi transformation.

REMOVES WATER BY QI TRANSFORMATION

The "dirty" part of fluids separated by the Small Intestine passes on to the Bladder which further transforms them into urine. The Bladder subsequently stores and excretes urine. The Bladder's function of transforming fluids requires Qi and heat which are provided by Kidney-Yang. In Chinese Medicine this is usually called Bladder's function of "Qi transformation", i.e. transformation of fluids by Qi.

Although it is the Bladder that performs this function, the energy to do this is derived from the Kidney. It is worth noting that the Small Intestine and Bladder work together to move fluids in the Lower Burner. This explains the use of certain Small Intestine points, such as Qiangu S.I.-2 in urinary diseases. The connection between the Small Intestine and the Bladder also explains how some Heart disharmonies can be transmitted to the Bladder via the Small Intestine (which is of course related to the Heart within the 5-Element model).

The Bladder can be seen as the Yang aspect of the Kidney and is therefore related to the Fire of the Gate of Vitality from which it derives its energy. For this reason symptoms of Bladder deficiency are similar to those of deficiency of the Gate of Vitality, i.e. abundant, clear-coloured urination.

Finally, the Bladder is assisted in its function of fluid transformation by the Triple Burner, or more precisely, the Lower Burner, which has the function of making sure the water passages in the lower part of the body are open and free.

DREAMS

The "Spiritual Axis" in chapter 43 says: *"When the Bladder is deficient one dreams of voyages"*.[17]

RELATIONSHIP WITH THE KIDNEYS

The relation between Bladder and Kidney is close. On the one hand, the Bladder derives the Qi necessary for its function of fluids transformation from the Kidney and the Gate of Vitality. On the other hand, the Kidneys rely on the Bladder to move and excrete some of their "dirty" fluids.

THE FUNCTIONS OF THE TRIPLE BURNER

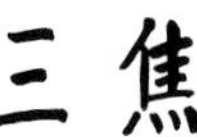

The Triple Burner is one of the most elusive aspects of Chinese Medicine and one which has been the subject of controversy for centuries.

Although it is "officially" one of the 6 Yang organs, Chinese doctors have always argued about the nature of the Triple Burner and in particular whether it has a "form" or not, i.e. whether it is an actual organ or a function. Rather than listing the functions of the Triple Burner, it is probably more appropriate to discuss three different views of the Triple Burner, which will throw light on its functions. These are:

The Triple Burner as one the six Yang organs

The Triple Burner as an "avenue for the Original Qi"

The Triple Burner as the three divisions of the body.

1 THE TRIPLE BURNER AS ONE OF THE SIX YANG ORGANS

Historically, this view is derived from the "Yellow Emperor's Classic". The "Simple Questions" in chapter 8 says: *"The Triple Burner is the official in charge of irrigation and it controls the water passages"*.[18] This comment about the Triple Burner is mentioned in the context of a list of functions of all the organs, from which it appears that the "Simple Questions" considers the Triple Burner as one of the 6 Yang organs. If this is the case, the Triple Burner has a "form", i.e. it is substantial, like all the other organs. Its function is similar to that of the other Yang organs, i.e. receiving food and drink, digesting and transforming it, transporting the nourishment and excreting the wastes. The function of the Yang organs in general is often expressed in the Chinese word *"tong"* 通 which means "making things go through" or "ensuring a free passage", etc. The function of the Triple Burner, in addition, is often expressed in the Chinese word *"chu"* 出 meaning "excreting" or rather "letting out". The Triple Burner performs this letting out function in relation to Defensive Qi in the Upper Burner, Nutritive Qi in the Middle Burner and Body Fluids in the Lower Burner. The "Spiritual Axis" in chapter 18 says: *"The person receives Qi from food, food enters the stomach, then spreads to the Lungs and the 5 Yin organs and the 6 Yang organs, the clear part goes to the Nutritive Qi, the dirty part to the Defensive Qi"*.[19] The capacity of the Nutritive and Defensive Qi to spread from the Stomach to the Lungs depends on the "letting out" function of the Triple Burner. In other words, the Triple Burner controls the movement of various types of Qi at the various stages of energy production, in particular ensuring that the various types of Qi are "let out" in a smooth way. Thus, the Triple Burner is a three-stage passage-way contributing to the production of Nutritive and Defensive Qi after the separation of food into a clear and dirty part and to the excretion of fluids. The Upper Burner lets out Defensive Qi (directing it to the Lung), the Middle Burner lets out Nutritive Qi (directing it to all the organs), the Lower Burner lets out Body Fluids (directing them to the Bladder).

The "Yellow Emperor's Classic" variously describes the function of the Triple Burner as "opening up", "discharging Qi", "letting Qi out". Malfunctions of the Triple Burner are variously described as "not flowing smoothly", "overflowing" or "being blocked". In practice this means that an impairment of the Triple Burner function will manifest as a blockage of the various types of Qi or fluids in the three stages: a blockage of Defensive Qi in the Upper Burner (impairment of the Lung dispersing function), a blockage of Nutritive Qi in the Middle Burner (impairment of the Spleen function of transportation) and a blockage of Body Fluids in the Lower Burner (impairment of the Bladder function of Qi transformation). These situations would cause sneezing, abdominal distention and retention of urine respectively.

2 THE TRIPLE BURNER AS AN "AVENUE FOR THE ORIGINAL QI"

This interpretation of the Triple Burner derives from the "Classic of Difficulties", chapter 66.[20] According to this classic, the Triple Burner "has a name but no form", i.e. it is not an organ but a collection of functions, it is insubstantial. The "Classic of Difficulties" states that the Original Qi resides in the lower abdomen, between the two Kidneys, it spreads to the 5 Yin and 6 Yang organs via the Triple Burner, it then enters the 12 channels and emerges at the Source (Yuan) points. From this came the interpretation of the Triple Burner as an "avenue for the Original Qi", i.e. the channel for expression of the Original Qi. Original Qi is also described in the same chapter as being the "motive force between the Kidneys", activating all physiological functions of the body and providing heat for the digestion. This "motive force between the Kidneys" can only carry out its functions through the intermediary of the Triple Burner. As mentioned before, Original Qi provides the heat necessary for the digestion and transformation of food. Because the Triple Burner is an "avenue for the Original Qi", it obviously has an influence on the process of digestion. This is clearly expressed in the "Classic of Difficulties" in chapter 31 which states that the "Triple Burner is the avenue of food and drink, the beginning and end of Qi".[21] It also states that the Upper Burner controls "receiving but not excreting", the Middle Burner "rotting and ripening of food and drink" and the Lower Burner "excreting but not receiving". All these expressions "receiving", "rotting and ripening" and "excreting" describe a process of transportation, transformation and excretion of food and fluids by the Triple Burner. From this point of view, there is therefore a convergence of views between the concept of Triple Burner in the "Yellow Emperor's Classic" and the "Classic of Difficulties", i.e. between the Triple Burner as an organ or a function, even though the starting point of these two classics is different. However, the "Yellow Emperor's Classic" emphasizes the role of the Triple Burner in its "letting out" function, seeing the three Burners as three avenues of excretion or "letting out". The "Classic of Difficulties", on the contrary, places emphasis on the work of "receiving", "rotting and ripening" and "excretion" of food and fluids, seeing digestion as a process of "Qi transformation" activated by the Original Qi through the intermediary action of the Triple Burner.

3 THE TRIPLE BURNER AS THE THREE DIVISIONS OF THE BODY

This view of the Triple Burner is derived from both the "Classic of Difficulties" (chapter 31) and the "Spiritual Axis" (chapter 18).[22] The three-fold division of the body is as follows: from the diaphragm upwards is the Upper Burner, between the diaphragm and the umbilicus is the Middle Burner, below the umbilicus is the Lower Burner. As far as organs and anatomical parts are concerned, the Upper Burner includes Heart, Lungs, Pericardium, throat and head; the Middle Burner includes Stomach, Spleen and Gall Bladder; the Lower Burner includes Liver, Kidneys, Intestines and Bladder.

a) The Upper Burner is like a mist

The main physiological process of the Upper Burner is that of distribution of fluids all over the body by the Lungs in the form of fine vapour. This is an aspect of the Lung dispersing function. For this reason the Upper Burner is compared to a "mist".[23]

The "Spiritual Axis" in chapter 30 says: *"The Upper Burner opens outwards, spreads the 5 tastes of the food essences, pervades the skin, fills the body, moistens the skin and it is like mist"*.[24]

b) The Middle Burner is like a maceration chamber

The main physiological processes in the Middle Burner are those of digestion and transportation of food and drink (described as "rotting and ripening") and the transportation of the nourishment extracted from food to all parts of the body. For this reason the Middle Burner is compared to a "maceration chamber" or a "bubbling cauldron".[25]

The "Spiritual Axis" in chapter 18 says: *"The Middle Burner is situated in the Stomach ... it receives Qi, expels the wastes, steams the body fluids, transforms the refined essences of food and connects upwards with the Lungs"*.[26]

c) The Lower Burner is like a ditch

The main physiological process in the Lower Burner is that of separation of the essences of food into a clean and dirty part, with the excretion of the dirty part. In particular, the Lower Burner directs the separation of the clean from the dirty part of the fluids and facilitates the excretion of urine. For this reason the Lower Burner is compared to a "drainage ditch".[27]

The "Spiritual Axis" in chapter 18 says: "*Food and drink first enter the stomach, the waste products go to the large intestine in the Lower Burner which oozes downwards, secretes the fluids and transmits them to the bladder*".[28]

In conclusion, the three-fold division of the Triple Burner is a summarization of the functions of all the Yang organs (but including also the Lungs and Spleen) in their work of receiving, digesting, transforming, absorbing, nourishing and excreting. The organs within each division are not separate from the Three Burners themselves. From acupuncture's perspective in particular, Lungs and Heart are the Upper Burner, Stomach and Spleen are the Middle Burner and Kidneys, Bladder and Intestines are the Lower Burner.

The three-fold division of the body can also be seen as a summarization of the mutual assistance and transformation into each other of the Gathering Qi (Upper Burner), Central Qi (Middle Burner) and Original Qi (Lower Burner).

RELATIONSHIP WITH THE PERICARDIUM

Although they are interiorly-exteriorly related, the relationship between Pericardium and Triple Burner is extremely tenuous. In the same way as for Heart and Small Intestine, the relationship between Triple Burner and Pericardium is more applicable to the channels, rather than to the interaction of the organs themselves. To add to the confusion, both the "Yellow Emperor's Classic" and the "Classic of Difficulties" always refer to the "5 Yin and 6 Yang organs" (omitting the Pericardium), but also to the 12 channels" (including the Pericardium). In terms of historical development, the concept of 5 Yin and 6 Yang organs preceded that of the 12 channels. Originally the Pericardium was not considered as separate from the Heart; the two were considered a single organ, which is perfectly logical considering their close anatomical relationship. In fact, when the "Spiritual Axis" lists the Source points of the 5 Yin organs in chapter 1, it lists Daling (Pericardium-7) as the Source point of the Heart.[29]

The "Classic of Difficulties" in chapter 38 says there are 6 Yang organs including the Triple Burner which "has a name but no form". It thus implies that the Triple Burner is different from the other regular Yang organs and their total only makes 6 by adding the Triple Burner.[30]

With the development of the channel theory, their number totalled 12, including the Triple Burner and Pericardium channels.

Although the Pericardium and Triple Burner channels are exteriorly-interiorly related within the 5-Element scheme, there is hardly a close relationship between these two organs. In fact, some Chinese teachers and doctors go so far as saying that the Pericardium and Triple Burner organs are not interiorly-exteriorly related as the other organs are.

The "Medicine Treasure" even says that the Triple Burner is interiorly-exteriorly related to the Gate of Vitality.[31] Since the Gate of Vitality is also called the "Ministerial Fire", this explains the attribution of Triple Burner to Fire in the 5-Elements context. The Pericardium is obviously closely connected to the Heart and naturally belongs to the Fire element, hence the connection between Pericardium and Triple Burner within the Fire Element.

NOTES

1 Simple Questions, p 58.
2 Simple Questions, p 78
3 Classic of Difficulties, p 80.
4 Simple Questions, p 126.
5 Syndromes and treatment of the Internal Organs, p 176
6 Syndromes and treatment of the Internal Organs, p 176
7 Syndromes and treatment of the Internal Organs, p 176
8 Simple Questions, p 126.
9 Spiritual Axis, p 85.
10 Simple Questions, p 58.
11 Simple Questions, p 103.
12 Spiritual Axis, p 85.
13 Spiritual Axis, p 85.
14 Simple Questions, p 58.
15 Spiritual Axis, p 85.
16 Simple Questions, p 59.

17 Spiritual Axis, p 85.
18 Simple Questions, p 59.
19 Spiritual Axis, p 51.
20 Classic of Difficulties, p 144.
21 Classic of Difficulties, p 79.
22 Spiritual Axis p 52 and Classic of Difficulties, p 79.
23 Medicine Treasure cited in Selected Historical Theories in Chinese Medicine, p 2.
24 Spiritual Axis, p 71.
25 Medicine Treasure, p 2.
26 Spiritual Axis, p 52.
27 Medicine Treasure, p 2.
28 Spiritual Axis p 52.
29 Spiritual Axis, p 3.
30 Classic of Difficulties, p 94. To add to the confusion, chapter 39 even says that there are 5 Yang organs (excluding the Triple Burner) and 6 Yin organs (not, as one would expect, counting the Pericardium, but counting the Kidneys as two organs).
31 Medicine Treasure, p 2.

14 The Functions of the Six Extraordinary Yang Organs

奇恒之腑

Besides the regular Yin and Yang organs, there are also 6 Extraordinary Yang Organs which complete the picture of Chinese physiology. They are called "Extraordinary Yang Organs" because they function like a Yin organ (i.e. storing Yin essence and not excreting), but have the shape of a Yang organ (i.e. hollow). They are: Uterus, Brain, Bones, Marrow, Gall-Bladder and Blood Vessels. The "Simple Questions" in chapter 11 says: *"Brain, Marrow, Bones, Blood Vessels, Gall-Bladder and Uterus all store Yin essences but have the shape of a Yang organ; they store the Essence and do not excrete, therefore they are called Extraordinary Yang organs".*[1]

All the 6 Extraordinary Yang Organs store some form of Yin essence, either the Kidney-Essence, or marrow or blood, and functionally they are all directly or indirectly related to the Kidneys.

THE UTERUS

The Uterus is the most important of the 6 Extraordinary Yang Organs. It has the function of regulating menstruation, conception and pregnancy. It is closely related to the Kidneys, the Directing Vessel (*Ren Mai*) and the Penetrating Vessel (*Chong Mai*) extraordinary vessels. Both the Directing and Penetrating Vessels originate from the Kidney and they have the function of regulating menstruation, conception and pregnancy, and both of them flow through the Uterus. In particular, the Directing Vessel provides Qi and the Penetrating Vessel provides Blood to the Uterus. Normal menstruation and pregnancy depend on the state of the Directing and Penetrating Vessels which, in turn, depend on the state of the Kidneys. If Kidney-Essence is abundant, the Directing and Penetrating Vessels are strong and the Uterus is therefore adequately supplied with Qi and Blood, so that there will be normal menstruation and pregnancy. If Kidney-Essence is weak, the Directing and Penetrating Vessels will be empty, and the Uterus will be inadequately supplied with Qi and Blood, so that there may be irregular menstruation, amenorrhoea or infertility.

Menstruation, conception and pregnancy also depend on the state of the Blood, upon which the Uterus depends. The functional relationship between Uterus and Blood is very close: the Uterus relies on an abundant supply of Blood at all times. Since the Heart governs the Blood, while the Liver stores the Blood and the Spleen controls the Blood, these three Yin organs are physiologically related to the Uterus. In particular, if the Spleen cannot produce enough Blood and Heart-Blood becomes deficient, the Uterus may lack Blood resulting in amenorrhoea. Similarly, if the Liver does not store enough Blood, the Uterus is starved of Blood and this may also cause amenorrhoea.

If the Blood stored by the Liver is hot, this may cause the Blood in the Uterus to flow out recklessly, causing menorrhagia or metrorrhagia. If Liver-Qi is stagnant, this may cause Liver-Blood stasis, which in turn, will affect the Blood of the Uterus, resulting in painful periods with dark clotted blood. In practice, the relationship between Uterus and Liver-Blood is extremely important and one which is very apparent in many pathological conditions. Because the Liver stores Blood and regulates the volume of Blood, menstrual irregularities are often due to a dysfunction of the Liver. For example, Liver-Qi stagnation often causes irregular periods; Liver-Blood stagnation often causes painful periods; Liver-Blood deficiency may cause scanty periods or absence of periods. Disorders of reproduction, on the other hand, are often due to a weakness of Kidney-Essence which should nourish the Uterus. Deficient Kidney-Essence may cause infertility or habitual miscarriage.

Among the Yang organs, the Uterus is closely related to the Stomach. This connection is via the Penetrating Vessel. This Vessel is closely related to the Stomach, and also flows through the Uterus, thus providing a link between Uterus and Stomach. Morning sickness during pregnancy and the nausea or vomiting which some women experience during menstruation are often caused by disruption of the Stomach because of changes in the Uterus.

Although the above obviously only applies to women, there is a corresponding connection in men. It is said in Chinese Medicine that *"The Uterus is related to the Kidneys, in males it is called Red Field (Dan Tian) or also Room of Essence, in females it is called Uterus* [literally Palace of the Child]".[2] The "Room of Essence" in men stores and produces sperm, and is closely related to Kidneys and Governing Vessel. If Kidneys and Governing Vessel are empty, the production and storage of sperm function of the Room of Essence will be affected, and this may cause impotence, premature ejaculation, clear and watery sperm, nocturnal emissions, spermatorrhoea, etc.

THE BRAIN

The Brain is also called the "Sea of Marrow". The "Spiritual Axis" in chapter 33 says: *"The Brain is the Sea of Marrow, extending from the top of the head to the point Fengfu (Du-16)"*.[3] The "Simple Questions" in chapter 10 says: *"The Marrow pertains to the Brain"*.[4]

In Chinese Medicine, the Brain controls memory, concentration, sight, hearing, touch and smell. The "Discussion on Stomach and Spleen" says: *"Sight, hearing, smelling, touch, intelligence all depend on the Brain"*.[5]

As we have seen, the Kidney-Essence produces Marrow which gathers to fill the Brain and spinal cord. Since Marrow originates from the Kidneys, the Brain is functionally related to this Yin organ. The brain also depends on the Heart, particularly Heart-Blood, for its nourishment, so that the physiological activities of the Brain depend on the state of Kidneys and Heart. The Kidneys store Essence and the Heart governs Blood: if both Essence and Blood are abundant, the brain is in good health, vitality is good, the ears can hear properly and the eyes can see clearly. If Kidney-Essence and Heart-Blood are empty, the Brain is sluggish, memory is poor, vitality is low, hearing and sight may be decreased. The relationship of the Brain with Kidneys and Heart explains how in practice certain symptoms such as poor memory and concentration, dizziness and blurred vision can be due to deficiency of the Sea of Marrow (i.e. the Kidneys) or deficiency of Heart-Blood.

The "Spiritual Axis" in chapter 33 says: *"If the Sea of Marrow is abundant, the vitality is good, the body feels light and agile and the span of life will be long; if it is deficient, there will be dizziness, tinnitus, blurred vision, fatigue and great desire to lie down"*.[6]

MARROW

"Marrow", the common matrix of Bone-marrow and Brain, is produced by the Kidney-Essence, it fills the Brain and spinal cord and forms Bone-marrow. The "Spiritual Axis" in chapter 36 says: *"The refined essence of food is changed into fat, it enters the bone cavities and fills the Brain with Marrow"*.[7]

The Chinese concept of "Marrow" should not be confused with bone-marrow as defined by Western Medicine. In Chinese Medicine, the function of Marrow is to nourish the Brain and spinal cord and to form Bone-Marrow. The "Simple Questions" in chapter 17 says: *"The bones are the residence of Marrow"*.[8]

Marrow is closely related to the Kidneys as the Kidney- Essence is the origin of Marrow. The "Simple Questions" in chapter 34 says: *"If the Kidneys are deficient, Marrow cannot be abundant"*.[9]

THE BONES

The Bones, like all the other Extraordinary Yang Organs, are also related to the Kidneys. They are considered one of the Extraordinary Yang Organs because they store Bone-Marrow. If Kidney-Essence and Marrow are deficient, the Bones lose nourishment, cannot sustain the body and there will be inability to walk or stand.

In clinical practice, the relationship between Kidneys and Bones can be exploited, by treating the Kidneys to speed up the healing of bone fractures.

THE BLOOD VESSELS

Blood vessels are considered one of the Extraordinary Yang Organs because they contain Blood. They are also indirectly related to the Kidneys because Kidney-Essence produces Marrow which contributes to producing Blood, and the Original Qi of the Kidneys also contributes to the transformation of the Food-Qi into Blood.

THE GALL BLADDER

The Gall Bladder is considered one of the Extraordinary Yang Organs because, unlike other Yang organs, it stores bile, which is a "pure" fluid. There is no particular significance in the Gall Bladder being one of the Extraordinary Yang Organs and its functions are the same as those of the Gall Bladder as an ordinary Yang organ which have already been discussed.

NOTES

1 Simple Question, p 77
2 1978 Fundamentals of Chinese Medicine (*Zhong Yi Ji Chu Xue* 中医基础学) Shandong Scientific Publishing House, Jinan.
3 Spiritual Axis, p 73.
4 Simple Question, p72.
5 Li Dong Yuan 1249 Discussion on Stomach and Spleen (*Pi Wei Lun* 脾胃论) cited in Concise Dictionary of Chinese Medicine, p 712.
6 Spiritual Axis, p 73.
7 Ibid. p 77.
8 Simple Question, p 100.
9 Ibid., p 198.

The Causes of Disease 15

病因

Identifying the cause of the patient's disharmony is an important part of Chinese medical practice. It is important not to consider the presenting disharmony as the cause of disease. For instance, if a person has loose stools, tiredness and no appetite, Spleen-Qi deficiency is not the cause of the disease, but simply an expression of the presenting disharmony. The cause of the disharmony itself is to be found in the person's dietary habits, life-style, exercise habits, etc.

Identifying the cause of the disharmony is important because, only by doing that, can we advise the patient on how to avoid it, minimize it or prevent its re-occurrence.

Chinese Medicine stresses balance as a key to health: balance between rest and exercise, balance in diet, balance in sexual activity, balance in climate. Any long-term imbalance can become a cause of disease. For example, too much rest (not enough exercise) or too much physical exercise, too much work, too much sex or not enough sex, an unbalanced diet, an unbalanced emotional life, extreme climatic conditions, can all become causes of disease. This balance is relative to each person. What is too much exercise for someone, may not be enough for another; what may constitute over-eating for someone engaged in mental work in a sedentary job, could be too little food to sustain someone engaged in heavy physical work.

We should not, therefore, have in mind an ideal and rigid state of balance to which each patient should conform. It is important (and sometimes difficult) to make an assessment of the person's constitution and body-mind condition and relate these to their diet, life-style and climatic conditions.

Identifying the cause of the disharmony is necessary otherwise it will not be possible to advise the patient on specific changes which will restore harmony. If a person suffers from abdominal pain and distension from stagnation of Liver-Qi very evidently caused by emotional problems, there is no point in subjecting him or her to very strict diets in order to avoid the abdominal pain. This would only add to the person's misery. On the other hand, if a person suffers from pain in the hands and wrists from exterior Damp-Cold caused by a lifetime of hard work cleaning and washing things in cold water, there is no point in delving deeply into his or her emotional life.

There is a saying in Chinese Medicine that goes :"*Examine the pattern to seek the cause*". This means that, generally speaking, the cause of the disease is found by examination of the pattern rather than by interrogation. This is because the nature of the pattern is often related to its specific cause of disease. This is especially true for the exterior, climatic causes of disease. If a person displays all the symptoms of an exterior attack of Wind-Heat, then we can say that Wind-Heat is the cause of the disease, no matter what climate the person was exposed to. In other words, identification of the cause (Wind-Heat) is achieved on the basis of the pattern, not the history.

In other cases, interrogation is necessary to identify the cause of disease. For example, if a person suffers from stagnation of Liver-Qi, we cannot know whether this is from emotional causes or from diet.

In trying to find a cause of the disease, it is convenient and useful to think of a person's life in three periods:

— the pre-natal period
— from birth to about 18
— adult life.[1]

Differing causes of disease tend to characterize each of these three periods, whilst within each of these three time spans, a person is likely to be affected by similar aetiological factors. For example, if a disease started during early childhood, it is very frequently due to dietary factors as the digestive system of new-born babies is very vulnerable.

Thus, if we can pin-point the beginning of the disharmony, we can have a first hint of what the likely cause might be.

1 *The pre-natal period*

Chinese Medicine stresses the importance of the parents' health in general, and at the time of conception specifically, for the health of the child. If the parents conceive when too old, or in poor health, the constitution of their child will be weak. This may also be the case if the mother suffered ill health or took excessive drugs during pregnancy.

If a mother suffers a shock during pregnancy, the health of the baby may be affected. This may manifest with a bluish tinge on the forehead and chin of the child and a Moving pulse (this is a pulse that is rapid, "trembles" and feels as if it is shaped like a bean).

2 *Childhood*

This is the period from birth to the teen-age years. A frequent cause of disease in early childhood is diet. Weaning a baby too early (as the tendency is more and more today) may cause Spleen deficiency. Feeding a child too much cow's milk may cause Dampness or Phlegm.

Emotions can be a cause of disease in childhood although in a slightly different way than for adults. Young children (under six) tend not to restrain their emotions, as they freely express them.

Children do suffer from emotional problems, but these are often caused by family situations, such as strain between the parents, a too strict upbringing, too demanding parents, too much pressure at school. All these situations can leave their mark on a child's psyche and be the cause for negative emotional patterns later in life. For example, headaches starting during childhood are often seen in bright children who are pushed too much by the parents to do well at school.

Accidents, traumas and falls are common causes of disease in childhood that can cause problems later in life. For example, a fall on the head in early childhood may cause headaches later, when another cause of disease is superimposed on the early one.

Excessive physical exercise at the time of puberty can cause menstrual problems in girls later in life, whilst too early sexual activity can cause urinary problems or painful periods in girls.

There are certain periods of life that are important watersheds as far as health is concerned: these are puberty for both sexes and, for women, childbirth and menopause. Particular care needs to be taken at those times, as they are important and delicate gateways when the body and mind are changing rapidly. The example of excessive physical exercise and sexual activity during puberty has already been mentioned. Childbirth, is a very important time for a woman: it is a time when she can be considerably weakened, but also strengthened if she takes care. For example, if a woman resumes work too soon after childbirth, this may seriously weaken the Spleen and

Kidneys. On the other hand, if she takes care to rest after childbirth, eat nourishing food and perhaps take herbal tonics, she can actually strengthen a previously weak constitution.

3 Adult life

Any of the usual causes of disease apply in this long period, paramount among them, emotional ones.

The causes of disease are usually divided into internal, external and others:

Internal: emotions
External: weather
Others: constitution, fatigue/over-exertion, excessive sexual activity, diet, trauma, epidemics, parasites and poisons, wrong treatment.

These are the causes of disease traditionally considered in Chinese Medicine. In our times we obviously have many new causes of disease which did not exist in the times when Chinese Medicine developed. For example, radiation, pollution or chemicals in food. In practice it is important to keep these new causes in mind as possible causes of disease, and it might therefore be necessary in certain cases to integrate Chinese diagnosis with other Western diagnostic tests to find the cause of the disease.

INTERNAL CAUSES

The view of the Internal Organs as physical-mental-emotional spheres of influence is one of the most important aspects of Chinese Medicine. Central to this is the concept of Qi as a matter-energy that gives rise to physical or mental and emotional phenomena at the same time. Thus, in Chinese Medicine, body, mind and emotions are an integrated whole with no beginning or end, in which the Internal Organs are the major sphere of influence.

For example, the "Kidneys" correspond to the actual kidney organ on an anatomical level, to the energies associated with the Kidneys on an energetic level, to the brain and thinking on a mental level, and to fear on an emotional level. All these levels simultaneously interact with each other.

This is one of the differences between Chinese and Western Medicine. While Western Medicine also recognizes the interaction between body and emotions, it does so in a completely different way than Chinese Medicine. In Western Medicine, the brain is at the top of the body-mind pyramid. The emotions affect the limbic system within the brain, nerve impulses travel down the hypothalamus, through to the sympathetic and parasympathetic nerve centres, finally reaching the internal organs. Thus a nerve impulse, triggered off by an emotional upset, is transmitted to the relevant organ.

The view of Chinese Medicine is entirely different. The body-mind is not a pyramid, but a circle of interaction between the Internal Organs and their emotional aspects.

Whereas Western Medicine tends to consider the influence of emotions on the organs as having a secondary or excitatory role rather than being a primary causative factor of disease, Chinese Medicine sees the emotions as an integral and inseparable part of the sphere of action of the Internal Organs.

The interaction of body and mind in Chinese Medicine is also expressed in the three "Treasures" Essence-Qi-Mind (see ch. 3). Essence is the material basis of Qi and Mind forming the foundation for a happy and balanced mental and emotional life.

It is important to put the role of the emotions in Chinese Medicine in perspective. First of all, emotions are a natural part of human existence and no human being ever escapes being sad, angry or worried sometimes. The emotions only become causes of disease when they are particularly intense and, most of all, when they are prolonged over a long period of time, especially when they are not expressed or acknowledged. Everyone is angry sometimes, but if someone harbours anger towards another person for years, this emotion becomes a cause of disease.

Secondly, Chinese Medicine is only concerned with the emotions when these are either the cause of disease, or when they themselves are the presenting symptoms. In other words, Chinese Medicine neither ignores the emotions as causes of disease, nor places too much emphasis on them to the exclusion of other causes.

Since the body and mind form an integrated and inseparable unit, the emotions can not only cause a disharmony, but they can also be caused by it. For example, a state of fear and anxiety over a long period of time may cause the Kidneys to become deficient; on the other hand, if the Kidneys become deficient through, say, having too many children too close together, this may cause a state of fear and anxiety. It is important, in practice, to be able to distinguish these two cases, as we should be able to advise and guide the patient. Patients are often reassured to know that their emotional state has a physical basis, or vice versa, that their disturbing physical symptoms are caused by their emotions. If we can make this distinction, then we can treat the disharmony properly and advise the patient accordingly.

Seven emotions are usually considered in Chinese Medicine, but this need not be interpreted too restrictively. The seven emotions are broad headings under which many other emotions can be included. This will be clarified and expanded on when discussing the emotions individually.

The seven emotions are:

Anger
Joy
Worry
Pensiveness
Sadness
Fear
Shock.

Each of the emotions has a particular effect on Qi and affects a certain organ:

— Anger makes Qi rise and affects the Liver
— Joy slows Qi down and affects the Heart
— Worry and Pensiveness knot Qi and affect the Spleen (Worry also affects the Lungs)
— Sadness dissolves Qi and affects the Lungs
— Fear makes Qi descend and affects the Kidneys
— Shock scatters Qi and affects the Kidneys and Heart.

Most of the emotions can, over a long period of time, give rise to Fire. There is a saying in Chinese Medicine: "The five emotions can turn into Fire". This is because most of the emotions can cause stagnation of Qi and when Qi is compressed in this way over a period of time it creates Fire, just as the temperature of a gas increases when its pressure is increased.

For this reason, when someone has suffered from emotional problems for a long time, there often are signs of Heat, which may be in the Liver, Heart, Lungs or Kidneys (Empty-Heat). This often shows on the tongue which becomes red or dark red and dry, and possibly has a red and swollen tip.

Finally, it should be mentioned here that in cases of severe and long-standing emotional problems, acupuncture alone may not be enough, and the patient may need the help and support of a skilled psychotherapist or counsellor.

ANGER

The term "anger", perhaps more than any of the other emotions, should be interpreted very broadly, to include several other allied emotional states, such as resentment, repressed anger, irritability, frustration, rage, indignation, animosity or bitterness.

Any of these emotional states can affect the Liver, if they persist for a long time, causing stagnation of Liver-Qi or Blood, rising of Liver-Yang or blazing of Liver-Fire. These are the three most common Liver disharmonies arising out of the above emotional problems.

Anger (intended in the broad sense outlined above) makes Qi rise and many of the symptoms and signs will manifest in the head and neck, such as headaches, tinnitus, dizziness, red blotches on the front part of the neck, a red face, thirst, a Red tongue and a bitter taste. One of the most common symptoms caused by anger is headache.

The "Simple Questions" in chapter 39 says: *"Anger makes Qi rise and causes vomiting of Blood and diarrhoea"*.[2] It causes vomiting of Blood because it makes Liver-Qi and Liver-Fire rise and it causes diarrhoea because it causes Liver-Qi to invade the Spleen.

Of course, someone who is angry may not

always display these symptoms, and he or she may appear subdued, depressed and pale. In particular, long-standing mental depression is often due to inner repressed anger or resentment. The state that one would associate with a depressed person judging by the appearance would be sadness, but, in fact, this is often not the case. When anger rather than sadness is the problem the tongue will be found to be red or dark-red and dry and the pulse Wiry (these two signs contradicting the appearance of the person). This depression is most likely due to long-standing resentment, often harboured towards a member of that person's family.

Anger often affects the Stomach and Spleen as well as the Liver. This can be due to stagnant Liver-Qi invading Stomach and Spleen. Such a condition is more likely to occur if someone gets angry at meal times. This is unfortunately a regular occurrence in certain families, when members of the family only meet at meal-times, and these become an occasion for family rows.

JOY

This term should also be interpreted broadly. Obviously joy is not in itself a cause of disease. In fact, the "Simple Questions" in chapter 39 says: *"Joy makes the Mind peaceful and relaxed, it benefits the Nutritive and Defensive Qi and it makes Qi relax and slow down"*.[3]

The "Simple Questions" in chapter 2 says: *"The Heart ... controls Joy, Joy injures the Heart, Fear counteracts Joy"*.[4]

What is meant here by "joy" is obviously not a state of healthy contentment but one of excessive excitement which can injure the Heart. In order to understand this, one can think of the fairly frequent situation when a migraine attack can be precipitated by a sudden excitement from good news.[5]

Joy can become a cause of disease when it is excessive as in those persons who are in a state of continuous mental stimulation (however pleasurable) or excessive excitement. In other words, a life of "hard playing". This leads to excessive stimulation of the Heart and, in time, can lead to Heart-Fire or Heart Empty-Heat, depending on the underlying condition.

SADNESS

This weakens the Lungs, but it also affects the Heart. In fact, according to the "Simple Questions", sadness affects the Lungs via the Heart. It says in chapter 39: *"Sadness makes the Heart cramped and agitated, this pushes towards the lungs' lobes, the Upper Burner becomes obstructed, Nutritive and Defensive Qi cannot circulate freely, Heat accumulates and dissolves Qi"*.[6]

According to this passage then, sadness primarily affects the Heart and the Lungs suffer in consequence since heart and lungs are both in the Upper Burner.

The Lungs govern Qi and sadness depletes Qi. This is often manifested on the pulse with a weakness of both Front positions (Heart and Lungs). In particular, the pulse has no "wave" and does not flow smoothly towards the thumb.

Sadness leads to deficiency of Lung-Qi and may manifest in a variety of symptoms, such as breathlessness, tiredness, depression or crying. In women, deficiency of Lung-Qi often leads to Blood deficiency and amenorrhoea.

Case history

A woman of 63 complained of anxiety, depression, sweating at night, feeling of heat in palms and chest and insomnia (waking up several times during the night). The tongue was dry and slightly peeled. The pulse was Floating-Empty especially in the Front position and without wave.

On interrogation, it transpired that all the symptoms appeared after three deaths in the family in a short space of time (of mother, father and husband).

In this case the profound sadness had "dissolved" Lung-Qi and, after some time, this developed into Lung-Yin deficiency. This was apparent from the night sweating, the Floating-Empty pulse, the feeling of heat of palms and chest and the slightly peeled tongue.

WORRY AND PENSIVENESS

Pensiveness means excessive thinking, excessive mental work or studying. This weakens the

Spleen and causes tiredness, loss of appetite and loose stools.

This is a very common cause of disease in our society, both in young people of school or university age, and adults in demanding intellectual occupations. Very often the Spleen deficiency induced by excessive mental work leads to impairment of the Spleen function of transformation and transportation and the formation of Phlegm. This is all the more likely if the person also has irregular meals or eats quickly at work, or discusses work while eating.

Worry depletes and knots both the Spleen and Lungs. Worry is also an extremely common emotion in our society. Different people worry about different things but life in industrialized societies is fraught with worry-inducing situations, such as financial worries, precariousness of employment, family worries.

Worry depletes Spleen-Qi causing much the same kind of damage as excessive mental work. Worry also knots Lung-Qi leading to anxiety, breathlessness and stiffness of the shoulders and neck. The breathlessness is the physical manifestation of the constraint of the Corporeal Soul induced by constant worrying. Many patients present with raised or arched shoulders and stiff neck with shallow breathing, typical of knotted Lung-Qi caused by chronic worry.

FEAR

Fear depletes Kidney-Qi, and it makes Qi descend. The "Simple Questions" in chapter 39 says: *"Fear depletes the Essence, it blocks the Upper Burner, which makes Qi descend to the Lower Burner"*.[7]

In my opinion, however, fear has a different effect in children and adults. In children, it makes Qi descend causing nocturnal enuresis. This common problem in children is often caused by fear or a feeling of insecurity in the child due to some family situation.

In adults, however, fear and chronic anxiety more often cause deficiency of Kidney-Yin and rising of Empty-Heat within the Heart, with a feeling of heat in the face, night sweating, palpitations and a dry mouth and throat.

SHOCK

Mental shock suspends Qi and affects the Heart and Kidneys. It suddenly depletes Heart-Qi and can lead to palpitations, breathlessness and insomnia. It is often reflected in the pulse with a so-called "Moving" pulse, i.e. a pulse that is short, slightly slippery and rapid and which "vibrates" as it pulsates.

The "Simple Questions" in chapter 39 says: *"Shock affects the Heart depriving it of residence, the Mind has no shelter and cannot rest, so that Qi becomes chaotic"*.[8]

Shock also affects the Kidneys because the body uses the Essence of the Kidneys to supplement the sudden depletion of Qi. For this reason, shock can cause such symptoms as night sweating, a dry mouth, dizziness or tinnitus.

EXTERNAL CAUSES

The external causes of disease are due to climatic factors, which are:

Wind
Cold
Summer-Heat
Dampness
Dryness
Fire.

They were called *"The Six Climates Excessively Victorious"*, and usually now called the *"Six Excesses"*. They are closely related to the weather and the seasons.

Under normal circumstances, the weather will have no pathological effect on the body, as this can adequately protect itself against exterior pathogenic factors. The weather only becomes a cause of disease when the equilibrium between the body and the environment breaks down, either because the weather is unseasonably excessive (for instance too cold in summertime or too hot in wintertime), or because the body is weak in relation to the climatic factor. Either way, one can say that climatic factors only become a cause of disease when the body is weak in relation to them. It is important to stress here that the body is only relatively weak, in relation to the climatic factor, not necessarily fundamentally weak. In other words, one does not need to be very weak to be invaded by exterior pathogenic factors. A relatively healthy person can also be attacked by exterior pathogenic factors, if they are stronger in relation to the body's energies at that particular time. So, the relative strength of climatic factors and Defensive Qi is all-important.

Climatic factors differ somewhat from other causes of disease, in so far as they denote both causes and patterns of disease. When we say that a certain condition is due to exterior attack of Wind-Heat, we are saying two things: firstly, that exterior Wind-Heat has caused it and secondly, that it manifests as Wind-Heat. In clinical practice, these descriptions are more important as expressions of pathological conditions than aetiological factors. For example, if a person has symptoms of a sore throat, sneezing, aversion to cold, slight sweating, tonsillitis, thirst, and a Floating-Rapid pulse, we can certainly diagnose an exterior invasion of Wind-Heat. This diagnosis is not made on the basis of interrogation, but through analysis of the symptoms and signs. In other words, if a person has the above symptoms and signs, these are Wind-Heat. We do not need to ask the patient whether he or she had been exposed to a hot wind in the hours previous to the arising of those symptoms. Hence, from this point of view, "Wind-Heat" indicates a pathological pattern, rather than an aetiological factor.

However, actual climatic elements do have a direct influence on the human body giving rise to the clinical manifestations observed by Chinese doctors over many centuries.

The underlying condition of the person also determines the type of exterior pattern that will arise. A person with tendency to Heat will most likely display symptoms of Wind-Heat if he or she is invaded by exterior Wind. On the other hand, a person with a tendency to deficiency of Yang will display symptoms of Wind-Cold if he or she is attacked by exterior Wind. This explains how one can have symptoms of Wind-Heat in the middle of the coldest Winter, or symptoms of Wind-Cold in the middle of the most torrid Summer.

Man-made climates can also cause disease. Air-conditioning can cause symptoms of attack of exterior Wind. For example, if someone enters an air-conditioned place coming from very hot outdoors, the person's skin pores will be open (from sweating) and the skin therefore more vulnerable to attack of Wind. The excessive heat and dryness of some centrally-heated places can cause symptoms of attack of Wind-Heat. Certain occupations are also prone to cause illness from exposure to artificial climates: for example those in the catering business who have to enter large refrigerated store-rooms many times a day, steel workers who are exposed to very high temperatures at work or cooks who spend the whole day in very hot kitchens. Climatic factors also include what the Chinese call exterior "Epidemic pathogenic factors". These are not qualitatively different from other climatic factors, but they are infectious and are often more virulent. They are usually associated with Heat and are called "Epidemic-Heat". In these cases, the exterior pathogenic factor is so strong that the majority of members or a community fall ill. Even in these cases, however, the strength of the body's Qi in relation to the pathogenic factor plays a role in the resistance to disease, as not all members of the community ever fall ill.

It is sometimes said that external climatic causes of disease do not affect people in affluent industrialized countries as people in these countries can afford better housing than in China. This is not entirely true because there are also pockets of poor housing in affluent industrialized countries where people have to contend with cold and damp conditions. In addition, due to the dictates of fashion, many people in industrialized countries display remarkably little common sense when it comes to dressing properly to protect oneself against climatic factors. In fact people often dress more appropriately and sensibly in China than in Western countries. As already discussed, the very improvement in housing in industrialized countries can in itself lead to exterior diseases as in the case of air-conditioning or excessive heat and dryness from central heating.

Exterior pathogenic factors enter the body either via the skin or via the nose and mouth. Chinese Medicine holds that exterior Heat is most likely to invade the body via the nose and mouth. This idea was developed during the late Ming dynasty by Dr Wu You Ke. When the pathogenic factor is in the skin or muscles, it is said to be in the Exterior energetic layers of the body and the resulting pattern of clinical manifestations is called an "exterior pattern". The definition of "exterior" is arrived at on the basis of the location of the pathogenic factor, not the aetiology. In other words a pattern is not called "exterior" because it is caused by an exterior pathogenic factor, but because the pathogenic factor is located in skin and muscles, i.e. the "Exterior" of the body. If an exterior pathogenic factor penetrates deeper to affect the internal organs (i.e. the "Interior"), the resulting pattern of clinical manifestations is defined as an "interior pattern", even though in this case it was caused by an exterior pathogenic factor.

Although exterior pathogenic factors usually invade the skin and muscles first (the Exterior of the body), the internal organs can also be affected to a certain extent, particularly if there is a pre-existing disharmony in a given organ. Each organ has a specific aversion to a certain climate. The "Simple Questions" in chapter 23 says: *"The Heart loathes heat, the Lungs loathe cold, the Liver loathes wind, the Spleen loathes dampness and the Kidneys loathe dryness"*.[9] This is in partial contradiction to statements in other books, where it is said that the Lungs loathe dryness and the Kidneys loathe cold.

Each of the six climatic factors is associated with a certain season during which it is more prevalent, i.e.

Wind-Spring
Heat-Summer
Dryness-Autumn
Cold-Winter
Dampness-Late Summer
Fire-Summer.

In fact, any of the climatic factors can arise in any season: it is not at all uncommon to have attacks of Wind-Heat in winter or Wind-Cold in summer. Living conditions also determine which climatic factor invades the body. For example, living in a damp house will cause invasion of exterior Damp irrespective of the season.

Once inside the body, exterior pathogenic factors can completely change their nature. For example, Wind-Cold can turn into Heat, Dampness can easily generate Heat, Fire and Heat can cause Dryness while extreme Heat can give rise to Wind.

Finally, some internally-generated pathogenic factors give rise to clinical manifestations which are similar to those caused by exterior climatic factors. For this reason, these will be discussed together.

Each of the climatic factors causes certain clinical manifestations which are typical of that particular climate. An experienced practitioner of Chinese Medicine will be able to infer the cause of the disease from the manifestations.

For example, exterior Wind causes symptoms and signs to arise suddenly and change rapidly.

Cold contracts and causes pain and watery discharges. Dampness invades the body gradually and causes turbid, sticky discharges. Dryness obviously dries the Body Fluids. Heat and Fire give rise to sensations of heat, thirst and mental restlessness.

Although the climatic causes of disease are important, in practice, exterior pathogenic factors such as Wind-Heat or Wind-Cold are clinically relevant as patterns of disharmony rather than causes. In other words, although the cause of a Wind-Heat pattern may be said to be in some cases climatic wind and heat, it is the pattern of Wind-Heat which is clinically significant and requiring treatment. For this reason, the clinical manifestations of these exterior pathogenic factors are discussed in the chapter on the Identification of Patterns according to Pathogenic Factors (see p. 293).

OTHER CAUSES OF DISEASE

The other causes of disease are:
— weak constitution
— over-exertion
— excessive sexual activity
— bad diet
— trauma
— parasites and poisons
— wrong treatment.

WEAK CONSTITUTION

Every person is born with a certain constitution which is dependent on the parents' health in general and their health at the time of conception specifically. It is also dependent on the mother's health during pregnancy.

The fusion of the parents' sexual essences at conception gives rise to a human being whose constitution is, to a large extent, determined at that time. The fetus is nourished by its Pre-Heaven Essence which is the determinant of that individual's constitution. By and large, the constitution of a human being cannot be changed: the immense power and stamina of certain of today's athletes is not only a matter of training but also of constitution, and those who are born with a relatively weak constitution can never hope to attain those outstanding athletic abilities. However, a person's constitution is not entirely fixed and immutable. It can be changed and improved within certain limits. A healthy and balanced life-style, together with breathing exercise to develop one's Qi, can lead to an improvement in one's constitution. As we know, the Essence, which is the basis of our inner strength and health, is not immutable, but is constantly replenished by Qi. Whilst it is quite easy to weaken one's constitution through inadequate rest, excessive work or excessive sexual activity, by taking care to achieve a balance in one's life it is possible to some extent to build up a weak constitution.

The broad field of Chinese Medicine (including breathing exercises and certain forms of martial arts of the "inner school" such as Tai Ji Quan), attaches great importance to the preservation of one's Essence and Qi and therefore the cultivation of one's constitution. This aim is implicit in the philosophy of and treatment by acupuncture and Chinese herbal medicine as well as the practice of traditional breathing exercises. These practices and ideas have their origin in the ancient Daoist preoccupation with longevity and immortality. Due to the Daoist masters research into herbal remedies, acupuncture and breathing exercises to attain "immortality" or longevity, we now have a rich inheritance of herbal and acupuncture treatments as well as breathing exercises aimed at strengthening a weak constitution.

The causes of poor constitution are to be found either in the parents' health in general, or in the parents' health at the time of conception. According to Chinese Medicine, if a woman conceives when she is too old, the child is more likely to have a poor constitution. Also, if she consumes alcohol or smokes during the pregnancy, this will adversely affect the child's constitution. The Chinese also believe this to be the case if the parents conceive in a state of drunkenness.

A severe shock to the mother during pregnancy will affect the constitution of the baby, particularly its Heart. This is often manifested with a bluish tinge on the forehead and on the chin.

The constitution of a person can be assessed by examining their history, pulse, face and tongue. A history of many childhood diseases, and in particularly whooping cough, indicates a weak constitution. Whooping cough in particular, is often indicative of an inherited weakness of the Lungs. An inherited weakness of the Lungs, or tendency to Lung diseases (especially Lung tuberculosis) in the family, is often manifested by two signs: a pulse in the Front position (either side or both) which can be felt going medially up towards the thenar eminence, and one or two cracks on the tongue in the Lung area (Fig. 48).

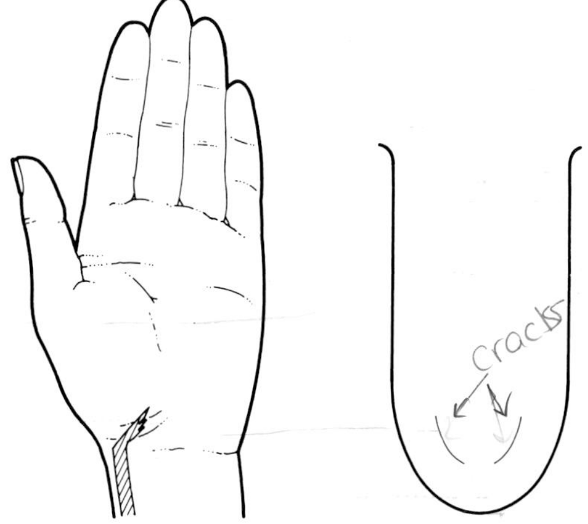

Fig. 48 Pulse and Tongue signs indicating weak Lungs

The face can show constitutional weaknesses especially the ears. Very small ears with short ear lobes show weak constitution.

A Scattered, Minute or Leather pulse (see p. 170) and a very Flabby tongue without "spirit" (see p. 150), are also indicative of a poor constitution.

An assessment of the constitution of a person is useful in clinical practice to make a realistic prognosis. It is always important to have a clear idea of what one can realistically expect to achieve with the treatment, and, more important, to advise patients with poor constitution about diet, proper rest, sexual activity and breathing exercises.

OVER-EXERTION

Over-exertion is a common cause of disease in Western societies. A proper balance between work/exercise and rest is obviously essential to health, and yet the overwhelming majority of people exceed in one direction or the other, taking too much or too little exercise, working too much and failing to take adequate rest.

The question of balance between activity and rest affects Qi directly. Whenever we work or exercise we are using up Qi; whenever we rest, Qi is restored.

There are actually two levels of Qi to be considered here. First there is the Essence which, being the foundation of our fundamental inner energy and vitality, determines our stamina and resistance to disease. Essence relates to long cycles (7 or 8 years) and so is only slowly affected by daily activities. On the other hand, Qi (the Post-Heaven Qi) which is formed by the Stomach and Spleen from food on a daily basis, and is constantly replenished, provides the energy for our daily activities.

In our daily activities of work and exercise, we normally use Qi, whilst Essence provides the physiological basis for long-term changes. Under normal circumstances, the Qi used up in normal work and exercise is quickly restored by proper diet and rest. If we take the pulse of a person who has been working very hard for a week, perhaps working towards exams, and who has been staying up until the early hours of the morning and eating poorly, the pulse will probably be very weak and deep. We may draw wrong conclusions from the pulse if we do not integrate this finding with the facts gleaned from the interrogation together with clues given by the appearance of the patient and observation of the tongue. In fact, if this person has adequate rest and a good diet, the pulse will return to normal in about two or three days. This shows that while Qi can be quickly used up, it can equally be rapidly restored by rest.

If, however, one works extremely hard and for very long hours over many months or years without adequate rest, then the body has no chance of restoring Qi fast enough: before it has made up the lost Qi, the person is working again, using up more Qi. When one overworks beyond the point that Qi can keep up with the demands, then one is forced to draw on the Essence to face the demands of this life-style. At this point, the Essence will begin to be depleted and symptoms of deficiency of Yin may appear. When this point is reached, even adequate rest will not help the situation very quickly, but only over a long period of time.

There are three types of over-exertion to be considered:

— mental overwork
— physical overwork
— excessive physical exercise.

1 Mental overwork

This type is extremely common in our fast, competitive and materialistic society. By mental overwork is meant working long hours in an intellectual occupation under conditions of stress. People may be driven to work very hard and very long hours in conditions of stress for various reasons. These could be poverty, greed, ambition or power hunger. Whatever the cause, working long hours eating irregular meals, working in condition of extreme stress, being always in a hurry, all these situations over a long period of time lead to exhaustion of Qi. They particularly tend to affect Stomach, Spleen and Kidneys. These conditions of work are usually associated with a very irregular diet which will tend to cause deficiency of Stomach-Qi or Stomach-Yin. Excessive mental work and concentration weakens the Spleen. Deficiency of Stomach-Yin in these conditions can eventually lead to Kidney-Yin deficiency.

2 Physical overwork

Physical overwork depletes mostly Spleen-Qi, as the Spleen dominates the muscles. Excessive use of one part of the body will also cause stagnation of Qi in that particular part. For example the constant repetitive movement which may be associated with a certain job, will tend to cause stagnation of Qi in that part. For example, the aching arm of a hairdresser or the aching elbow of a brick-layer.

Excessive lifting, as it happens so much in the building trade, weakens the Kidneys and the lower back.

Excessive standing also weakens the Kidneys. The "Simple Questions" in chapter 23 talks about the "five exhaustions": "*Excessive use of the eyes injures the Blood [i.e. the Heart]; excessive lying down injures Qi [i.e. the Lungs]; excessive sitting injures the muscles [i.e. the Spleen]; excessive standing injures the bones [i.e. the Kidneys]; excessive exercise injures the sinews [i.e. the Liver]*".[10]

3 Excessive physical exercise

A reasonable amount of exercise is of course beneficial and essential to good health. But exercise carried out to the point of exhaustion will deplete Qi. Excessive exercise is particularly harmful if carried out during puberty, especially for girls, who may later develop menstrual problems.

Certain types of exercise may also cause stagnation of Qi in a particular area. Weight-lifting affects the lower back, jogging the knees and tennis the elbows.

Lack of exercise is also a cause of disease. Regular exercise is essential for a proper circulation of Qi. Lack of exercise will lead to stagnation of Qi and, in some cases, Dampness. In particular, Oriental types of exercise such as Yoga or Tai Ji Quan aimed at developing Qi rather than just the muscles, are very beneficial and should be recommended to patients suffering from deficiency of Qi who do not have enough energy to undertake Western-type exercises.

EXCESSIVE SEXUAL ACTIVITY

Since ancient times in China excessive sexual activity has been considered a cause of disease because it tends to deplete the Kidney Essence. In the West, excessive sexual activity is hardly ever thought to be detrimental to health.

By "excessive sexual activity" is meant actual ejaculation for men and orgasm for women. Sexual activities not culminating in orgasm are not thought to be depleting to the Kidney Essence.

The sexual essences of both men and women are the outwards manifestation of the Kidney Essence. For this reason, the loss of these sexual essences leads to a temporary loss of Kidney-Essence. Under normal circumstances, however, this loss is quickly made up, and normal sexual activity does not lead to disease. It is only when it is excessive that the loss of Essence caused by sex is such that the body does not have time to recuperate and restore the Essence.

Of course, it is impossible to say what "normal" sexual activity is as this is entirely relative and dependent on the person's constitution and strength of Essence. What may constitute "excess sex" for a person with weak Kidneys, may be normal to another and vice versa. One can, however define sexual activity as "excessive" if it results in marked fatigue, and even more so if it causes certain other specific symptoms, such as dizziness, blurred vision, a lower back ache, weak knees and frequent urination. The important thing to realize is that sexual activity should be adjusted according to age, physical condition and even the seasons.

Sexual activity ought to be adjusted according to one's age, an idea which is often totally alien to most people in our society. The book "Classic of the Simple Girl" (Sui dynasty 581–618) gives an indication of recommended frequency of ejaculation for men according to age and health condition.[11]

Age	*In good health*	*Average health*
15	2x/day	Once/day
20	2x/day	Once/day
30	Once/day	Every other day
40	Every 3 days	Every 4 days
50	Every 5 days	Every 10 days
60	Every 10 days	Every 20 days
70	Every 30 days	None

Of course, this should not be taken literally, but only as a broad guideline.

Sexual activity should obviously be reduced if there is a deficiency of Qi or Blood, and particularly a deficiency of the Kidneys.

Finally, sexual activity should also be adjusted according to seasons, increasing in Spring and declining in Winter.

Although these "rules" should be interpreted loosely, as practitioners of Chinese Medicine, we should be able to advise our patients on this question.

In my practice I have seen patients who were engaging in levels of sexual activity which could not be described as "normal" by any standard and yet were totally astounded when the idea was suggested that their sexual activity might have something to do with their problems.

In fact, many sexual problems, such as impotence or premature ejaculation often require first of all, a decrease in sexual activity, if there is to be any chance of successful treatment.

Although excessive sexual activity affects both men and women, to a certain extent it affects men more, as women recover more quickly after it.

There are also some important differences between men and women's genital physiology from a Chinese medical perspective. It could be said that men's sexual energy is more directly related to the Kidney-Essence, whereas women's sexual energy is more directly related to Blood. The Red Field (*Dan Tian*) in men contains the Room of Essence, whereas in women it contains the Uterus.[12] It follows that ejaculation is a more direct loss of Kidney-Essence than orgasm is for women (even though there is some loss of Essence in women too). In women the Uterus is directly related to the Kidneys and any factor that weakens the Uterus eventually weakens the Kidneys, particularly Kidney-Yin. In particular, too many childbirths in too short a time, weaken the Uterus and the Kidneys in women. This is an important cause of depletion of Kidney Essence in women, somewhat equivalent to excessive sexual activity in men.

Chinese Medicine also considers the circumstances in which sexual activity takes place. For example, having sexual intercourse in a state of drunkenness is considered extremely harmful to any resulting fetus. Catching cold after sexual intercourse can severely weaken Kidney-Yang. As the energy of the Kidneys is temporarily weakened after intercourse, it is important not to be exposed to cold at this time.

Chinese Medicine also considers lack of sex as a cause of disease, even though this will never be mentioned in modern China. The "Classic of the Simple Girl" gives certain guidelines as to what the minimum recommended frequency of ejaculation should be according to age, such as every 4 days for a 20-year-old, every 8 days for a 30-year-old, every 16 days for a 40-year-old, every 21 days for a 50-year-old and every 30 days for a 60-year-old.[13] Of course, these guidelines too should not be taken literally either.

Sexual desire itself is also related to the Kidney energy. A healthy sexual desire reflects a good and strong Kidney energy. If the Kidneys are weak, and if, in particular Kidney-Yang is deficient, there may be a lack of sexual desire or inability to enjoy sex and reach an orgasm. On the other hand, if Kidney-Yin is severely deficient leading to the rising of Empty-Fire, there may be an excessive sexual desire with inability to be ever satisfied. The person may also have vivid sexual dreams resulting in nocturnal emissions in men and orgasms in women. For this reason, lack of sexual desire can be stimulated by strengthening Kidney-Yang and the Gate of Vitality, and excessive sexual desire can be dampened by nourishing Kidney-Yin.

Finally, it should be stressed that what has been said so far only concerns the relation between excessive sexual activity (with ejaculation and/or orgasm) and the Kidney energy, and that many other factors are involved in determining a happy sexual life. Although Chinese Medicine is mostly concerned with excessive sexual activity as a cause of disease, an unhappy sexual life with inability to reach an orgasm or lacking in warmth and affection is also an important and frequent cause of disease. This often causes deep unhappiness or anxiety which become causes of disease in themselves.

DIET

Diet is an important cause of disease, especially nowadays. A great many discoveries have been made in recent years to completely revolutionize our ideas on diet. For example, the role of vitamins and minerals in health and disease have only been discovered recently. On the other hand, food has never been subjected to so much chemical manipulation as in the past 30 years or so. Our food contains an incredible variety of chemicals, in the form of preservatives, flavourings, colourings, emulsifiers, etc. Even worse, some drugs, such as hormones and antibiotics, are present in certain foods. To complete the picture, agricultural growing methods have also undergone a complete revolution with the abandonment of traditional ways of preserving the soil's fertility and controlling pests, in favour of chemical pesticides and fertilizers. Residual amounts of these chemicals are inevitably present in food and water.

Because these changes in the production of food have been introduced relatively recently, Chinese ideas on diet do not take them into account. To give a very simple example, Chinese diet considers chicken meat to be beneficial to Blood. However, this does not take into account that battery chickens contain hormones and are raised in prison-like conditions, so that the nutritional value of their meat is certainly not the same as it would have been in China 1000 years ago.

All these modern changes in the production of food and modern research on food are important and need to be taken into account when considering diet as a cause of disease. However, a discussion of these aspects of foods would be entirely beyond the scope of this book, and I will therefore limit myself to a discussion of diet as a cause of disease from the traditional Chinese point of view.

Dietary habits can become a cause of disease if diet is unbalanced either from the quantitative or qualitative point of view.

First of all, malnutrition is an obvious cause of disease. In its broad sense, malnutrition exists not only in poor Third-World countries, but also in rich industrialized countries where it is present in certain less-obvious forms. For example, poor elderly people living alone often have a diet quite lacking in nutritive and caloric value. Other people may suffer from a mild form of malnutrition by adhering rigidly to very strict "diets", the number and variety of which is becoming mind-boggling. Some of those who adhere to such strict diets may unwittingly lack essential nutrients in their diet.

Another example of malnutrition in our society is in those who suffer from anorexia nervosa, and yet another in those who regularly starve themselves in order to slim. In passing, it is worth mentioning that some people who starve themselves to lose weight actually experience an increase in weight, whilst when they resume a balanced diet excess fat drops away. This apparent paradox is explained by the fact that starving weakens the Spleen, which fails to transform and transport food and fluids properly and this leads to weight gain. If proper food is eaten, the Spleen is strengthened, it transforms and transports food and fluids properly and this leads to loss of weight.

Malnutrition causes deficiency of Qi and Blood and weakens the Spleen function of transformation and transportation setting up a vicious circle because the lack of proper food weakens the Spleen while a weak Spleen fails to absorb the nutrients from what food is taken.

Over-eating is an even more common cause of disease in our society. Increasing affluence after the strictures of the Second World War, has produced a great abundance of food in rich industrialized countries and a dramatic increase in average weight of the population. From the point of view of Chinese Medicine, over-eating also weakens the Spleen and Stomach leading to accumulation of mucus, a feeling of fullness, belching, sour regurgitation, nausea and abdominal distension.

Excessive consumption of what Chinese Medicine considers to be cold-energy foods and raw foods (such as salads, ice-creams, iced drinks or fruit) may weaken the Spleen, in particular Spleen-Yang. The idea that an excessive consumption of salads and fruit can be detrimental to health runs counter to all modern ideas about diet, according to which, by eating raw vegetables and fruit, we can absorb all the vitamins and minerals contained in them. This is true to a certain extent and a moderate consumption of these foods can be beneficial. However, from the Chinese point of view, the Spleen likes dryness and warmth in food and dislikes excess of fluids and cold: an excessive consumption of the above foods will be very difficult to digest and may weaken Spleen-Yang causing diarrhoea, chilliness, cold mucus, abdominal pain and distension. Thus, particularly those who have a tendency to Spleen deficiency should not consume raw and cold foods in excess.

Excessive consumption of sweet foods and sugar, also extremely common in our society, blocks the Spleen function of transformation and transportation and gives rise to Dampness, with such symptoms as upper respiratory catarrh, abdominal distension and fullness, mucus in the stools and vaginal discharges.

Excessive consumption of hot energy and spicy foods (such as curry, alcohol, lamb, beef or spices) gives rise to Heat symptoms, especially of the Stomach or Liver, such as a bitter taste, a burning sensation in the epigastrium and thirst.

Excessive consumption of greasy and fried foods (such as any deep-fried foods, milk, cheese, butter, cream, ice-cream, banana, peanuts or fatty meats) gives rise to the formation of Phlegm or Dampness which in turn obstructs the Spleen function of transformation and transportation. This may cause various Phlegm symptoms, such as sinusitis, a nasal discharge, a "muzzy" feeling of the head, dull headaches, bronchitis and so on.

Chinese Medicine considers not only what one eats, but also how one eats it. One can eat the best-quality food available and perfectly balanced, but if it is eaten in the wrong circumstances, it will also lead to disease. For example, eating in a hurry, discussing work while eating, going straight back to work after eating, eating late in the evening, eating in a state of emotional tension, all these habits interfere with a proper digestion of food and, in particular, lead to deficiency of Stomach-Yin. This manifests with a tongue with rootless coating, or no coating in the centre, thirst, epigastric pain and dry stools.

TRAUMA

This refers to physical traumas, as mental shock is included among the emotional causes of disease.

Physical traumas cause local stagnation of Qi or Blood in the area. A slight trauma causes stagnation of Qi and a severe one causes stasis of Blood. In either case, it gives rise to pain, bruising and swelling. Although trauma may seem only a transient cause of disease, in practice, the effect of trauma can linger for a long time manifesting with local stagnation of Qi and/or Blood in the area affected.

Old accidents and falls, which the person may have completely forgotten, can often be the cause, or concurrent cause, of disease. This is especially true of headaches: as a rule of thumb, headaches which always occur in the same part of the head, are often caused by a previous injury to that part of the head. This means that local treatment aimed at removing stasis of Blood in that area is particularly applicable.

Old traumas can also become a concurrent cause of disease together with a later one. For example, a trauma to a knee may seem to have cleared up completely, but when the person later in life contracts Painful Obstruction Syndrome caused by exposure to cold and damp conditions, the exterior pathogenic factor often will settle in that knee.

PARASITES AND POISONS

Very little needs to be said about these as they are self-evident as causes of disease.

Infestation of intestinal worms is more common in children and although worms are an external cause of disease, Chinese Medicine regards poor diet as a contributory factor. An excessive consumption of greasy and sweet foods leads to Dampness which makes for a favourable breeding ground for worms.

The symptoms of worms depends on the type of worm, but in general they are: white vesicles on the face, sallow complexion, emaciation, small white spots inside the lips, purple spots inside the eyelids, loss of appetite or desire to eat strange objects (such as wax, leaves, raw rice), abdominal pain, itchy nose and anus.

WRONG TREATMENT

A complete discussion of iatrogenic diseases caused by the side-effects of medicinal (Western) drugs is well beyond the scope of this book.

As for Chinese Medicine, wrong treatment can obviously be a cause of disease. As for acupuncture, one of its great advantages as a form of treatment is that it is a relatively safe therapy. Even if a wrong treatment is applied, in most cases, the energy rebalances itself out in a few days. This is not to say, however, that ill-effects cannot arise from a wrong treatment.

As far as Chinese herbal treatment is concerned, the possibility of ill effects arising from a wrong treatment is greater. This is because Chinese herbs have a more definite and somewhat less "neutral" effect than acupuncture. For example, when tonifying the Kidneys with herbal treatment, it is essential to distinguish between Kidney-Yin and Kidney-Yang deficiency as the herbs used in each case would be entirely different and the incorrect use of hot herbs for Kidney-Yin deficiency or cold herbs for Kidney-Yang deficiency would lead to a definite aggravation. In contrast, with acupuncture, one can use such a point asTaixi KI-3 in both Kidney–Yin or Kidney-Yang deficiency without any ill effects.

One of the situations in which acupuncture can be used wrongly is when one fails to distinguish an exterior from an interior condition. For example, if one gives a tonifying treatment during an acute exterior condition, this may actually push the exterior pathogenic factor inwards and lead to an aggravation. This is all the more likely to happen if moxa is used.

NOTES

1 This method of investigation for the cause of disease was suggested by Dr J H F Shen during one of his London lectures, and I am indebted to him for the subsequent personal communications on this subject of which he is a true master.
2 Simple Questions, p 221.
3 Simple Questions, p 221.
4 Simple Questions, p. 38
5 There is a common story in Chinese Medicine which was related to me by two different teachers to illustrate this situation. According to this story, a certain promising young man had passed the examination to access the highest rank of the Imperial bureaucracy in the capital. As this man was walking in the Imperial palace, overjoyed for having passed the examination, a doctor friend of his saw him and, glancing at him, told him that he should immediately return to his native village because there was very bad news from his family there. The poor man became white in the face, and made preparations to leave straight away. Once he got to his village, his family told him that there was nothing wrong there and that they never sent for him. The young man returned to the capital and when he met his doctor friend again, he asked him in consternation, why on earth he had lied to him. The doctor told him that he saw on his face that he had had a sudden excitement and was overjoyed beyond measure: this could have seriously injured his heart. The only way to counteract this sudden excitement, was to instil fear in his heart, as fear counteracts joy.
6 Simple Questions, p 221.
7 Simple Questions, p 222.
8 Simple Questions, p 222.
9 Simple Questions, p 151.
10 Simple Questions, p 154.
11 1978 Classic of the Simple Girl (*Su Nu Jing* 素女经) French translation by Leung Kwok Po, Seghers, Paris, p 106. This book is a translation of a Chinese text of the same title published in 1908 (first published in 1903). This text itself, is a compilation from older texts on sexuality, the oldest dating back to the Tang dynasty
12 Fundamentals of Chinese Medicine, p 50.
13 Classic of the Simple Girl, p 107.

Diagnosis 16

診法

Chinese diagnosis is intimately related to Pattern Identification as it provides the diagnostic tools necessary to identify the patterns. Chinese diagnosis is based on the fundamental principle that signs and symptoms reflect the condition of the Internal Organs. The concept of signs and symptoms in Chinese Medicine is broader than in Western Medicine. Whilst Western Medicine mostly takes into account symptoms and signs as objective or subjective manifestations of a disease, Chinese Medicine takes into account many different manifestations, many of them not related to an actual disease process. It uses not only "symptoms and signs" but many other manifestations to form a picture of the disharmony present in a particular person. Many of the so-called symptoms and signs of Chinese Medicine would not be considered as such in Western Medicine. For example, absence of thirst (which confirms a Cold condition), incapacity of making decisions (which confirms a weakness of the Gall Bladder), a dislike of speaking (which confirms a weakness of the Spleen), a dull appearance of the eyes (which confirms a disturbed Mind), and so on. Whenever we refer to "symptoms and signs" it will be in the above context.

Over the centuries, Chinese diagnosis has developed an extremely sophisticated system of correspondences between outward signs and the Internal Organs. The correlation between outward signs and internal organs is summarized in the expression :"Inspect the exterior to examine the interior".

According to this basic idea underlying Chinese diagnosis, practically everything, such as skin, complexion, bones, channels, smells, sounds, mental state, preferences, emotions, tongue, pulse, demeanour, body build, reflects the state of the internal organs and can be used in diagnosis.

The second fundamental principle of Chinese diagnosis is that "*a part reflects the whole*". On the basis of this idea, and on the strength of centuries of accumulated clinical experience, a practitioner of Chinese Medicine can derive detailed information about the state of the whole organism, from examination of a small part of it. Chinese pulse diagnosis is, of course, a striking example of this, as so much information about the whole organism can be gleaned from palpation of a small section of the radial artery. Facial diagnosis, from which so much information about the whole body and mind is obtained from observation of the face, is another example.

In a way, discussing the clinical significance of isolated symptoms and signs contradicts the whole spirit of Chinese diagnosis. This, in fact, involves a synthesis of all symptoms and signs into a meaningful pattern of disharmony. The essence of the process of diagnosing and identifying the pattern is that all symptoms and signs must be considered in relation to the others. No symptom or sign can be considered in isolation. For example, thirst associated with a tongue with yellow coating and a Full-Overflowing pulse indicates Full-Heat, whereas thirst associated with a tongue without coating and a Floating-Empty pulse indicates Empty-Heat. For the purpose of learning, however, one normally has to consider the clinical significance of each symptom or sign one by one, keeping in mind that in practice the interrelationship of all the clinical manifestations is all-important.

Chinese diagnosis includes four methods traditionally described with four words:

Looking
Hearing (and smelling)
Asking
Feeling.[1]

These four methods are very old indeed as they were first mentioned in the "Annals" of Su Ma Qian, the famous historian of the early Han dynasty, in the chapter "Various Transmissions from Bian Que". In it he says: *"Feeling the pulse, observing the colours, listening to the sounds and observing the body, can reveal where the disease is"*.[2]

DIAGNOSIS BY LOOKING

This includes observation of the following elements:

Spirit
Body
Demeanour
Head and face
Eyes
Nose
Ears
Mouth
Teeth-gums
Throat
Limbs
Skin
Tongue
Channels.

SPIRIT

"Spirit" here means several different things. Firstly, it indicates the spirit of a person, his or her vitality and the state of his or her mental, emotional and spiritual being. It also indicates a general state of vitality; if this is thriving, the person "has spirit". The opposite, "not having spirit" indicates a state of lack of vitality. The "Simple Questions" says: *"If there is spirit the person thrives, if there is no spirit the person dies"*.[3]

The presence or absence of spirit can be observed in the complexion, the eyes, the state of mind and the breathing.

If the person has spirit, the complexion is healthy, the muscles are firm, the face colour is clear, the eyes have glitter and reveal inner vitality, the mind is clear, the breathing even.

If the person has no spirit, the complexion is unhealthy, the muscles are withered, the face colour is dark, the eyes move uncontrollably, show no inner vitality and are not clear, the mind is unclear and the breathing is stertorous.

BODY

There are three aspects to consider when examining the physical appearance of a patient. Firstly, the constitutional types, secondly long-term changes in physical appearance, and thirdly short-term changes.

Every individual is born with a certain constitution and consequently a certain body shape. There is a tremendous variety of body shapes even within the same race, not to mention that between races. It is therefore important not to consider as a diagnostic sign, a certain physical trait which is normal for that person.

Traditionally, five different constitutional body shapes are described, one for each element. These will be discussed in detail in chapter 23 ("The Principles of Treatment").

The Wood type has a tall and slender body. The Fire type has a small pointed head and small hands. The Metal type has broad and square shoulders, a strongly-built body and a triangular face. The Earth type has a slightly fat body, a large head, a large belly and thighs and wide jaws. The Water type has a round face and body and a long spine.

Besides these constitutional body shapes, there can be long-term changes in the body which can be important diagnostic signs. For example, a very large, barrel-like chest and epigastrium indicate an Excess condition of the Stomach. Very large upper thighs, out of proportion with the rest of the body which might even be thin, indicate Spleen deficiency. A thin and emaciated body usually indicates a long-standing deficiency of Blood or Yin. A fat body usually indicates deficiency of Spleen-Yang with tendency to retention of Dampness or Phlegm. All these body changes would only take place over a long period of time.

Finally, there can be short-term changes of diagnostic significance. Generally speaking, one can refer to the Five-Element correspondences between tissues and organs: for example, any change in the sinews (such as weakness or stiffness) would reflect a disharmony of the Liver, a change in the blood vessels (such as hardening of the vessels, which can be felt as a very hard and Wiry pulse) indicate a problem of the Heart, a change in the muscles (such as weak and flaccid muscles) would reflect a deficiency of the Spleen, a change in the skin (such as flaccid skin) would indicate a deficiency of Lung-Qi, and a change in the bones (such as brittle bones) would indicate a Kidney deficiency.

DEMEANOUR

This includes the way the person moves, and also movement of individual parts of the body, such as eyes, face, mouth, limbs, fingers.

The general principle is that an excess of movement, or rapid and jerky movements indicate Yang, Full or Hot patterns, while lack of movement, or slow movements indicate Yin, Empty or Cold patterns.

The way a person moves has to be considered also in relation to the 5-Element body type. For example, the Fire type should move quickly, if he or she moves slowly, then it indicates some problem. The Metal type should move slowly and deliberately, if she or he moves quickly, then it indicates some problem.

If a person moves very quickly and when in bed throws off the bedclothes, it may indicate an Excess pattern of Heat, often of the Liver or Heart. If a person moves very slowly and likes to lie down, it may indicate a Deficient pattern of Cold, usually of the Spleen.

Small movements and continuous fidgeting, especially of the legs, indicate a Deficient-Heat pattern of the Kidneys.

Movements such as tremors or convulsions always indicate the presence of interior Wind of the Liver. These could be convulsions of the whole body, or just tremors of an eyelid or cheek.

HEAD AND FACE

Hair

The state of the hair is related to the condition of Blood or Kidney-Essence. Falling hair may indicate a condition of Blood Deficiency, while prematurely greying hair indicates a decline of Kidney-Essence.

The thickness and lustre of the hair depends on the Lungs, and dull hair with a tendency to split indicates deficiency of Lung-Qi.

Face colour

Observation of the face colour is an extremely important part of visual diagnosis. The face colour reflects the state of Qi and Blood and is closely related to the condition of the Mind.

Various pathological colours are usually described, but before analysing the particular colour itself, one has to distinguish between a clear, shining type of colour, and a dull, dry type of colour. If the colour is clear and has a rather moist appearance it indicates that Stomach-Qi is still intact: this is a positive indication, even if the colour itself is pathological. If the colour has a rather dry and lifeless look, it indicates that Stomach-Qi is exhausted: this is always a negative indication and points to poor prognosis.

Green

A green colour of the face indicates any of the

following conditions: a Liver pattern, interior Cold, pain or interior Wind.

Red

Red indicates Heat. This can be Full or Empty Heat. In Full-Heat, the whole face is red, in Empty-Heat only the cheekbones are red.

Yellow

Yellow indicates Spleen deficiency or Dampness, or both. A bright orange-yellow colour indicates Damp-Heat, with the prevalence of Heat rather than Dampness. A hazy, smoky yellow indicates Damp-Heat, with the prevalence of Dampness. A withered, dried-up yellow indicates Heat in Stomach and Spleen. A sallow yellow colour indicates Stomach and Spleen deficiency. A dull-pale yellow colour indicates Cold-Damp in Stomach and Spleen. A pale yellow colour surrounded by red spots indicates Spleen deficiency and stasis of Liver-Blood. A clear and moist yellow colour in between the eyebrows indicates that Stomach-Qi is recovering after an illness affecting Stomach and Spleen. A dried-up and withered-looking yellow colour in the same area is a poor prognostic sign.

White

White indicates Deficiency, Cold, Blood Deficiency or Yang Deficiency. A dull-pale-white complexion indicates Blood deficiency, while bright-white complexion indicates Yang deficiency.

Black

Black complexion indicates Cold, pain, or Kidney disease, usually from Kidney-Yin deficiency. A black and moist-looking colour indicates Cold, while a dried-up and burned-looking colour indicates Heat, usually Empty-Heat from Kidney-Yin deficiency.

Finally, irrespective of the actual shade, the colour can be described as being deep or floating, clear or dull, thin or thick, scattered or concentrated and moist or dry.

A deep colour indicates an interior condition, while a floating colour indicates an exterior one.

A clear colour indicates a Yang condition, while a dull one indicates a Yin condition.

A thin colour indicates Qi deficiency and a thick one a Full condition.

A scattered colour indicates a new disease, while a concentrated one indicates an old disease.

A moist colour is a sign of good prognosis, while a dry colour is a sign of poor prognosis.

Face areas

Besides the colour, various areas of the face indicate the state of certain organs. There are two different arrangements of areas, one according to the "Simple Questions" chapter 32 and the other according to the "Spiritual Axis" chapter 49 (Figs 49 and 50).

Observation of the face colour should be integrated with the face areas. For example, a bluish colour in the centre of the forehead (which corresponds to the Heart according to the "Simple Questions") indicates that the Heart has suffered from a shock.

A red tip of the nose denotes Spleen deficiency. A very short chin indicates the possibility of Kidney deficiency.

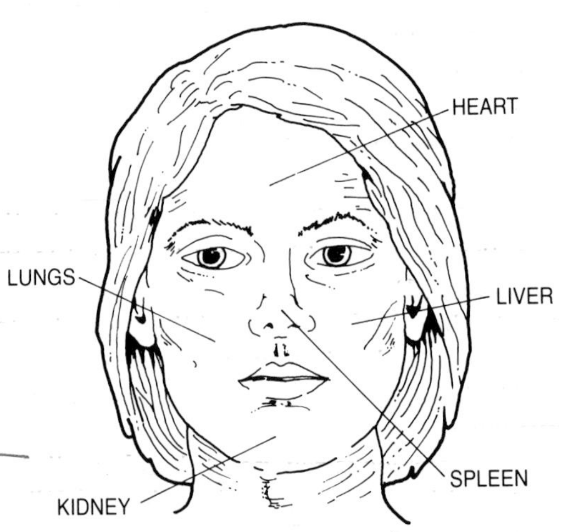

Fig. 49 Face diagnosis as from "Simple Questions"

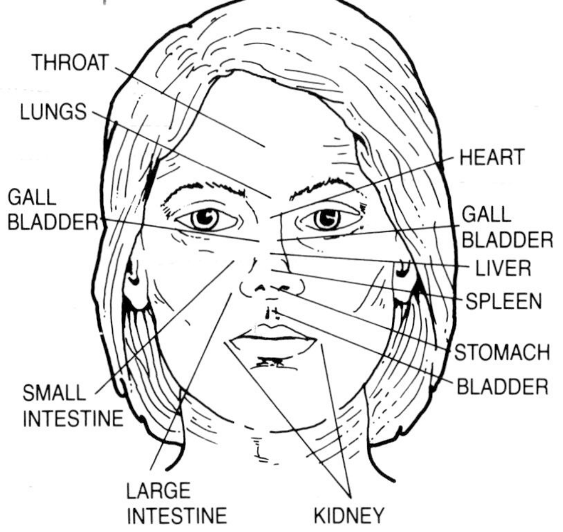

Fig. 50 Face diagnosis as from "Spiritual Axis"

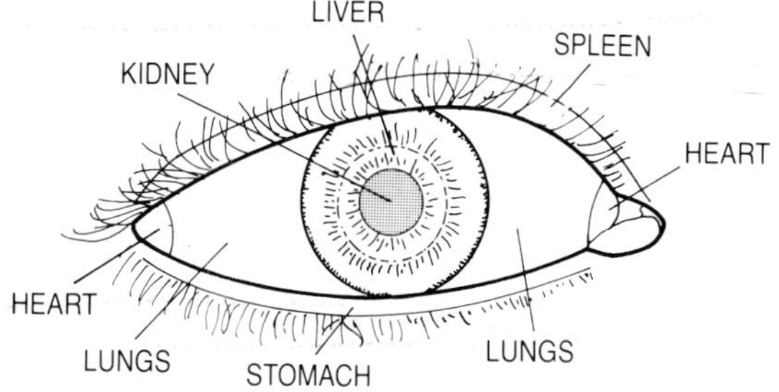

Fig. 51 Correspondence of eye areas to organs

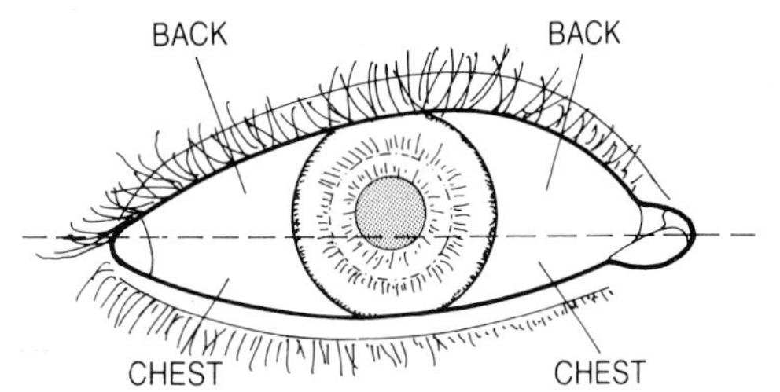

Fig. 52 Correspondence of eye areas to back or chest

EYES

Observation of the eyes is an extremely important part of diagnosis. The eyes reflect the state of the Mind and the Essence. The "Spiritual Axis" says: *"The Essence of the five Yin and the six Yang organs ascends to the eyes"*.[4]

If the eyes are clear and have glitter, they indicate that the Mind and the Essence are in a good state of vitality. If the eyes are rather dull or clouded, it shows that the Mind is disturbed and the Essence has been weakened. It is very common to see very dull and clouded eyes in people who have been suffering from deep emotional problems for a long time.

Different parts of the eye are related to different organs. The corners of the eye are related to the Heart, the upper eyelid to the Spleen (or to the Greater Yang channels), the lower eyelid to the Stomach, the sclera to the Lungs, the iris to the Liver and the pupil to the Kidney (Fig. 51).

A red colour in the corners of the eye indicates Heart-Fire; a red colour in the sclera indicates Lung-Heat. A yellow colour of the sclera indicates Damp-Heat.

If the whole eye is red, painful and swollen, it indicates either an exterior invasion of Wind-Heat or rising of Liver-Fire.

A dull white colour of the corners indicates Heat and a pale-white colour indicates Blood deficiency.

A swelling under the eyes indicates Kidney deficiency.

Finally, according to modern research carried out at the Fujian College of Traditional Chinese Medicine, the sclera of the eye can reflect lesions of the back or chest.[5] Injuries of back and chest, such as internal haematomas, can be reflected on the sclera. If one draws a horizontal line across the centre of the eye, the upper part reflects the back and the lower part reflects the chest; also the right eye will reflect lesions on the right side and the left eye those on the left side (Fig. 52).

Green, blue, purple or red spots appearing at the end of red veins with purple blood spots on them indicate lesions within the back or chest. Such spots that are not directly connected to the veins have no diagnostic significance. Grey and scattered spots like clouds indicate injuries of Qi, i.e. injuries causing only stagnation of Qi, without organic lesions. Deep-black spots like black sesame seeds, indicate injury of Blood, i.e. injuries causing stasis of Blood, a stage further than stagnation of Qi. Black spots surrounded by a grey, cloud-like halo indicate injuries of both Qi and Blood. If red veins are clearly visible and are spiral-shaped, they indicate pain.

NOSE

If the tip of the nose is green or blue it indicates abdominal pain. If it is yellow it indicates Damp-Heat. A white colour indicates Blood deficiency. If it is red it indicates Heat in Lung and Spleen. If it is grey it indicates an impairment of Water movement.

If the nose is slightly moist and shiny, it indicates that any disease there might be is not serious. If it is dry, it indicates Heat in the Stomach or Large Intestine. If it is dry and black, it indicates the presence of Fire-Poison.

A clear-watery discharge from the nose indicates a Cold pattern; a thick-yellow discharge indicates a Heat pattern.

Flaring of the nostrils in a person with high fever indicates extreme Heat in the Lungs.

EARS

A white colour of the ears indicates a Cold pattern while a Bluish or black colour indicates pain. If the ear lobes are dry, withered and black, they indicate extreme exhaustion of Kidney-Qi.

The ear lobes are an indicator in assessing prognosis: if they are shiny and slightly moist, the prognosis is good; if they are dry and withered, the prognosis is bad.

Swelling and pain in the ear (or middle ear) is usually due to Fire in the Lesser Yang channels.

The shape of the ear also helps to distinguish Full from Empty patterns: a swollen ear indicates the presence of a pathogenic factor, hence a Full pattern. A thin ear indicates deficiency of Qi or Blood.

Apart from the above signs, the shape and size of the ear lobe is related to one's constitution and Kidney energy in Chinese facial diagnosis. A long and full lobe is indicative of strong Kidneys and good constitution; a thin and small lobe is indicative of a rather poor constitution.

MOUTH AND LIPS

The normal colour of the lips should be pale-red and rather moist and shiny. If they are very pale, they indicate Emptiness of Blood or Yang. If they are too red and dry, they indicate Heat in the Spleen and Stomach.

If the lips are purple or bluish, they indicate stasis of Blood. If they are dry and red, it indicates that the Heat has begun to injure the body fluids.

If the mouth is always slightly open it is a sign of an Empty pattern. If the person only breathes through the mouth, it indicates a deficiency of Lung-Qi (unless of course, it is due to a blocked nose).

A greenish colour around the mouth indicates stasis of Liver-Blood and invasion of the Spleen by Liver-Qi.

TEETH AND GUMS

The teeth are considered an "extension of the bones" and are under the influence of the Kidneys. The gums are under the influence of the Stomach.

Moist teeth indicate a good state of the body fluids and Kidneys whilst dry teeth indicate exhaustion of fluids and deficiency of Kidney-Yin.

If the teeth are bright and dry like a stone, it indicates Heat in the Bright Yang (in the context of exterior diseases). If they are dry and greyish like bones, it indicates Empty-Heat from Kidney-Yin deficiency.

If the teeth are bleeding, it indicates extreme Heat in the Stomach.[6]

If the gums are swollen and painful and perhaps bleeding, it indicates Heat in the Stomach. If there is no pain, it indicates Empty-Heat.

If the gums are very pale, it indicates deficiency of Blood.

THROAT

Pain, redness and swelling of the throat indicates either invasion of exterior Wind-Heat or Fire in the Stomach.

If the throat is only sore and dry but not swollen and red, it indicates deficiency of Kidney-Yin with Empty-Heat.

LIMBS

A healthy colour and a firmness of the flesh around ankles and wrists indicates a good state of the body fluids. If the skin on these joints lacks lustre and is dry and the flesh shrivelled, it indicates exhaustion of Body Fluids.

Pale nails indicate deficiency of Blood; bluish nails indicate stasis of Blood (of the Liver).

The thenar eminence shows the state of the Stomach. A bluish colour of the venules on the thenar eminence of the thumb indicates Cold in the Stomach. Bluish and short venules indicate an Empty pattern. Red venules indicate Heat in the Stomach.

Examination of the venules on the index fingers of children under 2 is used for diagnosing infants. Usually the left index finger is examined in boys and the right one in girls. The creases at the metacarpo-phalangeal articulation and inter-phalangeal articulation are called "gates", the first one at the base being the "Gate of Wind", the second one the "Gate of Qi", and the third one the "Gate of Life" (Fig. 53).

If after rubbing the finger towards the body, venules appear only beyond the "Gate of Wind", this indicates an invasion by an exterior pathogenic factor and a mild disease. If the venules extend beyond the "Gate of Qi" this indicates an interior and rather more severe disease. If they extend beyond the "Gate of Life", this indicates a serious and life-threatening disease. Furthermore, if the venules are bluish they indicate a Cold pattern, if they are red they indicate a Heat pattern.

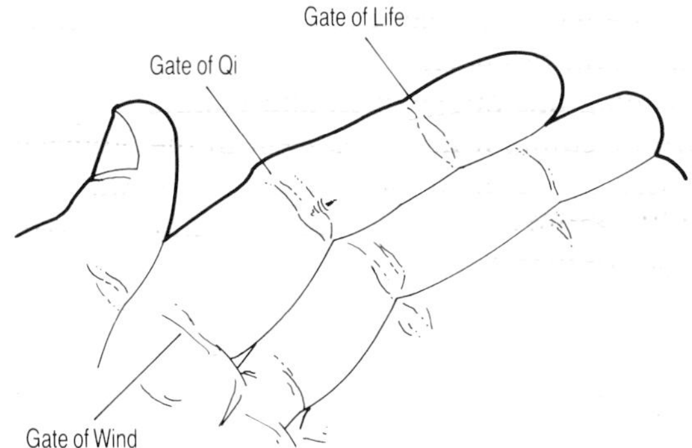

Fig. 53 The "Three Gates" on an infant's index finger

SKIN

The skin is physiologically related to the Lungs within the 5-Element model. However, it is also related to the condition of Blood and, through this, to the Liver. Hence, not all skin diseases are related to the Lungs. Many skin conditions are due to Heat or stasis of Blood and are related to the condition of the Liver. Furthermore, Heat in the Blood can also derive from Stomach-Heat so that some skin diseases are related to the Stomach.

Dry skin usually indicates deficiency of Liver-Blood, whilst itchy skin is due to Wind.

A swelling of the skin which leaves a mark on pressure with a finger indicates oedema. This is called true oedema in Chinese Medicine, or "Water oedema", and is due to deficiency of Kidney-Yang. If on pressure with a finger, no mark is left on the swollen skin, this is called "Qi oedema" and is not a true oedema. The swelling is caused by stagnation of Qi.

A yellow colour of the skin may indicate jaundice and two different shades are distinguished. A bright and clear yellow colour indicates "Yang jaundice" which is due to Damp-Heat. A dull-yellow colour indicates "Yin jaundice" which is due to Damp-Cold.

The venules which frequently appear on the skin are considered to be an exterior manifestation of the Blood-Connecting channels. They indicate a state of Fullness of the secondary Connecting channels. If they are red they indicate Heat, if bluish they indicate cold, if greenish they indicate pain and if purple they indicate stasis of Blood. They can be frequently seen behind the knees in older people.

TONGUE[7]

Observation of the tongue is a pillar of diagnosis

because it provides clearly visible clues to the patient's disharmony. Tongue diagnosis is remarkably reliable: whenever there are conflicting manifestations in a complicated condition, the tongue nearly always reflects the basic and underlying pattern.

Observation of the tongue is based on four main items: the tongue body colour, the body shape, the coating and the moisture.

— The body colour indicates the conditions of Blood, Nutritive Qi and Yin organs

— The body shape indicates the state of Blood and Nutritive Qi

— The coating indicates the state of the Yang organs

— The moisture indicates the state of the Body Fluids.

Various areas of the tongue reflect the state of the internal organs. A topography of the tongue in common use is as follows (Fig. 54):

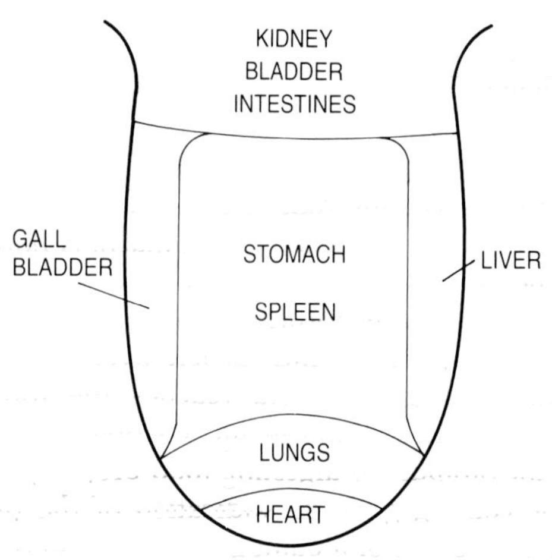

Fig. 54 Correspondence of tongue areas to organs

Tongue-body colour

The normal body colour should be pale-red. The body colour reflects the state of Blood and Nutritive Qi and the Yin organs. There are five pathological colours: Pale, Red, Deep-Red, Purple, and Blue.

Pale

A Pale body colour indicates either deficiency of Yang or deficiency of Blood. In deficiency of Yang the tongue is also usually slightly too wet and swollen, since deficient Yang Qi fails to transform and transport fluids. In deficiency of Blood the tongue tends to be somewhat dry.

If the sides of the tongue are especially Pale, or in severe cases slightly orangey, it indicates Deficiency of Liver-Blood.

Red

By "Red" is meant too red. A Red tongue body always indicates Heat. If the tongue has a coating, it indicates Full-Heat; if there is no coating, it indicates Empty-Heat.

A Red tip, usually on a Red tongue, indicates Heart-Fire or Heart Empty-Heat, according to whether the tongue has a coating or not. In severe cases, the tip can also be swollen and have red points on it.

Red sides indicate Liver-Fire or Gall-Bladder Heat. In severe cases they may also be swollen and display red spots. A Red centre indicates Stomach-Heat.

Red tongues are likely to have red points or spots. These are raised papillae and always indicate Heat; if they are rather large, in addition to Heat, they also indicate stasis of Blood.

Red points or spots are frequently seen on the tip (Heart-Fire), on the sides (Liver-Fire), on the root (Heat in the Lower Burner) and around the centre (Stomach-Heat).

Deep-red

This is simply a shade darker than Red and its clinical significance is the same as for the Red tongue, except that the condition is more severe.

Purple

A Purple tongue always indicates stasis of Blood. There are two types of Purple colour: Reddish-Purple and Bluish-Purple.

A Reddish-Purple tongue indicates Heat and stasis of Blood, and it develops from a Red tongue.

A Bluish-Purple tongue indicates Cold and stasis of Blood, and it develops from a Pale tongue.

A Purple colour is frequently seen on the sides indicating Liver-Blood stasis or in the centre, indicating stasis of Blood in the Stomach.

If the Purple colour is on the sides but only towards the middle section, and if the sides are swollen and the rest of the tongue is bluish-purple, this indicates stasis of Blood in the chest.

Blue

The significance of a Blue tongue is the same as a Bluish-Purple tongue, i.e. Interior Cold giving rise to stasis of Blood.

Tongue-body shape

The body shape of the tongue gives an indication of Blood and Nutritive Qi and it reflects the Full or Empty character of a condition.

Thin

A Thin body indicates either Blood deficiency if it is Pale, or Yin deficiency if it is Red and Peeled.

In both cases, it indicates that the condition is chronic.

Swollen

A Swollen tongue that is also Pale indicates retention of Dampness deriving from Yang deficiency. If it is Red or normal-coloured, it indicates retention of Damp-Heat.

Stiff

A Stiff tongue usually indicates Interior Wind.

Flaccid

A Flaccid tongue indicates deficiency of Body Fluids.

Long

A Long tongue indicates tendency to Heat, and in particular Heart-Heat.

Short

A Short tongue indicates interior Cold if it is Pale and wet, or extreme deficiency of Yin if it is Red and Peeled.

Cracked

Cracks indicate either Full-Heat or deficiency of Yin. Short horizontal cracks indicate Stomach-Yin deficiency. A long-deep midline crack reaching the tip indicates a tendency to a Heart pattern.

A shallow-wide crack in the midline not reaching the tip indicates Stomach-Yin deficiency.

Short transversal cracks on the sides, in the middle section of the tongue, indicate chronic Spleen-Qi deficiency.

Quivering

A Quivering tongue usually indicates Spleen-Qi deficiency.

Deviated

A Deviated tongue indicates interior Wind.

Toothmarked

A tongue with teethmarks indicates Spleen-Qi deficiency.

Tongue coating

The tongue coating reflects the state of the Yang organs and in particular the Stomach. A normal tongue should have a thin-white coating. The tongue coating is formed from some residual "dirty dampness" which is left over from the Stomach's digestion and reaches the tongue upwards. Thus a thin-white coating indicates that the Stomach is digesting food properly.

The coating gives an indication of the presence or absence of a pathogenic factor and of its strength. A thick coating always indicates the presence of a pathogenic factor and the thicker the coating the stronger the pathogenic factor. Such a pathogenic factor may be exterior or interior, such as exterior Wind, Dampness (interior of exterior), Cold, retention of Food, Phlegm, Heat, Fire. The absence of coating indicates deficiency of Stomach-Yin and/or Kidney-Yin. If the tongue is also Red all over, it is a definite indication of deficient Kidney-Yin.

The pathological coating colours can be: white, yellow, grey and black.

A white coating indicates a Cold pattern (unless of course, it is thin and white, in which case it is normal).

A yellow coating indicates a Full-Heat pattern. A grey and black coating can both indicate either extreme Cold or extreme Heat, according to whether the tongue is wet or dry.

Moisture

The amount of moisture on a tongue gives an indication of the state of Body Fluids. Whenever the tongue is Red or Deep-Red, one should check the moisture: if the tongue is also dry, it means that the Heat has begun to injure the Body Fluids.

A normal tongue should be very slightly moist, indicating that the Body Fluids are intact and are being properly transformed and transported.

If the tongue is too wet, it indicates that Yang-Qi is not transforming and transporting fluids and these accumulate to form Dampness.

If it is dry, it may indicate either Full-Heat or Empty-Heat, according to whether the tongue has a coating or not.

If the coating is sticky or slippery, it indicates retention of Dampness or Phlegm.

CHANNEL DIAGNOSIS

Manifestations occurring along the channels can be an important aid to diagnosis. Any findings arising from channel diagnosis, however, should always be integrated with all the others, and treatment should never be solely based on subjective or objective manifestations appearing along a channel.

Apart from the 14 main channels, there are a great number of other secondary channels which form an intricate web distributing Qi and Blood all over the body. Channels should not be seen as "lines" running in the body, but rather like areas of influence over a certain section of the body. The secondary channels are:
— the Connecting channels
— the Muscle channels
— the Cutaneous regions.

In addition, the Connecting channels branch out into three types of very minute channels, which are the Minute Connecting channels, the Blood Connecting channels and the Superficial Connecting channels.[8] It is these three types of capillary-like channels that are particularly important in producing the diagnostic signs which may appear along the course of a channel. For example, the small, purple distended venules appearing under the skin are, from the Chinese point of view, due to stasis of Blood in the Blood Connecting channels.

Channel diagnosis is based both on objective signs and subjective feelings experienced along the course of a channel. Objective signs include redness, white streaks, purple venules, purple spots, skin rashes following a definite channel pathway, flaccidity, hardness and a feeling of cold or heat. Anything that can be seen along a channel is due to the small Connective channels, such as the Minute, Blood or Superficial Connecting channels. Generally speaking, the appearance of the above signs along the course of a channel by itself indicates an Excess condition of the channel. For example, a greenish colour indicates retention of Cold in the channel or severe pain, a reddish colour indicates retention of Heat in the channels and a white colour indicates retention of Cold. Also the objective feeling of heat or cold along a channel indicate retention of Heat or Cold respectively. Flaccidity of the muscle along the course of a channel indicates a Deficient condition and that the channel is starved of Qi and Blood. This sign is often seen in Atrophy Syndrome. Rigidity or hardness of a muscle along the course of a channel indicates an Excess condition: this could be due to retention of Cold in the channel or to stagnation of Liver-Qi.

Subjective symptoms appearing along a channel include feelings of numbness, tingling, cold, heat, distension and, of course, pain or soreness. Generally speaking, dull sensations such as dull soreness or ache indicate an Empty condition of the channel, while sharp sensations such as sharp pain indicate a Full condition of the channel. However, this is not a general rule as a feeling of numbness, besides being due to Blood deficiency, can also be due to retention of internal Wind or Phlegm in the channel, both of which are Full conditions.

A subjective feeling of heat or cold obviously indicates a Cold or Hot condition of the channel.

DIAGNOSIS BY HEARING AND SMELLING

The same Chinese character *"wen"* means both "to hear" and "to smell". Both hearing and smelling are used in Chinese diagnosis.

DIAGNOSIS BY HEARING

Diagnosis by hearing includes listening to the sound and pitch of the voice, cough, breathing, vomiting, hiccup, borborygmi, groaning, and indeed any other sound emitted by a person.

As a general principle, a loud sound is indicative of a Full pattern, while a weak sound is indicative of an Empty pattern.

Voice

Sudden loss of voice is usually due to invasion of exterior Wind-Heat. A gradual loss of voice is due to deficiency of Lung-Qi or Lung-Yin.

A loud, coarse voice is indicative of an Excess pattern, while a weak and thin voice is indicative of a Deficiency pattern.

Reluctance to talk usually indicates a Cold pattern, while incessant talking indicates a Heat pattern.

The type of voice can also be diagnosed according to the 5-Element scheme of correspondences, so that a shouting voice is indicative of a Liver disharmony, a laughing voice of a Heart disharmony, a singing voice of a Spleen disharmony, a whimpering voice of a Lung disharmony and a groaning voice of a Kidney disharmony.

Breathing

A coarse, loud breathing sound indicates a Full pattern, while a weak, thin breathing sound indicates an Empty pattern.

Cough

A loud and explosive cough is indicative of a Full pattern, while a weak cough is indicative of an Empty pattern.

A dry cough indicates Lung-Yin deficiency.

DIAGNOSIS BY SMELLING

Body smell can be related to different organs within the 5-Elements system of correspondences: i.e. rancid for the Liver, burned for the Heart, sweetish for the Spleen, rank for the Lungs and putrid for the Kidneys.

Apart from the type of smell, as a general rule any strong, foul smell is indicative of Heat, while absence of smell is indicative of Cold.

Bad breath indicates Heat in the Stomach.

If the stools or urine have a strong, foul smell, it indicates Heat and, in the case of urine, also Dampness.

DIAGNOSIS BY ASKING

Diagnosis by interrogation is a very important part of Chinese diagnosis. In the process of identifying a pattern, not all the information is given by the patient. Indeed, even if it were, it would still have to be organized in order to identify the pattern. Very often the absence of a certain symptom or sign is diagnostically important, and patients, of course, would not report symptoms they do not experience. For example, in distinguishing between a Heat and a Cold pattern, it is necessary to establish whether a person is thirsty or not, and the absence of thirst would point to a Cold pattern. The patient would obviously not volunteer the information of "not being thirsty".

In a general sense, the interrogation is the talk between doctor and patient to find out how the problem arose, the living conditions of the patient, the environment, including the emotional environment and family environment. The aim of this investigation is, ultimately, to find the cause of the disease, in order for the patient and doctor to work together to try and eliminate it or minimize it.

In a specific sense, the interrogation aims at identifying the prevailing pattern in terms of 8 Principles, Internal Organs, Pathogenic Factors and Channels.

An added problem for practitioners in the West, is that the interrogation and the various expressions used to express symptoms are derived from Chinese experiences and culture and a Western patient would not necessarily use the same expressions. This is a problem, however, that can be overcome with experience. After some years of practice, we can learn to translate the Chinese way of expressing symptoms and find correlations more common to Western patients. For example, a Chinese person would spontaneously say that he or she has a "distending pain". A Western person, or at least an English person, would say that he or she feels "uncomfortably bloated", or has a "bursting sensation". The words are different, but the symptom they describe is the same.

The interrogation is traditionally carried out on the basis of ten questions. Although these are traditionally referred to in Chinese books as "questions", they represent more areas of questioning rather than actual questions. These varied a lot over the centuries, as different doctors placed the emphasis on different questions.

The most commonly used areas of questioning today are:

Chills and fever
Sweating
Head and body
Thorax and abdomen
Food and taste
Stools and urine
Sleep
Deafness and tinnitus
Thirst and drink
Pain.

Two areas of questioning are added for women and children:

Gynaecological condition
Children's problems.

It must be stressed that not all these questions need be asked in every situation. Nor are these the only possible questions since each situation requires an individual approach and other questions may be relevant.

Questions are not asked routinely, but following a lead, which may be provided by observation or symptoms or signs, from the very beginning of the meeting with a patient. Diagnosis and identification of patterns are closely interconnected and the various diagnostic methods are used to follow various leads so that a pattern may emerge.

1 CHILLS AND FEVER

In the context of exterior diseases, it is important to distinguish whether the patient has chilliness or fever or both. In this context, "chilliness" has a dual meaning: it means that the patient feels cold, but also that he or she has "aversion to cold", i.e. reluctance to go out in the cold.

If the person has aversion to cold and feels chilly, it indicates an exterior invasion of Wind-Cold or Wind-Heat. Aversion to cold is present in exterior invasions of both Wind-Cold and Wind-Heat because the pathogenic factor blocks the circulation of Defensive Qi which cannot warm the body and hence the patient feels cold. In invasions of Wind-Cold, fever may be present simultaneously with the aversion to cold. This is the pattern of Greater Yang within the 6-Stage Pattern Identification (see p. 479). If the fever is predominant and there is only slight aversion to cold, this indicates an exterior invasion not of Wind-Cold, but Wind-Heat. This is the pattern of Defensive Qi Level within the 4-Level Pattern Identification (see p. 481).

It is worth noting here that what is usually translated as "fever" from Chinese medical books indicates more a subjective feeling of heat rather than an actual temperature. Chinese Medicine was mostly unconcerned with objective measurements and relied primarily on observation of symptoms and signs. In other words, a person may have a pronounced feeling of heat without an actual fever. Conversely, one may have an actual temperature but have no feeling of heat.

If there is a fever without aversion to cold, this indicates an interior Heat pattern. This is the pattern of Bright Yang within the 6-Stage Pattern Identification.

If the patient suffers from alternating chills

and fever, this indicates an exterior invasion of Wind-Cold or Wind-Heat, and that the pathogenic factor is in the Lesser Yang (within the 6-Stage Pattern Identification).

In the context of interior diseases, if the patient feels chilly, it indicates Interior Cold from deficiency of Yang. Chilliness from deficiency of Yang can be distinguished from that from exterior Wind-Cold, is so far as the former is alleviated by covering oneself up and the latter is not. Most of us have experienced this during a severe attack of influenza or common cold with a temperature, when one feels chilly and shivers even in bed, no matter how many blankets one uses.

A low-grade fever getting worse in the afternoon, or only occurring in the afternoon, indicates Yin deficiency.

A constant low-grade temperature indicates a Damp-Heat pattern. A fever in the middle of the night in an adult indicates Yin deficiency, and in a child it indicates retention of food.

2 SWEATING

Evaluation of symptoms of sweating must be made by considering if it is part of an exterior or interior pattern.

In the context of Exterior conditions, sweating indicates a relatively deficient condition. For example, in exterior invasion of Wind-Cold, if there is sweating the condition is of a Deficient nature, if there is no sweating, it is of an Excess nature.

In the context of interior conditions, sweating may be caused by deficiency of Yang, deficiency of Yin, excess of Yang (i.e. Heat or Fire) or Damp-Heat.

One must distinguish sweating by the area of body, time of day, conditions and quality of sweat.

a) Area of body:

— Only on head: Heat in the Stomach or Damp-Heat
— Oily sweat on forehead: collapse of Yang
— Only on arms and legs: Stomach and Spleen deficiency
— Only on hands: Lung-Qi deficiency or nerves
— Whole body: Lung-Qi deficiency
— On palms, soles and chest: Yin deficiency (called 5-palm sweat").

b) Time of day:

— In day-time: Yang deficiency
— At night-time: Yin deficiency (in some cases it can also be from Damp-Heat).

c) Condition of illness:

— Profuse cold sweat during a severe illness: collapse of Yang
— Oily sweat on forehead, like pearls, not flowing: collapse of Yang, danger of imminent death.

d) Quality of sweat:

— Oily: severe Yang deficiency
— Yellow: Damp-Heat.

3 HEAD AND BODY

Head

The head is the area where all the Yang channels meet bringing clear Yang to the head and to the orifices, thus enabling the person to have clear sight, hearing, taste and smell.

Headache

This can be distinguished according to onset, time, location, character of pain, condition.

a) Onset:

— Recent onset, short duration: headache from exterior attack of Wind-Cold
— Gradual onset, in attacks: interior type.

b) Time of day:

— Day-time: Qi or Yang deficiency
— Evening: Blood or Yin deficiency

c) Location:

— Nape of neck: Greater Yang channels (can be from exterior invasion of Wind-Cold, or from interior Kidney deficiency)
— Forehead: Bright Yang channels (can be from Stomach-Heat or Blood deficiency)
— Temples and sides of head: Lesser Yang channels (can be from exterior Wind-Cold or Wind-Heat in the Lesser Yang, or from interior Liver and Gall Bladder Fire rising)
— Vertex: Terminal Yin channels (usually from deficiency of Liver-Blood)

— Whole head: exterior invasion of Wind-Cold.

d) Character of pain:

— Heavy feeling: Dampness or Phlegm
— Pain which is "inside" the head, "hurting the brain": Kidney deficiency
— Distending, throbbing: rising of Liver-Yang
— Boring, like a nail in a small point: stasis of Blood.

e) Condition:

— With aversion to wind or cold: exterior invasion
— Aggravated by cold: Cold pattern
— Aggravated by heat: Heat pattern
— Aggravated by fatigue, improved by rest: Qi deficiency.

Dizziness

Dizziness can be due to four factors which can be summarized as: Wind, Fire, Phlegm, Deficiency.

The main way to distinguish the various types of dizziness is by integration with the accompanying symptoms and signs.

Severe giddiness when everything seems to sway and the person loses the balance is usually due to internal Wind.

Slight dizziness accompanied by a feeling of heaviness and muzziness of the head indicates Phlegm obstructing the head and preventing the clear Yang from ascending to the head.

Slight dizziness aggravated when tired, indicates Qi deficiency.

A sudden onset of dizziness points to a Full pattern. A gradual onset points to an Empty pattern.

Body

Pain in the whole body

— Sudden onset, with chills and fever: exterior Wind-Cold
— Pain all over, with feeling of tiredness: Qi-Blood deficiency
— In women after childbirth: if the pain is dull, Blood deficiency. If the pain is severe, Blood stasis. Pain in arms and shoulders experienced only when walking: Liver-Qi stagnation
— Pain in all muscles, with hot sensation of the flesh: Stomach-Heat
— Pain with feeling of heaviness: Dampness obstructing muscles.

Pain in joints

— Wandering from joint to joint: from Wind
— Fixed and very painful: from Cold
— Fixed, with swelling and numbness: from Dampness.

Backache

— Continuous, dull: Kidney deficiency
— Recent onset, severe, with stiffness: sprain of back causing stasis of Blood
— Severe pain, aggravated during cold and damp weather, alleviated by application of heat: invasion of exterior Cold and Damp to the back channels
— Boring pain with inability to turn the waist: stasis of Blood
— Pain in the back extending up to the shoulders: exterior attack.

Numbness

— Numbness of arms and legs or only hands and feet on both sides: Blood deficiency
— Numbness of fingers, elbow and arm on one side only (especially of the first three fingers): internal Wind and Phlegm (this may indicate the possibility of impending Wind-stroke).

4 THORAX AND ABDOMEN

The thorax is under the influence of Heart and Lungs, while the flanks are under the control of the Liver and Gall-Bladder. The abdomen is influenced by the Liver, Intestines, Spleen, Kidneys and Bladder.

Pain in the chest is often due to stasis of Blood in the Heart, which, in turn is usually due to deficiency of Yang.

Chest pain accompanied by cough with profuse yellow sputum is due to Lung-Heat.

A feeling of distension and stuffiness of the

hypochondrium is due to stagnation of Liver-Qi. If the pain is severe there is stasis of Liver-Blood.

Epigastric pain can be due either to retention of food in the Stomach or to Stomach-Heat. If the pain is very dull and not very severe, it is due to Deficient-Cold in the Stomach. If the pain is alleviated by eating, it is of the Empty type; if it is aggravated by eating, it is of the Full type.

A feeling of fullness in the epigastrium is due either to Spleen deficiency or to Dampness.

Lower abdominal pain can be due to many different causes, the most common of which are internal Cold, stagnation of Liver-Qi or Liver-Blood, Damp-Heat, stasis of Blood in the Intestines or Uterus. These various conditions can only be differentiated on the basis of the accompanying symptoms and signs. An abdominal pain which is relieved by bowel movements is of a Full nature; if it is aggravated by bowel movements, it is of an Empty nature.

Hypogastric pain is usually due to Damp-Heat in the Bladder or sometimes Liver-Fire infusing downwards to the Bladder.

5 FOOD AND TASTE

These questions are aimed at establishing the state of Stomach and Spleen.

Food

In general, a condition that is relieved by eating is of an Empty nature; if it is aggravated by eating, it is of a Full nature.

Lack of appetite indicates Spleen-Qi deficiency. Being always hungry indicates Heat in the Stomach.

A feeling of fullness and distension after eating indicates retention of food. A preference for hot food (in terms of temperature) indicates a Cold pattern; preference for cold food indicates a Heat pattern.

Taste

A bitter taste indicates a Full-Heat pattern, either of Liver or Heart. If it is due to Liver-Fire, the bitter taste is more or less constant. If it is due to Heart-Fire, it is associated with insomnia, and is only present in the morning after a sleepless night, and not after a good night's sleep.

A sweet taste indicates either Spleen deficiency or Damp-Heat.

A sour taste indicates retention of food in the Stomach or disharmony of Liver and Stomach.

A salty taste indicates Kidney-Yin deficiency. Lack of taste sensation indicates Spleen deficiency.

A pungent taste indicates Lung-Heat.

VOMIT

— Sour vomiting: invasion of Stomach by Liver
— Bitter vomiting: Liver and Gall-Bladder Heat
— Clear-watery vomiting: Cold in the Stomach with retention of fluids
— Vomiting soon after eating: Heat pattern.

Any vomiting which is sudden and with a loud noise indicates a Full pattern. Any vomiting which is slow in coming and with a weak noise indicates an Empty pattern.

6 STOOLS AND URINE

These are two important questions to establish the Full or Empty and Hot or Cold character of a condition.

Stools

Constipation

Aggravation of a condition after a bowel movement suggests an Empty pattern; amelioration of a condition after a bowel movement suggests a Full condition.

Acute constipation with thirst and dry yellow coating indicates Heat in the Stomach and Intestines.

Constipation in old people or women after childbirth is due to deficiency of Blood.

Constipation with small, bitty stools like goat's stools indicates stagnation of Liver-Qi and Heat in the Intestines.

If the stools are not dry, difficulty in performing a bowel movement indicates stagnation of Liver-Qi.

Constipation with abdominal pain indicates internal Cold and deficiency of Yang.

Constipation with dry stools, without thirst, indicates Yin deficiency, usually of Kidneys and/or Stomach.

Alternation of constipation and diarrhoea indicates that stagnant Liver-Qi is invading the Spleen.

Diarrhoea

Pain accompanying diarrhoea always suggests involvement of the Liver or the presence of Heat.

The presence of a foul smell indicates Heat, while the absence of smell indicates Cold.

The most common cause of chronic diarrhoea is either Spleen-Yang, or Kidney-Yang deficiency or both. Chronic diarrhoea occurring every day in the very early morning is due to Kidney-Yang deficiency and is called "cock-crow diarrhoea" or also "5th-hour diarrhoea".

If the diarrhoea is accompanied by abdominal pain, it indicates the presence of interior Cold in the Intestines.

Diarrhoea with mucus in the stools indicates Dampness in the Intestines. If it has blood too, it indicates Damp-Heat in the Intestines.

Loose stools with undigested food indicate Spleen-Qi deficiency. A burning sensation in the anus while passing stools indicates Heat.

If the stools are not loose or only slightly loose but are very frequent and the person cannot hold them easily, it indicates deficiency of Middle Qi, i.e. the Qi of Stomach and Spleen: it also indicates sinking of Spleen-Qi.

Black or very dark stools indicate stasis of Blood. If the blood comes first, and is bright-red splashing in all directions, it indicates Damp-Heat in the Intestines.

If the blood comes first and is turbid and the anus feels heavy and painful, it indicates Heat in the Blood.

If the stools come first and then the blood, and this is watery, it indicates that Spleen-Qi is deficient and is unable to control Blood.

Borborygmi (gurgling sounds in the abdomen) with loose stools indicate Spleen deficiency.

Borborygmi with a feeling of abdominal distension and without loose stools, indicate stagnation of Liver-Qi.

Flatulence is generally due to stagnation of Liver-Qi. If there is a foul smell, it indicates Damp-Heat in the Spleen or Stomach-Heat. If there is no smell, it indicates interior Cold from Spleen-Yang deficiency.

Urine

The salient diagnostic features to be considered here are the function, pain, colour and amount of urine.

Function

Enuresis or incontinence indicate Kidney deficiency. Retention of urine indicates Damp-Heat in the Bladder.

Difficulty in urination indicates either Damp-Heat in the Bladder or deficiency of Kidney (the latter is more common in old people).

Very frequent and copious urination indicates Kidney deficiency, frequent and scanty urination is usually caused by Qi deficiency.

Pain

Pain before urination indicates stagnation of Qi in the Lower Burner, pain during urination indicates Heat in the Bladder and pain after urination indicates deficiency of Qi.

Colour

Pale urine indicates a Cold pattern, usually of the Bladder and Kidneys. Dark urine indicates a Heat pattern.

Turbid or cloudy urine indicates Dampness in the Bladder. Copious, clear and pale urination during an exterior invasion of Wind-Cold or Wind-Heat indicates that the pathogenic factor has not penetrated into the Interior (if it had, the urine would be dark).

Amount

Large amounts of urine indicate Kidney-Yang deficiency. Scanty urination indicates Kidney-Yin deficiency.

7 SLEEP

Insomnia

Sleep depends on the state of Blood and Yin. Blood and Yin are the "residence" of the Mind: without Blood and Yin, the Mind has no residence and it floats at night causing insomnia.

Insomnia in the sense of not being able to fall asleep, but sleeping well after falling asleep, indicates deficiency of Heart-Blood.

Insomnia in the sense of waking up many times during the night indicates deficiency of Kidney-Yin.

Dream-disturbed sleep indicates Liver-Fire or Heart-Fire. Restless sleep with dreams indicates retention of food.

Waking up early in the morning and failing to fall asleep again indicates deficiency of Gall-Bladder.

As people grow older, it is to some extent normal to wake early, due to the physiological decline of Qi and Blood.

Lethargy

Feeling sleepy after eating indicates Spleen-Qi deficiency. A general feeling of lethargy and heaviness of the body indicates retention of Dampness. If there is also dizziness, it indicates Phlegm.

Extreme lethargy and lassitude with a feeling of cold, indicates deficiency of Kidney-Yang.

Lethargic stupor with exterior Heat symptoms indicates invasion of Pericardium by Heat.

Lethargic stupor with rattling in the throat, a Slippery pulse and a sticky tongue coating, indicates blurring of the mind by Phlegm.

8 EARS AND EYES

The Kidneys open into the ears, but not every ear problem is related to the Kidneys. The Lesser Yang channels flow to the ear and some exterior Heat conditions can cause ear problems. In addition, Dampness and Phlegm obstruct the rising of clear Yang to the upper orifices and this can affect the ears.

Tinnitus

Onset

A sudden onset suggests a Full condition (usually Liver-Fire or Liver-Wind). A gradual onset suggests an Empty condition (usually deficiency of the Kidneys).

Pressure

If the noise is aggravated by pressing with one's hands on the ears, it suggests a Full condition; if it is alleviated, it suggests an Empty condition.

Character of noise

A loud, high-pitch noise like a whistle indicates Liver-Yang, Liver-Fire or Liver-Wind rising. A low-pitch noise like rushing water indicates Kidney deficiency.

Deafness

A sudden onset suggests a Full condition (of the same type as for tinnitus) and a gradual onset suggests an Empty condition.

In chronic cases, apart from Kidney deficiency, deafness can also be due to:

— Heart-Blood deficiency
— Deficiency of Qi of the Upper Burner
— Yang Qi deficiency.

Eyes

Pain

Pain like a needle and with redness of the eye associated with headache indicates Fire-Poison in the Heart channel.

Pain, swelling and redness of the eye indicate either invasion of the eye channels by exterior Wind-Heat, or interior Liver-Fire.

Blurred vision and "floaters" in the eyes indicate Liver-Blood deficiency. Photophobia also indicates Liver-Blood deficiency.

A feeling of pressure in the eyes indicates Kidney-Yin deficiency.

Dryness

Dryness of the eyes indicates Liver and/or Kidney Yin deficiency.

9 THIRST AND DRINK

Thirst with desire to drink large amounts of cold water indicates a Full-Heat pattern, which can be of any organ.

Absence of thirst indicates a Cold pattern, usually of the Stomach or Spleen.

Thirst but with no desire to drink indicates Damp-Heat (the Heat gives rise to the thirst, but the Dampness makes one reluctant to drink).

Thirst with desire to sip liquids slowly, or to sip warm liquids indicates Yin deficiency (usually of Stomach or Kidneys).

Desire to drink cold liquids suggests a Heat pattern; desire to drink warm liquids suggests a Cold pattern.

10 PAIN

Pain can be caused by Full or Empty conditions. The Full or Empty character of pain should always be ascertained, especially with relation to pain experienced in the head, chest or abdomen.

Aetiology and pathology of pain

Pain can be due to the following Excess conditions:

— Invasion of exterior pathogenic factors
— Interior Cold or Heat
— Stagnation of Qi or Blood
— Obstruction by Phlegm
— Retention of food.

All these conditions cause an obstruction to the circulation of Qi in the channels and therefore pain. These are all Full types of pain. There is a saying in Chinese Medicine that goes: *"If the channels are free there is no pain; if the channels are obstructed there is pain"*.

Pain can also be due to Deficiency conditions:

— Deficiency of Qi and Blood
— Consumption of Body Fluids from Yin deficiency.

These conditions cause malnourishment of the channels and hence pain. This is an Empty type of pain and would tend to be duller than the previous type (Table 2).

Stagnation of Qi causes distention more than pain, or a distending pain, having no fixed location.

Stasis of Blood causes a severe, boring pain, with a fixed location in a small area.

WOMEN

Special questions need to be asked of women regarding menstruation, discharges, pregnancy and childbirth.

Menstruation

The condition of menstruation gives a very vivid idea of a woman's state of Qi and Blood. One must ask about the cycle, amount of bleeding, colour of blood, quality and pain.

Table 2 Characters of pain

	Empty	Full	Cold	Heat
Pressure	alleviated	aggravated	—	—
Food	alleviated	aggravated	—	—
Type	dull-lingering	sharp	cramping	burning
Temperature	—	—	better with heat	better with cold
Bowel movement	aggravated	alleviated	aggravated	alleviated
Posture	better lying down	better sitting	—	—
Onset	slow, gradual	sudden	—	—
Vomiting	aggravated	alleviated	aggravated	alleviated
Rest/movement	better with rest	better with movement	better with movement	worse with movement

Cycle

If the periods always come early it indicates either Heat in the Blood or Qi deficiency.

If the periods always come late, it indicates either Blood deficiency of stagnation of Blood or Cold.

If the periods are irregular, coming sometimes early and sometimes late, it indicates stagnation of Liver-Qi or Liver-Blood, or Spleen deficiency.

Amount

A heavy loss of blood indicates either Heat in the Blood or Qi deficiency (see under colour of blood below).

Scanty periods indicate either Blood deficiency or stagnation of Blood or Cold.

Colour

A dark-red or bright-red colour indicates Heat in the Blood. Pale blood indicates Blood deficiency.

Purple or blackish blood indicates stasis of Blood or Cold. Fresh-red blood indicates Empty-Heat from Yin deficiency.

Quality

Congealed blood with clots indicates stasis of Blood or Cold. Watery blood indicates Blood or Yin deficiency.

Turbid blood indicates Blood-Heat or stagnation of Cold.

Pain

Pain before the periods indicates stagnation of Qi or Blood.

Pain during the periods indicates Blood-Heat or stagnation of Cold. Pain after the periods indicates Blood deficiency.

These questions and their answers have limited value with regard to women who take the contraceptive pill, or had an intra-uterine device fitted, or in multiparous women.

Leucorrhoea

This must be distinguished according to colour, consistency and smell.

Colour

A white discharge indicates a Cold pattern. This could be from Spleen or Kidney-Yang deficiency, or exterior Cold-Damp, or sometimes from stagnation of Liver-Qi.

A yellow discharge indicates a Heat pattern, usually Damp-Heat in the Lower Burner.

A greenish discharge indicates Damp-Heat in the Liver channel. A red and white discharge also indicates Damp-Heat.

A yellow discharge with pus and blood in a woman after menopause indicates toxic Damp-Heat in the uterus.

Consistency

A watery consistency suggests a Cold-Damp pattern, whilst a thick consistency suggests a Damp-Heat pattern.

Smell

A fishy smell indicates Damp-Cold; a leathery smell indicates Damp-Heat.

Pregnancy

Infertility can be due to Empty conditions such as Blood or Kidney-Essence deficiency, or to Full conditions such as Damp-Heat in the Lower Burner or stasis of Blood in the uterus.

Vomiting during pregnancy indicates Stomach and Penetrating Vessel deficiency.

Miscarriage before three months indicates Blood or Essence deficiency and is associated with a Kidney deficiency; after three months it indicates Liver-Blood stasis or sinking of Spleen-Qi.

Childbirth

Nausea and heavy bleeding after delivery indicates exhaustion of the Penetrating Vessel.

Sweating and fever after delivery indicate exhaustion of Qi and Blood.

Post-natal depression is usually due to Blood deficiency leading to Heart-Blood deficiency.

CHILDREN

Interrogation of children does not differ substantially from that of adults, except that it needs to be carried out mostly with the child's parents.

There are several questions, however, which are peculiar to children's problems.

First of all, one needs to ask about the pregnancy as emotional shocks or physical traumas can affect the constitution of the baby. Also the consumption of alcohol, smoking and use of drugs (of the medicinal or "recreational" kind) all affect the health of the baby adversely.

Traumas at birth, such as Caesarian or very long birth will affect the baby, particularly the baby's Lungs.

One also needs to ask about breast-feeding and weaning. Weaning too early can lead to the retention of food and some skin diseases.

It is also important to ask about vaccinations as, in some cases, these may cause problems. Finally, in older children, one must ask about childhood diseases such as whooping cough or measles. Whooping cough usually leaves the Lungs quite weakened especially if it occurs in a severe form.

Persistent sore throats and/or a runny nose in children often indicates too early weaning or too rich food consumed too early.

DIAGNOSIS BY FEELING

Diagnosis by feeling includes palpation of the pulse, skin, limbs, hand, chest, abdomen and points.

PULSE DIAGNOSIS

Pulse diagnosis is an extremely complex subject with many ramifications, and the following will only be a simple discussion of it in the context of Chinese diagnosis.

Pulse diagnosis is important for two reasons: because it can give very detailed information on the state of the internal organs, and because it reflects the whole complex of Qi and Blood. The pulse can be seen as a clinical manifestation, a sign like any other such as thirst, insomnia or a red face. The important difference is that, besides giving certain specific indications, the pulse also reflects the organism as a whole, the state of Qi, Blood and Yin, the Yin and Yang organs, all parts of the body, and even the constitution of a person. The tongue can reflect these phenomena too, but less so than the pulse.

The main drawback of pulse diagnosis is that it is an extremely subjective form of diagnosis, probably more than any other element of Chinese diagnosis. If a face is red, or if a tongue is red, these are quite objective signs, and anyone can see them. Feeling the pulse is an extremely subtle skill and is very difficult to learn. Most students will be familiar with the frustrating experience of not being able to feel that a certain pulse is "choppy" or "slippery".

The pulse can give very detailed information on the state of the internal organs, but it is also subject to external, short-term influences, which make its interpretation very difficult indeed and fraught with pitfalls. For example, if a person has been running upstairs the pulse becomes rapid very quickly, and it would be wrong to interpret that as a sign of a "Heat pattern". If a person has had an emotional upset or shock, the pulse will also change quickly. If a person works very hard and has very little sleep for a week or so, the pulse can become very weak and deep, but it is quickly restored with just a few days' rest. From this point of view, the tongue is less subject to such short-term influences.

The practice of taking the pulse on the radial artery was started by the "Classic of Difficulties". Before that, the pulse was felt at nine different arteries, three on the head, three on the hands and three on the legs, reflecting the state of the energy of the Upper, Middle and Lower Burner respectively. This location for pulse-taking was described in the "Simple Questions" in chapter 20.[9] These positions for pulse-taking are all on acupuncture points which are situated near arteries. They are shown in Table 3.

Table 3 The "9 Regions" of the pulse from the "Simple Questions"

		Point	Artery	Area or organ
HEAVEN	Upper	Extra-point Taiyang	Temporal artery	Sides of head
	Middle	Ermen TB-21	Temporal artery	Ear and eyes
	Lower	Juliao ST-3	Facial artery	Teeth and mouth
PERSON	Upper	Taiyuan LU-9	Radial artery	Lungs
	Middle	Shenmen HE-7	Ulnar artery	Heart
	Lower	Hegu L.I.-4	Radial artery	Chest
EARTH	Upper	Taichong LIV-3	Dorsal m. artery	Liver
		Wuli LIV-10	Femoral artery	Liver
	Middle	Chongyang ST-42	Dorsal artery	Spleen
		Jimen SP-11	Femoral artery	Spleen
	Lower	Taixi KI-3	Tibial artery	Kidneys

As can be seen from the table, Taichong LIV-3 and Chongyang ST-42 have an alternative position for pulse-taking at Wuli LIV-10 and Jimen SP-11 respectively.

The "Classic of Difficulties" established the practice of feeling the pulse at the radial artery, dividing it into three areas and feeling it at three different levels, i.e superficial, middle and deep. The three sections of the pulse at the radial artery were called "inch", "barrier" and "cubit". In this book they will be called "Front", "Middle" and "Rear" respectively. Three levels at each of the three sections made the so-called "nine regions".[10]

The "Classic of Difficulties" clearly relates the three sections of the pulse to the three Burners. It says: *"There are three positions, inch, bar and cubit and nine regions [each position being] superficial, middle and deep. The upper [distal] position corresponds to Heaven and reflects diseases from the chest to the head; the middle position corresponds to Person and reflects diseases between the diaphragm and umbilicus; the lower [proximal] position corresponds to Earth and reflects diseases from below the umbilicus to the feet"*.[11]

Over the centuries, there have been several different attributions of organs to individual pulse positions. The two most commonly used today are derived from the "Pulse Classic" (A.D. 280) of Wang Shu He and the "Pulse Study of Bin-hu lake explained simply" (1564) by Li Shi Zhen.

The pulse positions adopted in the "Pulse Classic" are:

	Left	*Right*
FRONT	Heart/Small Intestine	Lungs/Large Intestine
MIDDLE	Liver/Gall Bladder	Spleen/Stomach
REAR	Kidney/Bladder	Fire of Gate of Vitality/Lower Burner

The pulse positions adopted in the "Pulse Study of Bin-hu lake explained simply" are:

	Left	*Right*
FRONT	Heart/Thorax	Lungs/Chest
MIDDLE	Liver/Gall Bladder	Spleen/Stomach
REAR	Kidneys/Small Intestine	Kidneys/Large Intestine

Another widely used arrangement comes from the "Golden Mirror of Medical Tradition" (1742) by Wu Qian. This includes positions for the Yang organs:

	Left	*Right*
FRONT	Heart/Pericardium	Lungs/Chest
MIDDLE	Liver/Gall Bladder	Spleen/Stomach
REAR	Kidney/Bladder/Small Intestine	Kidney/Large Intestine

The left Rear position is usually thought to reflect the Qi of Kidney-Yin and the right Rear position that of Kidney-Yang.

Contradictory though these different arrangements might seem, there is actually a common strand running through them. First of all, there is general agreement that the Front positions reflect the state of Qi in the Upper Burner, the Middle positions the Middle Burner and the Rear positions the Lower Burner (apart from Wang Shu He's positioning of Large Intestine and Small Intestine in the Front positions, which will be explained shortly).

However, with regard to the Yang organs, there seem to be the most discrepancies. In fact, some doctors did not even consider that the state of the Yang organs could be reflected on the pulse.

In my opinion the differences are reconcilable because different pulse arrangements reflect the different therapeutic approaches of the herbalist and acupuncturist. Given that the pulse reflects the Qi of both organ and channel, the acupuncturist working on the channels would naturally assign the Small Intestine and Large Intestine to the same position as the Heart and Lungs to which their channels are connected. The herbalist, on the other hand, would give more importance to the internal organs rather than channels, and assign the Small Intestine and Large Intestine to the Rear position, i.e. the Lower Burner, which is where these organs are situated.

Another reason for the discrepancies is that the Small Intestine and Large Intestine organs are much less closely related to their respective channels than the other organs. These two organs are situated in the Lower Burner while their channels are in the arms (all other organs in the Upper Burner have their respective channels on the arms, and those of the Middle or Lower Burner have their respective channels on the legs). Moreover, the functions of the actual intestinal organs and their respective channels do not closely correspond for, although the Small Intestine and Large Intestine channel points can be used for their corresponding organ problems, they are much more frequently used to treat diseases of the Upper Burner areas (shoulders, neck, head) and invasions of exterior pathogenic factors affecting the shoulders, neck and head.

This aside, another aspect of pulse diagnosis also explains why we should not make too much of the different pulse positions assumed by different doctors. The pulse essentially reflects the state of Qi in the different Burners and at different energetic levels which are dependent on the pathological condition. The pulse needs to be interpreted dynamically rather than mechanically. For this reason, we should not attach undue importance to the organ (or channel) positions on the pulse. The most important thing is to appraise how Qi is flowing; what is the relationship of Yin and Yang on the pulse; at what level Qi is flowing (i.e. is the pulse superficial or deep); whether the body's Qi is deficient and whether there is an attack by an exterior pathogenic factor.

Each pulse position can reflect different phenomena in different situations. For example, let us consider the left Middle pulse (Liver position): in a state of health, the Liver and Gall Bladder Qi will be balanced or, to put it differently, Yin and Yang within the Liver/Gall Bladder sphere are balanced. In this case, the pulse will be relatively soft and smooth and not particularly superficial or deep and the Gall Bladder influence on the pulse will not be felt. But if Liver-Yang is in excess and rises upwards affecting the Gall Bladder channel (causing severe temporal headaches), the rising Qi will be reflected on the pulse which will be Wiry (harder than normal) and more superficial (it will be felt pounding under the finger). In interpreting this pulse we can say that Liver-Yang is rising, or, to put it differently, that the Gall Bladder Qi is in Excess.

To give another example, if the right Front pulse (Lung pulse) is quite full, bigger than normal and rapid, it could indicate an emotional problem affecting the Lungs. Here, the pulse would reflect the state of the Lungs. But on another occasion exactly the same type of pulse may indicate something quite different when for example the patient has an acute, large, purulent tooth abscess. In such a case, the pulse reflects the state of the Large Intestine channel (where the abscess is) rather than a problem with the Lung organ.

When feeling the pulse, one should assess it at

three different depths: a superficial, middle and deep level. The superficial level is felt by just resting the fingers on the artery very gently; the deep level is felt by pressing quite hard to the point of nearly obliterating the pulse and then releasing very slightly; the middle level is felt in between these two pressures.

The three levels of the pulse give an immediate idea of the level of Qi in the pulse and therefore the kind of pathological condition that might be present. In particular:
— the Superficial level reflects the state of Qi (and the Yang organs)
— the Middle level reflects the state of Blood
— the Deep level reflects the state of Yin (and the Yin organs).

Thus, by examining the strength and quality of the pulse at the three levels, one can have an idea of the pathology of Qi, Blood or Yin, and also of the relative state of Yin and Yang.

The clinical significance of the three levels was interpreted differently by different doctors but all these approaches are equally valid and should be borne in mind.

For example, besides reflecting Qi, Blood and Yin, the three levels also reflect the following:
— Superficial level: Exterior diseases
— Middle level: Stomach and Spleen diseases
— Deep level: Interior diseases.

Li Shi Zhen gives yet another interpretation of the three levels as follows:
— the Superficial level reflects the state of Heart and Lungs
— the Middle level reflects the state of Stomach and Spleen
— the Deep level reflects the state of Liver and Kidneys.

With this slant, the Qi of the internal organs is not only reflected at the various positions, but also depths. The idea is that the Heart and Lungs (particularly the Lungs) can be said to control the Exterior of the body and their Qi is therefore felt at the superficial level. The Stomach and Spleen make Blood and their Qi can therefore be felt at the Blood (middle) level. The Liver and Kidneys (particularly the Kidneys) control the Yin energies and their Qi is therefore felt at the Yin (deep) level.

Thus, the clinical significance of the three levels of depth on the pulse can be interpreted in three different ways, each of them meaningful (Table 4).

Conversely one can interpret the three positions Front, Middle and Rear as reflecting the energies Qi, Blood and Yin respectively, as well as the three body areas of Upper, Middle and Lower and their respective organs (Table 5).

Method for taking the pulse

Time

Traditionally, the best time for taking the pulse is in the early morning when the Yin is calm and the Yang has not yet come forth.

This is of course not always possible to

Table 4 Clinical significance of the three pulse levels

Level	Energy types	Energy levels	Organs
Superficial	Qi (and Yang organs)	The exterior	Heart and Lungs
Middle	Blood	Stomach and Spleen	Stomach and Spleen
Deep	Yin (and Yin Organs)	The interior	Kidneys

Table 5 Clinical significance of pulse positions

Pulse positions	Energy type	Burner	Organs
Front	Qi	Upper	Heart-Lungs
Middle	Blood	Middle	Stomach-Spleen
Rear	Yin	Lower	Kidneys

achieve when patients are seen throughout the day.

Levelling the arm

The patient's arm should be horizontal and should not be held higher than the level of the heart.

Placing the fingers

The practitioner's fingers are all placed on the pulse, which is felt with the first three fingers. To assess individual positions, it may be necessary to lift two of these fingers slightly, but, generally, it is better to keep all the fingers in place to get a better idea of Qi and Blood in general.

Equalizing the breathing

It is traditionally important for the practitioner to regulate and balance his or her own breathing pattern in order to be better attuned to the patient's Qi better and to become more receptive.

Another reason for doing this was that the patient's pulse was correlated with the practitioner's breathing cycles in order to determine whether it is slow or rapid.

Factors to take into account

Several factors should be taken into account in order to evaluate each pulse in its context and in relation to an individual patient.

Seasons

These influence the pulse, it being deeper in wintertime and more superficial in summertime.

Sex

Men's pulses are naturally slightly stronger than women's. Also, in men the left pulse should be very slightly stronger, and in women the right pulse should be slightly stronger. This is in accordance with the symbolism of Yin and Yang, following which the left side is Yang (hence male) and the right side is Yin (hence female).

In men, the Front position should be very slightly stronger, while in women the Rear position should be so. This also follows the Yin-Yang symbolism according to which upper is Yang (hence male) and lower is Yin (hence female).

Occupation

The pulse of those who are engaged in heavy physical work should be stronger than those who are engaged in mental work.

The normal pulse

The pulse should have three qualities which are described as having Stomach-Qi, having spirit and having a root.

Stomach Qi

A pulse is said to have Stomach Qi, when it feels "gentle", "calm" and is relatively slow (4 beats per respiratory cycle).

A pulse with Stomach Qi is not rough. The Stomach is the Sea of Food, the Root of the Post-Heaven Qi and the origin of Qi and Blood. For this reason, it gives "body" to the pulse. If the pulse feels too rough or hard, it indicates that the Stomach function is impaired. The "Simple Questions" in chapter 19 says: *"The Stomach is the Root of the 5 Yin organs; the Qi of the Yin organs cannot reach the Lung channel [i.e. the radial artery on the Lung channel] by itself but it needs Stomach-Qi . . . if the pulse is soft it indicates that it has Stomach-Qi and the prognosis is good"*.[12]

This particular quality of being "soft" (but not too soft), "gentle", "calm" and "not rough" is important: beginners often take a rough and hard quality of the pulse as being "healthy".

Spirit

The pulse is said to have spirit when it is soft but with strength, neither big or small and regular. It should also be regular in its quality, i.e. it should not change quality very easily and frequently. A pulse that has these qualities reflects a good state of Heart Qi and Blood.

Root

A pulse is said to have root in two different senses. It has a root when the deep level can be felt clearly, and also when the Rear position can be felt clearly. Having a root indicates that the Kidneys are healthy and strong.

Thus a pulse that has spirit, Stomach Qi and root indicates a good state of the Mind, Qi and Essence respectively.

When interpreting the pulse one should therefore pay attention to the following elements and in this order:

Feel the pulse as a whole

Feel whether the pulse has spirit, Stomach Qi and root

Feel the three levels and the three positions

Feel the strength of the pulse

Feel the quality of the pulse.

There are 28 pulse qualities, as follows.

1 Floating (or superficial) pulse

Feeling

This pulse can be felt with a light pressure of the fingers, just resting the fingers on the artery.

Clinical significance

This quality indicates the presence of an exterior pattern from invasion by an exterior pathogenic factor, such as Wind-Cold or Wind-Heat. If it is Floating and Tight it indicates Wind-Cold; if it is Floating and Rapid it indicates Wind-Heat.

If the pulse is Floating at the superficial level but Empty at the deep level, it indicates deficiency of Yin.

In rare cases, the pulse can be Floating in Interior conditions, such as anemia or cancer. In these cases, the pulse is Floating because Qi is very deficient and "floats" to the surface of the body.

2 Deep pulse

Feeling

This pulse is the opposite to the preceding one: it can only be felt with a heavy pressure of the fingers and is felt near the bone.

Clinical significance

This quality indicates an Interior condition, which could assume many different forms. It also indicates that the problem is in the Yin organs.

If it is Deep and Weak it indicates deficiency of Qi and Yang. If it is Deep and Full, it indicates stasis of Qi or Blood in the Interior, or interior Cold or Heat.

3 Slow pulse

Feeling

This pulse has three beats per respiration cycle (of the practitioner). In the old times the rate was referred to the practitioner's respiration cycle, but nowadays the pulse rate can also be counted conventionally using a watch.

Normal rates vary but they are roughly:

Age (year)	*Rate (beat/min)*
1-4	90 or more
4-10	84
10-16	78/80
16-35	76
35-50	72/70
50+	68

Clinical significance

A Slow pulse indicates a Cold pattern. If it is Slow and Empty it indicates Empty-Cold from deficiency of Yang. If it is Slow and Full, it indicates Full-Cold.

4 Rapid pulse

Feeling

This pulse has more than 5 beats per each respiration cycle, or has a higher rate than the ones indicated above.

Clinical significance

A Rapid pulse indicates a Heat pattern. If it is Empty and Rapid, it indicates Empty-Heat from Yin deficiency. If it is Full and Rapid, it indicates Full-Heat.

5 Empty pulse

Feeling

The Empty pulse feels rather big but soft. "Empty" may suggest that nothing can be felt, but this is not so: this pulse is actually rather big but it feels empty on a slightly stronger pressure and is soft.

Clinical significance

The Empty pulse indicates Qi deficiency.

6 Full pulse

Feeling

This pulse feels full, rather hard and rather long. "Full" is often used in two slightly different ways. On the one hand, it indicates a specific type of pulse as described above; on the other hand, this term is often used to indicate any pulse of the Full type.

Clinical significance

The Full pulse indicates a Full pattern. A Full and Rapid pulse indicates Full-Heat, and a Full and Slow pulse indicates Full-Cold.

7 Slippery pulse

Feeling

A Slippery pulse feels smooth, rounded, slippery to the touch, as if it were oily. It slides under the fingers.

Clinical significance

The Slippery pulse indicates Phlegm, Dampness, retention of food or pregnancy.

Generally speaking, the slippery pulse is Full by definition, but in some cases it can also be Weak, indicating Phlegm or Dampness with a background of Qi deficiency.

8 Choppy pulse

Feeling

This pulse feels rough under the finger: instead of a smooth pulse wave, it feels as if it had a jagged edge to it.

Choppy also indicates a pulse that changes rapidly both in rate and quality.

Clinical significance

A Choppy pulse indicates deficiency of Blood. It may also indicate exhaustion of fluids and it may occur after profuse and prolonged sweating or vomiting.

9 Long pulse

Feeling

This pulse is basically longer than normal: it extends slightly beyond the normal pulse position.

Clinical significance

It indicates a Heat pattern.

10 Short pulse

Feeling

This pulse is the opposite of the previous one: it occupies a shorter space than the normal position.

Clinical significance

The Short pulse indicates severe deficiency of Qi. It frequently appears on the Front positions of left or right.

It also specifically denotes deficiency of Stomach-Qi.

11 Overflowing

Feeling

This pulse feels big, it extends beyond the pulse position, it is superficial and generally feels as if it overflows the normal pulse channel, like a river overflows during a flood.

Clinical significance

The Overflowing pulse indicates extreme Heat. It frequently appears during a fever, but it is also felt in chronic diseases characterized by interior Heat.

If it is Overflowing but Empty on pressure, it indicates Empty-Heat from Yin deficiency.

12 Fine (or thin) pulse

Feeling

This pulse is thinner than normal.

Clinical significance

A Fine pulse indicates deficiency of Blood. It may also indicate internal Dampness with severe deficiency of Qi.

13 Minute pulse

Feeling

This pulse is basically the same as the Fine one, just more so. It is extremely thin, small and difficult to feel.

Clinical significance

The Minute pulse indicates severe deficiency of Qi and Blood.

14 Tight pulse

Feeling

This pulse feels twisted like a thick rope.

Clinical significance

A Tight pulse indicates Cold which may be interior or exterior, such as in invasion of exterior Wind-Cold. If it is Tight and Floating it indicates exterior Cold; if it is Tight and Deep it indicates interior Cold.

This pulse is frequently felt in asthma from Cold in the Lungs, and in Stomach conditions from Cold.

The Tight pulse may also indicate pain from an interior condition.

15 Wiry pulse

Feeling

This pulse feels taut like a guitar string. It is thinner, more taut and harder than the Tight pulse. The Wiry pulse really hits the fingers.

Clinical significance

The Wiry pulse can indicate three different conditions:

- Liver disharmony
- Pain
- Phlegm.

16 Slowed-down pulse

Feeling

This pulse has 4 beats for each respiration cycle.

Clinical significance

This is generally a healthy pulse and has no pathological significance.

17 Hollow pulse

Feeling

This pulse can be felt at the superficial level, but if one presses slightly harder to find the middle level it is not there; it is then felt again at the deep level with a stronger pressure. In other words, it is empty in the middle.

Clinical significance

This pulse appears after a haemorrhage. If the pulse is rapid and slightly Hollow it may indicate a forthcoming loss of blood.

18 Leather pulse

Feeling

This pulse feels hard and tight at the superficial level and stretched like a drum, but it feels completely empty at the deep level. It is a large pulse, not thin.

Clinical significance

The Leather pulse indicates severe deficiency of the Kidney-Essence or Yin.

19 Firm pulse

Feeling

The Firm pulse is felt only at the deep level and it feels hard and rather wiry. It could be described as a Wiry pulse at the deep level.

Clinical significance

The Firm pulse indicates interior Cold (if it is also Slow) or interior stagnation and pain.

20 Weak-floating (or soft) pulse

Feeling

The Weak-Floating pulse can be felt only on the superficial level. It feels very soft and is only slightly floating, i.e. not as much as the Floating pulse. It disappears when a stronger pressure is applied to feel the deep level. It is similar to the Floating-Empty pulse, but it is softer and not so Floating.

Clinical significance

The Weak-Floating pulse indicates deficiency of Yin and Essence.

It may also indicate the presence of Dampness, but only when this pathogenic factor is present in combination with a very Empty condition.

21 Weak pulse

Feeling

A Weak pulse cannot be felt on the superficial level, but only at the deep level. It is also soft.

Clinical significance

The Weak pulse indicates deficiency of Yang.

22 Scattered pulse

Feeling

This pulse feels very small and is relatively superficial. Instead of feeling like a wave, the pulse feels as if it were "broken" in small dots.

Clinical significance

This pulse indicates very severe deficiency of Qi and Blood, and in particular of Kidney-Qi. It always indicates a serious condition.

23 Hidden pulse

Feeling

This pulse feels as if it were hidden beneath the bone. It is very deep and difficult to feel. It is basically an extreme case of a Deep pulse.

Clinical significance

The Hidden pulse indicates extreme deficiency of Yang.

24 Moving pulse

Feeling

The Moving pulse has a round shape like a bean, it is short and it "trembles" under the finger. It has no definite shape, having no head or tail, just rising up in the centre. It feels as if it is shaking and is also somewhat slippery.

Clinical significance

This pulse indicates shock, anxiety, fright or

extreme pain. It is frequently found in persons with deep emotional problems particularly from fear, or in those who have suffered an intense emotional shock, even if many years previously.

25 Hasty pulse

Feeling

This pulse is Rapid and it stops at irregular intervals.

Clinical significance

The Hasty pulse indicates extreme Heat and a deficiency of Heart-Qi. It is also felt with conditions of Heart-Fire.

26 Knotted pulse

Feeling

This pulse is Slow and it stops at irregular intervals.

Clinical significance

The Knotted pulse indicates Cold and deficiency of Heart-Qi or Heart-Yang.

27 Intermittent pulse

Feeling

This pulse stops at regular intervals.

Clinical significance

This pulse always indicates a serious internal problem of one or more Yin organs. If it stops every 4 beats or less, the condition is serious.

It can also indicate a serious heart problem (in a Western medical sense).

28 Hurried

Feeling

This pulse is very rapid, but it also feels very agitated and urgent.

Clinical significance

This pulse indicates an Excess of Yang, with Fire in the body exhausting the Yin.

The 28 pulse qualities can be grouped into six groups of pulses with similar qualities:
a) The Floating kind: Floating-Hollow-Leather
b) The Deep kind: Deep-Firm-Hidden
c) The Slow kind: Slow-Knotted
d) The Rapid kind: Rapid-Hasty-Hurried-Moving
e) The Empty kind: Empty-Weak-Fine-Minute-Weak/Floating- Short-Scattered
f) The Full kind: Full-Overflowing-Wiry-Tight-Long.

PALPATING THE SKIN

This includes feeling the temperature, moisture and texture of the skin.

Temperature

A subjective feeling of heat of a person does not always correspond to an objective heat feeling of the skin. If the skin actually feels hot to the touch it often indicates the presence of Damp-Heat.

A cold feeling of the skin indicates a Cold pattern. This is often felt in the loins, lower abdomen or lower back, where it indicates a deficiency of Kidney-Yang.

If the skin feels hot on first touch and if the pressure of the fingers is maintained it ceases to feel hot, it indicates invasion of exterior Wind-Heat with the pathogenic factor still only on the Exterior.

If the skin over a blood vessel feels hot on medium pressure but not on heavy pressure, it indicates interior Heat in the Middle Burner or Heart.

If the skin feels hot on heavy pressure which nearly reaches the bone, it indicates Empty-Heat from Yin deficiency.

Moisture and texture

A moist feeling of the skin may indicate invasion of the Exterior by Wind-Cold or, more usually, by Wind-Heat.

If the skin feels moist in the absence of exterior symptoms, it indicates spontaneous sweating from deficiency of Lung-Qi.

If the skin feels dry, it indicates Blood deficiency or Lung-Yin deficiency.

Skin which feels rough may indicate Painful Obstruction Syndrome from Wind. If the skin is scaly and dry, it indicates exhaustion of body fluids.

If the skin is swollen and a pit is left visible after pressing with one's finger, it indicates oedema. If no pit is formed on pressing a swollen area, it indicates retention of Dampness, and the swelling is called "Qi swelling" as opposed to the former called "Water swelling".

PALPATING THE LIMBS

If the hands and feet feel cold to the touch it indicates deficiency of Yang. If the whole arm and leg feel cold, it indicates a Kidney-Yang deficiency. If only the forearm and lower leg (or only hands and feet) feel cold, it may indicate interior Cold from stagnation of Qi. Thus the former indicates Empty-Cold, the latter Full-Cold. If only the hands and feet feel cold, it may be due to stagnation of Qi. This is sometimes called the *Si Ni San* Syndrome because this formula is used to treat it.

If the limbs feel hot, it indicates a Heat pattern. If the hands are hot on the dorsum, it indicates Full-Heat. If they are hot on the palms, it indicates Empty-Heat from Yin deficiency.

PALPATING THE HAND

The palm of the hand reflects the state of most internal organs in a pattern similar to that found in the ear. The correspondence of various areas to internal organs can be visualized by superimposing the figure of a small baby to the palm of the hand (Fig. 55).[13]

The major areas of correspondence are (Fig. 56):

1. Chest cavity organs

2 and 3. Abdominal cavity organs

4. Reproductive and urinary organs
5. Respiratory organs
6. Intestines, rectum.

A more detailed representation of the correspondence with internal organs is shown in Fig. 56.

Diagnosis is made by gently pressing the relevant areas: a sharp pain indicates a Full condition and a dull soreness indicates an Empty condition of the relevant organ.

PALPATING THE CHEST

First of all, one should palpate the area over the left ventricle apex of the heart, where the pulsation of the heart can be felt and sometimes even seen. This area is called "Interior Emptiness" (*Xu Li*) in Chinese Medicine.

Traditionally, this area is considered to be the end of the Stomach Great Connective Channel, starting in the stomach itself (see p. 347). It is also considered to reflect the state of the Gathering Qi of the chest (*Zong Qi*). If the pulsation under this area is regular, and not tight nor rapid, it indicates a good state of the Gathering Qi. If the pulsation is faint but clear, it indicates deficiency of Gathering Qi.

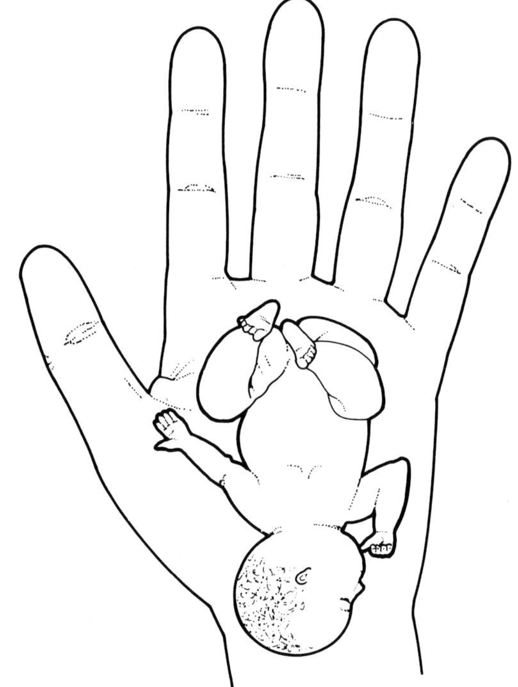

Fig. 55 Hand diagnosis areas

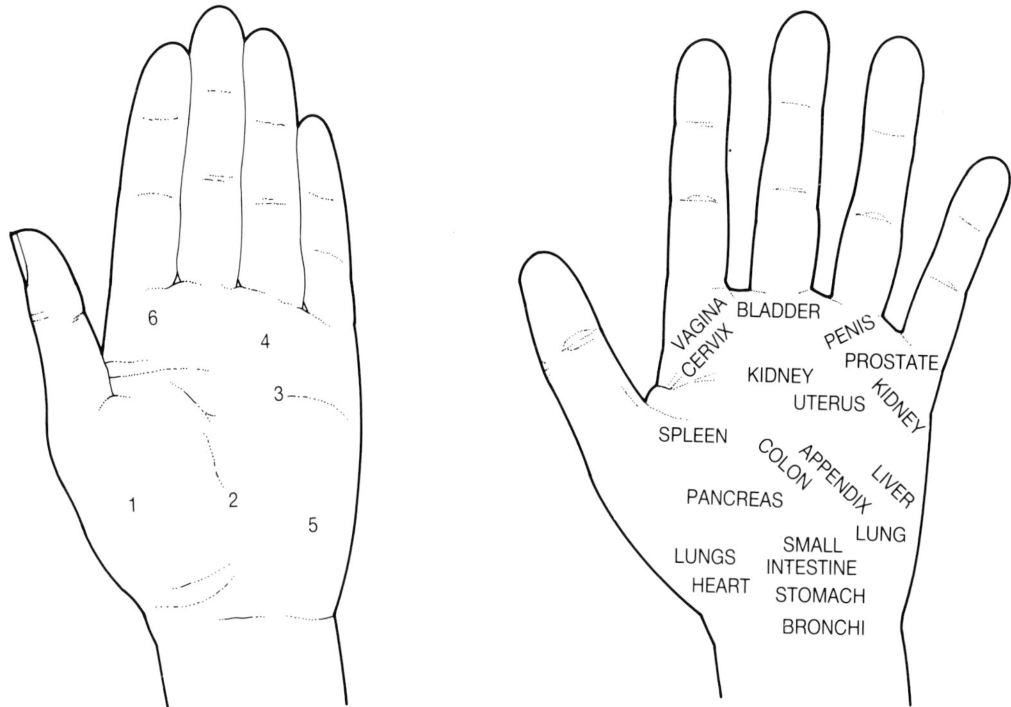

Fig. 56 Organ positions in hand diagnosis

If the pulsation is too strong it indicates "outpouring of Gathering Qi", i.e. a state of hyperactivity due to pushing oneself too much.

If the pulsation cannot be felt, it indicates Phlegm or hiatus hernia.

If the area just below the xyphoid process feels full and is painful on pressure, it indicates a Full pattern. It is often caused by bottled-up emotional problems which affect the chest and give rise to stagnation of Qi in this area.

PALPATING THE ABDOMEN

If the abdomen feels full on touch and no pain is elicited on pressure it indicates an Empty pattern; if pain is elicited, it indicates a Full pattern.

The elasticity and strength of the abdomen is important: it should feel solid but not hard, resilient but not tight, elastic but not soft. If it feels like this it indicates the good state of the Original Qi. If it feels too soft and flabby, it indicates deficiency of Original Qi.

The relative tightness or softness of the upper and lower part of the abdomen is significant. The upper part of the abdomen just below the xyphoid process reflects the state of the Upper Burner Qi, i.e. Lung and Heart Qi and Gathering Qi. This area should be relatively softer than the rest, indicating a smooth flow of Lung and Heart Qi. If it feels hard and knotted, it indicates a constraint of Lung and Heart Qi and a constriction of the Corporeal Soul due to emotional tension.

The lower part of the abdomen below the umbilicus should feel relatively tenser (but elastic) than the rest, indicating a good state of the Original Qi of the Kidneys. If it feels soft and flabby, it indicates a weakness of the Original Qi.

Abdominal masses that move under the fingers indicate stagnation of Qi: if they do not move and feel very hard, they indicates stasis of Blood.

PALPATING POINTS

Channel and points diagnosis is based on

objective or subjective reactions appearing at certain points. Generally speaking, any point can be used in diagnosis, following the general principles outlined above for the channels. However, certain points are particularly useful in diagnosis: these are the Back Transporting points (see ch. 38), the Front Collecting points (see ch. 38), the Lower-Sea points (see ch. 38) and Ah Shi points.

The Back Transporting points are the places where the Qi and Blood of a particular organ "infuses": they are directly related to their respective organ and very often manifest certain reactions when the organ is diseased.

As a general principle, any sharp pain (either spontaneous or on pressure) on these points indicates a Full condition of the relevant organ, and a dull soreness (either spontaneous or on pressure) indicates an Empty condition. Each Back Transporting point can reflect the condition of its relevant organ, e.g. Weishu BL-21 for the Stomach, etc. In addition, Gaohuangshu BL-43 reflects the state of the Lungs, Zhishi BL-53 is often sore in Kidney-diseases and Shangliao BL-31, Ciliao BL-32, Zhongliao BL-33 and Xialiao BL-34 reflect the state of the reproductive system particularly in women.

The Front Collecting points are particularly reactive to pathological changes of the internal organs and are useful for diagnostic purposes. Each Front Collecting point reflects the state of an internal organ and a list is given in chapter 38.

The Lower-Sea points are also useful in diagnosing stomach or intestinal diseases: Zusanli ST-36 for the stomach, Shangjuxu ST-37 for the Large Intestine and Xiajuxu ST-39 for the Small Intestine. In addition, there is a special point between Zusanli ST-36 and Shangjuxu ST-37 which reflects the state of the appendix. Its location is variable and is situated wherever there is a soreness in between those two points. If this special point (called "*Lanweixue*" meaning "appendix point") is painful on pressure, it indicates inflammation of the appendix. If the appendix is healthy, there will be no reaction at this point.

Finally, Ah Shi points can be used for diagnosis. The theory of Ah Shi points was developed by Sun Si Miao (581-682) during the Tang dynasty. He said very simply that wherever there is soreness on pressure (whether on a channel or not), there is a point. This is obviously because the channel network is so dense that every area of the body is irrigated by a channel. As we have already seen, dull soreness on pressure indicates an Empty condition of the channel influencing that area, while a sharp pain on pressure indicates a Full condition of the channel.

NOTES

1 I have chosen to name these four methods of examination using simple words to express the actions, rather than the more formalized medical expressions of "observation", "auscultation", "interrogation" and "palpation". These terms, familiar in Western Medicine, can suggest a Western medical procedure. For example, "auscultation" suggests listening to chest sounds through a stethoscope, a procedure very different from the Chinese diagnostic method of listening.

2 Su Ma Qian (145 BC -?) Annals, cited in History of Chinese Medicine, p 19.

3 Simple Questions, ch 13, p 86.

4 Spiritual Axis, ch 80, p 151-152.

5 Guangdong College of Traditional Chinese Medicine 1964 A Study of Diagnosis in Chinese Medicine (*Zhong Yi Zhen Duan Xue* 中医诊断学)Shanghai Scientific Publishing House, p 34-35.

6 Nanjing College of Traditional Chinese Medicine, 1978 A Study of Warm Diseases (*Wen Bing Xue* 温病学) Shanghai Scientific Publishing House, p 53.

7 This is only a brief account of tongue diagnosis. For a detailed discussion of tongue diagnosis in clinical practice see Maciocia G 1987 Tongue Diagnosis in Chinese Medicine Eastland Press, Seattle.

8 Comprehensive Text, p 90.

9 Simple Questions, p 129-135.

10 Classic of Difficulties, ch 18, p 46.

11 Ibid., p 46

12 Simple Questions, p 127-128.

13 Li Wen Chuan-He Bao Yi 1987 Practical Acupuncture (*Shi Yong Zhen Jin Xue* 实用针灸学)People's Health Publishing House, Beijing, p 37.

Identification of Patterns 17

辨證

Identification of patterns indicates the process of identifying the basic disharmony that underlies all clinical manifestations. This is the essence of Chinese medical diagnosis and pathology. Identifying a pattern involves discerning the underlying pattern of disharmony by considering the picture formed by all symptoms and signs.

Rather than analysing symptoms and signs one by one in trying to find a cause for them as Western Medicine does, Chinese Medicine forms an overall picture taking all symptoms and signs into consideration to identify the underlying disharmony. In this respect, Chinese Medicine does not look for causes but patterns. Thus, when we say that a certain patient presents the pattern of Deficient Kidney-Yin, this is not the cause of the disease (which has to be looked for in the person's life), but the disharmony underlying the disease or the way the condition presents itself. Of course, in other respects, after identifying the pattern, Chinese Medicine does go a step further in trying to identify a cause for the disharmony.

"Symptoms and signs" in Chinese Medicine have a rather different meaning than in Western Medicine. They are different from the relatively narrow area explored by Western Medicine despite its battery of clinical tests. Instead, the doctor of Chinese Medicine widens his or her view to assess changes in a broad range of common bodily functions such as urination, defecation, sweating, thirst and so on. Furthermore, the doctor of Chinese Medicine takes into account many clinical manifestations ranging from certain facial and bodily signs to psychological and emotional traits which are not really "symptoms" or "signs" as such, but rather expressions of a certain disharmony. Many of the clinical manifestations contributing to form a picture of an underlying disharmony would not be considered as "symptoms" or "signs" in Western Medicine. For example, absence of thirst, inability to make decisions, a dull appearance of the eyes or thirst with desire to drink in small sips, all meaningful manifestations in Chinese Medicine, would not be considered as such in Western Medicine. Thus, whenever the words "symptoms" and "signs" occur, they should be interpreted in this broad way. Over many centuries of accumulated clinical experience by countless doctors, Chinese Medicine has developed a comprehensive and extremely effective diagnostic system and symptomatology to identify disease patterns and the underlying disharmonies.

Identifying patterns also follows the typical way of Chinese natural philosophy which looks for relationships rather than causes. Each symptom and sign has a meaning only in relation to all the others: one symptom can mean different things in different situations. For example, a dry tongue accompanied by a feeling of cold, absence of thirst, cold hands and profuse pale urination indicates Yang deficiency, while a dry tongue accompanied by a feeling of heat, thirst, night-sweating and a rapid pulse indicates Yin deficiency.

Identifying the pattern of disharmony blends diagnosis, pathology and treatment principle all in one. When we say that a certain syndrome is characterized by deficiency of Spleen-Yang with retention of Dampness, we are defining the nature of the condition, the site and, by implication, the treatment principle. In this example, the treatment principle would be to tonify Spleen-Yang and transform Dampness. In the particular case of exterior patterns, by identifying the pattern we also identify the "cause". For example, if we say that a certain complex of clinical manifestations forms the pattern of exterior invasion of Wind-Cold, we are simultaneously identifying the cause (Wind-Cold), the type of pattern and by implication the treatment principle, which in this case would be to release the Exterior and scatter Cold.

Identifying the pattern allows us to find the nature and character of the condition, the site of the disease, the treatment principle and the prognosis.

As the "Essentials of Chinese Acupuncture" points out "identification [of the pattern] is made not from a simple list of symptoms and signs, but from a reflection on the pathogenesis of the disease".[1]

In other words, we should not only identify the pattern but also understand how it arose and how different aspects of it interact with each other. For example, if we identify the pattern of Liver-Qi stagnation and also one of Spleen-Qi deficiency, we should go a step further and find out how these two patterns interact and whether one can be considered the cause of the other.

There are several methods used to identify patterns. These are applicable in different situations and were formulated at different times in the development of Chinese Medicine. The various modes of identifying patterns are:

Identification of patterns according to the 8 Principles

Identification of patterns according to Qi, Blood and Body Fluids

Identification of patterns according to the Internal Organs

Identification of patterns according to Pathogenic Factors

Identification of patterns according to the 5 Elements

Identification of patterns according to the Channels

Identification of patterns according to the 6 Stages

Identification of patterns according to the 4 Levels

Identification of patterns according to the 3 Burners.

Each of these is applicable in different cases.

1 IDENTIFICATION OF PATTERNS ACCORDING TO THE EIGHT PRINCIPLES

Elements of this identification are found throughout Chinese medical texts starting from the "Yellow Emperor's Inner Classic" and the "Discussion on Cold-induced Diseases". In its present form, this method of identifying patterns was formulated by Cheng Zhong Ling in the early Qing dynasty (see following chapter).

The identification according to the 8 Principles is based on the categories of Interior/Exterior, Hot/Cold, Full/Empty and Yin/Yang. It is the summarization of all other modes of identification and is applicable in all cases, for both interior and exterior diseases. This method of identification of patterns is discussed in chapter 18.

2 IDENTIFICATION OF PATTERNS ACCORDING TO QI, BLOOD AND BODY FLUIDS

This method of identification of patterns describes the basic disharmonies of Qi, Blood and Body Fluids, such as deficiency, stagnation and rebellion of Qi, deficiency, stasis, Heat and loss of Blood and deficiency of fluids, oedema and Phlegm.

This particular method is very important and constantly used in clinical practice especially for internal diseases. It is integrated with the method of identification according to the Internal Organs. This method of identification is discussed in chapter 19.

3 IDENTIFICATION OF PATTERNS ACCORDING TO THE INTERNAL ORGANS

Again, elements of this process of identification of patterns are found throughout Chinese medical text from the earliest times, but, in its present form, it was formulated during the early Qing dynasty.

This method of identification is based on the pathological changes occurring in the Internal Organs, and is the most important of all the various systems for the diagnosis and treatment of internal diseases.

In a way, it consists in the application of the 8 Principles to specific Internal Organs. For example, according to the 8 Principles, a condition may be due to Full-Heat, but, applying the process of identification according to the Internal Organs, we can identify the organ affected by the Full-Heat. This identification is discussed in chapter 20.

4 IDENTIFICATION OF PATTERNS ACCORDING TO PATHOGENIC FACTORS

This method of pattern identification is based on the pathological changes occurring when the body is invaded by pathogenic factors such as Wind, Dampness, Cold, Heat, Dryness and Fire. Each of these pathogenic factors may be exterior or interior. This method of identification is discussed in chapter 32.

5 IDENTIFICATION OF PATTERNS ACCORDING TO THE FIVE ELEMENTS

This method of identification of patterns is based on the interpretation of clinical manifestations according to the generating, over-acting and insulting sequences of the 5 Elements. These will be described in chapter 33.

6 IDENTIFICATION OF PATTERNS ACCORDING TO THE CHANNELS

This is the oldest of all modes of identification of patterns. Reference to it occurs in the "Spiritual Axis".[2] This method of identification of patterns describes the symptoms and signs related to each channel, rather than the organ (see ch. 34).

This way of identifying patterns comes into its own when an acupuncturist treats a condition which is caused by damage to a channel rather than an internal organ or even by damage to an internal organ manifesting along its corresponding channel. For this reason, it is not used much for the treatment of internal conditions, as it does not give the doctor enough information to make a diagnosis or formulate a method of treatment. When treating an internal condition, i.e. a disease of an internal organ, the identification of patterns according to the Internal Organs is the preferred method.

7 IDENTIFICATION OF PATTERNS ACCORDING TO THE SIX STAGES

This was formulated by Zhang Zhong Jing (born c. AD 158) in his "Discussion on Cold-induced Diseases". This method of identification is used not only for the diagnosis and treatment of diseases from exterior Cold, but also for hot, internal conditions as many of its recommended herbal prescriptions can treat interior conditions (see App. 1).

This method of identification has been the bible of Chinese doctors, especially in North China, for about 16 centuries, to be supplanted, especially in South China, by the method of identification according to the 4 Levels and 3 Burners.

8 IDENTIFICATION OF PATTERNS ACCORDING TO THE FOUR LEVELS

This was devised by Ye Tian Shi (1667-1746) in his book "Discussion of Warm Diseases" and it describes the pathological changes caused by exterior Wind-Heat. It is the most important and most widely used method of identification of patterns for the treatment of febrile infectious diseases that start with invasion of exterior Wind-Heat (see App. 2).

9 IDENTIFICATION OF PATTERNS ACCORDING TO THE THREE BURNERS

This was formulated by Wu Ju Tong (1758–1836) in his book "A Systematic Identification of Febrile Diseases". This method of identification of patterns is usually combined with the previous one for the diagnosis and treatment of febrile infectious diseases starting with invasion of Wind-Heat (see App.3).

These last three methods of identifications of patterns are deeply rooted in the tradition of herbal medicine, rather than acupuncture: they can only really be understood and put into perspective within the context of herbal medicine. A brief sketch of their clinical manifestations is given in Appendices 1, 2 and 3. They will not be fully discussed in the present book as I have given a full account of them elsewhere.[3]

NOTES

1 Essentials of Chinese Acupuncture, p 60.
2 Spiritual Axis, ch 10, p 30 to 39.
3 The interested reader can refer to the author's book Tongue Diagnosis in Chinese Medicine.

Identification of Patterns According to the Eight Principles

18 八綱辨証

The identification of patterns according to the 8 Principles is the foundation for all the other methods of pattern formulation. It is the basic groundwork of pattern identification in Chinese Medicine, allowing the practitioner to identify the location and nature of the disharmony, as well as establish the principle of treatment.

Although the term "8 Principles" is relatively recent in Chinese Medicine (early Qing dynasty), their main aspects were discussed both in the "Yellow Emperor Classic of Internal Medicine" and in the "Discussion on Cold-induced Diseases". Both these classics contain many references to Interior/Exterior, Hot/Cold, Full/Empty and Yin/Yang characters of diseases.

Doctor Zhang Jing Yue (also called Zhang Jie Bin) (1563-1640) discussed the identification of patterns according to the above principles and called it the "Six Changes" (*Liu Bian* 六变), these being Interior/Exterior, Full/Empty and Hot/Cold.

During the early Qing dynasty, at the time of Emperor Kang Xi (1661–1690), doctor Cheng Zhong Ling wrote the "Essential Comprehension of Medical Studies" (*Yi Xue Xin Wu* 医学心悟), in which he, for the first time, used the term "8 Principles" (*Ba Gang* 八纲).

The method of identification of patterns according to the 8 Principles differs from all the others in so far as it is the theoretical basis for all of them and is applicable in every case. For example, the method of identification of patterns according to the Channels is only applicable in channel problems, and that according to the Internal Organs in organ problems, but the identification of patterns according to the 8 Principles is applicable in every case because it allows us to distinguish Exterior from Interior, Hot from Cold and Full from Empty. It therefore allows us to decide which method of identification of patterns applies to a particular case. No condition is too complex to fall outside the scope of identification according to the 8 Principles.

It is important to realize that identifying a pattern according to the 8 Principles does not mean rigidly "categorizing" the disharmony in order to "fit" the clinical manifestations in pigeon holes. An understanding of the 8 Principles, on the contrary, allows us to unravel complicated patterns and identify the basic contradictions within them, reducing the various disease manifestations to the bare relevant essentials.

Although this process might seem rigid and somewhat forced in the beginning, after a few years of practice, it will become completely natural and spontaneous.

The 8 Principles should not be seen in terms of "either-or". It is not at all unusual to see conditions that are Exterior and Interior simultaneously, or Hot and Cold, or Full and Empty or Yin and Yang. It is even possible for a condition to be all of these at the same time. The purpose of applying the 8 Principles is not to categorize the disharmony, but to understand its genesis and nature. It is only by understanding this that we can decide on treatment for a particular disharmony.

Moreover, not every condition need have all four characteristics (Interior or Exterior, Hot or Cold, Full or Empty and Yin or Yang). For example, a condition need not necessarily be either hot or cold. Deficiency of Blood is a case in point as it does not involve any Hot or Cold symptoms.

The 8 Principles are:

Interior-Exterior
Full-Empty
Hot-Cold
Yin-Yang.

INTERIOR-EXTERIOR

The differentiation of Exterior and Interior is not made on the basis of what caused the disharmony (aetiology), but on the basis of the location of the disease. For example, a disease may be caused by an exterior pathogenic factor, but if this is affecting the Internal Organs, the condition will be classified as interior.

EXTERIOR

An Exterior condition affects the skin, muscles and channels. An Interior condition affects the Internal Organs and bones. Skin, muscles and channels are also called the "Exterior" of the body, and the Internal Organs the "Interior". In the context of exterior diseases from Wind, the Exterior is sometimes also called the "Lung-Defensive Qi portion", as the Lung controls both the skin and the Defensive Qi which circulates in the skin and muscles.

The clinical manifestations arising from invasion of the Exterior by a pathogenic factor are also called an "exterior pattern", while the manifestations arising from a disharmony of the Internal Organs is called an "interior pattern".

When we say that an exterior condition affects the skin, muscles and channels, we mean that these areas have been invaded by an exterior pathogenic factor, giving rise to typical "exterior" clinical manifestations. However, it would be wrong to assume that any problem manifesting on the skin, is an "exterior pattern". In fact, most chronic skin problems are due to an interior pattern manifesting on the skin.

There are two types of exterior conditions: those that affect skin and muscles and are caused by an exterior pathogenic factor having an acute onset (such as in invasion of Wind-Cold or Wind-Heat); and those that affect the channels and have a slower onset (such as in Painful Obstruction Syndrome).

When an exterior pathogenic factor invades skin and muscles it gives rise to a typical set of symptoms and signs which are described as an "exterior pattern". It is difficult to generalize as to what these symptoms and signs are, as it depends on the other characters, i.e. whether they are of the Cold or Hot type, and the Empty or Full type. However, fever and aversion to cold occurring simultaneously always indicate an invasion from an exterior pathogenic factor.

Generally speaking, we can say that the main symptoms of an exterior pattern are fever, aversion to cold, aching body, a stiff neck and a Floating pulse. The onset is acute and the correct treatment will usually induce a swift and marked improvement of the condition.

If the condition is one of Cold (such as Wind-Cold) the symptoms are a slight or absent fever, aversion to cold, severe aches in the body, severe stiff neck, chilliness, no sweating, no thirst, a Floating-Tight pulse and a thin-white tongue coating.

If the condition is one of Heat (such as Wind-Heat) the symptoms are fever, aversion to cold, slight sweating, thirst, a Floating-Rapid pulse and a thin-yellow tongue coating. In this case the body aches are not so pronounced.

The main factors in differentiating the Hot or Cold character of an exterior pattern are:

— thirst (Hot) or its absence (Cold)
— white (Cold) or yellow (Hot) tongue coating
— Tight (Cold) or Rapid (Hot) pulse
— Fever (Hot) or its absence (Cold).

The character of an exterior pattern will further depend on its Full or Empty character. If a person has a tendency to deficiency of Qi or Blood, the exterior pattern will have an Empty character. This is also described as an exterior pattern from Wind-Cold with prevalence of Wind.

The clinical manifestations of an Exterior-Empty pattern are slight or no fever, sweating, aversion to wind, slight body-aches, a Floating-Slow pulse and a thin-white tongue coating.

If a person has a tendency to Fullness, the exterior pattern will have a Full character.

The clinical manifestations of such an Exterior-Full pattern are fever, no sweating, severe body-aches, aversion to cold, a Floating-Tight pulse and a thin-white tongue coating.

The main factors in differentiating an Empty from Full Exterior condition are:
— sweating (Empty) or its absence (Full)
— Pulse (Slow in Empty and Tight in Full)
— severity of body aches (severe in Fullness, less severe in Emptiness).

It must be stressed that "Full" and "Empty" describing the character of an exterior condition are only relative, and do not represent actual Fullness and Emptiness. In fact, an exterior pattern is characterized by Fullness by definition as it consists in an invasion by an exterior pathogenic factor. The person's Qi is still relatively intact and the pathogenic factor fights against the body's Qi. It is precisely this that defines a Full condition: i.e. one characterized by the presence of a pathogenic factor and the resulting struggle with the body's Qi. Thus an exterior condition must, by definition be Full. However, according to a person's pre-existing condition, one can further differentiate an exterior condition between Full and Empty, but only in relative terms.

Case history

A young girl of 13 fell ill with what was described as "influenza". She had a temperature of 102 F, a sore throat, cough, headache, aches in all joints, slight thirst and slight sweating. Her tongue was slightly red on the sides and the Pulse was Floating in both Front positions.

This is a clear example of invasion of exterior Wind-Heat.

The second kind of exterior pattern is that occurring when an exterior pathogenic factor invades the channels in a gradual way causing Painful Obstruction Syndrome. This is characterized by obstruction to the circulation of Qi in channels and joints by a pathogenic factor, which can be Cold, Dampness, Wind or Heat.

In obstruction from Cold, usually only one joint is affected, the pain is severe and is relieved by application of heat. In obstruction from Wind, the pain moves from joint to joint. In obstruction from Dampness, there will be swelling of the joints, while in obstruction from Heat, the pain is severe and the joints are swollen and hot.

INTERIOR

A disharmony is defined as interior when the Internal Organs are affected. This may or may not have arisen from an exterior pathogenic factor, but once the disease is located in the Interior, it is defined as an interior pattern, and treated as such.

It is impossible to generalize to give the clinical manifestations of interior conditions as these will depend on the organ affected, and whether the condition is Hot or Cold and Full or Empty.

Most of the Internal Organs patterns described in Chapters 20–31 are internal ones.

Interior patterns of the Hot or Cold and Full or Empty type will be described shortly.

HOT-COLD

Hot and Cold describe the nature of a pattern and their clinical manifestations depend on whether they are combined with a Full or Empty condition.

HOT

Full-Heat

The main manifestations are fever, thirst, red

face, red eyes, constipation, scanty-dark urine, a Rapid-Full pulse, and a Red tongue with yellow coating.

This is a description of an Interior Full-Heat pattern as Exterior Heat has already been discussed above.

These are only the general symptoms of Full-Heat, as many others are possible depending on which organ is mostly affected. Fever need not always be present as many conditions of Interior-Full-Heat such as Liver-Fire or Heart-Fire do not involve fever.

Aside from the above clinical manifestations, there are other diagnostic guides which indicate Heat.

Any raised, red skin eruption which feels hot, indicates Heat. For example, acute urticaria normally takes this form. As for pain, any burning sensation indicates Heat. For example, the burning sensation of cystitis, or a burning feeling in the stomach. Any loss of blood with large quantities of dark-red blood, indicates Heat in the Blood. As far as the mind is concerned, any condition of extreme restlessness or manic behaviour, indicates Heat in the Heart.

Full-Heat arises when there is an Excess of Yang energies in the body. Common causes of this are the excessive consumption of hot-energy foods or long-standing emotional problems, when the stagnation of Qi generates Heat. The former will mostly cause Stomach or Liver Heat, while the latter will mostly cause Liver or Heart Heat.

Full-Heat can also develop from the invasion of an exterior pathogenic factor which turns into Heat once in the body. Most pathogenic factors, including Cold, are likely to turn into Heat once in the body. A typical example of this is when exterior Cold or Heat turns into Heat and settles in the Stomach, Lung or Intestines causing high fever, sweating and thirst. The Bright Yang pattern of the 6-Stage Pattern Identification and the Qi Level of the 4-Level Pattern Identification describe such situations.

From the Yin-Yang point of view, Full-Heat arises from Excess of Yang (Fig. 57).

Case history

A woman of 50 suffered from burning pain in the epigastrium. She also complained of nausea with occasional vomiting, bleeding of the gums, bad breath, thirst and insomnia. Her tongue was Red, had a crack in the centre with a spiky yellow coating and was dry. Her pulse was Full and slightly Rapid.

These manifestations indicate Full-Heat in the Stomach.

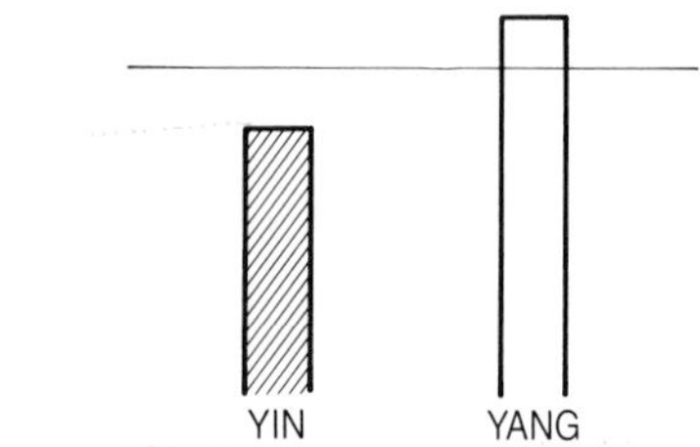

Fig. 57 Full-Heat from Excess of Yang

Empty-Heat

The main manifestations are afternoon fever or a feeling of heat in the afternoon, a dry mouth, a dry throat at night, night sweating, a feeling of heat in the chest and palms and soles (also called "5-palm heat"), dry stools, scanty-dark urine, a Floating-Empty and Rapid pulse and a Red-Peeled tongue.

Again, these are only the general symptoms and signs; others depend on which organ is mostly affected.

Aside from these manifestations, Empty-Heat can easily be recognized from a typical feeling of mental restlessness, fidgeting and vague anxiety. The person feels that something is wrong, but is unable to describe what or how. Empty-Heat restlessness is quite different from that of Full-Heat, and one can almost visually perceive the Emptiness underlying the Heat.

From the Yin-Yang point of view, Empty-Heat arises from Deficiency of Yin (Fig. 58). If the Yin energy is deficient for a long period of time, the Yin is consumed and the Yang is relatively in Excess.

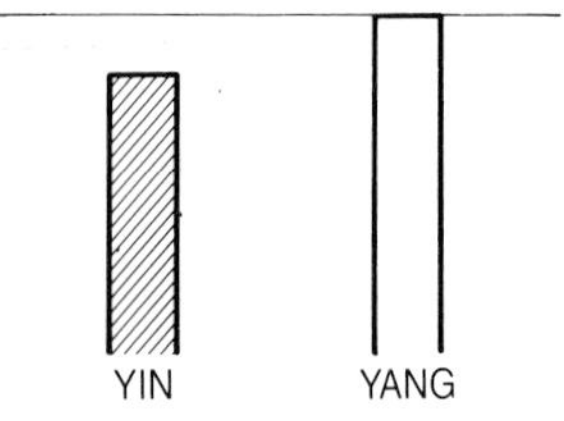

Fig. 58 Empty-Heat from Deficiency of Yin

Table 6 Comparison between Full-Heat and Empty-Heat

	Full-Heat	Empty-Heat
Face	Whole face red	Malar flush
Thirst	Desire to drink cold water	Desire to drink warm water, or cold water in small sips
Eyelid	Red all over inside eyelid	Thin red line inside eyelid
Taste	Bitter taste	No bitter taste
Feeling of heat	All day	In the afternoon or evening
Fever	High fever	Low-grade fever in the afternoon
Mind	Very restless and agitated	Vague anxiety, fidgeting
Bowels	Constipation, abdominal pain	Dry stools, no abdominal pain
Bleeding	Profuse	Slight
Sleep	Dream-disturbed, very restless	Waking up frequently during the night or early morning
Skin	Red-hot-painful skin eruptions	Scarlet-red, not raised, painless skin eruptions
Pulse	Full-Rapid-Overflowing	Floating-Empty, Rapid
Tongue	Red with yellow coating	Red and Peeled or Thin
Treatment method	Clear Heat	Nourish Yin, clear empty Heat

Empty-Heat frequently arises from deficiency of Kidney-Yin. Because Kidney-Yin is the foundation for all the Yin energies of the body, when this is deficient it can affect the Yin of the Liver, Heart and Lungs. A long-standing deficiency of Yin in any of these organs can give rise to Empty-Heat manifesting with various symptoms, such as mental restlessness and insomnia when Heart-Yin is deficient, irritability and headaches when Liver-Yin is deficient and malar flush and dry cough when Lung-Yin is deficient.

In practice, it is important to differentiate Full-Heat from Empty-Heat as the treatment method in the former case is to clear the Heat, while in the latter case is to nourish Yin (Table 6).

Case history

A woman of 54 suffered from severe anxiety, insomnia, dizziness, tinnitus, soreness of the lower back, a feeling of heat in the evening, a dry mouth and night sweating. Her face was flushed on the cheek-bones. Her pulse was Floating-Empty and slightly Rapid and her tongue was Red and Peeled.

This is an example of Empty-Heat (dry mouth, feeling of heat, flushed cheek-bones, night sweating, Rapid pulse and Red-Peeled tongue) arising from Kidney-Yin deficiency (soreness of the back, dizziness and tinnitus). The Empty-Heat was affecting the Heart as indicated by the anxiety and insomnia.

COLD

Full-Cold

The main manifestations are chilliness, cold limbs, no thirst, pale face, abdominal pain aggravated on pressure, desire to drink warm liquids, loose stools, clear-abundant urination, Deep-Full-Tight pulse and a Pale tongue with thick white coating.

These are the clinical manifestation of Interior Full-Cold as Exterior Cold has already been described above.

Cold contracts and obstructs and this often causes pain. Hence pain, especially abdominal pain, is a frequent manifestation of Full-Cold. Also, anything that is white, concave (as opposed to raised), bluish-purple may indicate Cold. For example, a pale face or pale tongue, a white tongue coating, concave very pale spots on the tongue, a bluish-purple tongue and bluish lips or fingers and toes.

From the Yin-Yang point of view, Full-Cold arises from Excess of Yin (Fig. 59).

Interior Full-Cold can arise from direct invasion of exterior Cold into the Interior. In particular, exterior Cold can invade the Stomach

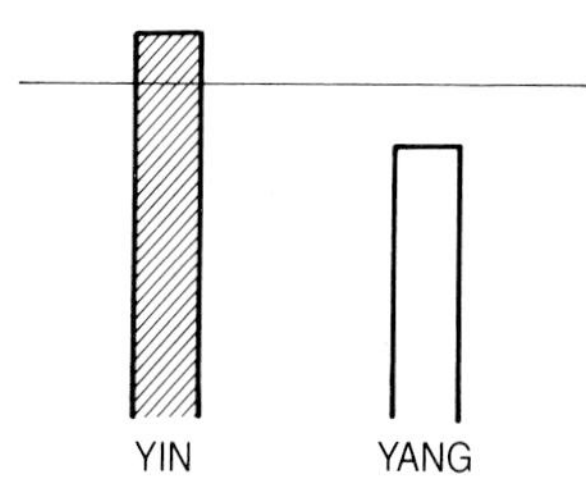

Fig. 59 Full-Cold from Excess of Yin

causing vomiting and epigastric pain, the Intestines causing diarrhoea and abdominal pain and the Uterus causing dysmenorrhoea. All these conditions would have an acute onset.

Cold can also invade the Liver channel causing swelling and pain of the scrotum.

One of the main manifestations of interior Full-Cold is abdominal pain as Cold contracts and obstructs the circulation of Yang Qi, giving rise to pain.

Case history

A woman of 24 had had a sudden attack of severe, spastic abdominal pain. Her stools became loose, her tongue had a thick-white-sticky coating, and her pulse was Deep andTight.

These manifestations clearly indicated an attack of exterior Cold and Damp.They are a case of Full-Cold. The severity and sudden onset of the pains indicates a Full condition, as does the thick tongue coating (in case of Empty- Cold it would have been thin). The Cold and Damp come from the exterior but have attacked the Interior directly, in this case the Intestines. The Cold character of the pattern is apparent from the white coating and the Tight pulse. The presence of Dampness with the Cold is indicated by the stickiness of the tongue coating and the loose stools (due to Dampness obstructing the Spleen function of transformation).

Empty-Cold

The main manifestations are chilliness, cold limbs, a dull-pale face, no thirst, listlessness, sweating, loose stools, clear-abundant urination, a Deep-Slow or Weak pulse and a Pale tongue with thin white coating.

From the Yin-Yang point of view, Empty-Cold arises from deficiency of Yang (Fig. 60).

Empty-Cold develops when Yang-Qi is weak and fails to warm the body. It is mostly related to Spleen-Yang, Kidney-Yang, Heart-Yang or

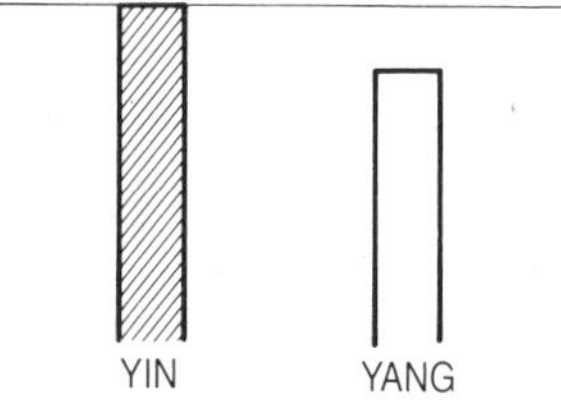

Fig. 60 Empty-Cold from Deficiency of Yang.

Lung-Qi deficiency. The most common cause is Spleen-Yang deficiency. When this is deficient, the Spleen fails to warm the muscles, hence the chilliness. The Spleen needs heat for its function of transformation of food, and when Yang is deficient, food is not transformed properly and loose stools result.

Case history

A woman of 31 suffered from tiredness, weight-gain, constipation and chilliness. In the past, she had also developed a swelling of the thyroid gland. Her tongue was very Pale and Swollen, and the pulse was very Fine, Deep and Slow.

This is a clear case of Yang deficiency with internal Empty-Cold. The tiredness, chilliness, Pale and Swollen tongue and Deep-Slow pulse, all indicate deficiency of Spleen-Yang. The deficiency of Spleen-Yang has given rise to internal Dampness, manifested by weight-gain, the Swollen tongue and the swelling of the thyroid gland. The constipation is, in this case, due to deficiency of Yang, since deficient Yang Qi is unable to promote the descending function of the Intestines. This is a less common type of constipation, as normally deficiency of Yang will cause loose stools.

COMBINED HOT AND COLD

A condition can often be characterized by the presence of both Heat and Cold. These can be Cold on the Exterior and Heat in the Interior, Heat on the Exterior and Cold in the Interior and Heat above and Cold below. Furthermore, in some cases, some of the symptoms and signs may point to a false appearance of Heat while the true condition is Cold or vice versa.

Cold on the exterior—heat in the interior

This condition is found when a person has a pre-existing condition of interior Heat and is subsequently invaded by exterior Wind-Cold.

The symptoms and signs would include a fever with aversion to cold, no sweating, a headache and stiff neck, aches throughout the body (manifestations of exterior Cold), irritability and thirst (manifestations of interior Heat).

This situation also occurs in attacks of Latent Heat combined with a new invasion of Wind-Cold. According to the theory of Warm diseases

Table 7 Comparison between Full-Cold and Empty-Cold

	Full-Cold	Empty-Cold
Face	Bright-white	Sallow-white
Pain	Sharp, worse on pressure	Dull, better on pressure
Bowels	Better after bowel movement	Worse after bowel movement
Pulse	Full-Tight-Deep	Weak-Slow-Deep
Tongue	Thick-white coating	Thin-white coating

(from exterior Wind-Heat), a person can be attacked by Cold in wintertime without developing any manifestations of it. The Cold can lie dormant in the Interior and change into Heat. In the Spring, with the rising of Yang energy, the interior Heat may be pulled towards the Exterior especially in combination with a new attack of Wind-Cold. Because of this, the person would have symptoms and signs of an attack of Wind-Cold, but also signs of interior Heat such as a thirst, irritability and a Fine-Rapid pulse, as described above.

Heat on the exterior—cold in the interior

This situation simply occurs when a person with a Cold condition is attacked by exterior Wind-Heat. There will therefore be some symptoms of exterior invasion of Wind-Heat (such as a fever with aversion to cold, a sore throat, thirst, a headache and a Floating-Rapid pulse) and some symptoms of interior Cold (such as loose stools, chilliness and profuse-pale urine).

Heat above—cold below

In some cases there is Heat above (as Heat tends to rise) and Cold below. The manifestations of this situation might be thirst, irritability, sour regurgitation, bitter taste, mouth ulcers (manifestations of Heat above), loose stools, borborygmi and profuse-pale urine (manifestations of Cold below).

True cold — false heat and true heat — false cold

In some cases there may be contradictory signs and symptoms, some pointing to Heat and some to Cold. This usually only happens in extreme conditions and is quite rare. It is important not to confuse this phenomenon with common situations when Heat and Cold are simply combined. For example, it is perfectly possible for someone to have a condition of Damp-Heat in the Bladder and Cold in the Spleen. This is simply a combination of Hot and Cold signs in two different organs, and does not fall under the category of False Heat and True Cold or vice versa.

In cases of False Heat and False Cold, tongue diagnosis shows its most useful aspect as the tongue-body colour nearly always reflects the true condition. If the tongue-body colour is Red it indicates Heat, if it is Pale it indicates Cold.

It is worth mentioning here that False Heat and False Cold are not the same as Empty-Heat and Empty-Cold. Empty-Heat and Empty-Cold arise from deficiency of Yin or Yang respectively, but there is nevertheless Heat or Cold. In False Heat and False Cold, the appearance is false, i.e. there is no Heat or Cold respectively.

The clinical manifestations of False Heat and False Cold are best illustrated by a table (Table 8).

FULL-EMPTY

The differentiation between Fullness and Emptiness is an extremely important one. The distinction is made according to the presence or absence of a pathogenic factor and to the strength of the body's energies.

A Full condition is characterized by the presence of a pathogenic factor (which may be interior or exterior) of any kind and by the fact that the body's Qi is relatively intact. It therefore battles against the pathogenic factor and this results in the rather plethoric character of the symptoms and signs.

An Empty condition is characterized by weakness of the body's Qi and the absence of a pathogenic factor.

If the body's Qi is weak but a pathogenic factor

Table 8 Clinical manifestations of False Heat and False Cold

Diagnostic signs	True Cold-False Heat	True Heat-False Cold
By looking	Red cheeks, but red colour is like powder, rest of face white; irritability but also listlessness, desire to lie with body curled-up; Pale and wet tongue	Dark face, bright eyes with "spirit', red-dry lips, irritability, strong body tongue-body colour Red-dry
By hearing	Breathing quiet; low voice.	Breathing noisy, loud voice
By asking	Thirst but no desire to drink, or desire to drink warm fluids, body feels hot but he or she likes to be covered: sore throat but without redness or swelling; pale urine	Thirst with desire to drink cold fluids: scanty-dark urine, constipation, burning sensation in anus
By feeling	Pulse Rapid, Floating and Big but Empty	Pulse Deep, Full. Cold limbs but chest is hot

lingers on, the condition is of Empty character complicated with Fullness.

The distinction between Full and Empty is one which is more than any other made on the basis of observation. A strong, loud voice, an excruciating pain, a very red face, profuse sweating, restlessness, throwing off the bedclothes, outbursts of temper, are all signs of a Full condition. A weak voice, a dull-lingering pain, a very pale face, slight sweating, listlessness, curling up in bed, quiet disposition, are all signs of an Empty condition.

The main clinical manifestations of an Empty condition are chronic disease, listlessness, apathy, lying curled up, a weak voice, weak breathing, low-pitch tinnitus, pain alleviated by pressure poor memory, slight sweating, frequent urination, loose stools and a pulse of the Empty type.

The main clinical manifestations of a Full condition are acute disease, restlessness, irritability, a red face, a strong voice, coarse breathing, pain aggravated by pressure, high-pitch tinnitus, profuse sweating, scanty urination, constipation and a pulse of the Excess type.

As usual, it is difficult to generalize and some of the above symptoms cannot, strictly speaking, be categorized as Full symptoms. Just to give one example, constipation is included among the Full symptoms because it is often caused by stagnation or by Heat, but there are also Deficient causes of constipation, such as Blood or Yin deficiency.

Moreover, the above symptoms are broad generalizations, indeed too general to be of use in clinical practice.

Many examples could be given of Full conditions. First of all, any exterior condition due to invasion of exterior Cold, Wind, Damp or Heat is Full by definition, as it is characterized by the presence of those exterior pathogenic factors.

Any interior pathogenic factor also gives rise to a Full condition, provided the body's Qi is strong enough to engage in a struggle against such pathogenic factors. Examples of these are interior Cold, Heat, Dampness, Wind, Fire and Phlegm. Stagnation of Qi and Stasis of Blood are also Full conditions.

Conditions characterized by a combination of Emptiness and Fullness arise when there is a pathogenic factor but its influence is not very strong while the body's Qi is weak and not reacting properly against it. Examples of conditions of Emptiness complicated with Fullness are: Kidney-Yin deficiency with rising of Liver-Yang, Kidney-Yin deficiency with flaring up of Heart Empty-Heat, Spleen-Qi deficiency with retention of Dampness or Phlegm, deficiency of Blood with stasis of Blood, deficiency of Qi with stasis of Blood.

We can distinguish four types of Emptiness:

Empty Qi
Empty Yang
Empty Blood
Empty Yin.

EMPTY QI

The clinical manifestations are a pale face, a weak voice, slight sweating (in daytime), slight breathlessness, tiredness, lack of appetite and an Empty pulse.

These are only the symptoms of Lung and Spleen Qi Emptiness, which are those customarily given in Chinese books, as it is the Spleen that produces Qi and the Lungs that govern Qi. However, there can be many other symptoms of Emptiness of Qi, according to which organ is involved, in particular Heart or Kidneys. These will be described in the chapter on the Identification of Patterns according to the Internal Organs (see ch. 20).

Emptiness of Qi is the first and least severe deficiency from which one can suffer. Most of the above symptoms arise from weakness of Lung-Qi failing to control breathing, and weakness of Spleen-Qi failing to transform and transport.

Case history

A man of 30 suffered from tiredness, lack of appetite and persistent catarrh in the nose and throat. His pulse was Empty and the tongue was slightly Pale and slightly Swollen.

These manifestations indicate Spleen-Qi deficiency, complicated by the presence of Dampness (causing the mucus).

EMPTY YANG

The main clinical manifestations are, in addition to those of Emptiness of Qi: chilliness, a bright-pale face, cold limbs, no thirst, a desire for hot drinks, loose stools, frequent-pale urination, a Weak pulse and a Pale-Wet tongue.

Qi is part of Yang, and Emptiness of Qi is similar in nature to Emptiness of Yang. In fact, the two are practically the same, just emphasizing different aspects of the functions of Qi. In Emptiness of Qi, it is the Qi function of transformation that is mostly at fault, while in Emptiness of Yang, it is the Qi function of warming and protecting that is impaired.

The organs which most commonly suffer from Yang deficiency are the Spleen, Kidneys, Lung, Heart and Stomach. The patterns for each of these are discussed in the chapter on the Internal Organs patterns (see ch. 20).

Case history

A woman of 30 suffered from tiredness, chilliness, chronic soreness of the lower back, frequent and pale urination and loose stools. Her pulse was Weak, especially on the right side, and her tongue was Pale and wet.

These manifestations clearly indicate Deficiency of Spleen and Kidney-Yang.

EMPTY BLOOD

The main manifestations of Emptiness of Blood are a dull-pale face, pale lips, blurred vision, dry hair, depression, tiredness, poor memory, numbness, insomnia, scanty periods or amenorrhoea, a Fine or Choppy Pulse and a Pale-Thin tongue.

The above symptoms are due to dysfunction of various organs. Emptiness of Liver-Blood causes blurred vision, depression, tiredness, numbness, scanty periods. Emptiness of Heart-Blood causes pale face, pale lips, Pale tongue, insomnia.

Blood is part of Yin and a long-standing Emptiness of Blood gives rise to dryness, causing dry hair.

The organs which are most likely to suffer from Blood Emptiness are the Liver, Heart and Spleen. These patterns are described in chapters 20–25.

Case history

A woman of 27 suffered from tiredness, poor memory, scanty menstruation, constipation and insomnia. Her pulse was Choppy and her tongue was Pale and Thin.

These manifestations indicate deficiency of Blood of the Liver (scanty menstruation, tiredness, constipation) and the Heart (poor memory, insomnia).

EMPTY YIN

The main manifestations of Emptiness of Yin are low-grade fever or a feeling of heat in the afternoon, 5-palm heat, a dry throat at night, night sweating, emaciation, a Floating-Empty pulse and a Red-Peeled and dry tongue.

Again, the above are only the general symptoms of Emptiness of Yin, other symptoms depending on which organ is mostly involved. The organs most likely to suffer from Yin Emptiness are the Kidneys, Lung, Heart, Liver and Stomach.

Yin Qi has the function of cooling, hence the heat symptoms (Empty-Heat) such as a low-grade fever, a feeling of heat, night sweating, 5-palm heat and a Red tongue.

Yin also moistens, hence the symptoms of dryness such as dry throat and tongue.

Case history

A woman of 45 suffered from dizziness, night sweating, soreness of the lower back and a slight tinnitus. Her pulse was Fine and her tongue was of a normal colour with a rootless coating.

These manifestations point to deficiency of Kidney-Yin and Stomach-Yin (the "rootless" coating indicates deficiency of Stomach-Yin).

Case history

A young woman of 31 had had a severe abdominal and hypogastric pain 6 months prior to examination. During that attack she doubled up in spasms and had a slight temperature. Afterwards her stools became loose and she felt very weak. The abdominal pain would occasionally return after exertion, felt in the right iliac fossa and being worse for pressure. She also developed a vaginal discharge. Her appetite was poor and her legs felt weak and she was exhausted in general. During the last two months she had experienced some bleeding in between periods and a slight swelling of the ankles. The tongue was peeled except for some thin yellow coating in the centre. There were ice-floe cracks on the root while the tongue body was thin. Her pulse was Rapid, Slippery, slightly Floating-Empty and both Rear positions were Fine but also slightly Wiry. Her voice was very weak and she generally appeared weak and withdrawn.

This rather complicated case is introduced here to illustrate the intricate web of Emptiness and Fullness appearing simultaneously. First of all, the sudden onset of abdominal pain with slight temperature probably indicated an invasion of exterior Damp-Heat. However, she must have obviously suffered from previous Spleen-Qi deficiency: this is apparent by the Empty and Fine pulse, the general exhaustion and the weak voice. The Spleen-Qi deficiency had led to the formation of Dampness, hence the vaginal discharge.

Besides the Spleen deficiency she must have also suffered from Kidney-Yin deficiency: this is apparent from the peeled tongue, the cracks on the root of the tongue, the Floating-Empty and Rapid pulse and the swollen ankles. This last sign is usually a sign of Kidney-Yang deficiency, but as explained before, it is not at all unusual to have a mixture of symptoms and signs from Kidney Yin and Yang deficiency: this happens because Kidney-Yin and Kidney-Yang share the same root and a deficiency of one often causes a secondary deficiency of the other. In this case there is a primary deficiency of Kidney-Yin and a secondary deficiency of Kidney-Yang (swollen ankles). How can a young person of 31 suffer from such severe Kidney-Yin deficiency? On interrogation, it became apparent that, for many years she had worked very hard and long hours. Her work also involved a lot of lifting which, over a long period of time injured the Kidneys while overworking injured Kidney-Yin. However, lifting can also cause stagnation of Qi in the Lower Burner. This concurrent factor (together with the exterior Damp-Heat) accounts for her severe abdominal pain. Had the pain been caused only by Damp-Heat, it would have been less severe.

The bleeding in between periods more recently was due to deficiency of Qi and Yin failing to hold Blood.

To summarize, this case shows a mixture of Emptiness of Qi (Spleen) and Yin (Kidneys) with Fullness in the form of Damp-Heat. It also shows a mixture of exterior and interior conditions, as the Damp-Heat originally arose from an exterior invasion, but due to the previously present Spleen-Qi deficiency, was transformed into interior Dampness.

YIN-YANG

The categories of Yin and Yang within the 8 Principles have two meanings: in a general sense, they are a summarization of the other six, whilst in a specific sense they are used mostly in Emptiness of Yin and Yang and Collapse of Yin and Yang.

Yin and Yang are a generalization of the other six Principles since Interior, Emptiness and Cold are Yin and Exterior, Fullness and Heat are Yang in nature.

In a specific sense, the categories of Yin and Yang can define two kinds of Emptiness and also two kinds of Collapse. Emptiness of Yin and Yang have already been described above.

Collapse of Yin or Yang simply indicates an extremely severe state of Emptiness. It also implies a complete separation of Yin and Yang from each other. Collapse of Yin or Yang is often, but not necessarily, followed by death.

COLLAPSE OF YIN

The main manifestations are abundant perspiration, skin hot to the touch, hot limbs, a dry mouth with desire to drink cold liquids in small sips, retention of urine, constipation, a Floating-Empty and Rapid pulse and a Red-Peeled, Short and Dry tongue.

COLLAPSE OF YANG

The main manifestations are chilliness, cold limbs, weak breathing, profuse sweating with an oily sweat, no thirst, frequent-profuse urination or incontinence, loose stools or incontinence, a Minute-Deep pulse and a Pale-Wet-Swollen-Short tongue.

The following are two rather complicated case histories to illustrate the interaction of the 8 Principles in the same condition.

Case history

A woman of 45 suffered from persistent and profuse uterine bleeding. The bleeding started with each period and then continued for 3 weeks. The blood was dark at first and then clear-coloured and there was pain. She also experienced pre-menstrual tension, irritability (she said "she could kill someone") and swelling of the breasts. She felt very tired most of the time, did not sleep well and sweated at night. She also complained of frequent urination, having to pass water twice at night. Her bowels had been loose for 3 years and she felt thirsty. Asked whether she felt either hot or cold she answered "both". She was overweight. Her pulse was Deep, Weak and both Rear positions were very Weak. Her tongue was slightly Red tending to Purple, but also slightly Pale on the sides. It was peeled in the centre and there was a rootless coating on the root, and the root itself had no "spirit". There were cracks in the centre and root.

These clinical manifestations paint a very complicated picture. What is apparent from the pulse and tongue first is deficiency of Stomach and Kidney-Yin: the absence of "spirit" on the root, the rootless coating on the root, the cracks on the root, the night-sweating, the thirst, all point to Kidney-Yin deficiency. The peeled and cracked centre indicates Stomach-Yin deficiency. The Kidney deficiency is also confirmed by the very Deep and Weak pulse on the Rear positions. Contradicting the Yin deficiency are: frequent urination, pale sides of the tongue, sometimes feeling cold and the diarrhoea. The frequent urination, nocturia, feeling cold and diarrhoea are due to Kidney-Yang deficiency. It is not at all uncommon to have both Kidney Yin and Yang deficiency as they share the same root and a deficiency of one often causes a lesser deficiency of the other. In this case, the deficiency of Kidney-Yin is predominant at the moment (judging from tongue and pulse). The deficiency of both Kidney Yin and Yang explains why she feels hot sometimes and cold other times.

The reddish-purple colour of the tongue, the painful periods with dark blood initially and pre-mentrual tension indicate stagnation of Liver Qi and Blood. The stasis of Liver-Blood was probably a consequence of a long-standing deficiency of Liver-Blood which is apparent from the pale colour of the sides of the tongue and her tiredness.

The profuse and persistent bleeding is caused by deficiency of Qi and Yin unable to hold blood. This is a Deficient type of bleeding, hence the clear colour of the blood after the initial darkness.

In conclusion, this case shows Deficiency (of Kidneys, Stomach and Liver-Blood), Excess (stasis of Blood), Yin deficiency (of Kidneys and Stomach), Yang deficiency (of Kidneys too), Cold symptoms (diarrhoea, frequent urination, feeling cold) and Hot symptoms (feeling hot, night sweating). Thus it shows Deficiency and Excess, Heat and Cold, Yin and Yang simultaneously.

Case history

A young man of 18 had suffered from epilepsy since the age of 11. The attacks were characterized by severe convulsions and passing out with foaming at the mouth. He also suffered from migraine headaches, tinnitus and irritability. His pulse was Fine, Rapid and slightly Wiry. His tongue was Red, redder at the sides, Stiff and with a thick-sticky yellow coating.

There was some contradiction between the pulse, the tongue and the symptoms. The tongue indicates a Full-Heat condition (Red with coating) and the presence of Phlegm (sticky coating). It also indicates Liver-Fire (redder on the sides). Both of these are Excess patterns (Liver-Fire and Phlegm). The pulse is Fine, which indicates deficiency of Blood.

The Phlegm originates from long-standing deficiency of Spleen-Qi. Spleen-Qi deficient fails to produce Blood and this causes Liver-Blood deficiency (hence the Fine pulse). The deficiency of Liver-Blood leads to the rising of Liver-Yang and the stirring of Liver-Wind, hence the epileptic convulsions. His epilepsy is therefore traceable to two concurrent causes: the stirring up of Liver-Wind and Phlegm misting the brain. The stirring of Liver-Wind causes the convulsions, while the Phlegm misting the brain causes unconsciousness during the attacks.

In conclusion, this condition is characterized by Emptiness (of Spleen-Qi and Liver-Blood) and Fullness (Liver-Wind and Phlegm).

19 Identification of Patterns According to Qi-blood-body Fluids

氣血津液辨証

The Pattern Identification according to Qi, Blood and Body Fluids is based on the possible pathological changes of these vital substances. These patterns describe the clinical manifestations arising when Qi, Blood or Body Fluids are either deficient or stagnant.

There is some overlap between these patterns and those according to the 8 Principles and Internal Organs. For example, the pattern of Qi Deficiency is essentially the same as Qi Deficiency according to the 8 Principles. The patterns according to Qi, Blood and Body Fluids are important as they complete the clinical picture emerging from the 8-Principle and Internal Organ patterns.

QI PATTERN IDENTIFICATION

These can be:

- Deficiency of Qi
- Sinking of Qi
- Stagnation of Qi
- Rebellious Qi.

QI DEFICIENCY

Clinical manifestations

Breathlessness, weak voice, spontaneous sweating, no appetite, loose stools, tiredness, Empty pulse.

These are the symptoms and signs of Lung and Spleen Qi deficiency. Obviously, there can be Qi deficiency of other organs too. Heart-Qi deficiency is marked by palpitations, whilst Kidney-Qi deficiency leads to frequent urination. As mentioned in the chapter on the 8 Principles, it is customary to list only the symptoms of Lung and Spleen Qi deficiency, firstly because they are more common, and secondly because the Lungs govern Qi and the Spleen is the source of Qi through its activity of transformation and transportation.

QI SINKING

Clinical manifestations

Feeling of bearing down, tiredness, listlessness, mental depression, prolapse of organs (stomach, uterus, intestines, anus, vagina or bladder), Empty pulse.

In addition to the above symptoms, there can be any of the other symptoms of Qi deficiency. "Qi sinking" is, in fact, only a particular aspect of Qi deficiency and not essentially separate from it.

This distinction needs to be made, however, as when it comes to treatment, it is necessary not only to tonify but also to raise Qi. There are particular herbs and acupuncture points (such as Du-20 with moxa) that have this effect.

QI STAGNATION

Clinical manifestations

Feeling of distension, distending pain that moves from place to place, abdominal masses that appear and disappear, mental depression, irritability, gloomy feeling, frequent mood swings, frequent sighing, Wiry or Tight pulse, slightly Purple tongue.

These are only the general but essential and distinctive symptoms of Qi stagnation. The feeling of distension, which can affect the hypochondrium, epigastrium, throat, abdomen and hypogastrium, is the most characteristic and important of the symptoms of Qi stagnation.

Emotional symptoms are also very characteristic and frequent in stagnation of Qi, particularly of Liver-Qi.

Other symptoms and which part of the body is mostly affected depend on which organ is involved. The Liver is the organ that is most affected by stagnation of Qi, and these symptoms are described under the Pattern Identification according to the Internal Organs (see page 215).

REBELLIOUS QI

The symptoms of Rebellious Qi have to be distinguished according to the organ involved.

"Rebellious Qi" occurs when Qi flows in the wrong direction, i.e. a direction different than its normal physiological one. This varies from organ to organ, as each has its own normal direction of flow of Qi. These have been described in chapter 4.

There are two types of rebellious Qi, a Deficient and Excess type. Generally speaking, rebellious Qi is of the Excess type by definition, but there is one example of a Deficiency type of rebellious Qi, and that is Spleen-Qi sinking (instead of rising).

The different kinds of rebellious Qi are summarized in Table 9.

As in the case of sinking Qi, the identification of Rebellious Qi is important from the point of view of treatment as there are herbs and specific acupuncture points to subdue rebellious Qi.

Table 9 Rebellious Qi types

Organ	Normal Qi direction	Pathological Qi direction	Symptoms and signs
Stomach	Downwards	Upwards	Belching, hiccup, nausea, vomiting
Spleen	Upwards	Downwards	Diarrhoea, prolapse
Liver	Upwards	i) Excessive upwards	Headache, dizziness, irritability
		ii) Horizontally:	
		— to Stomach	Nausea, belching, vomiting
		— to Spleen	Diarrhoea
		— to Intestines	Dry stools
		iii) Downwards	Burning urination
Lungs	Downwards	Upwards	Cough, asthma
Kidneys	Downwards	Upwards	Asthma
Heart	Downwards	Upwards	Mental restlessness, insomnia

BLOOD PATTERN IDENTIFICATION

These can be:
- Deficiency of Blood
- Stasis of Blood
- Heat in the Blood
- Loss of Blood.

DEFICIENCY OF BLOOD

Clinical manifestations

Sallow complexion, pale lips, dizziness, poor memory, numbness, blurred vision, insomnia, Pale and slightly dry tongue, Choppy or Fine pulse.

Deficiency of Blood usually arises from Spleen-Qi deficiency since Spleen-Qi initiates the first steps in the production of Qi and Blood.

Once Blood becomes deficient, it affects particularly the Liver and Heart. The above symptoms are mixed symptoms of Liver (numbness, blurred vision, dizziness) and Heart Blood deficiency (sallow complexion, poor memory, insomnia, Pale tongue).

In addition to the above symptoms, others are possible mostly in the gynaecological and mental-emotional sphere; for instance, amenorrhea or scanty periods and depression, anxiety or lack of spirit of initiative.

In severe and long-standing cases, deficiency of Blood can further lead to pronounced dryness as Blood is part of Yin. This manifests with a particularly dry tongue, dry skin, dry hair and withered nails. In even more severe cases, the long-standing dryness of the Blood can give rise to interior Liver-Wind which, combined with dryness, can cause some skin diseases characterized by dry and itchy skin.

STASIS OF BLOOD

Clinical manifestations

Dark complexion, purple lips, pain which is boring, fixed and stabbing in character, abdominal masses that do not move, purple nails, bleeding with dark blood and dark clots, Purple tongue, Wiry, Firm or Choppy pulse.

These are only the general symptoms of stasis of Blood, without specific reference to particular organs. One of the main distinguishing symptoms of stasis of Blood is pain that is fixed in one place, and is of a boring or stabbing character. It is useful here to compare and contrast stagnation of Qi with stasis of Blood (Table 10).

The organ that is most frequently affected by stasis of Blood is the Liver. Other affected organs are the Heart, Lungs, Stomach, Intestines and Uterus.

The symptoms and signs for each of these organs are as follows:

Liver

Purple nails, dark face, painful periods with dark menstrual blood with dark clots, abdominal pain, premenstrual pain, Purple tongue especially on the sides, Wiry or Firm pulse.

Heart

Purple lips, stabbing or pricking pain in the chest, mental restlessness, Purple tongue on

Table 10 Comparison between Stagnation of Qi and Stasis of Blood

	Stagnation of Qi	Stasis of blood
Pain/distension	More distension than pain	More pain than distension
Location	Moving pain	Fixed pain
Character	Distending pain, feeling of fullness	Boring or stabbing pain
Abdominal masses	Appearing and disappearing	Fixed
Skin	Not appearing on skin	May manifest with purple blotches or bruises
Face	May be unchanged	Dark colour or bluish-green
Tongue	Normal colour or slightly purple	Definitely purple and possibly with purple spots
Pulse	Only slightly Wiry	Wiry, Firm or Choppy

the sides towards the front, purple and distended veins under the tongue, Choppy or Knotted pulse.

Lungs

Feeling of oppression of the chest, coughing of dark blood, tongue purple in the front part or the sides in the centre section, purple and distended veins under the tongue.

Stomach

Epigastric pain, vomiting of dark blood, dark blood in stools, tongue Purple in the centre.

Intestines

Severe abdominal pain, dark blood in stools.

Uterus

Dysmenorrhea, pre-menstrual pain, menstrual blood dark with clots, amenorrhea, abdominal masses, Purple tongue.

Stasis of Blood can derive from:

1 *Stagnation of Qi*: this is the most common cause of stasis of Blood. Qi moves Blood, if Qi stagnates Blood congeals.

2 *Deficiency of Qi*: deficiency of Qi over a long period of time may cause stasis of Blood as Qi becomes too weak to move Blood.

3 *Heat in the Blood*: Heat in the Blood may cause the Blood to coagulate and stagnate.

4 *Blood deficiency*: if Blood is deficient over a long period of time, it will induce Qi deficiency and subsequently stasis of Blood, from impairment of the Qi moving function.

5 *Interior Cold*: this slows down the circulation of Blood.

HEAT IN THE BLOOD

Clinical manifestations

Feeling of heat, skin diseases with red eruptions, dry mouth, bleeding, Red tongue, Rapid pulse.

These are only the general symptoms of Blood Heat. Others may be present according to the organ involved.

If Heart-Blood has Heat, there will be anxiety, mental illness (such as manic-depression) and mouth ulcers. If Liver-Blood has Heat, there will be skin diseases characterized by itching, heat and redness. This is one of the most common types of skin diseases.

If the Blood-Heat affects the Uterus and the Penetrating Vessel, there will be excessive blood loss during the periods.

LOSS OF BLOOD

Clinical manifestations

Epistaxis, haematemesis, haemoptysis, melaena, menorrhagia, metrorrhagia, haematuria.

Loss of Blood can occur from two main causes: either because deficient Qi is unable to hold Blood, or because Blood-Heat pushes blood out of the vessels. The former is a Deficiency type, the latter an Excess type of loss of Blood. Two other causes for loss of Blood are stasis of Blood and Yin deficiency. These can be differentiated (Table 11).

BODY-FLUID PATTERN IDENTIFICATION

These are:

Deficiency of Body Fluids
Oedema
Phlegm.

DEFICIENCY OF BODY FLUIDS

Clinical manifestations

Dry skin, mouth, nose, cough, lips, dry Tongue.

Body Fluids are part of Yin and their deficiency always causes a condition of dryness. This is not quite the same as Yin deficiency as it can precede it. It may, however, be considered as a mild form of Yin deficiency.

Deficiency of Body Fluids can also, on the other hand, derive from Yin deficiency: if Yin is deficient over a long period of time, Body Fluids will become deficient too.

Deficiency of Body Fluids can also be caused by a heavy and prolonged loss of fluids such as

Table 11 Differentiation of causes of haemorrhage

Cause	Colour of blood	Quantity
Heat in blood	Fresh red or dark	Heavy loss
Stasis of blood	Very dark with clots	Scanty loss
Qi deficiency	Pale	Heavy loss,prolonged
Yin deficiency	Bright-red	Scanty

in sweating (as during a febrile disease), vomiting and diarrhoea.

As there is a constant interchange between fluids and Blood, deficiency of fluids can also derive from a heavy loss of Blood, such as during childbirth.

Finally, severe and chronic deficiency of Blood can cause dryness and deficiency of fluids.

Deficiency of fluids affects mostly the Lungs, Stomach, Kidneys and Large Intestine.

Lungs

The main symptoms are dry skin and dry cough.

Stomach

The Stomach is the origin of fluids and a deficiency of Stomach-Qi and particularly Stomach-Yin will induce a deficiency of Body Fluids. The main symptoms are a dry tongue with horizontal cracks and a dry mouth but without desire to drink, or with a desire to drink in small sips.

Kidneys

The Kidneys govern Water and deficiency of Kidney-Yin causes dryness and deficiency of Body Fluids. The main symptoms are scanty urination, a dry mouth at night and a dry throat.

Large Intestine

The Large Intestine is related to the Stomach within the Bright Yang and a deficiency of fluids of the Stomach is easily transmitted to the Large Intestine. The main symptoms are dry stools.

OEDEMA

Oedema arises from deficiency of either Spleen, Lungs or Kidneys or all three of them. Lungs, Spleen and Kidneys are the three organs that are mostly involved in the transformation and transportation of fluids. If one or two or three of these organs is deficient, the Body Fluids are not transformed properly, they overflow out of the channels and settle in the space under the skin. This is the origin of oedema.

If oedema is caused by Lung-Qi deficiency it will affect the top part of the body, such as the face and hands. This type of oedema can also be caused by invasion of exterior Wind-Cold interfering with the Lung function of dispersing and descending Body Fluids.

Oedema from Spleen-Qi deficiency tends to affect the middle part of the body, such as the abdomen (ascites).

If oedema is caused by Kidney-Yang deficiency, it will affect the lower part of the body, such as the legs and ankles.

PHLEGM

The concept of Phlegm is very wide-ranging and important in Chinese Medicine. It is extremely frequent in clinical practice. Phlegm is at the same time a pathological condition and an aetiological factor. Phlegm which is retained over a long period of time becomes itself a cause of disease.

The main cause for the formation of Phlegm is Spleen deficiency. If the Spleen fails to transform and transport Body Fluids, these will accumulate and change into Phlegm. The Lungs and Kidneys are also involved in the formation of Phlegm. If the Lungs fail to disperse and lower fluids and if the Kidneys fail to transform and excrete fluids, these may accumulate into Phlegm. However, the Spleen is always the primary factor in the formation of Phlegm.

The essential signs of Phlegm are a slippery or sticky tongue coating and a Slippery or Wiry pulse.

There are two types of Phlegm, one "substantial", one "non-substantial". In the old classics, these were described as Phlegm "having a form" and Phlegm "without a form".

Substantial Phlegm can be seen, such as the sputum that collects in the Lungs and is spat during bronchitis or other Lung diseases.

Non-substantial Phlegm can be retained subcutaneously or in the channels. It can obstruct the Heart-orifices or the Gall-Bladder or Kidneys in the form of stones. It can settle in the joints in the form of arthritic bone deformities.

The two types of Phlegm can be summarized as follows.

Substantial Phlegm

Phlegm in the Lungs.

Non-substantial Phlegm

Under the skin

This takes the form of lumps under the skin (although not all lumps are due to Phlegm), nerve-ganglia swellings, swelling of lymph-nodes, swelling of the thyroid, some fibroids and lipomas.

In the channels

Phlegm in the channels is not visible as a swelling, but it causes numbness. This is more common in old people and is frequently seen in Wind-stroke.

Misting the Heart

Non-substantial Phlegm can obstruct the Heart-orifices and mist the Mind. This gives rise to some types of mental illness such as schizophrenia and manic-depression and also to epilepsy.

In Gall-Bladder or Kidneys

Gall-Bladder or Kidney stones are considered as a form of Phlegm, arising from the "steaming and brewing" of Phlegm by Heat over a long period of time.

In the joints

The bone deformities that occur in chronic rheumatoid arthritis are seen as a form of Phlegm. When the fluids are not transformed and accumulate in the joints over a long period of time, they can give rise to Phlegm and this can further condense to form bone growths.

To summarize, Phlegm can affect the internal organs or the channels and skin.

Phlegm (substantial or non-substantial) can assume different forms, according to its associations with other pathogenic factors.

Wind-Phlegm

This causes dizziness, nausea, vomiting, numbness of the limbs, coughing of phlegm, a rattling sound in the throat and aphasia.

This form of Phlegm is seen in Wind-stroke.

Phlegm-Heat

This is manifested with expectoration of yellow-sticky phlegm, a red face, dry mouth and lips, restlessness, a Red tongue with sticky-yellow coating and a Rapid-Slippery pulse.

This form of Phlegm affects the Lungs, the Stomach or the Heart.

Cold-Phlegm

This is manifested with expectoration of white-watery phlegm, a cold feeling in limbs and back, nausea, a Pale tongue with white-wet coating and a Deep-Slippery-Slow pulse.

This form of Phlegm is often seen in Stomach or Lung patterns.

Damp-Phlegm

This is manifested with expectoration of very profuse phlegm which is white and sticky, no appetite, no thirst, a feeling of oppression of chest

Table 12 Types of Phlegm

	Area affected
Damp-Phlegm in the Lungs Phlegm-Fire in the Stomach Phlegm misting the Heart	Internal Organs
Phlegm blocking the channels Phlegm under the skin Phlegm in the joints	Limbs

and epigastrium, a sticky tongue coating and a Slippery pulse.

This form of Phlegm is seen in Lung patterns.

Qi-Phlegm

This type of Phlegm is non-substantial and is manifested with a feeling of swelling in the throat (but no actual swelling), a difficulty in swallowing and a feeling of oppression of chest and diaphragm.

This form of Phlegm is usually associated with stagnation of Qi in the throat. It is caused by emotional problems giving rise to (or deriving from) stagnation of Liver-Qi. The typical feeling of constriction of the throat is called "plum-stone syndrome" in Chinese Medicine and this feeling appears and disappears according to mood swings.

Phlegm-Fluids

Finally, another form of Phlegm is called "Yin" in Chinese Medicine which simply means "fluids" or "watery". This is a type of substantial Phlegm characterized by very watery and thin fluids. It can actually be heard splashing in the body.

There are four kinds of Phlegm-Fluids:

1 Phlegm-Fluids in Stomach and Intestines

This is manifested with abdominal fullness and distention, vomiting of watery fluids, a dry tongue and mouth without desire to drink, a splashing sound in the stomach, a feeling of fullness of the chest, loose stools, loss of weight, a Deep-Slippery pulse and a Swollen tongue with sticky coating.

2 Phlegm-Fluids in the hypochondrium

This is manifested with hypochondriac pain which is worse on coughing and breathing, a feeling of distension of the hypochondrium, shortness of breath, a sticky tongue coating and a Deep-Wiry pulse.

3 Phlegm-Fluids in the limbs

This is manifested with a feeling of heaviness of the body, a pain in the muscles, no sweating, no desire to drink, a cough with abundant-white sputum, a sticky-white coating and a Wiry or Tight pulse.

4 Phlegm-Fluids above the diaphragm

This is manifested with a cough, asthma, oedema, dizziness, abundant-white sputum, a sticky-thick-white tongue coating and a Wiry pulse. All the symptoms are aggravated by exposure to cold.

Case history

A man of 32 suffered from tiredness, poor appetite, a feeling of muzziness and heaviness of the head. He also experienced a feeling of oppression of the chest, lack of concentration and dizziness. His pulse was Empty but also slightly Slippery and his tongue was Pale with a sticky coating.

These manifestations are due to deficiency of Spleen-Qi leading to the formation of Phlegm (the non-substantial kind). The Phlegm causes the muzziness, heaviness, dizziness and inability to think clearly, as it obstructs the rising of clear Yang Qi to the head.

20 Identification of Patterns According to the Internal Organs

脏腑辨証

The Identification of Patterns according to the Internal Organs is based on the symptoms and signs arising when the Qi and Blood of the internal organs is out of balance.

This method of identification of patterns is used mostly for interior and chronic conditions, but it also includes a few exterior and acute patterns.

The internal organs patterns are an application of the 8-Principle method of pattern identification to the particular disharmony of a specific internal organ. For example, according to the 8-Principle identification the symptoms and signs of Qi deficiency are shortness of breath, a weak voice, a pale face, lassitude and lack of appetite. Although useful to diagnose a condition of Qi deficiency, this is not detailed enough and does not identify which organ is involved. It is therefore too general to give an indication of the treatment needed. According to the Internal-Organ pattern identification, the above symptoms can be further classified as Lung-Qi deficiency (shortness of breath and weak voice) and Spleen-Qi deficiency (lassitude and lack of appetite). This is more useful in clinical practice because it gives concrete indications as to which organ needs to be treated.

The identification of patterns according to the internal organs is the most important one in clinical practice, particularly for interior chronic diseases.

Let us now look at some of the characteristics of this method of identification of patterns.

1) In the following pages the patterns of each organ will be described in detail. It is important to realize that, in practice, not all the symptoms and signs described need necessarily appear simultaneously. What these patterns describe are actually advanced cases of a particular organ disharmony. In some cases, even only two symptoms will be sufficient to identify a specific internal organ pattern. In fact, the real art of Chinese diagnosis consists in being able to detect a certain disharmony from a minimum of symptoms and signs.

2) The organ patterns are not "pigeon holes" into which we fit certain symptoms and signs. In practice, it is essential to have an understanding of the aetiology and pathology of a given disharmony. The aim of this method, therefore, is not to "classify" symptoms and signs according to organ patterns, but to understand how the symptoms and signs arise and how they interact with each other, in order to identify the prevailing organ disharmony.

3) The organ patterns are not diseases in a Western medical sense. Patterns are not just a collection of symptoms and signs, but an expression of the disharmony prevailing in a person. Symptoms and signs are used to identify the character and nature of the disharmony which, in itself, gives an indication as to the strategy and method of treatment needed.
4) Organ patterns appear in different degrees of severity, and the symptoms and signs listed under each pattern usually only describe the advanced cases of a given organ disharmony. In practice, if a pattern is only just developing, its symptoms and signs will be few and mild. Identifying an organ pattern as it is arising with only a few symptoms and signs releases the full potential of Chinese Medicine in the prevention of disease. For example, the symptoms and signs of Kidney-Yin deficiency are tinnitus, dizziness, night sweating, a dry mouth at night, malar flush, insomnia, backache, a Red-peeled tongue and a Floating-Empty and Rapid Pulse. In fact, what this picture of symptoms and signs describes, is quite an advanced case of Kidney-Yin deficiency. In practice, if a Kidney-Yin deficiency is just developing, a patient might only suffer from backache, slight night sweating and have a tongue with a slightly rootless coating: these manifestations would be enough to warrant a diagnosis of Kidney-Yin deficiency.
5) In practice several patterns may occur simultaneously.
The combinations can be:
a) two or more patterns from the same Yin organ (e.g. Liver-Qi stagnant and Liver-Fire);
b) two or more patterns from different Yin organs (e.g. Liver-Fire and Heart-Fire);
c) one or more patterns of a Yin organ with one or more patterns of a Yang organ (e.g. Spleen-Qi deficiency and Bladder Damp-Heat);
d) an interior and an exterior pattern (e.g. retention of Damp-Phlegm in the Lungs and exterior attack of Wind-Cold in the Lungs);
e) an interior organ pattern and a Channel pattern (e.g. Lung-Qi deficiency and Painful Obstruction Syndrome of the Large Intestine channel).
6) There is no correspondence between the organ patterns of Chinese Medicine and organ diseases of Western Medicine. For example, a patient can suffer from Kidney-Yin deficiency without any recognizable kidney disease from the Western medical point of view. Vice versa, a patient may suffer from a kidney inflammation from a Western point of view not corresponding to a Kidney pattern from the Chinese medical point of view.

In the discussion of each organ pattern the following points will be discussed:
A brief summary of the functions of the organ
The clinical manifestations
The pathology (explanation of how the manifestations arise)
The aetiology
The treatment.

With regard to treatment, the most useful acupuncture points will be mentioned for each pattern. However, it should be understood that these are not point prescriptions, but simply the best points to use according to their functions. Not all the points mentioned, therefore, would ever be used in each case.

Furthermore, when the functions of each point are explained, only those functions which are relevant to the pattern in question will be mentioned. For example, in the pattern of Heart-Yang collapse Baihui Du-20 is recommended for its function of restoring consciousness, even though it has many other functions which are not listed under that pattern. The functions of the points are described in detail in chapter 40.

Finally, with regard to needling method, whenever the reducing method is indicated, it is understood that this is to be replaced by the even method in all the usual cases, i.e.
— when the illness is chronic
— when the patient is in a very weak condition or is very old
— when there is a mixed pattern of Deficiency and Excess.

Heart Patterns 21

心脏病証

The most important Heart functions are those of governing Blood and housing the Mind. Most of the pathological changes of the Heart reflect this and involve the Blood and the Mind.

Governing Blood and housing the Mind are complementary functions, mutually influencing each other. Blood and Yin are the "residence" for the Mind: if Blood and Yin are flourishing, the Mind will be in a good state and the person will feel mentally happy and vital. If Blood and Yin are deficient, the Mind will suffer, the person will feel unhappy, depressed and lack vitality. Conversely, if the Mind is disturbed from emotional upsets, this can induce a weakness of Blood or Yin and therefore lead to symptoms of Heart-Blood or Heart-Yin deficiency.

GENERAL AETIOLOGY

EXTERIOR PATHOGENIC FACTORS

Generally speaking, exterior climatic factors do not affect the Heart directly. Of all the climatic factors, Fire and Heat are the ones that most affect the Heart, but even those, not directly. Chinese Medicine maintains that exterior pathogenic factors do not affect the Heart directly, but the Pericardium instead. The "Spiritual Axis" in chapter 71 says: *"If exterior pathogenic factors attack the Heart, they penetrate the Pericardium instead"*.[1] Thus, if exterior Heat invades the body, it will easily affect the Pericardium. Among all the patterns in Chinese Medicine, the only one pertaining to the Pericardium is that of Heat invasion. This is especially significant in the context of the Chinese herbal treatment of infectious diseases caused by exterior Heat. It denotes a condition of rapid invasion of exterior Heat at the Nutritive-Qi level manifesting with very high temperature, delirium and, in severe cases, coma. Invasion of the Pericardium by Heat mists the Mind and causes coma.

However, in the context of acupuncture, the scope of the Pericardium channel in treatment is much broader than this, and it is very widely used for a great variety of conditions and patterns.

EMOTIONS

Joy

The Heart is related to "joy" within the 5 Element correspondence scheme. Under normal circumstances, a happy state of mind is obviously beneficial to the Mind and the body. It is only when joy is excessive that it becomes a cause of disease and it can injure the Heart. The significance of "joy" as a cause of disease was discussed in the chapter on the causes of disease (see p. 131).

Excess joy–excessive excitement–can injure the Heart and, more specifically, makes Heart Qi slow down and become deficient, and it dilates the Heart. However, this is not an important or common cause of Heart disharmony.

Sadness

Although related to the Lungs within the 5-Element scheme, sadness deeply affects Heart-Qi. Lungs and Heart are very closely related as one governs Qi and the other Blood, and they mutually assist each other. Sadness induces Qi deficiency of the Lungs which, in time, affects the Heart and makes Heart-Qi deficient. The "Simple Questions" in chapter 39 says: *"Sadness dissolves Qi"*.[2]

Sadness is a very common cause of Heart-Qi deficiency and when it affects both Lungs and Heart, it can often be manifested on the pulse with a very weak pulse on both Front positions (i.e. Heart and Lung positions).

Prolonged sadness, and its deriving deficiency of Qi, over a long period of time, can lead to stagnation of Qi which, in turn, can turn into Fire. When this happens, it will cause Heart-Fire.

Anger

What is termed "anger" in Chinese Medicine includes feelings of frustration, resentment and depression (see chapter "The Causes of Disease", p. 127).

Although anger affects the Liver directly, it may also affect the Heart indirectly. Anger causes the rising of Liver-Yang or Liver-Fire, and this can easily be transmitted to the Heart causing Heart-Fire. This is manifested on the tongue with a Red body colour on the sides and tip and possibly with red points on the tip.

The Heart patterns discussed are:

- Deficiency patterns
  - Heart-Qi deficiency
  - Heart-Yang deficiency (and Heart-Yang Collapse)
  - Heart-Blood deficiency
  - Heart-Yin deficiency
- Excess patterns
  - Heart-Fire blazing
  - Phlegm-Fire agitating within
  - Phlegm misting the Heart
- Deficiency-Excess pattern
  - Heart-Blood stagnant.

HEART-QI DEFICIENCY

Clinical manifestations

Palpitations, shortness of breath on exertion, sweating, pallor, tiredness, listlessness.

Tongue: Pale or normal colour. In severe cases the tongue could have a midline crack reaching the tip and with a swelling on each side of it.

Pulse: Empty. In severe cases, the Heart pulse could feel slightly Overflowing and Empty (i.e. it feels very superficial and somewhat pounding with a light pressure of the finger but empty with a heavier pressure).

Key symptoms: palpitations, tiredness, Empty pulse.

Pathology

This pattern includes general signs of Qi deficiency (such as shortness of breath, sweating, pallor, tiredness and Empty pulse) and palpitations, which is the cardinal sign of Heart-Qi deficiency. In this case the palpitations will be only light and occasional.

Aetiology

1 Blood loss

This pattern may be caused by a chronic illness,

particularly after a serious haemorrhage or after a prolonged chronic haemorrhage (such as from menorrhagia).The Heart governs Blood and any severe or prolonged blood loss will cause a deficiency of Heart-Blood which, in turn, will lead to deficiency of Heart-Qi, given the close interrelationship between Blood and Qi.

2 Emotional problems

Emotional problems, particularly from sadness, can lead to deficiency of Heart-Qi.

Treatment

Principle of treatment: tonify Heart-Qi.

Points: Tongli HE-5, Neiguan P-6, Xinshu BL-15, Shanzhong Ren-17, Qihai Ren-6.

Method: all with reinforcing method.

Explanation

HE-5 tonifies Heart-Qi. It is preferable to HE-7 in this case, as HE-7 also tonifies Heart-Blood and pacifies the Mind.

P-6 also tonifies Heart-Qi and it would be particularly useful if sadness is the cause of pattern.

BL-15 is the Back Transporting point and it tonifies Heart-Qi. Direct moxa could be used on this point.

Ren-17 is the Gathering point for Qi and it tonifies the Qi of the Upper Burner and therefore Heart-Qi. This point would also be particularly useful if sadness is the cause of disease as it will tonify both Lung and Heart-Qi.

Ren-6 tonifies the whole body's Qi and will therefore strengthen Heart-Qi. This point would be particularly useful in case the Heart deficiency derives from a chronic illness with general deficiency of Qi.

HEART-YANG DEFICIENCY

Clinical manifestations

Palpitations, shortness of breath on exertion, tiredness, listlessness, sweating, feeling of stuffiness or discomfort in the heart region, feeling of cold, bright-pale face, cold limbs (especially hands).

Tongue: Pale, wet, Swollen.

Pulse: Deep-Weak or Knotted.

Key symptoms: palpitations, feeling of cold, cold limbs, Deep pulse.

Pathology

Some of the symptoms are the same as for Heart-Qi deficiency (palpitations, shortness of breath, tiredness, sweating and pale face): this is because Heart-Qi deficiency could be considered as included within Heart-Yang deficiency. In other words, it is not possible to have a deficiency of Yang without a deficiency of Qi.

The feeling of cold and cold hands are due to Heart-Yang not transporting Defensive Qi to the extremities to warm them. The feeling of stuffiness in the chest region is due to Heart-Yang not moving Qi in the chest and hence leading to a slight stagnation of Qi in the chest.

The bright-pale face is typical of Yang deficiency (in Blood deficiency the face would be dull-pale).

The tongue is Pale because Heart-Yang cannot transport enough Blood to the tongue, and it is wet and swollen because Heart-Yang cannot transform the fluids which therefore accumulate on the tongue.

The Deep and Weak pulse reflects the deficiency of Yang. A Knotted pulse (a Slow pulse that stops at irregular intervals) might be found in severe cases.

Aetiology

This is basically the same as for Heart-Qi deficiency. In addition, Heart-Yang deficiency may also derive indirectly from a chronic deficiency of Kidney-Yang as Kidney-Yang is the source of all Yang energies of the body. Heart-Yang deficiency may therefore be indirectly caused by any of the causes of Kidney-Yang deficiency (see p. 253).

Treatment

Principle of treatment: tonify and warm Heart-Yang.

Points: Tongli HE-5, Neiguan P-6, Xinshu BL-15, Shanzhong Ren-17, Qihai Ren-6, Dazhui Du-14.

Method: all with reinforcing method, moxa is applicable.

Explanation

HE-5 and P-6 tonify Heart-Qi (see above).

BL-15 tonifies Heart-Yang if moxa is used.

Ren-17 also tonifies Heart-Yang if moxa is used. This point would be particularly useful if there is stuffiness of the chest.

Ren-6 with moxa also tonifies all Yang energies of the body and is particularly useful if the Heart-Yang deficiency results from Kidney-Yang deficiency.

Du-14 with direct moxa tonifies Heart-Yang.

HEART-YANG COLLAPSE

Clinical manifestations

Palpitations, shortness of breath, weak and shallow breathing, profuse sweating, cold limbs, cyanosis of lips, in severe cases coma.

Tongue: Very Pale or Bluish-Purple, Short.

Pulse: Hidden-Minute-Knotted.

Key symptoms: cyanosis of lips, Hidden-Minute pulse, cold limbs.

Pathology

This pattern is an extreme case of Heart-Yang deficiency and is not substantially different from it. The clinical manifestations are basically the same as for Heart-Yang deficiency, only more severe. In addition to these, there is cyanosis of lips which is due to Yang Qi deficient not moving the Blood, hence resulting in severe stasis of Blood.

The coma is caused by the complete collapse of Heart-Qi, hence the Mind has no "residence". This coma is of the Deficiency type.

The Tongue may be Short (i.e. cannot be extended much out of the mouth) because the deficiency of Yang is so severe that Yang Qi cannot move the tongue muscle at all. Also, the deficiency of Yang generates internal Cold which contracts the muscles, hence the tongue cannot be stuck out.

The Hidden pulse is an extreme case of the Deep pulse and reflects the severe deficiency of Yang. The Knotted pulse reflects the severe deficiency of Yang not giving the Heart enough energy to beat regularly.

Aetiology

This is the same as for Heart-Yang Deficiency. Heart-Yang Collapse however, always derives from a chronic and severe deficiency of Kidney-Yang. The total collapse of Qi (whether it is Yin or Yang Qi) always derives from the collapse of Kidney energy (whether Kidney-Yin or Kidney-Yang), which is the foundation of all energies of the body. Thus, any of the causes of Kidney-Yang deficiency, are indirectly causes of Heart-Yang Collapse: these can be excessive sexual activity, overwork over a long period of time and a chronic illness.

Treatment

Principle of treatment: rescue Yang, restore consciousness, stop sweating.

Points: Qihai Ren-6, Guanyuan Ren-4, Shenque Ren-8, Mingmen Du-4, Zusanli ST-36, Neiguan P-6, Shenshu BL-23, Baihui Du-20, Dazhui Du-14, Xinshu BL-15.

Method: all with reinforcing method, no retention of needle, moxa is applicable.

Explanation

Ren-4, Ren-6 and Ren-8 rescue Yang Qi and stop sweating if indirect moxibustion on ginger or aconite is applied.

Du-4 with moxa tonifies Kidney-Yang.

ST-36 and P-6 strengthen Heart-Yang.

BL-23 with moxa strengthens Kidney-Yang.

Du-20 is the meeting point of all the Yang channels: it rescues Yang and promotes resuscitation if used with direct moxibustion.

Du-14 and BL-15 combined together can tonify Heart-Yang if direct moxibustion is applied.

It is important to stop sweating because profuse sweating will further weaken the Heart in

Table 13 Summary of Qi deficiency, Heart-Qi and Heart-Yang deficiency

Qi Deficiency	Heart-Qi Deficiency	Heart-Yang Deficiency
Tiredness	Tiredness	Tiredness
Shortness of breath	Shortness of breath	Shortness of breath
Pale face	Pale face	Pale face
Empty pulse	Empty pulse	Weak pulse
Pale tongue	Pale tongue	Pale tongue
	Palpitations	Palpitations
		Chilliness
		Cold limbs
		Stuffiness of the chest

two ways. Firstly, a loss of sweat implies loss of Defensive Qi, which represents a further loss of Yang. Secondly, a loss of fluids from sweating leads to a deficiency of Blood because of the interchange relation between Body Fluids and Blood. The resulting deficiency of Blood will further weaken the Heart.

HEART-BLOOD DEFICIENCY

Clinical manifestations

Palpitations, dizziness, insomnia, dream-disturbed sleep, poor memory, anxiety, propensity to be startled, dull-pale complexion, pale lips.

Tongue: Pale, Thin, slightly dry.

Pulse: Choppy or Fine.

Key symptoms: palpitations, insomnia, poor memory, Pale tongue.

Pathology

The Heart governs Blood, if Blood is deficient the Heart suffers and the Mind is deprived of its "residence", hence the insomnia, dream-disturbed sleep, anxiety and propensity to be startled. The Heart also controls the mental faculties and if Heart-Blood is deficient thinking will be dull and the memory poor.

Blood is the mother of Qi: if Heart-Blood is deficient, Heart-Qi also becomes deficient causing palpitations. There is a subtle difference between the palpitations from Heart-Qi or from Heart-Blood deficiency. In the former case, it is the Qi of the Heart which is deficient and fails to control the Blood. In the latter case, it is the Blood of the Heart which is deficient and fails to nourish Qi. Although they are both described as palpitations, the clinical appearance of the symptoms will be different in each case. In the case of Heart-Qi deficiency, the palpitations will occur more in the daytime and maybe on exertion without any other particular feeling. In the case of Heart-Blood deficiency, the palpitations will occur more in the evening, even at rest and with a slight feeling of uneasiness in the chest or anxiety.

Dizziness is a general symptom of Blood deficiency and is caused by Blood not nourishing the brain.

Dull-pale complexion reflects the deficiency of Blood (in deficiency of Yang, it is bright-pale).

The tongue is the offshoot of the Heart and when Heart-Blood is deficient, not enough Blood reaches the tongue which becomes Pale. The slight dryness (related to the deficiency of Blood) distinguishes this tongue from that of Heart-Yang deficiency which is wet. When not enough Blood reaches the tongue over a long period of time, this becomes also Thin. This is another factor which distinguishes this tongue from that of Heart-Yang deficiency which is Swollen.

The Choppy or Fine pulse reflects deficiency of Blood.

Aetiology

1) A diet which has not enough nourishment or is lacking in Blood-producing foods, can lead to Spleen-Qi deficiency. Food-Qi produced by the Spleen is the basis for the production of Blood, hence Spleen-Qi deficiency, over a long period of time, may lead to Blood deficiency. Blood deficiency, in turn, can weaken the Heart and cause Heart-Blood deficiency. For this reason, Heart-Blood deficiency is often associated with Spleen-Qi deficiency.

2) Anxiety and worry over a long period of time can disturb the Mind which, in turn, can depress the Heart function. Since the Heart governs Blood, this eventually leads to Heart-Blood deficiency.

3) A severe haemorrhage (such as during childbirth) can lead to Blood deficiency; since the

Heart governs Blood. This, in time, can lead to Heart-Blood deficiency. In fact, Chinese Medicine holds this to be the cause of post-natal depression and mental confusion.

Treatment

Principle of treatment: tonify Blood, tonify Heart, pacify the Mind.

Points: Shenmen HE-7, Neiguan P-6, Juque Ren-14, Jiuwei Ren-15, Guanyuan Ren-4, Geshu BL-17, Pishu BL-20.

Method: all with reinforcing method. Moxa can be used.

Explanation

HE-7 tonifies Heart-Blood and pacifies the Mind.

P-6 tonifies Heart-Qi and pacifies the Mind.

Ren-14 and Ren-15 tonify Heart-Blood and pacify the Mind. They are particularly useful if there is pronounced anxiety.

Ren-4, BL-17 and BL-20 tonify Blood. BL-17 is the Gathering point for Blood and BL-20 is the Back Transporting point for the Spleen and it tonifies Spleen-Qi to produce more Blood.

Case history

A 51 year old lady suffered from poor circulation in hands and feet, poor memory, dizziness, numbness of fingers, dull headaches on the vertex, palpitations and insomnia. Her tongue was pale, slightly orangey on the sides and her pulse was Choppy.

This is a clear example of deficiency of Blood of both Heart and Liver (the orangey colour of the tongue on the sides indicates long-standing deficiency of Liver-Blood).

HEART-YIN DEFICIENCY

Clinical manifestations

Palpitations, insomnia, dream-disturbed sleep, propensity to be startled, poor memory, anxiety, mental restlessness, "uneasiness", "fidgetiness", malar flush, low-grade fever or feeling of heat especially in the evening, "feeling hot and bothered", night sweating, dry mouth and throat, 5-palm heat.

Tongue: Red, no coating, tip redder and swollen with red points, deep midline crack reaching the tip.

Pulse: Floating-Empty and Rapid or Fine-Rapid. It may also be Overflowing in both Front positions and Weak in both Rear positions.

Key symptoms: palpitations, mental restlessness, feeling of heat, malar flush, Red-Peeled tongue with deep midline crack.

Pathology

As can be noticed, the pattern of Heart-Yin deficiency includes that of Heart-Blood deficiency. In other words, it is not possible to have Heart-Yin deficiency without Heart-Blood deficiency because Yin embodies Blood. The symptoms common to Heart-Blood deficiency are: insomnia, dream-disturbed sleep, propensity to be startled, poor memory and anxiety. There is a slight difference in the insomnia, however. In Heart-Blood deficiency the patient will find it difficult to fall asleep, but once asleep, will sleep well. In Heart-Yin deficiency the patient will find it difficult to fall asleep *and* will wake up many times during the night.

"Mental restlessness" is a loose translation of a typical Chinese Medicine expression which is always applied to this pattern and which literally means "heart feels vexed". It indicates the feeling of mental irritability or uneasiness typical of Yin deficiency. The patient feels uneasy, fidgety or fretful without any apparent reason. This is accompanied by a feeling of heat in the face, typically in the late evening.

The mental restlessness, malar flush, 5 palm-heat (a feeling of heat in palms, soles and chest), low-grade fever or feeling of heat, dry mouth and throat and night-sweating are all due to Empty-Heat deriving from Yin deficiency. Heart-Yin deficiency is often accompanied or caused by Kidney-Yin deficiency. This causes the Water to be deficient so that Kidney-Yin cannot rise to nourish and cool the Heart. Since Heart-Yin loses the nourishment of Kidney-Yin, this leads to the flaring up of Empty-Heat of the Heart.

This pattern is more common in middle-aged or old people as Yin deficiency usually arises then. The pattern of Heart-Blood deficiency is more common in young people, especially young women.

The tongue is Red and Peeled: Peeled from deficiency of Yin and Red from the flaring up of Empty-Heat. The red and swollen tip with red points reflects the flaring of Empty-Heat within the Heart (the tip reflects the condition of the Heart). The midline crack can appear in any of the Heart patterns. A shallow midline crack without any change in the tongue-body colour indicates a slight constitutional weakness of the Heart and does not necessarily indicate any pathological change. If the midline crack is deep and the tip is red or redder than the rest, or even swollen, this indicates that the Heart is not only constitutionally weak, but that there is a pathological change in the Heart energy from various causes. In this case, the midline crack on a Red and Peeled tongue indicates Heart-Yin deficiency. The Heart fluids are deficient so that the tongue (which is the offshoot of the Heart), does not receive enough fluids and becomes cracked, much like the soil cracks during a drought.

The Floating-Empty pulse reflects Yin deficiency. The pulse is often Weak on both Rear positions reflecting the deficiency of Kidney-Yin, and Overflowing on both Front positions reflecting the flaring up of Heart Empty-Heat.

Aetiology

Long-standing anxiety, worry and an excessively busy life "always on the go", can damage Yin Qi. If this situation which leads to Yin deficiency is accompanied by deep emotional problems and anxiety, the Mind becomes disturbed and Heart-Yin deficiency develops. This is a very common situation in the type of patients we see in the West where our hectic life-style is particularly conducive to Yin deficiency.

Heart-Yin deficiency can also arise after an attack of exterior Heat consuming the Body Fluids and exhausting the Yin of the Heart. However, this usually only happens in very hot countries.

Treatment

Principle of treatment: tonify and nourish Heart-Yin, nourish Kidney-Yin if necessary, pacify the Mind.

Points: Shenmen HE-7, Neiguan P-6, Juque Ren-14, Jiuwei Ren-15, Guanyuan Ren-4, Yinxi HE-6, Sanyinjiao SP-6, Fuliu KI-7, Zhaohai KI-6.

Method: all with reinforcing method, no moxa.

Explanation

HE-7 tonifies Heart-Blood and Heart-Yin and pacifies the Mind.

P-6 pacifies the Mind.

Ren-14 and Ren-15 pacify the Mind. In particular, Ren-15 is an excellent point to pacify the Mind if there is marked anxiety and mental restlessness.

Ren-4 tonifies Yin and "grounds" the Mind when there is Empty-Heat.

HE-6 tonifies Heart-Yin and stops night sweating.

SP-6 tonifies Yin and calms the Mind.

KI-7 tonifies Kidneys and stops night sweating in combination with HE-6.

KI-6 tonifies Kidney-Yin and promotes sleep.

Table 14 Comparison between Heart-Blood and Heart-Yin deficiency.

Pattern	Common Manifestations	Differentiation
Heart-Blood Deficiency	Palpitations, poor memory, insomnia, dream-disturbed sleep, anxiety, Fine pulse	Dull-pale face, Choppy pulse, Pale Tongue
Heart-Yin Deficiency		Malar flush, feeling of heat, Floating-Empty pulse, Red-peeled tongue

Case history

A 50 year old lady suffered from night sweating, lower backache, a feeling of heat in the face in the evenings and dry mouth at night. Her tongue was Red, redder on the tip and Peeled and her pulse was Weak and very Deep and Weak in both Rear positions.

This is a case of Yin deficiency of Heart and Kidneys with Empty-Heat in the Heart.

HEART-FIRE BLAZING

Clinical manifestations

Palpitations, thirst, mouth and tongue ulcers, mental restlessness, feeling agitated, "impulsiveness", feeling of heat, insomnia, red face, dark urine or blood in urine and bitter taste.

Tongue: Red, tip redder and swollen with red points, yellow coating. There may be a midline crack reaching to the tip.

Pulse: Full-Rapid-Overflowing especially on the left Front position. It could also be Hasty (Rapid and stopping at irregular intervals).

Key symptoms: tongue ulcers, thirst, palpitations, Red tongue.

Pathology

This is an Excess pattern of Full-Heat in the Heart, and it contrasts with the previous one of Heart-Yin deficiency where there is Empty-Heat in the Heart. There are several symptoms of Heat, such as thirst, red face, feeling of heat, Red tongue and Rapid-Overflowing or Hasty Pulse.

The tongue is the offshoot of the Heart and when this has Fire, the excess Heat may flare upward to the tongue causing ulcers. These ulcers will have a red and raised rim around them and will be very painful (ulcers with a white rim around them can be due to Empty-Heat from Yin deficiency).

The mental restlessness is very pronounced and is due to the excess Heat in the Heart disturbing the Mind. This "mental restlessness" differs from that of Heart-Yin deficiency in that it is more severe and the patient appears more restless, more agitated, hotter and generally more plethoric.

The insomnia is due to Heat in the Heart disturbing the Mind at night. The patient will wake up frequently and have disturbing dreams, typically of fires and flying.

The red face is due to the flaring of Heat upwards and manifesting on the complexion, which is the outward manifestation of the Heart. This can be differentiated from the redness of Heart-Yin deficiency when only the cheek-bones are flushed (malar flush), whereas in the case of Heart-Fire blazing, the whole face is red.

The bitter taste is a symptom of Full-Heat in the Heart since the Heart opens into the tongue and controls taste. The bitter taste of Heart-Fire can be differentiated from that of Liver-Fire by the fact that the former appears only in the morning and is related to the quality of sleep: if the patient has a sleepless night there will be bitter taste in the morning, if he or she has a better night there will be no bitter taste.

The dark urine or blood in the urine are due to the transmission of Heart-Fire to the Small Intestine (to which the Heart is interiorly-exteriorly related), and from this to the Bladder (to which the Small Intestine is related within the Greater Yang).

The tongue is Red with a coating, reflecting Full-Heat. The red and swollen tip shows the localization of the Heat in the Heart.

The Rapid pulse shows Heat and its Overflowing quality especially in the Front position, shows the presence of Heart-Fire.

Aetiology

Emotional problems such as chronic anxiety, constant worrying and depression can lead to Heart-Fire. These emotions, over a long period of time, can lead to stagnation of Qi, and when Qi stagnates over many years, it may give rise to Fire.

In particular, long-term stagnation of Qi associated with mental depression can turn into Fire causing the appearance of the pattern of Heart-Fire blazing. Many patients suffering from chronic mental depression will display the symptoms and signs of this pattern, even though they may look very subdued and slow. In other words, their look may point to a Deficiency pattern, while all the other symptoms and signs point to the Excess pattern of Heart-Fire blazing.

Heart-Fire is often transmitted from Liver-Fire. It can therefore be indirectly caused by any of the causes of Liver-Fire, such as anger, frustration and resentment.

Treatment

Principle of treatment: clear the Heart, pacify the Mind.

Points: Shaochong HE-9, Shaofu HE-8, Shenmen HE-7, Jiuwei Ren-15, Sanyinjiao SP-6, Zhaohai KI-6.

Method: All with reducing method, except SP-6 and KI-6 to be reinforced. No moxa.

Explanation

HE-9 and HE-8 clear Heart-Fire.

HE-7 pacifies the Mind.

Ren-15 pacifies the Mind and clears Heat.

SP-6 and KI-6 are used to promote Yin and cool Fire, even though there may be no Yin deficiency.

Table 15 Comparison between Heart-Fire blazing and Heart-Yin deficiency

	Heart-Fire blazing	Heart-Yin deficiency
Face	Whole face red	Malar flush
Bitter taste	Yes	No
Dark urine	Yes	No
Tongue	With yellow coating	No coating
Pulse	Full-Overflowing	Floating-Empty or Fine

Case history

A woman of 34 suffered from severe anxiety, insomnia, worrying and brooding, palpitations and mental restlessness. She also had headaches affecting the right eye and side of the head along the Gall Bladder channel. The headaches were severe and throbbing in character. Her periods came irregularly, sometimes late and sometimes early, were heavy and the blood was dark with clots. She also experienced pre-menstrual irritability. Her pulse was Wiry but Fine and her tongue was Deep-Red with red points along the sides and the tip, the tip was redder and swollen and there was a thick yellow coating.

These manifestations are rather complicated. The pattern on the whole is one of Full-Heat as the tongue is Red and has a coating. There is Liver-Fire which is causing the headaches. This is evident also from the Wiry quality of the pulse and the Red colour of the tongue with red points on the sides. Liver-Fire over a long period of time can easily be transmitted to the Heart and cause Heart-Fire: this was the cause of the anxiety, insomnia, palpitations, worrying, mental restlessness and a red and swollen tip of the tongue with red points. In addition, there was also stasis of Liver-Blood as evidenced by the pre-menstrual irritability and the irregularity of her periods with dark-clotted blood.

PHLEGM-FIRE HARASSING THE HEART

Clinical manifestations

Mental restlessness, palpitations, bitter taste, insomnia, dream disturbed sleep, propensity to be startled, incoherent speech, mental confusion, rash behaviour, tendency to hit or scold people, uncontrolled laughter or cry, agitation, shouting, muttering to oneself, mental depression and dullness; in severe cases aphasia and coma.

Tongue: Red, yellow-sticky coating, midline crack with yellow prickles in it. The tip may be redder and swollen with red points.

Pulse: Full-Rapid-Slippery or Rapid-Overflowing-Slippery or Rapid-Full-Wiry.

Key symptoms: all the various mental symptoms and the Red tongue with sticky-yellow coating.

Pathology

This is an Excess pattern characterized by the presence of Fire and Phlegm obstructing the Heart. All the mental symptoms are due to Phlegm obstructing the Heart orifices and disturbing the Mind. Although the main manifestations derive from dysfunction of the Heart, this pattern is also characterized by deficient Spleen-Qi being unable to transform and transport fluids which accumulate into Phlegm. The interior Heat facilitates this process by condensing the fluids into Phlegm. There are actually two separate aspects to this pattern which may appear separately or alternately (as in manic-depression):

1) Mental depression and dullness, muttering to oneself: this is called DIAN in Chinese, meaning "insanity".

2) Uncontrolled laughter or cry, shouting, violent behaviour, hitting or scolding people, incoherent speech: this is called KUANG in Chinese, meaning "violent behaviour".

Both these patterns are of the Excess type and are caused by Phlegm and Fire obstructing the Heart and Mind. It is important not to be misled by the Yin nature of the symptoms in the DIAN type and think that it is a Deficiency pattern requiring tonification.

The obstruction of the Heart orifices can, in

extreme cases, blur the Mind entirely and lead to aphasia and coma. In Chinese medical terminology this is described as "Phlegm obstructing the Heart orifices". This coma is of the Excess type (contrary to that from Heart-Yang Collapse) as is caused by obstruction by Phlegm.

The yellow-sticky coating on the tongue reflects the presence of Phlegm and the Red body colour reflects the presence of Heat. The yellow prickles inside the midline crack also indicate the presence of Phlegm in the Heart.

The Slippery quality of the Pulse indicates Phlegm.

Aetiology

1) Severe emotional problems and depression leading to stagnation of Qi which, over a long period of time, turns into Fire.
2) Excessive consumption of hot-greasy foods creates Heat and Phlegm.
3) This pattern can also appear during fevers from exterior Heat invading the Pericardium. In this case there would not be all the mental symptoms, but only mental confusion and unconsciousness. Exterior Heat can also be a contributing factor to the formation of Interior Phlegm-Fire.

Treatment

Principle of treatment: clear Heart-Fire, resolve Phlegm, pacify the Mind.

Points: Jianshi P-5, Shenmen HE-7, Shaofu HE-8, Shaochong HE-9, Daling P-7, Jiuwei Ren-15, Xinshu BL-15, Zhongwan Ren-12, Fenglong ST-40, Sanyinjiao SP-6, Taichong LIV-3, Xingjian LIV-2, Pishu BL-20, Baihui Du-20, Benshen GB-13, Toulinqi GB-15, Shenting Du-24.

Method: all with reducing method, except Ren-12 and BL-20 which should be reinforced. No moxa.

Explanation

P-5 resolves Phlegm from the Heart and clears orifices.

HE-7 clears Heat and pacifies the Mind.

HE-8 and HE-9 clear Heart-Fire and restore consciousness.

P-7 pacifies the Mind and clears Heart-Fire.

Ren-15 pacifies the Mind.

BL-15 clears Heart-Fire.

Ren-12 tonifies the Spleen to resolve Phlegm.

ST-40 resolves Phlegm.

SP-6 resolves Phlegm and pacifies the Mind.

LIV-3 pacifies the Mind and subdues Fire (it brings Fire down, away from the top part of the body).

LIV-2 subdues Fire (the same way as LIV-3).

Du-20 restores consciousness in case of coma.

GB-13 and Du-24 pacify the Mind.

GB-15 pacifies the Mind and balances the mental state (when it oscillates between mania and depression).

Ancient prescription

There is an ancient prescription for manic behaviour from Sun Si Miao (581-682), the eminent doctor of the Tang dynasty, author of the "Thousand Golden Ducat Prescriptions". This is: Renzhong Du-26, Shaoshang LU-11, Yinbai SP-1, Daling P-7, Shenmai BL-62, Fengfu Du-16, Jiache ST-6, Chengjiang Ren-24, Laogong P-8, Shangxing Du-23, Huiyin Ren-1, Quchi L.I.-11, Shexia (the two points on the veins under the tongue), Jianshi P-5, Houxi S.I.-3. These points should be needled one by one in this order, without retention of needle with reducing method.

Case history

A 37 year-old woman suffered from what had been diagnosed as manic-depression since her teen-age years. The symptoms differed according to whether she was at the manic or depressive phase.

Manic phase: palpitations, uncontrolled activity, "cannot stop", talking very fast, over-excited, uncontrolled laughter, obsessional thoughts.
Depressive phase: frightened of failure, frustration, depressed mood, does not want to see people, tiredness, inability to work, mentally unclear. The tongue was Red, with a tip redder and swollen with red points, and a thick-sticky yellow coating.
The Pulse was Full and Overflowing.

All these manifestations point to obstruction of the Heart orifices and misting of the Mind by Fire and Phlegm. The Red tongue, Overflowing pulse and the mental symptoms all indicate Fire, while the sticky tongue coating denotes the presence of Phlegm.

Case history

A woman of 67 had been suffering from manic depression for a long time. She had bouts of depression alternating with bouts of manic behaviour. These symptoms appeared after the death of her husband. During the depressive phase she felt extremely gloomy, had no interest in life, did not wash or speak to anyone. During the manic phase she would have lots of energy, go for several days without sleep and spend money uncontrollably. Her pulse was Wiry and Overflowing on the Front positions. Her tongue was red with a sticky-yellow coating all over, and the tip was redder and swollen.

All the manifestations point to Phlegm and Fire stirring the Heart and obstructing the Heart orifices, causing her mental symptoms.

PHLEGM MISTING THE MIND

Clinical manifestations

Mental confusion, unconsciousness, lethargic stupor, vomiting, rattling sound in the throat, aphasia.

Tongue: Thick-sticky-slippery coating, midline crack reaching the tip with prickles in it. Tongue-body Swollen.

Pulse: Slippery.

Key symptoms: mental confusion, rattling sound in throat, sticky-slippery tongue coating.

Pathology

This pattern is also called "Phlegm obstructing the Heart orifices". This pattern is of the Excess type and is very similar to the previous one, except for the absence of Fire. Although similar, the two patterns occur in different types of patients and situations. The pattern of Phlegm misting the Mind is seen either in children, when it can be a cause of mental retardation or speech difficulties, and in adults after an attack of Wind-stroke when Wind associates with Phlegm causing coma, paralysis and aphasia. In both these cases all the severe mental symptoms of the previous pattern are absent.

The mental confusion, lethargic stupor, unconsciousness, are all due to Phlegm obstructing the Heart and therefore the Mind.

The Heart opens into the tongue and the Phlegm prevents the tongue from moving, hence the aphasia. The obstructive effect of the Phlegm on the Heart prevents Heart-Qi from opening into the tongue and Heart-Blood from housing the Mind: hence the Heart "orifices" (Mind and tongue) are obstructed.

Vomiting and rattling sound in the throat are due to Phlegm obstructing the chest.

The sticky-slippery coating and Slippery pulse reflect the presence of Phlegm.

Aetiology

1) In children, constitutional.
2) In adults this pattern can be caused by excessive consumption of greasy-cold-raw foods leading to the formation of Phlegm. However, for the Phlegm to obstruct the Heart, the dietary origin of this pattern is usually combined with severe emotional problems such as long-standing anxiety.

Treatment

Principle of treatment: open the Heart, resolve Phlegm, restore consciousness (if unconscious).

Points: Shaochong HE-9, Jianshi P-5, Xinshu BL-15, Fenglong ST-40, Renzhong Du-26, Zhongwan Ren-12, Pishu BL-20.

Method: all with reducing method except for Zhongwan Ren-12 and Pishu BL-20 which should be reinforced.

Explanation

HE-9 clears the Heart and opens its orifices. In case of unconsciousness it could be bled.

P-5 resolves Phlegm from the Heart. This is the main point for this pattern.

BL-15 clears the Heart and is particularly useful in children to clear Phlegm from the Heart: it will stimulate the child's intellectual capacities and speech.

ST-40 resolves Phlegm.

Du-26 is used to restore consciousness if necessary.

Ren-12 and BL-20 tonify the Spleen to resolve Phlegm.

HEART-BLOOD STAGNANT

Clinical manifestations

Palpitations, pain in the heart region which may radiate to the inner aspect of the left arm or to the shoulder, discomfort or feeling of oppression or constriction of the chest, cyanosis of lips and nails, cold hands.

Tongue: Purple.

Pulse: Knotted.

Key symptoms: pain in the heart region, cyanosis of lips, purple tongue.

Pathology

This pattern does not occur on its own, but is derived from other Heart patterns, mostly Heart-Yang deficiency, Heart-Blood deficiency or Heart-Fire. The symptoms and signs will therefore vary according to the origin of the pattern. The symptoms and signs described above are only those related to the stasis of Heart-Blood and in practice, there would be in addition some symptoms of Heart-Yang deficiency or Heart-Blood deficiency or Heart-Fire, according to which pattern is involved.

If it is due to Heart-Yang or Heart-Blood deficiency, this pattern is a combined Deficiency/ Excess pattern. If it is due to Heart-Fire, it is an Excess pattern. In most cases, it is derived from Heart-Yang deficiency.

Yang Qi moves and transports. If Heart-Yang is deficient, it cannot move the Blood in the chest, hence the Blood stagnates in this area and causes the pain and feeling of tightness. The intensity of the pain can vary from a mild pricking sensation to a really intense stabbing pain. Chest pain is the key symptom of this pattern, which other Heart patterns do not have. The pain typically comes in repeated bouts and is elicited by exertion or cold weather.

If the stasis of Blood is derived from Heart-Fire, its mechanism is different. In this case the stasis is caused by Heat congealing Blood in the chest.

In any case, this pattern closely resembles the Western medical disease entity of angina pectoris.

The cyanosis of lips and nails and the cold hands are due to stagnant Heart-Blood not reaching the face and hands. The stasis of Blood in the chest also obstructs the circulation of Gathering Qi, which normally has the function of helping the movement of Lung and Heart Qi to the hands resulting in cold hands.

The Purple colour of the tongue body reflects the stasis of Blood. In most cases, this will be Bluish-Purple reflecting the Internal Cold from Deficiency of Yang causing stasis of Blood. It can also be Reddish-Purple if it is associated with Heart-Fire.

The Knotted pulse is Slow and stops at irregular intervals and reflects the presence of interior Cold. The irregularity of it is due to the stagnation of Blood which prevents it from circulating properly.

Aetiology

Emotional problems, particularly anxiety, grief, resentment or bottled-up anger over a long period of time can lead to stagnation of Blood in the chest. The chest is the most likely part of the body where pent-up emotions are kept and they therefore easily lead to impairment in the circulation of Qi or Blood in this area. Furthermore, all these emotions disturb the Mind. Heart-Blood is the physiological basis for the Mind and any emotional problem that constrains the Mind may lead to stagnation of Qi and/or Blood of the Heart.

This pattern may be derived from other Heart patterns, particularly Heart-Yang deficiency. Therefore, any of the causes leading to Heart-Yang deficiency can, in the long run, lead to Heart-Blood stagnation.

Treatment

Principle of treatment: regulate Blood, remove stasis, tonify and warm Heart-Yang, pacify the Mind.

Points: Neiguan P-6, Ximen P-4, Shenmen HE-7, Shanzhong Ren-17, Jueyinshu BL-14, Geshu BL-17, Xuehai SP-10, Shencang KI-25.

Method: all with reducing method during an

attack, or even method in between the attacks. Moxa is applicable if there is Heart-Yang deficiency.

Explanation

P-6 regulates Heart-Blood and opens the chest. This is the main point.

P-4 is the Accumulation point and is particularly useful to stop heart-pain during an acute attack.

HE-7 pacifies the Mind.

Ren-17 regulates Qi and Blood in the chest and stimulates the circulation of Gathering Qi. Moxa after needling can be used if there is Heart-Yang deficiency.

BL-14 regulates Heart-Blood.

BL-17 regulates Blood if needled. If used to regulate Blood, moxa cannot be used.

SP-10 regulates Blood.

KI-25 is a local chest point to move Qi and Blood in the chest. It is particularly useful if the Heart-Yang deficiency is associated with Kidney-Yang deficiency.

Case history

A 52-year-old lady had been suffering from bouts of severe palpitations and stabbing pain in the chest radiating to the left arm for 30 years. During the attacks her lips became cyanotic and she felt cold. The tongue was Bluish-Purple and the pulse Knotted.

This is an example of stagnation of Heart-Blood from deficiency of Heart-Yang.

Case history

A 77-year-old man suffered from a more or less permanent sensation of constriction of the chest elicited by exertion. The tongue was Reddish-Purple and the pulse was Wiry.

This is an example of stasis of Heart-Blood from Heart-Fire.

NOTES

1 Spiritual Axis, p 128.
2 Simple Questions, p 221.

Liver Patterns 22

肝脏病証

The main function of the Liver is that of ensuring the smooth flow of Qi. This function was discussed in detail in the chapter on the organ's functions. Its influence extends all over the body and to many different Yin or Yang organs. It helps the Spleen to transform and transport food essences and the Stomach to rot and ripen food. Liver-Qi also helps Spleen-Qi to ascend and Stomach-Qi to descend.

It stimulates the Gall-Bladder secretion of bile and it ensures the smooth flow of Qi in the Intestines and the Uterus, thus influencing menstruation. Moreover, it has a paramount influence on the emotional state: the smooth flow of Liver-Qi ensures a "smooth flow" of our emotional life. If Liver-Qi is constrained over a long period of time, our emotional life will be characterized by depression, frustration, irritability and emotional tension generally.

As the Liver ensures the smooth flow of Qi but has no part in the actual production and supply of Qi, it does not have patterns involving deficiency of Qi (although it does have patterns of deficiency of Blood and Yin). In relation to Qi, the most important and common pattern is that of Stagnation of Liver-Qi. A frequent consequence of stagnation of Liver-Qi is loss of harmony in the function of various organs so that Stomach-Qi cannot descend, Spleen-Qi cannot transform, the Gall-Bladder cannot secrete bile freely, the Qi of the Intestines becomes "stagnant", the Qi of the Uterus stagnates causing period pain and the emotional life is constrained. From a pathological point of view, the most striking and apparent symptom of stagnation of Liver-Qi is distension. When Liver-Qi cannot flow smoothly, Qi accumulates and gives rise to a characteristic feeling of distension, which could manifest in the epigastrium, hypochondrium, abdomen or hypogastrium.

Liver pathology is also characterized by rapid changes such as skin rashes that appear quickly, sudden tinnitus, sudden outbursts of anger, or in severe cases, sudden collapse and coma.

Whilst Liver-Qi can never be deficient, Liver-Blood and Liver-Yin can. The Liver stores Blood and this can easily be depleted leading to symptoms of Blood deficiency and scanty periods. Liver-Blood can also become stagnant: this is usually a consequence of stagnation of Liver-Qi. Qi is the "commander of Blood", when Qi stagnates, Blood congeals.

The functional relationship between the Liver and the sinews often manifests in pathological circumstances with physical tiredness and weakness or contraction of the tendons.

GENERAL AETIOLOGY

EXTERIOR PATHOGENIC FACTORS

The two pathogenic factors which affect the Liver are Wind and Dampness.

Exterior Wind can easily interfere with the Liver functions of ensuring the smooth flow of Qi and storing Blood. Exterior Wind does not attack the Liver directly (it does attack the Lung-Defensive Qi portion) but it can aggravate a situation of Interior Wind of the Liver; it could, for instance, precipitate an attack of Interior Liver-Wind causing a Wind-stroke.

In some cases, exterior Wind can aggravate an internal Liver disharmony causing stiff neck and headaches.

Exterior Wind can also stir the Blood stored in the Liver and manifest with skin rashes which start suddenly and move quickly, such as in urticaria. In such cases, the Wind usually combines with Heat to cause Heat in Liver-Blood at the superficial levels of the Blood-Connecting channels.The sudden onset and quick changes are typical of Wind as a pathogenic factor.

EMOTIONS

Anger

This is the emotion which is most related to the Liver function. As mentioned before (see chapter 15 "Causes of Disease", p. 127), "anger" is a broad term used in Chinese Medicine which includes feelings of frustration, repressed anger, resentment, and irritation. As always in Chinese Medicine, the relationship between a certain emotion and organ is mutual: the Liver function of ensuring a smooth flow of Qi has a profound influence on the emotional state, and conversely, the emotional state will influence the Liver function.

Thus if the Liver is functioning well and its Qi flowing smoothly, the emotional state will be happy and free-going and the person will be in good spirits and freely express his or her emotions. If Liver-Qi stagnates and does not flow freely and unimpeded, it will stagnate and affect the emotional state causing anger, and irritability. Over a long period of time, stagnation of Liver-Qi will severely impair the circulation of Qi giving rise to a gloomy emotional state of constant resentment, repressed anger or depression. On a physical level, these constrained emotions could be "carried" in the chest, hypochondrium, epigastrium or throat. The person will then experience a feeling of tightness of the chest and perhaps sigh frequently, or distension of the hypogastrium, or tension in the stomach area or a feeling of lump in the throat with difficulty in swallowing. These feelings are particularly related to stagnation of Liver-Qi.

If Liver-Qi rebels upward causing the rising of Liver-Yang, the person will be very irritable, "fly off the handle" very easily and suffer from headaches.

Stagnation of Qi over a long period of time can lead to Fire as the implosion of Qi caused by emotional constraint generates Heat. This situation is often manifested on the tongue with red sides and tip, possibly with red points on the tip.

DIET

An excessive consumption of greasy and "hot" foods can lead to Liver-Fire. From the point of view of Chinese dietary principles, hot foods are lamb, beef, curries, spices and alcohol. Deep-fried foods are also hot.

An inadequate consumption of warming foods, such as meat and grains, can lead to a state of Blood deficiency which can lead to deficiency of Liver-Blood. This is more common in women who particularly need an adequate supply of Blood-forming foods at certain times of their life, such as at puberty and after childbirth, as well as, to a lesser degree, after each period. A severe blood loss after childbirth can also lead to deficiency of Liver-Blood.

The Liver patterns to be discussed are:

- Excess patterns
  - Stagnation of Liver-Qi
  - Stagnation of Liver-Blood

Liver-Fire blazing upwards
Liver-Wind agitating within
Damp-Heat in Liver and Gall-Bladder
Stagnation of cold in the Liver channel
Deficiency pattern
Liver-Blood deficiency
Deficiency-Excess pattern
Liver-Yang rising.

STAGNATION OF LIVER-QI

Clinical manifestations

a) Feeling of distension of hypochondrium and chest, hypochondriac pain, sighing, hiccup.
b) Melancholy, depression, moodiness, fluctuation of mental state.
c) Nausea, vomiting, epigastric pain, poor appetite, sour regurgitation, belching, feeling of pulsation in epigastrium, "churning feeling in the stomach", abdominal distension, borborygmi, diarrhoea.
d) Unhappiness, "feeling wound-up", feeling of lump in the throat, feeling of difficulty in swallowing.
e) Irregular periods, painful periods, distension of breasts before the periods, pre-menstrual tension and irritability.

Tongue: the body colour may be normal.

Pulse: Wiry, especially on the left side.

Key symptoms: hypochondriac and chest distension, depression, moodiness, Wiry pulse.

Pathology

This is by far the most common of the Liver patterns and also one of the most common patterns in general. Obviously not all the above manifestation need be present to warrant a diagnosis of Liver-Qi stagnation. I have arranged the manifestations in five different groups to highlight the different pathology of each group. Stagnation of Liver-Qi is very far-reaching and manifests its influence in a wide range of symptoms and signs.

a) On a physical level, stagnation of Liver-Qi manifests primarily in the hypochondrium, i.e. the area just below the rib-cage, on either side. The stagnation may be manifested with pain, but even more with a characteristic feeling of distension which is predominant to the pain. When Liver-Qi stagnates in the chest, the person will experience a feeling of distension of the chest.

Sighing is a spontaneous way to release the stagnant Qi in the chest and hiccup is due to Liver-Qi stagnant in the diaphragm.

b) The second group of symptoms includes several emotional manifestations which are very common and typical of Liver-Qi stagnation.

c) Most of these manifestations (nausea, vomiting, epigastric pain, no appetite, belching, etc.) are due to stagnant Liver-Qi invading the Stomach horizontally and preventing Stomach-Qi from descending. Borborygmi is due to stagnation of Liver-Qi in the Intestines impairing their transportation function. Diarrohea is due to stagnant Liver-Qi invading the Spleen and impairing its function of transportation and transformation. In these situations when Liver-Qi invades Stomach and Spleen, there is a certain overlap of patterns between the Stomach/Spleen and Liver and is often difficult to know where one starts and the other ends.

d) The stagnation of Liver-Qi in the throat (where the Liver channel also flows), gives rise to the feeling of lump in the throat (this is described in Chinese Medicine as like a feeling "of plum stone in the throat"). The feeling comes and goes according to the emotional state.

e) Finally, stagnation of Liver-Qi can impair the movement of Blood in the Directing and Penetrating Vessels, thus affecting the Uterus, resulting in irregular and painful periods and pre-menstrual tension with distension of the breasts (which are also under the influence of the Liver channel).

This pattern is of the Excess type and, as mentioned in the case of Heart-Fire, one should not be misled by the emotional state of the person which may appear to be "deficient" (i.e. the person is depressed, moody and quiet). In spite of its appearance, it is caused by an "implosion" of Qi due to the stagnation of Liver-Qi and, as such, it is to be treated as an Excess pattern.

Typically, the emotional symptoms fluctuate a lot: the person goes through periods of depression when all the physical symptoms also appear, and periods when the depression is lifted and the physical symptoms disappear. This fluctuation is typical of Liver-Qi stagnation.

As Qi "is the commander of Blood and when Qi stagnates Blood congeals", stagnation of Liver-Qi over a long period of time can easily induce stagnation of Liver-Blood. This will be discussed as a separate pattern.

Aetiology

Emotional problems

Problems in the emotional life are by far the most important (if not the only) cause of Liver-Qi stagnation. As mentioned before, a state of frustration, repressed anger or resentment over a long period of time can cause the circulation to be impeded so that Qi does not flow smoothly and it becomes stuck resulting in stagnation of Liver-Qi.

Treatment

Principle of treatment: disperse the Liver and regulate Qi.

Points: Yanglingquan GB-34, Taichong LIV-3, Zhangmen LIV-13, Qimen LIV-14, Zhigou T.B.-6, Neiguan P-6.

Method: reducing method, no moxa.

Explanation

GB-34 regulates Liver-Qi and it particularly influences the hypochondriac region.

LIV-3 also regulates Liver-Qi and it particularly affects the throat.

LIV-13 regulates Liver-Qi in the Middle Burner, particularly when it invades the Spleen.

LIV-14 regulates Liver-Qi in the Middle Burner, particularly when it affects the Stomach.

T.B.-6 regulates Liver-Qi and it particularly affects the sides of the body.

P-6 regulates Liver-Qi (by virtue of the relationship between Liver and Pericardium channels within the Terminal Yin). This point would be particularly well indicated when the stagnation of Liver-Qi is caused by emotional problems.

Case history

A woman of 50 suffered from tiredness, depression, pronounced mood swings, pre-menstrual depression and irritability, distension of the breasts before the periods and a swelling of the thyroid gland with a feeling of constriction in the throat. The pulse was Wiry, the tongue-body colour was normal and only slightly Purple on the sides.

The above manifestations indicate stagnation of Liver-Qi manifesting more in the throat, rather than the hypochondrium. The depression, mood-swings and pre-menstrual irritability with distension of the breasts, the Wiry pulse, the slightly purple colour on the sides of the tongue, all clearly point to stagnation of Liver-Qi. Had the periods been painful with dark-clotted blood and the tongue been more purple, one would have diagnosed stasis of Liver-Blood.

Case history

A young woman of 34 suffered from epigastric and abdominal pain of a spastic character, indigestion, belching, a feeling of fullness and distension of the abdomen and nausea. Her bowel movements alternated between constipation with small, bitty stools and diarrhoea. The pulse was Wiry and the tongue was Red with redder sides and a yellow coating.

These symptoms and signs show stagnation of Liver-Qi, with Liver-Qi invading the Stomach (epigastric pain and distension, belching, nausea), the Spleen (diarrhoea, abdominal pain and distension) and the Intestines (constipation with small bitty stools). The Wiry pulse and red colour of the sides of the tongue confirms the involvement of the Liver. Thus, in this case, the symptoms and signs appear in three organs (Stomach, Spleen and Intestines) but all stem from the primary factor of Liver-Qi stagnation. The Red colour of the tongue shows that the stagnation of Liver-Qi is beginning to transform into Fire, as it often happens after a prolonged period.

STASIS OF LIVER-BLOOD

Clinical manifestations

Vomiting of blood, epistaxis, painful periods, irregular periods, menstrual blood dark and clotted, abdominal pain, "masses" in abdomen, purple nails, purple lips, purple complexion, dry skin (in severe cases), petechiae.

Tongue: Purple especially on the sides, with purplish spots. Pulse: Wiry.

Key symptoms: dark and clotted menstrual blood, Purple tongue.

Pathology

This pattern always derives from that of stagnation of Liver-Qi. When Qi stagnates, in the long run it leads to stasis of Blood. The Liver stores Blood and is particularly affected by stasis of Blood.

When Liver-Blood stagnates, the Blood in the Directing and Penetrating Vessels will also stagnate and affect the menstrual function. The chief manifestation of stasis of Blood in the uterus is dark and clotted menstrual blood. Blood stasis always leads to pain, and in this pattern, pain is predominant in relation to distension (whereas in stagnation of Liver-Qi the distension is predominant in relation to pain).

Stasis of Blood of the Liver may cause pain not only during (or before) the periods, but also generally in the abdomen at other times and it affects men too. The pain from stasis of Blood is usually fixed in one place and is boring or stabbing in character. This may also be accompanied by a swelling or mass in the abdomen which is fixed (stagnation of Qi can also be manifested with abdominal masses but which would come and go).

Vomiting of blood and epistaxis are caused by stasis of Blood in the Liver channel.

The Purple colour of the tongue body reflects stasis of Blood. In severe cases there will also be purplish spots, usually on the sides.

The Liver manifests on the nails and their purple colour reflects the stasis of Blood in the Liver. General stasis of Blood also causes purple lips and complexion. In severe cases, stagnant Blood obstructs the circulation of fluids (due to the interchange between Body Fluids and Blood) and the skin becomes dry. Petechiae (of a purple colour) are due to bleeding under the skin caused by Blood stasis in the Blood Connecting channels.

Aetiology

This is the same as for stagnation of Liver-Qi, i.e. from emotional problems. Stasis of Liver-Blood is usually a consequence of long-standing stagnation of Liver-Qi.

Treatment

Principle of treatment: disperse the Liver, regulate Blood.

Points: Yanglingquan GB-34, Taichong LIV-3, Ganshu BL-18, Geshu BL-17, Xuehai SP-10, Qihai Ren-6.

Method: reducing method, no moxa.

Explanation

GB-34 regulates Liver-Qi; in order to regulate Blood, it is necessary to regulate Qi first.

LIV-3 regulates Liver-Qi and Blood.

BL-18 regulates Liver-Blood.

BL-17 is the Gathering point for Blood and it can regulate Blood (when used with needle only, without moxa).

SP-10 regulates Blood.

Ren-6 regulates Qi (apart from tonifying Qi) and is used to regulate Qi and move Blood in the abdomen, in cases of abdominal pain.

Case history

A 35-year old woman suffered from very painful periods with dark, clotted blood, pre-menstrual distension of breasts, a thin-white vaginal discharge, a feeling of heaviness and bearing down sensation, chilliness, floaters in eyes and dizziness. She also experienced abdominal pain in mid-cycle. Her pulse was Deep and Choppy and her tongue was Bluish-Purple and Swollen and had a dirty-sticky coating.

The pain during and before the periods with dark clotted blood and the purple colour of the tongue body indicated stasis of Blood. With stasis of Liver-Blood there was also some stagnation of Liver-Qi as indicated by the pre-menstrual distension of breasts. Pre-existing to the stasis of Liver-Blood, there was also deficiency of Liver-Blood as indicated by the Choppy pulse, Pale tongue (a Bluish-Purple colour develops from a Pale colour), the floaters and the dizziness.

Besides this Liver disharmony, there was also Spleen-Yang deficiency leading to the retention of Dampness, as indicated by the chilliness, the white vaginal discharge, the Swollen tongue body, the feeling of heaviness and bearing down sensation and the dirty-sticky tongue coating. Deficient Spleen-Yang generated internal Cold which congealed Blood. Stasis of Blood is, in this case, caused by internal Cold, and the chilliness and Bluish-Purple tongue are important factors in determining this. Had the tongue been Reddish-Purple, the diagnosis would have been different.

Case history

A woman of 43 had a very large sub-serous fibroid in the uterus. She experienced pain before and sometimes during the periods which were heavy and the blood was dark with clots. She also had headaches before her periods. For 6 weeks the previous year she suffered from what was diagnosed as thyroiditis manifesting with a rapid pulse, a swelling of the neck and an earache. Her pulse was Deep and Wiry and her tongue was Reddish-Purple and Stiff.

All these symptoms and signs are due to stasis of Liver-Blood, which is further confirmed by the pulse and tongue. The fibroid is also a manifestation of stasis of Liver-Blood: when Liver-Qi stagnates over a long period of time, Liver-Blood becomes stagnant, and this affects the Directing and Penetrating Vessels which flow through the uterus. The "thyroiditis" is also a manifestation of stasis of Liver Qi and Blood affecting the neck.

LIVER-FIRE BLAZING UPWARDS

Clinical manifestations

Irritability, propensity to outbursts of anger, tinnitus, deafness, temporal headache, dizziness, red face and eyes, thirst, bitter taste, dream-disturbed sleep, constipation with dry stools, dark-yellow urine, epistaxis, haematemesis, haemoptysis.

Tongue: Red body, redder on the sides, yellow coating, dry.

Pulse: Full-Wiry-Rapid.

Key symptoms: irritability, red face, red eyes, Red tongue with yellow coating.

Pathology

This pattern is characterized by Full-Heat in the Liver. Liver-Fire has a natural tendency to flare upwards, hence many of the symptoms and signs reflect the rising of Liver-Fire towards the head, such as red face and eyes, temporal headache, dizziness, dream-disturbed sleep and irritability.

Liver-Fire ascends to the ears and clouds the ear-orifices causing tinnitus and deafness which, in this case, will be characterized by a sudden onset. The tinnitus will be experienced as a high-pitch whistle.

The headache is caused by the rising upwards of Liver-Qi and Liver-Fire and will be very intense, throbbing in character, usually on the temple or in the eye.

The bitter taste is caused by the rising of Liver-Fire towards the throat and mouth. Bitter taste can also be caused by Heart-Fire in which case, it manifests only in the mornings after a bad night's sleep (it will not be present after a good night's sleep). If bitter taste is caused by Liver-Fire it will be present the whole day and not just in the morning.

Liver-Fire dries up Body Fluids resulting in constipation with dry stools and a concentrated, dark urine.

In a few cases, Liver-Fire heats the Blood and causes it to extravasate, resulting in epistaxis or vomiting or coughing of blood.

The Red tongue body reflects the Heat and the redder colour of the sides reflects the location of Heat in the Liver.

The Full-Rapid quality of the Pulse reflects Full-Heat and its Wiry quality reflects the location of Heat in the Liver.

Aetiology

The most common cause of this pattern is a long-standing emotional state of anger, resentment, repressed anger or frustration. The emotional repression makes Qi stagnate and implode giving rise to Heat.

From a dietary point of view, the excessive consumption of alcohol, fried foods and meat (especially lamb and beef), can contribute to the formation of Heat in the Liver.

Treatment

Principle of treatment: sedate the Liver, clear Fire.

Points: Xingjian LIV-2, Taichong LIV-3, Fengchi GB-20, Taiyang, Benshen GB-13, Quchi L.I.-11.

Method: reducing method, no moxa.

Explanation

LIV-2 is the main point to use: it is specific to clear Liver-Fire.

LIV-3 sedates the Liver.

GB-20 clears Liver-Fire and subdues ascending Liver-Qi. A very important point to use in case of problems with the eyes or headaches caused by Liver-Fire.

Taiyang (extra point) clears Liver-Fire and is used for temporal headache.

GB-13, Quchi L.I.-11 subdues ascending Liver-Yang and calms the Mind.

L.I.-11 clears Heat.

LIVER-WIND AGITATING WITHIN

There are three distinct types of Liver-Wind from three different causes. These are:

Extreme Heat generating Wind

Deficiency of Liver-Yin with rising of Liver-Yang leading to Liver-Wind

Deficiency of Liver-Blood leading to Liver-Wind.

The general clinical manifestations of Liver-Wind are : tremor, tic, numbness, dizziness and convulsions or paralysis. Internal Wind signs are characterized by movement or the absence of it, hence the tremor and convulsions or paralysis (as in Wind-stroke).

Each of the above three types of Liver-Wind will be discussed separately.

1 EXTREME HEAT GENERATING WIND

Clinical manifestations

High temperature, convulsions, rigidity of the neck, tremor of limbs, opisthotonos, in severe cases coma. STROKE

Tongue: Deep-Red, Stiff, thick yellow coating.

Pulse: Wiry-Rapid-Full.

Key symptoms: high temperature, convulsions, Stiff tongue.

Pathology

This is a pattern encountered only in acute febrile diseases, when the exterior pathogenic Heat has penetrated deeply into the Blood level and given rise to internal Wind of the Liver. It is more common in children when it is seen as a complication of such febrile diseases as measles, encephalitis and meningitis. This is an Excess type of Internal Wind.

Internal Wind causes signs which are characterized by movement hence the tremor of limbs and the convulsions. On the other hand, internal Wind prevents the Liver from moistening the sinews, which causes rigidity of the neck and opisthotonos. In severe cases, the extreme Heat and Wind can cloud the Mind and cause coma.

Aetiology

Wei Qi Ying Blood

This is due to invasion of exterior Heat or Wind-Heat penetrating to the Blood level (which is the deepest level) and generating internal Wind.

Treatment

Principle of treatment: clear Heat, disperse the Liver, subdue Wind.

Points: Taichong LIV-3, Xingjian LIV-2, Shixuan extra points, Houxi S.I.-3, Baihui Du-20, Fengfu Du-16, Fengchi GB-20.

Method: reducing method, bleeding of the Shixuan points.

Explanation

LIV-3 and LIV-2 disperse the Liver and subdue Wind. In addition, LIV-2 is particularly indicated to clear Heat.

Shixuan points (ten points on each of the fingertips) clear Heat, subdue Wind and restore consciousness.

S.I.-3 expels interior Wind from the Governing Vessel.

Du-20, Du-16 and GB-20, all subdue Internal Wind.

Note: This pattern may correspond to acute diseases such as meningitis and it is given here for reference only: in such cases, the patient obviously needs urgent Western medical treatment.

Case history

An 11-month old baby girl developed a high temperature of unknown origin which went on for three days. At the end of the three days she had an epileptic fit with strong convulsions, and continued to have such fits ever since.

This is a clear example of Liver-Wind stirred by intense Heat. It is more common in children. This baby had obviously contracted some kind of viral infection which, from the Chinese point of view, is described, in its beginning stages, as invasion of exterior Wind-Heat. The exterior Heat, if not treated, penetrates in the Interior going through successive stages which are clearly set out in the Identification of Patterns according to the 4 Levels: the four levels are the Defensive Qi, Qi, Nutritive Qi and Blood level. At the Blood level, which is the deepest, Heat enters the Blood and stirs Wind in the Liver: the convulsions are due to such internal Wind.

2 LIVER-YANG RISING CAUSING WIND

Clinical manifestations

Sudden unconsciousness, convulsions, deviation of eye and mouth, hemiplegia, aphasia or difficult speech, dizziness.

Tongue: Red-Peeled, Deviated.

Pulse: Floating-Empty or Wiry-Fine and Rapid.

Key symptoms: sudden unconsciousness, convulsions, deviation of eye and mouth.

Pathology

This condition arises from deficiency of Liver-Yin which, over a long period of time, causes the rising upwards of Liver-Yang. Under certain circumstances, Liver-Yang can generate internal Wind. In these cases Wind-stroke may occur. This is internal Wind from a combination of Deficiency and Excess.

Aetiology

This pattern needs two factors to appear: deficiency of Liver-Yin and ascending Liver-Yang. The causes of Liver-Yin deficiency are usually to be found in excessive sexual activity or excessive exercise and physical exertion over a long period of time. In a woman, Liver-Yin deficiency can arise as a consequence of Liver-Blood deficiency (such as from chronic menorrhagia) over a long period of time.

Ascending Liver-Yang is usually caused by emotional factors and most of all, a continuous state of anger, resentment, frustration, etc.

Treatment

Principle of treatment: nourish Liver-Yin, subdue Liver-Yang, subdue Wind.

Points: Ququan LIV-8, Taichong LIV-3, Ganshu BL-18, Sanyinjiao SP-6, Taixi KI-3, Fengfu Du-16, Fengchi GB-20.

Method: reinforcing on LIV-8, SP-6 and KI-3; reducing on LIV-3, Du-16, GB-20; even method on BL-18.

Explanation

LIV-8 tonifies Liver-Yin.

LIV-3 subdues Liver-Yang and Liver-Wind.

SP-6 and KI-3 tonify Yin.

Du-16 and GB-20 subdue Wind.

BL-18 can tonify Liver-Yin and also subdue Liver-Yang.

3 DEFICIENT LIVER-BLOOD CAUSING WIND

Clinical manifestations

Numbness of limbs, tic, shaking of head, tremor of limbs.

Tongue: Pale, Deviated

Pulse: Choppy

Key symptoms: shaking of head, tremors, Pale tongue.

Pathology

This pattern is caused by deficiency of Liver-Blood creating an emptiness in the blood vessels which is "filled" by internal Wind. This is a Deficient type of internal Wind. The shaking of the head, tic and tremor are all due to the internal Wind. The numbness is due to deficient Blood not nourishing muscles and sinews. The tremor of the limbs in this case is quite fine, not real convulsions as in the previous two cases.

Aetiology

This is due to a chronic deficiency of Liver-Blood and can therefore be caused by any of the causes of Liver-Blood deficiency.

Treatment

Principle of treatment: tonify Liver-Blood, subdue Wind.

Points: Ququan LIV-8, Taichong LIV-3, Sanyinjiao SP-6, Taixi KI-3, Ganshu BL-18, Geshu BL-17, Pishu BL-20, Shenshu BL-23, Hegu L.I.-4, Fengchi GB-20, Fengfu Du-16, Baihui Du-20.

Method: reducing on LIV-3, L.I.-4, GB-20, Du-16, Du-20, reinforcing on the others.

Explanation

LIV-8 tonifies Liver-Blood.

LIV-3 subdues Liver-Wind.

SP-6, KI-3, BL-20 and BL-23 tonify Blood.

BL-17 (with direct moxa) tonifies Blood.

BL-18 tonifies Liver-Blood and subdues Liver-Wind.

GB-20, Du-16 and Du-20 subdue Liver-Wind.

L.I.-4 (in combination with LIV-3) eliminates Wind from the face. It is particularly indicated for facial tic.

DAMP-HEAT IN LIVER AND GALL BLADDER

Clinical manifestations

Fever, scanty-dark urine, fullness and pain of chest and hypochondrium, jaundice, bitter taste, nausea, vomiting, loss of appetite, abdominal distention, vaginal discharge, pain-redness-swelling of scrotum, vaginal itching.

Tongue: Red body, sticky-yellow coating.

Pulse: Slippery-Wiry-Rapid.

Key symptoms: fever, fullness chest and hypochondrium, nausea, sticky yellow coating, Slippery pulse.

Pathology

This pattern arises from a combination of Heat in the Liver and Dampness arising from Spleen deficiency. The Spleen deficiency is therefore a pre-condition for this pattern to manifest.

The accumulation of Dampness in the Liver and Gall-Bladder channel obstructs the smooth flow of Qi and causes stagnation of Liver-Qi resulting in distension and pain of the hypochondrium and chest. Dampness can obstruct the flow of bile which accumulates and overflows under the skin causing jaundice.

The stagnation of Liver-Qi deriving from the accumulation of Damp, causes Liver-Qi to invade the Stomach and gives rise to nausea, vomiting, loss of appetite and abdominal distension.

Damp-Heat causes low-grade continuous fever. This is easily distinguished from the Yin-deficiency fever (which is also low-grade) because the fever from Damp-Heat is continuous, whereas that from Yin deficiency only arises in the afternoon and evening. Bitter taste is caused by Liver Heat.

Dampness has a tendency to infuse downwards and if it flows down and settles in the Lower Burner it will cause vaginal discharge and itching or pain-swelling and redness of the scrotum in men.

The stickiness or greasiness of the tongue coating is highly indicative of the presence of Dampness.

Aetiology

Firstly, since Spleen deficiency leading to the formation of Dampness is the pre-condition for this pattern, any of the causes which lead to Spleen deficiency can be present. These are the excessive consumption of greasy foods or an irregular diet and life-style (see pattern of Spleen-Qi deficiency, p. 242).

Long-term stagnation of Liver-Qi can lead to Liver Heat which combines with the Dampness. Any of the causes of Liver-Qi stagnation (excessive anger, etc.), therefore, can lead to this pattern.

Finally, Damp-Heat can also be caused by external, climatic Damp-Heat. This is very common in tropical countries, but is not altogether unknown to happen in temperate or cold countries, especially in summertime.

Treatment

Principle of treatment: resolve Dampness, disperse the Liver and Gall-Bladder, clear Heat.

Points: Qimen LIV-14, Riyue GB-24, Yanglingquan GB-34, Ganshu BL-18, Danshu BL-19, Zhiyang Du-9, Zhongwan Ren-12, Yinlingquan SP-9, Sanyinjiao SP-6, Taibai SP-3, Quchi L.I.-11, Xingjian LIV-2.

Method: reducing method on all points except Ren-12 which should be tonified.

Explanation

LIV-14 regulates Liver-Qi in the hypochondrium and epigastrium.

GB-24 regulates Liver-Qi, soothes the Gall-Bladder and resolves Dampness.

GB-34, BL-18 and BL-19 move stagnant Liver-Qi and resolve Dampness.

Du-9 resolves Dampness from the Gall-Bladder channel.

Ren-12 tonifies the Spleen to resolve Dampness.

SP-9, SP-6 and SP-3 resolve Dampness. In particular, SP-9 and SP-6 resolve Dampness from the Lower Burner.

L.I.-11 resolves Dampness and clears Heat.

LIV-2 clears Liver-Heat.

STAGNATION OF COLD IN THE LIVER CHANNEL

Clinical manifestations

Fullness and distension of the hypogastrium (just over the bladder) with pain which refers to the scrotum and testis. Straining of the testis or contraction of the scrotum. In women there can be shrinking of the vagina. The pain is alleviated by warmth.

Tongue: Pale, wet, white coating.

Pulse: Wiry-Deep-Slow.

Key symptoms: hypogastric pain referring to scrotum, Wiry-Deep-Slow Pulse.

Pathology

This is caused by invasion of the Liver channel by cold. The Liver channel flows around the external genitalia, hence the pain and contraction of the scrotum (Cold contracts).

The Pulse is Deep reflecting the presence of interior Cold, Wiry reflecting affection of the Liver and Slow reflecting the presence of Cold.

Aetiology

This is due to invasion of exterior Cold.

Treatment

Principle of treatment: sedate the Liver, disperse the Cold.

Points: Zhongji Ren-3, Ligou LIV-5, Dadun LIV-1.

Method: reducing method, moxa is applicable.

Explanation

Ren-3 with moxa disperses Cold from the Lower Burner.

LIV-5, Connecting point of the Connecting channel which flows around the genitals, can disperse Cold from the Liver-channel.

LIV-1 clears Liver channel and removes obstruction of Cold from the Lower Burner.

DEFICIENCY OF LIVER-BLOOD

Clinical manifestations

Dizziness, numbness of limbs, insomnia, blurred vision, "floaters" in eyes, scanty menstruation or amenorrhoea, dull-pale complexion, pale lips, muscular weakness, muscle spasms, cramps, withered and brittle nails, dry hair and skin.

Tongue: Pale body especially on the sides which, in extreme cases, can assume an orange colour, and Dry.

Pulse: Choppy or Fine.

Key symptoms: blurred vision, scanty periods, dull-pale complexion, Pale tongue.

Pathology

The Liver stores Blood and any deficiency of Blood often manifests in the Liver sphere. As the Liver opens into the eyes, when Liver-Blood is deficient the eyes will lack nourishment and moisture so that they cannot see clearly.

The Liver controls the sinews and when Liver-Blood is deficient these will lack nourishment and moistening and the person will experience muscular weakness or cramps.

Dizziness, pale lips, dull-pale complexion are all signs of general Blood deficiency. As the Liver manifests in the nails, when Liver-Blood is deficient they will lose nourishment and become withered and brittle.

Liver-Blood is closely related to the Directing and Penetrating Vessels which are dependent on the Liver for their Blood supply. Thus, when Liver-Blood is deficient, the Directing and Penetrating Vessels will also lack Blood, resulting in scanty periods or no periods at all.

The tongue is of course Pale and in severe cases it becomes slightly orange on the sides.

Aetiology

A diet poor in nourishment or lacking in protein can weaken the Spleen which, in turn, cannot make enough Blood. When not enough Blood is produced by the Spleen, not enough Blood is stored by the Liver.

A serious haemorrhage (such as during childbirth) can also lead to deficiency of Liver-Blood.

The Kidneys play a role in the formation of Blood and a deficiency of Kidney-Qi or Kidney-Essence can lead to deficiency of Blood. Therefore, any of the causes of Kidney deficiency, can also lead to deficiency of Liver-Blood.

Treatment

Principle of treatment: tonify the Liver, nourish Blood

Points: Ganshu BL-18, Pishu BL-20, Shenshu BL-23, Geshu BL-17, Ququan LIV-8, Sanyinjiao SP-6, Zusanli ST-36, Guanyuan Ren-4.

Method: reinforcing, moxa can be used.

Explanation

BL-18 tonifies Liver-Blood.

BL-20 tonifies the Spleen to produce Blood.

BL-23 tonifies the Kidneys to produce Blood.

BL-17 with direct moxa, tonifies Blood.

LIV-8 tonifies Liver-Blood.

ST-36 and SP-6 tonify the Post-Heaven Qi to produce Blood.

Ren-4 tonifies Blood (with direct moxa).

Case history

A woman of 38 suffered from poor memory, tiredness, a tingling sensation in the limbs, dry hair and constipation with slightly dry stools. Her pulse was Choppy and her tongue was Pale, Thin and slightly dry.

All these symptoms and signs are due to deficiency of Liver-Blood.

LIVER-YANG RISING

Clinical manifestations

Headache which may be on the temples, eyes or lateral side of the head, dizziness, tinnitus, deafness, dry mouth and throat, insomnia, irritability, feeling worked-up, shouting in anger.

Tongue: Red, especially on the sides.

Pulse: Wiry.

Key symptoms: headache, irritability, Wiry Pulse.

Pathology

This is a mixed Deficiency/Excess pattern as it derives from deficiency of Liver-Yin and/or Kidney-Yin causing the rising of Liver-Yang. In 5-Element terms, Water is deficient and fails to nourish and "submerge" Wood, which becomes too dry and causes the rising upwards of Liver-Yang.

This pattern is therefore characterized by an imbalance between Liver-Yin (which is deficient) and Liver-Yang (which is in excess). The manifestations described above are only those of the rising of Liver-Yang. In practice, they would normally appear together with some symptoms and signs of Liver and/or Kidney Yin deficiency. The symptoms of Liver-Yin deficiency (not usually described as a pattern in itself) are basically the same as Liver-Blood deficiency, with the only addition of dry eyes. In addition to the signs of Liver-Yin (and Liver-Blood) deficiency, there may also be signs of Kidney-Yin deficiency.

Usually Liver-Yang rising is a result of Kidney/Liver Yin deficiency, but in practice, it can also arise from Kidney-Yang deficiency. This is because Kidney-Yin and Kidney-Yang have the same root, and a deficiency of one always implies a deficiency of the other (albeit to a lesser degree). Therefore, when Kidney-Yang is deficient, Kidney-Yin will also be deficient to a certain extent and may give rise to symptoms of rising of Liver-Yang.

The main difference between the pattern of Liver-Yang rising and that of Liver-Fire blazing is that in Liver-Fire blazing there is "solid" Fire drying up the Body Fluids and causing symptoms and signs of dryness such as constipation, scanty-dark urine, red eyes and face and bitter taste which are absent in Liver-Yang rising. Liver-Fire blazing is a purely Excess pattern, while Liver-Yang rising is a combined De-

Table 16 Comparison and differentiation of Liver-Yang rising and Liver-Fire blazing

	Liver-Yang Rising	Liver-Fire Blazing
Common symptoms	Irritability, propensity to anger, tinnitus, deafness,headache, dizziness, insomnia, Red tongue body with redder sides, Wiry pulse	
Differentiating symptoms		Red face and eyes, thirst, bitter taste, constipation, dark urine, Rapid pulse

ficiency/Excess pattern characterized by an imbalance between Yin and Yang, without "solid" Fire.

Most of the manifestations are due to the rising of Liver-Yang to the head: tinnitus, deafness (both of sudden onset), propensity to outbursts of anger and headache. The headache is one of the most common and distinctive signs of rising of Liver-Yang. Typically, it would be on either temple, but it can also be on the lateral side of the head (Gall-Bladder channel) or in or just above the eye. It is usually unilateral. With regard to headaches, Chinese Medicine holds that an Excess condition more often manifests on the right side, whereas a Deficient condition more often manifests on the left side. In case of Liver-Yang rising, therefore, it would manifest more often on the right side, but this is by no means an absolute rule.

The tongue and pulse reflect the rising of Liver-Yang. However, it should be emphasized that, in practice, they can often be very different. This happens when the pulse and tongue reflect the underlying Deficient condition of Liver-Blood or Liver-Yin deficiency rather than the rising of Liver-Yang itself. In these cases, the tongue is often Pale (rather than Red) and the pulse is often Choppy and Fine (rather than Wiry), if there is Liver-Blood deficiency. In case of Liver and Kidney Yin deficiency, the tongue would be Red and Peeled, and the pulse would be Floating-Empty.

Aetiology

The most common cause of rising of Liver-Yang is from emotional problems, in particular anger, frustration and resentment over a long period of time.

Treatment

Principle of treatment: subdue Liver-Yang, tonify Yin.

Points: Taichong LIV-3, Waiguan T.B.-5, Sanyinjiao SP-6, Taixi KI-3, Ququan LIV-8, Xiaxi G.B.-43, Yangfu G.B.-38, Zanzhu BL-2, Taiyang extra point, Fengchi GB-20, Tianchong G.B.-9, Shuaigu G.B.-8, Xuanli G.B.-6.

Method: reducing method on points to subdue Liver-Yang and tonifying method on points to tonify Yin.

Explanation

LIV-3 subdues Liver-Yang. This is the main distal point to use.

T.B.-5 subdues Liver-Yang and is particularly indicated for headaches along the Gall-Bladder channel.

SP-6 and KI-3 tonify Kidney-Yin.

LIV-8 tonifies Liver-Yin.

G.B.-43 subdues Liver-Yang. Being near the toe, it can be used to treat the opposite end of the channel, i.e. headaches on the Gall-Bladder channel.

G.B.-38 subdues Liver-Yang and Liver-Fire and is often used for chronic and stubborn migraine headaches.

BL-2 subdues Liver-Yang and is used as a local point for headaches around the eye.

Taiyang subdues Liver-Yang and is used as a local point for headaches on the temple.

G.B.-20 subdues Liver-Yang and is used as a local or adjacent point for headaches on the occiput and around the eyes.

G.B.-9, G.B.-8 and G.B.-6 subdue Liver-Yang and are important local points for headaches on the lateral side of the head.

Case history

A woman of 35 had suffered from headaches since the age of 14. The headaches occurred on the right temple and in the eye socket, were of a throbbing character and were accompanied by nausea and blurred vision. Her periods were rather scanty and she felt often tired. She also had dry hair, poor memory and insomnia. Her pulse was Choppy but slightly Wiry on the left, and her tongue was Pale, but with red spots on the sides.

This case illustrates well the rising of Liver-Yang caused by deficiency of Liver-Blood. Her symptoms of Liver-Yang rising are headache, nausea, a Wiry pulse on the left and red spots on the sides of the tongue. Her symptoms of Liver-Blood deficiency are scanty periods, dry hair, poor memory, insomnia, a Choppy pulse and a Pale tongue. The poor memory and insomnia also show that the deficiency of Blood has affected the Heart.

LIVER COMBINED PATTERNS

The combined patterns of the Liver are:

- Liver and Kidney Yin Deficiency
- Liver invading the Spleen
- Liver invading the Stomach
- Liver-Fire insulting the Lungs.

The pattern "Liver and Kidney Yin Deficiency" will be discussed under the Kidney patterns.

LIVER INVADING THE SPLEEN

Clinical manifestations

Irritability, abdominal distension and pain, alternation of constipation and diarrhoea, stools sometimes dry and bitty and sometimes loose, flatulence, tiredness.

Tongue: Red on the sides or Pale.

Pulse: Weak on the right and Wiry on the left.

Key symptoms: alternation of constipation and diarrhoea, abdominal distension and pain.

Pathology

The Liver is responsible for the smooth flow of Qi throughout the body. When Liver-Qi stagnates in the abdomen, it often disturbs the Spleen function of transformation and transportation: in Chinese Medicine terms, it is said that the "Liver invades the Spleen", or that "Liver and Spleen are not harmonized". In 5-Element terms, it corresponds to Wood overacting on Earth. In 8-Principle terms, it is a pattern of mixed Deficiency and Excess: Excess of the Liver (stagnation of Liver-Qi) and Deficiency of Spleen-Qi.

When the stagnation of Liver-Qi predominates there is constipation with dry, difficult and bitty stools. When the deficiency of the Spleen predominates, there are loose stools. The distension and pain of the abdomen are caused by the stagnation of Liver-Qi in the abdomen. Distension is the most characteristic symptom of stagnation of Qi. There may be some pain too (typically "distending pain"), but not severe.

This pattern can present itself with two different situations characterized by a different emphasis. In one situation the Liver is primarily in Excess and stagnant and it actively "invades" the Spleen interfering with its transformation and transportation function. This pattern is therefore primarily an Excess pattern: there is constipation more frequently than diarrhoea and the abdominal distension and pain are quite marked.

In another situation the Spleen is primarily deficient and "allows" itself to be invaded by the Liver. This pattern is primarily a Deficiency pattern: there are loose stools more often than constipation and the abdominal pain is only slight.

This explains why the tongue could either be Red on the sides or Pale. In the first case, when the Liver actively invades the Spleen, it would be Red on the sides. In the latter case, when the Spleen is weak and allows itself to be invaded by the Liver, the tongue would be Pale.

Aetiology

This pattern is usually caused by emotional problems which affect the Liver, such as anger, frustration and resentment. These emotions, over a long period of time, cause Liver-Qi to stagnate and this interferes with the Spleen functions.

However, the emotional factors are usually combined with other factors that cause Spleen deficiency, such as irregular diet and overwork.

Treatment

Principle of treatment: harmonize the Liver and tonify the Spleen.

Points: Qimen LIV-14, Zhangmen LIV-13, Yanglingquan G.B.-34, Taichong LIV-3, Qihai Ren-6, Zhongwan Ren-12, Zusanli ST-36, Sanyinjiao SP-6.

Method: reducing for points to harmonize the Liver (LIV-14, LIV-13, G.B.-34, LIV-3), reinforcing for points to tonify the Spleen.

Explanation

LIV-14 harmonizes the Liver and promotes the smooth flow of Liver-Qi.

LIV-13 harmonizes Liver and Spleen.

G.B.-34 promotes the smooth flow of Liver-Qi and calms abdominal pain in combination with Qihai Ren-6.

LIV-3 promotes the smooth flow of Liver-Qi and calms abdominal pain.

Ren-6 stops abdominal pain and moves Qi in the abdomen (in combination with Yanglingquan G.B.-34).

Ren-12 and ST-36 tonify the Spleen.

SP-6 tonifies the Spleen, regulates the Liver, harmonizes Liver and Spleen and stops abdominal pain.

LIVER INVADING THE STOMACH

Clinical manifestations

Irritability, distension and pain in epigastrium and hypochondrium, fullness in epigastrium, sour regurgitation, belching, nausea, vomiting.

Tongue: Red on the sides or Pale.

Pulse: Weak on the right and Wiry on the left.

Pathology

This pattern is characterized by stagnation of Liver-Qi invading the Stomach and interfering with the descending of Stomach-Qi: this results in the ascending of Stomach-Qi, hence the belching, nausea and vomiting.

The stagnation of Liver-Qi in the Middle Burner also interferes with the Stomach rotting and ripening of food resulting in fullness in the epigastrium and sour regurgitation.

The stagnation of Liver-Qi causes distension, pain and irritability. The same things that were said about Liver invading the Spleen apply to this pattern with regard to the two possible situations. For this reason, the tongue could be Red on the sides if it is Liver-Qi that primarily invades the Stomach, or Pale if the Stomach is primarily weak and allows itself to be invaded by the Liver.

Aetiology

This is also caused by emotional problems, as for the previous pattern, combined with irregular diet and overwork.

Treatment

Principle of treatment: harmonize the Liver and tonify the Stomach.

Points: Qimen LIV-14, Zhangmen LIV-13, Yanglingquan G.B.-34, Shangwan Ren-13, Xiawan Ren-10, Zusanli ST-36, Weishu BL-21.

Method: reducing for points to harmonize the Liver (LIV-14, LIV-13, G.B.-34) and reinforcing for points to tonify the Stomach.

Explanation

LIV-14 and LIV-13 harmonize the Liver in the Middle Burner. In particular, LIV-14 harmonizes Liver and Stomach.

G.B.-34 harmonizes the Liver, stimulates the smooth flow of Liver-Qi particularly in the hypochondrium.

Ren-13 subdues rebellious ascending Stomach-Qi.

Ren-10 stimulates the descending of Stomach-Qi.

ST-36 tonifies the Stomach.

BL-21 tonifies the Stomach and is particularly important in chronic cases.

LIVER-FIRE INSULTING THE LUNGS

Clinical manifestations

Breathlessness, asthma, fullness and stuffiness of the chest and hypochondrium, cough, yellow or blood-tinged sputum, headache, dizziness, red face, thirst, bitter taste, scanty-dark urine, constipation.

Tongue: Red, redder on the sides, swollen in the front part, yellow coating.

Pulse: Wiry and Slippery.

Key symptoms: breathlessness, asthma, fullness of hypochondrium, headache, Wiry pulse.

Pathology

The Liver controls the smooth flow of Qi: this has an influence on the descending of Lung-Qi. If Liver-Qi stagnates over a long period of time, it turns into Liver-Fire. Fire tends to rise and therefore Liver-Qi rebels upwards towards the chest. Here it prevents Lung-Qi from descending resulting in breathlessness and asthma.

The stagnation of Liver-Qi causes hypochondriac and a feeling of distension of the chest.

The rising of Liver-Fire causes headache, dizziness, red face, thirst and bitter taste. Fire in the body causes scanty-dark urine, constipation and blood-tinged sputum.

From the 5-Element point of view, this pattern is described as Wood insulting Metal.

The deep-red colour of the sides of the tongue reflects the presence of Liver-Fire. The swelling in the front part reflects the stagnation of Qi and Fire in the chest area.

Aetiology

This pattern is caused by anger which causes the formation of Liver-Fire, usually after a prolonged time of Liver-Qi stagnation.

It is also compounded by the excessive consumption of hot and greasy foods which tend to create Heat.

Treatment

Principle of treatment: clear Liver-Fire, harmonize the Liver, stimulate the descending of Lung-Qi.

Points: Xingjian LIV-2, Qimen LIV-14, Shanzhong Ren-17, Tiantu Ren-22, Neiguan P-6, Lieque LU-7, Quchi L.I.-11.

Method: reducing.

Explanation

LIV-2 clears Liver-Fire.

LIV-14 harmonizes Liver-Qi in the chest.

Ren-17 and Ren-22 stimulate the descending of Lung-Qi.

P-6 harmonizes Liver-Qi in the chest (by virtue of the relation between Liver and Pericardium within the Terminal Yin) and stimulates the descending of Lung-Qi.

LU-7 stimulates the descending of Lung-Qi.

L.I.-11 clears Heat.

Lung Patterns 23

肺脏病証

The main Lung function is that of governing Qi and deficiency of Qi is the most important Deficiency pattern of the Lungs.

The Lungs also have a dispersing and descending function and they are the most "exterior" organ controlling the skin and Defensive Qi. This means that the Lungs are the first organ to be affected by exterior pathogenic factors such as Wind-Cold and Wind-Heat.

All the Deficiency patterns of the Lung revolve around Deficiency of Qi and most of the Excess patterns revolve around invasion of the Lungs by exterior pathogenic factors.

GENERAL AETIOLOGY

EXTERIOR PATHOGENIC FACTORS

The Lungs control the skin, they are the most "exterior" of the organs and influence Defensive Qi: for all these reasons, the Lungs are the organ which is most easily and directly affected by exterior pathogenic factors, particularly Wind, Heat, Fire, Cold, Dampness and Dryness. The Lungs are sometimes called the "delicate" organ because of their susceptibility to invasion by exterior pathogenic factors.

Exterior pathogenic factors engage in a fight with Defensive Qi and impair the Lung dispersing and descending functions. All the symptoms and signs arising from these Excess patterns are a reflection of the impairment of the Lung dispersing and descending functions (headache, aches of the body, aversion to cold, sneezing, stuffed nose, etc.).

Wind usually combines with other pathogenic factors notably Cold and Heat to form Wind-Cold and Wind-Heat: these are the two most common exterior pathogenic factors to attack the Lungs. When the Lungs are attacked by these exterior pathogenic factors, it is the Lung Exterior portion (or Lung-Defensive Qi portion) which is invaded, not the Lung organ itself. The pattern is therefore an exterior one, even though there may be such symptoms as cough.

The Lungs are also easily injured by Dryness as it is an organ that needs a certain amount of moisture to function properly (one can think of the moistening fluid in the pleural cavity). Excessively dry weather can therefore cause the Lungs to become dry resulting in such symptoms as a dry cough, a dry throat, dry skin.

Dampness does not usually attack the Lungs directly, except when combined with Wind, in which case it will impair not only the Lung dispersing and descending function giving rise to the usual exterior symptoms mentioned above, but also its function of regulating the Water passages, giving rise to facial oedema.

DIET

Diet has an important influence on the Lung function. The excessive consumption of cold and raw foods can generate internal Dampness which affects the Spleen and is often "stored" in the Lungs. It is said in Chinese Medicine that "the Spleen creates Phlegm and the Lungs store it". In this case there would be profuse sputum in the Lungs. For this reason, an excessive consumption of cold and raw foods is contraindicated in cases of asthma due to retention of Damp-Phlegm in the Lungs.

Apart from cold and raw foods, an excessive consumption of milk, cheese and butter (but particularly milk) have the same effect on the Lungs, giving rise to Phlegm.

EMOTIONS

The emotions pertaining to the Lungs are sadness and worry. Prolonged sadness disperses Qi and prolonged worry knots Qi. Both these emotions have an effect on the Lungs if they persist over a long period of time. In particular, sadness causes deficiency of Lung-Qi and worry causes stagnation of Qi in the chest which affects the Lungs. Prolonged sadness is often reflected on the pulse which becomes weak on both left and right Front position (Lungs and Heart).

LIFE-STYLE

Sitting for long periods of time bent over a desk to read or write can weaken Lung-Qi (because the chest is impeded and proper breathing impaired).

The patterns discussed are:

- Deficiency patterns
  - Lung-Qi Deficiency
  - Lung-Yin Deficiency
  - Lung Dryness
- Excess patterns
  - Invasion of Lungs by Wind-Cold
  - Invasion of Lungs by Wind-Heat
  - Invasion of Lungs by Wind-Water
  - Damp-Phlegm obstructing the Lungs
  - Phlegm-Heat obstructing the Lungs
  - Phlegm-Fluids obstructing the Lungs.

LUNG-QI DEFICIENCY

Clinical Manifestations

Shortness of breath, cough, watery sputum, weak voice, daytime sweating, dislike to speak, dislike of cold, bright-white complexion, propensity to catching colds, tiredness.

Tongue: Pale or normal-coloured.

Pulse: Empty, particularly in the right Front position.

Key symptoms: shortness of breath, weak voice, bright-white complexion, Empty Pulse.

Pathology

The Lungs govern Qi and respiration, and when Qi is deficient, breathing is short especially on exertion. The shortness of breath in this case is only slight (not like the one seen in bronchitis or asthma) and mostly on exertion.

The Lungs send Qi downwards and if Lung-Qi is deficient, Qi cannot descend and will cause cough.

The watery sputum is caused by impairment of the Lung function of regulating the Water passages, so that fluids cannot be transformed in the Upper Burner and turn into sputum.

The tone and strength of voice is an expression of the strength of the Gathering Qi which, in turn, depends on Lung-Qi, hence the weak voice and dislike to speak in this pattern.

Lung-Qi influences the skin and controls Defensive Qi which regulates the opening and closing of the pores. When Lung-Qi is weak, the Defensive Qi is weak on the skin layers and the pores become flaccid and let sweat out.

Defensive Qi also has the function of warming the skin and muscles, hence the dislike of cold in the Lung-Qi deficiency pattern.

The bright-white complexion reflects deficiency of Yang (which in the case of the Lungs is synonymous with deficiency of Qi).

Finally, Defensive Qi protects the body from exterior pathogenic factors and when Lung-Qi is deficient, Defensive Qi is not strong enough to perform its protective function and the body is easily prone to invasion of exterior Cold.

The Empty Pulse reflects the deficiency of Qi.

Aetiology

First of all, this pattern could be due to hereditary weakness, particularly if one of the parents suffered from tuberculosis of the Lungs. In these cases the tongue often has one or two small transversal cracks in the Lung area (just behind the tip), and the Pulse can be felt further up the wrist in a position medial to the normal Front position. When the pulse can be felt in this position, it often has a Slippery and slightly Wiry quality (see Fig. 48, p. 135).

Lung-Qi deficiency can also be induced by prolonged stooping over a desk for long hours. This constricts breathing and, in the long run, will cause Lung-Qi deficiency.

This pattern can also be the result of an exterior attack of Wind-Cold or Wind-Heat which is not treated properly, so that some pathogenic factor remains in the body and, in the long run, causes Lung-Qi deficiency. In this case the tongue often has a very thin yellow coating in the Lung area. This is often seen when a person develops a chronic cough after an exterior attack of Wind-Cold or Wind-Heat.

This situation is particularly aggravated when antibiotics are taken for a cold or a flu with the result of "locking" the Cold in the chest and interfering with the Lung dispersing and descending functions.

Treatment

Principle of treatment: tonify Lung Qi, warm Yang.

Points: Taiyuan LU-9, Lieque LU-7, Qihai Ren-6, Feishu BL-13, Shenzhu Du-12, Zusanli ST-36.

Method: reinforcing method, moxa is applicable.

Explanation

LU-9 is the Source point of the Lung and it tonifies Lung-Qi.

LU-7 tonifies Lung-Qi and stimulates the Lung descending function. For this reason, it is particularly useful if there is a cough or a residual pathogenic factor from a previous attack of Wind-Cold or Wind-Heat.

Ren-6 tonifies Qi.

BL-13 tonifies Lung-Qi.

Du-12 tonifies Lung-Qi and is particularly important to use in chronic cases.

ST-36 tonifies Stomach and Spleen Qi. It is often necessary to tonify the Stomach and Spleen in order to nourish the Lungs. In 5-Element terms this corresponds to "Tonifying Earth to nourish Metal".

LUNG-YIN DEFICIENCY

Clinical Manifestations

Cough which is dry or with a little sticky sputum, blood-tinged sputum, low-grade fever in the afternoon, feeling of heat in the afternoon or evening, malar flush, night sweating, 5-palm heat, insomnia, dry mouth and throat, hoarse voice, tickly throat.

Tongue: Red, Peeled, cracks in the Lung area, dry.

Pulse: Floating-Empty and Rapid.

Key symptoms: dry cough, feeling of heat in the afternoon, Red-Peeled tongue.

Pathology

This is characterized by deficiency of Body Fluids and ensuing dryness. Hence the dry cough, dry throat and mouth, tickly throat and hoarse voice.

When Yin deficiency is pronounced, Empty-Heat is produced causing a low-grade fever, a feeling of heat, malar flush, 5-palm heat (a feeling of heat of the chest, palms of hands and soles of feet), night sweating and a Rapid pulse.

The Red and Peeled tongue is indicative of Yin deficiency with Empty-Heat. It must be emphasized that a Red and completely Peeled tongue only appears in the late stages of Yin deficiency, whereas in the beginning stages and in a young person, the tongue may not be completely Peeled. The transversal cracks in the Lung area are even more likely to appear in Lung-Yin deficiency than in Lung-Qi deficiency.

Aetiology

This pattern can develop from Lung-Qi deficiency after a long period of time. Any of the causes of Lung-Qi deficiency, therefore, can lead to Lung-Yin deficiency.

Lung-Yin deficiency is often associated with Stomach and/or Kidney-Yin deficiency. An irregular diet such as eating late at night or eating in a hurry, can cause Stomach-Yin deficiency , while overwork over a long period of time can cause Kidney-Yin deficiency.

Lung-Yin deficiency can also develop from a condition of dryness of the Lungs which, in turn, may originate internally or externally.

Treatment

Principle of treatment: tonify Lung-Yin, nourish Body Fluids, clear Empty-Heat.

Points: Taiyuan LU-9, Shanzhong Ren-17, Gaohuangshu BL-43, Feishu BL-13, Shenzhu Du-12, Guanyuan Ren-4, Zhaohai KI-6, Zhongwan Ren-12, Yuji LU-10.

Method: reinforcing on all points except LU-10 which should be reduced, no moxa.

Explanation

LU-9 is the Source point and it can tonify Lung-Yin.

Ren-17 tonifies Qi and Lung-Yin.

BL-43 tonifies Lung-Yin and is particularly important in chronic cases.

BL-13 and Du-12 tonify Lung Qi and Yin.

Ren-4 tonifies Kidney-Yin and is particularly necessary when the Lung-Yin deficiency is associated with Kidney-Yin deficiency. Ren-4 also conducts Empty-Heat downwards.

KI-6 tonifies Kidney-Yin and benefits the throat. It is particularly useful if there is a dry throat and cough. It can be combined with Lieque LU-7 to open the Directing Vessel. The combination of these two points tonifies Lung-Qi and Lung-Yin, stimulates the descending function of the Lungs, tonifies Kidney-Yin, benefits the throat and reestablishes the communication between Lungs and Kidneys.

Ren-12 tonifies the Stomach and nourishes fluids (as the Stomach is the origin of fluids).

LU-10 is used with reducing method to clear Empty-Heat from the Lungs.

LUNG DRYNESS

Clinical Manifestations

Dry cough, dry skin, dry throat, dry mouth, thirst, hoarse voice.

Tongue: dry.

Pulse: Empty, especially on right Front position.

Key symptoms: dry cough, dry throat, hoarse voice, dry tongue which is not Red.

Pathology

This is a state of dryness of the Lungs, with deficiency of Body Fluids. It is a stage preceding Yin deficiency. It is characterized by dryness but not yet Yin deficiency.

Aetiology

This can be either exterior or interior. It can be caused by exterior dryness, during long spells of dry and hot weather.

It can also be internally produced, usually from Stomach-Yin deficiency in persons who have an irregular diet with irregular meal times, eating late at night, worrying about work while eating, etc.

Treatment

Principle of treatment: moisten the Lungs, nourish fluids.

Points: Taiyuan LU-9, Guanyuan Ren-4, Zhaohai KI-6, Sanyinjiao SP-6, Zhongwan Ren-12.

Method: reinforcing method.

Explanation

LU-9 moistens the Lungs.

Ren-4 tonifies Kidney-Yin and nourishes fluids.

KI-6 nourishes fluids and benefits the throat.

SP-6 nourishes fluids.

Ren-12 tonifies the Stomach and nourishes fluids.

INVASION OF LUNGS BY WIND-COLD

Clinical Manifestations

Cough, fever, itchy throat, stuffed nose or runny nose with clear-watery mucus, sneezing, aversion to cold, occipital headache, body aches.

Tongue: thin-white coating.

Pulse: Floating especially in the Front position.

Key symptoms: aversion to cold, sneezing, Floating pulse.

Pathology

This corresponds to the Greater Yang stage of the 6 Stage Pattern Identification, from the "Discussion on Cold-induced Diseases" by Zhang Zhong Jing (See App. 1).[1]

At this stage the exterior Wind-Cold attacks the Defensive-Qi layer of the Lung system and the exterior Cold engages in a fight with the Defensive Qi. Fever results from this fight. However, if the pathogenic factor is not too strong, or if the Defensive Qi does not react to it, there may not be a fever.

The exterior Cold obstructs the Lung system and impairs the Lung descending function causing a cough and a stuffed or runny nose, and the Lung dispersing function causing sneezing.

The exterior Cold also obstructs the circulation of Defensive Qi resulting in occipital headache, body aches and aversion to cold, as it prevents Defensive Qi from warming the muscles.

The headache is typically on the occiput along the Greater Yang channels (Small Intestine and Bladder), or it could be in the whole head.

The tongue may not show much at all in the beginning stages. The body colour will be unchanged and there might only be a thin-white coating, white indicating Cold, and thin indicating that the pathogenic factor is at the beginning stage.

The Pulse will be Floating reflecting the rush of the body's Qi to the exterior layers to fight the pathogenic factor. It might be Floating in all positions, or only in the Front ones, or even only in the right Front position (Lungs).

Aetiology

This is due to exposure to Wind and Cold. As was discussed in chapter 15 "The Causes of Disease", diagnosis of this pattern is not done according to aetiology but to pathology. In other words, if a patient displays all or some of the above symptoms and signs, we can diagnose an invasion of Lung by Wind-Cold and we do not need to enquire about the person's probable exposure to wind and cold.

Furthermore, invasion of the Lungs by Wind-Cold is due to the relative weakness of the body's Qi in relation to the pathogenic factor at that particular time. Thus the person need not have been exposed to extremes of wind and cold to develop the above symptoms and signs. This explains why we can catch a cold in any season, even during a hot summer, and not just in wintertime.

Finally, as previously discussed (see "The Causes of Disease" p. 127), there are artificial sources of Wind-Cold such as air conditioning, draughts or refrigerated store-rooms which can cause this pattern.

As the body's Qi is only relatively weak in comparison to the pathogenic factor, this pattern is of Excess nature which calls for a reducing treatment method. To think that we need to tonify the body's Qi because it has succumbed to the exterior pathogenic factor due to its weakness would be wrong and would make the patient worse.

Table 17 Comparison between invasion of Wind-Cold and invasion of Wind-Heat

Aetiology/ Pathology	Fever	Aversion to cold	Aches	Thirst	Urine	Tongue	Pulse	Treatment
WIND-COLD on Exterior obstructing Defensive Qi	Light	Heavy	Heavy	No	Clear	Body normal, coating thin-white	Floating Tight	Release Exterior, scatter Cold
WIND-HEAT on Exterior obstructing Defensive Qi and drying fluids	Heavy	Light	Light	Yes	Dark	Tip and sides Red, thin-white coating	Floating Rapid	Release Exterior clear Heat

Treatment

Principle of treatment: release the Exterior, scatter Cold, stimulate the Lung descending and dispersing function.

Points: Lieque LU-7, Fengmen BL-12, Fengfu Du-16.

Method: reducing method, moxa is applicable after needling.

Explanation

LU-7 disperses Wind-Cold, releases the Exterior and stimulates the Lung descending and dispersing functions.

BL-12 releases the Exterior and expels Wind. Moxa can be used on this point after needling. Cupping this point is extremely effective to expel Wind.

Du-16 expels Wind, and is particularly useful if there is headache.

INVASION OF LUNGS BY WIND-HEAT

Clinical Manifestations

Cough, fever, aversion to cold, sore throat, stuffed or runny nose with yellow mucus, headache, body aches, slight sweating, thirst, swollen tonsils.

Tongue: body Red on the sides or tip, the coating is thin and either white or yellow.

Pulse: Floating-Rapid.

Key symptoms: fever, aversion to cold, sore throat, Floating-Rapid pulse.

Pathology

This is the same as for Invasion of Wind-Cold, with the only difference that Wind in this case combines with Heat. In invasion of Wind-Heat there is more often a fever.

Contrary to what one would expect, in invasion of Wind-Heat the person also experiences an **aversion to cold, similarly to Invasion of Wind-Cold. This is due to the fact that the pathogenic** factor obstructs the circulation of the Defensive Qi which therefore cannot warm the muscles.

Exterior Heat dries up Body Fluids resulting in thirst and a sore throat.

The tongue coating can be white (even though white usually indicates Cold) because in the very beginning stage of invasion of Wind-Heat there is not enough time for the Heat to turn the coating yellow.

Aetiology

This is due to exposure to climatic wind and heat. Similarly as for Wind-Cold, there are many artificial factors which may cause invasion of Wind-Heat, such as central heating and certain other artificial sources of heat at the place of work (such as for cooks or steel-workers).

Treatment

Principle of treatment: release the Exterior, clear Heat, stimulate the Lung descending and dispersing functions.

Points: Hegu L.I.-4, Quchi L.I.-11, Shaoshang LU-11, Dazhui Du-14, Fengmen BL-12, Fengfu Du-16, Fengchi GB-20.

Method: reducing method, no moxa.

Explanation

L.I.-4 and L.I.-11 release the Exterior and clear Heat. LU-11 is especially indicated for a sore throat and swollen tonsils.

Du-14 clears Heat.

BL-12, Du-16 and GB-20 expel exterior Wind.

INVASION OF LUNGS BY WIND-WATER

Clinical Manifestations

Sudden swelling of eyes and face, gradually spreading to the whole body, bright-shiny complexion, scanty and pale urination, aversion to Wind, fever, cough, breathlessness.

Tongue: White-slippery coating.

Pulse: Floating-Slippery.

Key symptoms: sudden swelling of face, aversion to Wind, Floating-Slippery pulse.

Pathology

This is an exterior pattern due to attack of Wind-Cold and Dampness. It differs from a normal attack of Wind-Cold in that it impairs the Lung function of controlling Water passages resulting in facial oedema.

Since the Lung-Defensive Qi portion is obstructed by the exterior Wind-Cold-Damp, the Lungs cannot direct fluids downwards: this also causes facial oedema and scanty urination.

The bright-shiny complexion and pale urine reflect deficiency of Yang, as Defensive Qi is obstructed by the exterior Wind-Cold-Damp.

Aversion to Wind is due to failure of Defensive Qi to warm the muscles. "Aversion to wind" is basically the same as "aversion to cold" except for a difference of degree of intensity, aversion to cold being stronger. Some doctors say that aversion to cold is experienced even indoors, whereas aversion to Wind is only experienced outdoors.

The fever reflects the struggle between the Defensive Qi and the exterior Wind-Cold-Damp.

The cough and breathlessness are due to the impairment of the Lung descending function.

The slippery tongue coating and pulse reflect the presence of Dampness.

The Floating Pulse reflects the presence of a pathogenic factor on the Exterior.

Aetiology

This is due to exposure to exterior Wind-Cold and Dampness.

Treatment

Principle of treatment: release the Exterior, scatter Cold, resolve Dampness, restore the Lung descending function and open the Water passages.

Points: Lieque LU-7, Pianli L.I.-6, Wenli L.I.-7, Hegu L.I.-4, Fengmen BL-12, Shuifen Ren-9, Feishu BL-13.

Method: reducing method.

Explanation

LU-7 releases the Exterior, stimulates the Lung descending function and opens the Water passages.

L.I.-6 opens the Lung Water passages.

L.I.-7 is the Accumulation point of the Large Intestine channel and is used for acute conditions.

L.I.-4 releases the Exterior and opens the Water passages.

BL-12 and BL-13 release the Exterior and stimulate the descending of Lung-Qi.

Ren-9 opens the Water passages and resolves oedema.

DAMP-PHLEGM OBSTRUCTING THE LUNGS

Clinical Manifestations

Chronic cough coming in bouts, profuse white sputum which is easy to expectorate, white-pasty complexion, feeling of oppression of the chest, feeling "clogged-up", shortness of breath, dislike of lying down.

Tongue: thick-sticky white coating.

Pulse: Slippery or Weak-Floating and Fine.

Key symptoms: Chronic cough with profuse white sputum, thick-sticky white tongue coating.

Pathology

This is an Excess pattern of a chronic nature. From the 8-Principle point of view, it is an Excess-Interior-Cold pattern. It is characterized by the presence of Phlegm retained in the Lungs. However, this is seldom a purely Excess pattern because the Phlegm usually arises from a chronic dysfunction of the Spleen in transforming and transporting fluids, which accumulate to form Phlegm. As mentioned before, the Spleen produces Phlegm and the Lungs store it.

The presence of Phlegm is clearly indicated by the profuse sputum and the sticky tongue coating.

Phlegm obstructs the Lungs and impairs their descending function, hence the cough.

The white complexion reflects deficiency of Yang of the Spleen and Lung, whilst its pasty quality reflects the presence of Phlegm and Dampness.

The stuffiness of the chest is caused by the obstruction of Phlegm in the chest.

The patient dislikes to lie flat and prefers to sit up or lie propped up because the obstruction of Phlegm in the chest is made worse by the horizontal position. This is a typical sign of Excess pattern.

The Pulse would be Slippery in a purely Excess pattern when the person's Qi is not weakened. However, in chronic cases, when the person's Qi has been weakened, the Pulse would be Weak-Floating reflecting the presence of Dampness and weakness of Qi. The Weak-Floating Pulse is also described as Soft.

Aetiology

First of all, a deficiency of Spleen-Qi or Spleen-Yang is a pre-condition for the arousal of this pattern. Therefore, any of the causes of Spleen deficiency may also lead to this pattern.

Recurrent attacks of exterior pathogenic factors may weaken the Lungs and Spleen leading to the formation of Phlegm which settles in the Lungs. In children it is often a result of whooping cough.

Excessive consumption of greasy foods and/or cold and raw foods leads to the formation of Phlegm and can therefore contribute to the arousal of this pattern.

Treatment

Principle of treatment: resolve Phlegm, restore the Lung descending function.

Points: Chize LU-5, Lieque LU-7, Zhongfu LU-1, Shanzhong Ren-17, Fenglong ST-40, Neiguan P-6, Tiantu Ren-22, Zhongwan Ren-12, Shuifen Ren-9, Pishu BL-20, Feishu BL-13.

Method: reducing method on all points except BL-20 Pishu and Ren-12 Zhongwan which should be tonified.

Explanation

LU-5 expels Phlegm from the Lungs.

LU-1 stops cough and resolves Phlegm.

Ren-17 stimulates the Lung descending function.

LU-7 stimulates the Lung descending function and stops cough.

ST-40 resolves Phlegm.

P-6 opens the chest and expels Phlegm from the chest.

Ren-22 expels Phlegm from the throat and stimulates the Lung descending function.

Ren-12 tonifies the Spleen to resolve Phlegm.

Ren-9 stimulates the Spleen function of transformation and transportation and resolves Dampness.

BL-20 tonifies the Spleen to resolve Phlegm.

BL-13 stimulates the Lung descending function.

PHLEGM-HEAT OBSTRUCTING THE LUNGS

Clinical Manifestations

Barking cough, profuse yellow or green or dark, and foul smelling sputum, shortness of breath, asthma, feeling of oppression of the chest.

Tongue: Red body, thick-sticky yellow coating.

Pulse: Slippery-Rapid-Full.

Key symptoms: cough, yellow or green sputum, thick-sticky yellow coating, Rapid-Slippery pulse.

Pathology

This is a chronic condition, similar to the previous one of Damp-Phlegm, but accompanied by Heat. In chronic conditions, Phlegm can easily combine with Heat. The underlying condition is also in this case a deficiency of Spleen-Qi leading to the formation of Phlegm.

From the 8-Principle point of view, this is an Excess-Hot-Interior condition.

Aetiology

This can be due to excessive consumption of greasy and hot foods (such as fried meats, alcohol, greasy and pungent foods) leading to the formation of Phlegm and Heat.

Smoking can also be a factor leading to the pattern since tobacco has a hot energy from the point of view of Chinese Medicine.

This pattern can also be precipitated or aggravated by invasion of exterior Wind-Heat.

Treatment

Principle of treatment: resolve Phlegm, clear Heat, stimulate the Lung descending function.

Points: Chize LU-5, Lieque LU-7, Yuji LU-10, Quchi L.I.-11, Zhongfu LU-1, Feishu BL-13, Zhongwan Ren-12, Fenglong ST-40.

Method: reducing method, except for Ren-12.

Explanation

LU-5 clears Heat and Phlegm from the Lungs.

LU-7 restores the Lung descending function and stops cough.

LU-10 clears Heat from the Lung.

L.I.-11 clears Heat.

LU-1 restores the Lung descending function and clears Lung-Heat.

BL-13 can clear Lung-Heat.

Ren-12 resolves Phlegm (with even method).

ST-40 resolves Phlegm.

PHLEGM-FLUIDS OBSTRUCTING THE LUNGS

Clinical Manifestations

Cough, breathlessness, splashing sounds in the chest, vomiting of white-watery-frothy sputum, chilliness, cough which may be elicited by a scare.

Tongue: Pale body, thick-sticky white coating.

Pulse: Fine and Slippery or Weak-Floating.

Key symptoms: cough with white-watery-frothy sputum.

Pathology

This is a chronic condition of Phlegm in the Lungs. This pattern is characterized by a particular kind of Phlegm which is very watery, dilute and frothy. This is called "Phlegm-Fluid" and it always indicates that the condition is chronic and that the body is weak. It is also characterized by deficiency of Yang of the Spleen and Lung (hence the chilliness and Pale tongue body).

This pattern is only seen in old or middle-aged people.

Aetiology

The underlying condition for this pattern is a chronic deficiency of Spleen-Yang and this can be caused by over-exertion and poor diet over a long period of time.

The excessive consumption of greasy and cold-raw foods also leads to the formation of Phlegm.

Treatment

Principle of treatment: resolve Phlegm, tonify Spleen- and Lung-Qi.

Points: Chize LU-5, Taiyuan LU-9, Shanzhong Ren-17, Feishu BL-13, Fenglong ST-40, Gaohuangshu BL-43, Zhongwan Ren-12, Zusanli ST-36, Shuifen Ren-9.

Method: reducing on LU-5, ST-40 and Ren-9; tonifying on all the other points. Moxa is applicable.

Explanation

LU-5 clears Phlegm from the Lungs.

LU-9 tonifies Lung- Qi and resolves Phlegm. It is particularly indicated for chronic conditions.

Ren-17 tonifies Lung-Qi and stimulates the Lung descending function.

BL-13 tonifies Lung-Qi.

ST-40 resolves Phlegm.

BL-43 tonifies Lung-Qi and is indicated in chronic conditions.

Ren-12 resolves Phlegm.

ST-36 tonifies Spleen-Qi.

Ren-9 resolves Phlegm.

COMBINED PATTERNS

The combined patterns of the Lungs are:

Lung-Qi and Kidney-Yang Deficiency

Lung- and Kidney-Yin Deficiency

Liver-Fire invading the Lungs

Spleen- and Lung-Qi Deficiency

All these combined patterns have already been discussed under the relevant other organs, i.e. Kidneys, Liver, Spleen. In particular, the pattern of Lung-Qi and Kidney-Yang Deficiency can appear either as "Kidney Deficient, Water overflowing to Lungs" or "Kidneys failing to receive Qi", both of them discussed under the Kidney patterns.

NOTES

1 Nanjing College of Traditional Chinese Medicine, Shang Han Lun Research Group 1980 Discussion of Cold-induced Diseases (*Shang Han Lun* 伤寒论), Shanghai Scientific Publishing House.

Spleen Patterns 24

脾脏病証

The most important Spleen function is that of transporting and transforming food and fluids. Any Spleen disharmony will therefore always influence the digestive process, with such symptoms as abdominal distension, lack of appetite and loose stools.

The Spleen controls muscles and is responsible for transporting Food-Qi to the muscles throughout the body and in particular to the four limbs. A disharmony in this sphere often causes tiredness, which is an extremely common symptom of Spleen deficiency.

Finally, the Spleen controls Blood and a weakness of Spleen-Qi often causes bleeding.

GENERAL AETIOLOGY

EXTERIOR PATHOGENIC FACTORS

The Spleen is easily attacked by external Dampness. This can invade the body in different ways due to environmental circumstances or life habits, such as living in a damp area or a damp house, living in foggy mountain areas, wearing wet clothes after swimming or exercising, sitting on damp surfaces, wading in water. Women are particularly prone to exterior Dampness especially at certain times of their life, i.e. during each period and after childbirth.[1]

An invasion of the Spleen by exterior Dampness will give rise to abdominal distension, lack of appetite, nausea, feeling of heaviness, thick-white tongue coating and a Slippery pulse.

Exterior Dampness can be combined with Heat or Cold giving rise to symptoms of Damp-Heat or Damp-Cold.

MENTAL FACTORS

The excessive use of the mind in thinking, studying, concentrating and memorizing over a long period of time tends to weaken the Spleen. This also includes excessive pensiveness and constant "brooding".[2]

DIET

Since the Spleen is in charge of transforming and transporting food, diet plays an extremely important role in Spleen disharmonies. The Spleen is said to prefer warm and dry foods. By "warm" is meant warm in terms of both temperature and food energy. All foods can be classified as warm (or hot) or cool (or cold). Examples of warm foods are meat, ginger and pepper. Examples of cold foods are all raw foods (salads), fruit (with few exceptions), vegetables and icy-cold drinks.

An excessive consumption of cold foods will impair the Spleen transformation and transportation function causing digestive problems and interior Dampness.

The Spleen patterns discussed are:
- Deficiency patterns
  - Spleen-Qi deficiency
  - Spleen-Yang deficiency
  - Spleen not controlling Blood
  - Spleen-Qi sinking
- Excess patterns
  - Cold-Dampness invading the Spleen
  - Damp-Heat invading Spleen.

SPLEEN-QI DEFICIENCY

Clinical manifestations

No appetite, abdominal distension after eating, tiredness, lassitude, sallow complexion, weakness of the limbs, loose stools.

If Spleen-Qi deficiency gives rise to Dampness, there may also be nausea, a feeling of oppression of the chest and epigastrium and a feeling of heaviness.

Tongue: Pale or normal-coloured, in chronic cases the sides will be swollen sometimes with transversal cracks. Pulse: Empty.

Key symptoms: no appetite, tiredness, loose stools.

Pathology

This is by far the most common Spleen disharmony and probably the most common pattern in general, no doubt because of our irregular dietary habits and excessive use of the mind in studying, working, etc.

The pattern of Spleen-Qi deficiency is also central to all Spleen disharmonies as all its other Deficiency patterns are but a variation of it.

The impairment of the Spleen transformation and transportation function causes the various digestive symptoms, such as abdominal distension, loose stools and lack of appetite. As the Spleen is responsible for transporting Food-Qi to the four limbs, when Spleen-Qi is deficient, the limbs will be deprived of nourishment and feel weak. The Spleen also transports Food-Qi throughout the body, hence the tiredness and lassitude experienced when Spleen-Qi is deficient.

If Spleen-Qi is deficient over a long period of time, the inability of Spleen-Qi in transforming fluids can give rise to Dampness which obstructs the chest and epigastrium resulting in the typical sensation of "oppression".

Dampness is heavy and difficult to get rid of: it accumulates in the muscles causing a feeling of heaviness (which could be of the head or limbs). Nausea is caused by the obstruction of Dampness in the epigastrium preventing Stomach-Qi from descending.

On the tongue, a chronic deficiency of Spleen-Qi is often manifested with a swelling of the sides, but only in the middle section of the tongue (as opposed to the swelling from Liver-Yang or Liver-Fire which is all along the sides of the tongue). In even more severe cases, the sides will be swollen and have small transversal cracks.[3]

The Empty pulse reflects deficiency of Qi.

Aetiology

Diet

As mentioned before, excessive consumption of cold and raw foods can hinder the Spleen function of transformation and transportation and lead to Spleen-Qi deficiency. Eating at irregular times or excessive eating can also strain the Spleen capacity and lead to Spleen-Qi deficiency. Eating too little or eating a protein-deficient diet can also cause Spleen deficiency.

Mental strain

Excessive thinking or mental strain over a long period of time can cause Spleen-Qi deficiency. This is common in students or business people who spend long periods of time every day in mental work. This is particularly harmful if one goes back to work straight after a hurried lunch, or even worse, conducts business over lunch.

Climate

Prolonged exposure to dampness (either from weather or from the place of living) can weaken the Spleen and lead to Spleen-Qi deficiency.

Chronic disease

Any protracted disease will tend to weaken the Spleen and lead to Spleen-Qi deficiency. This is the reason why catarrh is such a frequent consequence of protracted diseases, as Spleen-Qi is weakened and this leads to the formation of Phlegm.

Treatment

Principle of treatment: tonify Spleen-Qi.

Points: Zhongwan Ren-12, Zusanli ST-36, Taibai SP-3, Sanyinjiao SP-6, Pishu BL-20, Weishu BL-21.

Method: reinforcing method.

Explanation

Ren-12 tonifies Spleen-Qi.

ST-36 tonifies Spleen-Qi. The Stomach and Spleen are very closely related and points on the Stomach channel are often used to tonify the Spleen.

SP-3 is the Source point of the Spleen and tonifies Spleen-Qi.

SP-6 tonifies Spleen-Qi.

BL-20 and BL-21 can tonify Spleen-Qi. The combination of these two points is particularly important to treat chronic conditions of both Spleen and Stomach deficiency.

SPLEEN-YANG DEFICIENCY

Clinical manifestations

Lack of appetite, abdominal distension after eating, tiredness, sallow or bright-white complexion, weakness of the four limbs, loose stools, oedema, chilliness, cold limbs.

Tongue: Pale, Swollen, wet.

Pulse: Weak, Slow, Deep.

Key symptoms: loose stools, chilliness, cold limbs and tiredness.

Pathology

This pattern is substantially the same as Spleen-Qi deficiency with the addition of Cold symptoms, such as chilliness and cold limbs. These are due to the failure of Spleen-Yang to warm the body.

The oedema is due to the impairment of the Spleen function in transforming and transporting fluids; when fluids cannot be transformed, they accumulate under the skin giving rise to oedema.

The tongue is Pale from the deficiency of Yang, and wet because the impairment in the Spleen function of fluid transportation leads to accumulation of fluids on the tongue.

The Pulse is Deep and Slow reflecting the deficiency of Yang.

Aetiology

The aetiology of this pattern is exactly the same as for Spleen-Qi deficiency, the only difference being that this pattern is more likely to be caused by exposure to a cold and damp environment.

Treatment

Principle of treatment: tonify and warm Spleen-Yang.

Points: the same as for Spleen-Qi deficiency, with the addition of Yinlingquan SP-9, Shuifen Ren-9, Shuidao ST-28, Sanjiaoshu BL-22 which should all be reduced if there is Dampness.

Method: reinforcing method. Moxa must be used.

Explanation

SP-9 resolves Dampness in the Lower Burner.

Ren-9, ST-28 and BL-22 can all stimulate the Spleen to transform and transport fluids and resolve oedema.

SPLEEN-QI SINKING

Clinical manifestations

Any of the symptoms and signs of Spleen-Qi deficiency with the addition of: bearing down sensation in the abdomen, prolapse of stomach, uterus, anus or vagina, frequency and urgency of urination.

Tongue: Pale.

Pulse: Empty or Weak. When the stomach is prolapsed, this can be felt on the middle right position on the pulse. If we divide the Stomach position on the pulse in three parts, the upper part will simply not be felt when the stomach is prolapsed.

Key symptoms: bearing down sensation, Weak Pulse.

Pathology

This is exactly the same as for Spleen-Qi deficiency. The main difference is that this pattern reflects the impairment of the Spleen function of raising Qi.

Haemorrhoids and varicose veins are also partly due to the sinking of Spleen-Qi not being able to keep the veins in their proper place.

The frequency and urgency of urination are due to the sinking of Qi unable to control urine.

Aetiology

Again, this is the same as for Spleen-Qi deficiency. In addition, persons who, because of their work, have to stand long hours every day, are more prone to this pattern if there are other factors in their life that cause Spleen-Qi deficiency.

Treatment

Principle of treatment: tonify Spleen-Qi, raise Qi.

Points: all the same as for Spleen-Qi deficiency, plus Baihui Du-20, Qihai Ren-6, Liangmen ST-21, Chengqiang Du-1.

Method: reinforcing. Moxa is applicable.

Explanation

Du-20 raises Qi. When used to raise Qi, moxa cones should be applied. It is particularly useful for prolapse of the uterus.

Ren-6 tonifies and raises Qi. It is used for all prolapses.

ST-21 tonifies Stomach and is used for prolapse of stomach.

Du-1 is used for prolapse of anus.

SPLEEN NOT CONTROLLING BLOOD

Clinical manifestations

Any of the Spleen-Qi deficiency manifestations, plus: purpura, blood spots under the skin, blood in the urine or stools, menorrhagia or metrorrhagia, sallow complexion and shortness of breath.

Tongue: Pale.

Pulse: Fine.

Key symptoms: Fine Pulse, Pale tongue and bleeding.

Pathology

All these symptoms are due to the impairment of the Spleen function of controlling Blood. When Spleen-Qi is deficient, it cannot hold the blood in the vessels and bleeding appears from various sources, such as under the skin, in the stools or urine or from the uterus. This is bleeding of Deficient nature, as opposed to the bleeding from Heat in the Blood which is of an Excess nature.

Aetiology

This is the same as for Spleen-Qi deficiency.

Treatment

Principle of treatment: tonify Spleen-Qi.

Points: the same as for Spleen-Qi deficiency, plus: Xuehai SP-10, Geshu BL-17, Yinbai SP-1.

Method: reinforcing, moxa is applicable.

Explanation

SP-10 strengthens the Spleen function of controlling Blood and returns blood to the blood vessels.

BL-17 tonifies Blood and stops bleeding, if needled. No moxa.

SP-1 with moxa cones, strengthens the Spleen function of controlling Blood and stops uterine bleeding. Moxa can only be applied to this point to stop bleeding, if this is of a Deficient nature.

COLD-DAMP INVADING THE SPLEEN

Clinical manifestations

No appetite, feeling of oppression of the chest and epigastrium, feeling of cold in the epigastrium which improves with the application of warmth, feeling of heaviness of the head, sweetish taste in the mouth or absence of taste, no thirst, loose-thin stools, white vaginal discharge, lassitude and feeling of heaviness.

Tongue: sticky-thick-white coating.

Pulse: Slippery-Slow.

Key symptoms: feeling of oppression of chest-epigastrium, feeling of heaviness and sticky tongue coating.

Pathology

This is an Excess pattern occurring when the Spleen is invaded by exterior Dampness. The above manifestations correspond to the acute stage, but the pattern can also be chronic.

Dampness obstructs the chest and epigastrium and prevents the normal movement of Qi causing the typical feeling of stuffiness and heaviness. Dampness also prevents the clear Yang from ascending to the head causing the feeling of heaviness of the head.

The Spleen opens into the mouth and when Dampness obstructs the Spleen, it affects the taste.

Dampness is heavy and has a tendency to infuse downwards: when this happens, it will cause vaginal discharge.

The sticky or slippery tongue coating is highly indicative of Dampness, as is the Slippery Pulse.

The pattern presented here derives from invasion of the Spleen by exterior Dampness, but very similar manifestations can arise from a chronic deficiency of Spleen-Qi which leads to the formation of Dampness. The main differentiating features will be the pulse and tongue. In case of Dampness from chronic Spleen-Qi deficiency, the pulse would be Fine or Weak and only slightly Slippery (rather than Full-Slippery), and the tongue would be Pale and have a thin coating (rather than a thick coating).

Aetiology

This is from exposure to exterior Dampness, which would derive either from the weather or living conditions.

Treatment

Principle of treatment: resolve Damp.

Points: Yinlingquan SP-9, Sanyinjiao SP-6, Zhongwan Ren-12, Taibai SP-3, Touwei ST-8.

Method: reducing or even.

Explanation

SP-9 resolves Dampness from the Lower Burner.

SP-6 resolves Dampness.

Ren-12 tonifies the Spleen to resolve Dampness.

ST-8 resolves Dampness from the head. It is particularly indicated for feeling of heaviness of the head or headache from Dampness.

DAMP-HEAT INVADING THE SPLEEN

Clinical manifestations

Stuffiness of the epigastrium and lower abdomen, no appetite, feeling of heaviness, thirst without desire to drink or with a desire to drink in small sips, nausea, vomiting, abdominal pain, loose stools with offensive odour, burning sensation of the anus, scanty and dark-yellow urination, low-grade fever, headache.

Tongue: sticky-yellow coating.

Pulse: Slippery-Rapid.

Key symptoms: sticky-yellow coating, loose stools with offensive odour and low-grade fever.

Pathology

The pathology is essentially the same as for Cold-Damp invading the Spleen, with the difference that in this case there is Heat. Most of the symptoms can be analysed in the same way as those of Damp-Cold.

The low-grade fever is caused by the steaming of Damp-Heat and is constant throughout the day (contrary to the low-grade fever from Yin deficiency which only appears in the afternoon or early evening).

The offensive odour of the stools, the burning sensation of the anus and the scanty dark-yellow urination are indicative of Heat.

Aetiology

This is usually due to exterior Damp-Heat, i.e. exposure to hot and humid weather.

It can also be due to eating unclean or contaminated food.

Treatment

Principle of treatment: resolve Dampness, clear Heat.

Points: Yinlingquan SP-9, Sanyinjiao SP-6, Zhiyang Du-9, Quchi L.I.-11, Pishu BL-20, Yanglingquan G.B.-34.

Method: reducing method, no moxa.

Explanation

SP-9 and SP-6 resolve Dampness and Damp-Heat from the Lower Burner.

Du-9 resolves Damp-Heat.

L.I.-11 clears Heat and resolves Dampness.

BL-20 resolves Dampness.

G.B.-34 resolves Damp-Heat.

COMBINED PATTERNS

The combined patterns are:

Spleen and Lung Qi Deficiency

Spleen and Liver Blood Deficiency

Spleen obstructed by Dampness with stagnation of Liver Qi.

SPLEEN AND LUNG QI DEFICIENCY

Clinical manifestations

No appetite, tiredness, loose stools, weak voice, slight breathlessness, bright-white complexion, slight spontaneous sweating.

Tongue: Pale.

Pulse: Empty, especially on the right side.

Key symptoms: no appetite, tiredness and breathlessness.

Pathology

Both Spleen and Lungs are involved in the production of Qi and they influence each other in health and disease.

The Spleen is the source of Food-Qi from which all Qi is produced; the Lungs control breathing and the taking in of air which combines with Food-Qi to produce True Qi. Thus they both determine the crucial stages of the production of Qi. There is a saying in Chinese Medicine: "The Spleen is the source of Qi and the Lungs are the pivot of Qi".[4]

In pathological situations, deficiency of one often affects the other: a diet poor in nourishment or excessive in cold and raw foods will weaken the Spleen and eventually affect the Lungs, because they will not receive enough Food-Qi. On the other hand, poor breathing, lack of exercise, excessive stooping over a desk for many years, all weaken Lung-Qi: not enough air is taken in, Lung-Qi weakens and therefore not enough Qi from the Lungs is available to produce True Qi.

Aetiology

As mentioned before, this pattern is caused by a diet lacking in nourishment or from lack of proper exercise or excessive sedentary work at a desk.

Treatment

Principle of treatment: tonify Lung and Spleen Qi.

Points: Zusanli ST-36, Taibai SP-3, Pishu BL-20, Weishu BL-21, Taiyuan LU-9, Feishu BL-13, Shenzhu DU-12.

Method: reinforcing.

Explanation

ST-36 tonifies Spleen-Qi.

SP-3, BL-20 and BL-21 tonify Spleen-Qi.

LU-9 and BL-13 tonify Lung-Qi.

Du-12 tonifies Lung-Qi, particularly for chronic conditions.

SPLEEN AND LIVER BLOOD DEFICIENCY

Clinical manifestations

Dizziness, tiredness, sallow complexion, loose stools, no appetite, blurred vision, numbness or tingling of limbs.

Tongue: Pale, paler on the sides. In severe cases the sides could have a slight orange colour.

Pulse: Choppy.

Key symptoms: dizziness, loose stools and pale or orangey sides of the tongue.

Pathology

The Spleen is the origin of Blood because Food-Qi produced by the Spleen is the basis for the formation of Blood. If Spleen-Qi is deficient, not enough Blood is produced. Since the Liver stores Blood, when this is deficient, there will be lack of Blood in the Liver. This will cause dizziness, blurred vision, numbness and a pale or orangey colour of the sides of the tongue.

The other symptoms are typical of Spleen-Qi deficiency.

Aetiology

This pattern is usually due to dietary factors: either a diet lacking in nourishment or excessive in cold and raw foods.

Treatment

Principle of treatment: tonify Spleen-Qi, promote Blood, tonify Liver-Blood.

Points: Zusanli ST-36, Taibai SP-3, Pishu BL-20, Weishu BL-21, Ququan LIV-8, Ganshu BL-18, Geshu BL-17, Sanyinjiao SP-6.

Method: reinforcing, moxa is applicable

Explanation

ST-36, SP-3, BL-20 and BL-21 tonify Spleen-Qi.

LIV-8 tonifies Liver-Blood.

BL-18 and BL-17 promote Blood and tonify Liver-Blood (moxa is applicable on BL-17).

SP-6 tonifies Spleen-Qi and promotes Blood.

OBSTRUCTION OF SPLEEN BY DAMPNESS WITH STAGNATION OF LIVER-QI

Clinical manifestations

Stuffiness and fullness of the epigastrium, nausea, no appetite, loose stools, feeling of heaviness, thirst with desire to drink in small amounts, sallow complexion, hypochondriac pain, jaundice, bitter taste.

Tongue: thick-sticky-yellow coating.

Pulse: Slippery and Wiry.

Key symptoms: stuffiness and fullness of epigastrium, hypochondriac pain and a thick-sticky-yellow tongue coating.

Pathology

When the Spleen is deficient and fails in its function of transformation and transportation, fluids accumulate into Dampness. Dampness obstructs the flow of Qi in the Middle Burner interfering with the proper direction of flow of Qi (ascending Spleen-Qi, descending Stomach-Qi or smooth flow of Liver-Qi). After a long period of time, the obstruction of Dampness gives rise to Heat. Dampness begins to interfere with the smooth flow of Liver-Qi and the flow of bile: Liver-Qi stagnates in the Middle Burner and the Gall-Bladder cannot secrete bile.

Aetiology

This pattern is caused by the excessive consumption of greasy foods which tend to create Dampness in the Spleen.

Treatment

Principle of treatment: tonify the Spleen to resolve Damp, promote the smooth flow of Liver-Qi, clear Heat.

Points: Zhongwan Ren -12, Sanyinjiao SP-6, Taibai SP-3, Pishu BL-20, Zhangmen LIV-13, Qimen LIV-14, Riyue G.B.-24, Yanglingquan G.B.-34.

Method: reducing for points of Liver and Gall-Bladder channels as well as for SP-6, LIV-13 and SP-3 (to resolve Dampness); reinforcing for the other points (to tonify the Spleen).

Explanation

Ren-12 tonifies the Spleen to resolve Dampness.

SP-6 resolves Dampness.

SP-3 resolves Dampness.

BL-20 tonifies the Spleen to resolve Dampness.

LIV-13 promotes the smooth flow of Liver-Qi, resolves Dampness from the Middle Burner.

LIV-14 promotes the smooth flow of Liver-Qi.

G.B.-24 promotes the smooth flow of Liver-Qi and the secretion of bile.

G.B.-34 promotes the smooth flow of Liver-Qi in the Middle Burner.

NOTES

1 The idea that women should pay great attention to not catching dampness during each period and particularly after childbirth is deeply rooted in Chinese culture. Even today, in rural areas some women follow the custom of not washing at all for one month after childbirth. In all parts of China, both rural areas and cities, women often do not wash their hair at the time of menstruation.

2 Some modern Chinese textbooks, such as the "Essentials of Chinese Acupuncture" call the emotion related to the Spleen "meditation". This is obviously a mistranslation of the Chinese character which simply indicates "thinking" or "pensiveness". Far from being a cause of disease, meditation is very beneficial to the Spleen and Heart.

3 Tongue Diagnosis in Chinese Medicine, p 70-71.

4 Differentiation and Treatment of the Internal Organs, p 291.

Kidney Patterns 25

腎脏病証

The main Kidney function is that of storing Essence and governing birth, growth and reproduction. Since the Essence of the Kidneys can never be in excess but can only be deficient, Chinese medical theory holds that the Kidneys do not have Excess patterns but only Deficiency ones. There is, however, an exception as acute Damp-Heat can affect Bladder and Kidneys. In chronic conditions, though, all Kidney patterns are either of the Deficiency type or the combined Deficiency/Excess type.

Central to any Kidney pathology is the duality of Kidney-Yin and Kidney-Yang. Although this duality can be observed both in physiology and pathology, it is in disease that it becomes very apparent.

Kidney-Yin represents the Essence and the fluids within the Kidneys. Kidney-Yang is the motive force of all physiological processes and it is the root of transformation and movement. Kidney-Yin is the material foundation for Kidney-Yang, and Kidney-Yang is the exterior manifestation of Kidney-Yin.

Every pathological condition of the Kidneys will necessarily manifest itself as a deficiency of Kidney-Yin or Kidney-Yang. However, as mentioned in the chapter on the Kidney functions (see p. 95), Kidney-Yin and Kidney-Yang have the same root and they are but two manifestations of the same entity. It follows that in pathological conditions, a deficiency of Yin of the Kidneys will also necessarily imply, to a lesser degree, a deficiency of the Yang of the Kidneys and vice versa. However, it must be stressed that the deficiency will always be primarily either of Yin or Yang: it can never be 50% Yin and 50% Yang deficient. This can be expressed in diagrammatic form (Fig. 61).

It will be noted that this diagram differs from those presented in other acupuncture books in so far as the column for Yin is below the normal mark in Yang deficiency, and the column for Yang is below the normal mark in Yin deficiency. This is a visual representation of the fact that Kidney-Yin and Kidney-Yang have the same origin and one cannot be deficient without the other also being slightly (but to a lesser degree) deficient.

This situation would be very familiar to those who have clinical experience. How often do we see a patient who has a malar flush, dark urine, night sweating, tinnitus (Kidney-Yin deficiency) but also swollen ankles (Kidney-Yang deficiency)? Or how often do we see a patient whose urination is frequent and pale, he or she feels chilly, has a lower back ache (Kidney-Yang deficiency) but also suffers from night sweating (Kidney-Yin deficiency)?

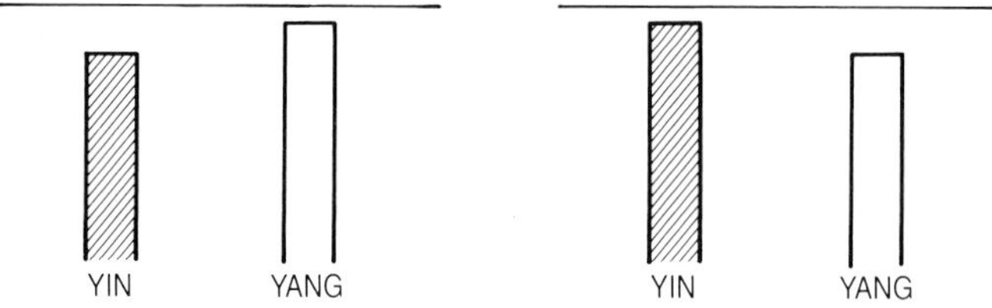

Fig. 61 Deficiency of Kidney-Yin and Kidney-Yang

The Kidneys are called the "Root of Pre-Heaven Qi" because they store Essence. The Kidneys are nearly always affected in chronic diseases. There is a saying in Chinese Medicine: *"A chronic disease will inevitably reach the Kidneys"*.

The Kidneys are also the root of all the other organs, as Kidney-Yin is the foundation for the Yin of Liver and Heart, whilst Kidney-Yang is the foundation for the Yang of Spleen and Lungs. Thus most chronic diseases will eventually manifest with a Kidney disharmony, either Kidney-Yin or Kidney-Yang deficiency. Since the Kidneys are the foundation for the Yin and Yang energies of all other organs, the combined patterns of the Kidneys with other organs will be discussed in this chapter.

GENERAL AETIOLOGY

HEREDITARY WEAKNESS

The Pre-Heaven Qi of each person is formed at conception from the union of the parents' Kidney-Essences (sperm and ova are but an external manifestation of Kidney-Essence). It follows that the inherited constitution will depend on the strength and quality of the parents' Essences in general and at the time of conception in particular.

Chinese Medicine has always placed great emphasis on the relation between the parents' Essences and the hereditary constitution of their offspring. Some ancient texts even stated the most auspicious or unfavourable times of conception in great detail.[1]

If the parents' Essences are weak, the child's Kidneys will also be weak. This may manifest with poor bone development, some mental retardation, a pigeon-chest, a weak back, incontinence, enuresis, loose teeth and thin hair.

One of the most important factors in the parents' condition is their age. As Kidney-Essence declines with age, if the parents conceive when they are too old, their child's constitution might suffer. Similarly, if the parents are in a state of exhaustion at the time of conception, this may also induce a hereditary weakness of their child. This may explain the sometimes striking difference in physical appearance and personality amongst siblings.

EMOTIONS

The emotion pertaining to the Kidneys is fear. This includes fear, anxiety and shock. It is said in Chinese Medicine that fear makes Qi descend. In children this will be manifested with enuresis: in fact, very often enuresis is caused by a situation of anxiety or insecurity in the family for the child.

In adults, however, very often fear and anxiety do not make Qi descend but rise. Very often a long-standing situation of anxiety may induce Empty-Fire within the Kidneys, which rises to the head causing dry mouth, malar flush, mental restlessness and insomnia.

EXCESSIVE SEXUAL ACTIVITY

This is modestly referred to in Chinese books as "unregulated affairs of the bedroom" or "excessive labours of the bedroom". Traditionally, the idea that excessive sexual activity can weaken the Kidneys is very old and can be found in the Yellow Emperor's Classic.[2]

As mentioned in the chapter "Causes of Disease" (see p. 127), excessive sexual activity weakens the Kidney energy because sexual energy is a manifestation of the Kidney-Essence, and the orgasm quite simply tends to deplete the Kidney-Essence. It should be clarified here that by "excessive sexual activity" is meant actual ejaculation for men and orgasm for women. Sexual activity without ejaculation or orgasm does not have a depleting effect on the Kidney-Essence. "Excessive sexual activity" also includes masturbation which affects the Kidney energy as much as sex with a partner.

Apart from the Kidneys, other organs, notably the Heart and Liver, contribute to a normal and happy sexual life.

The Heart is directly related to the Kidneys as the two must support and nourish each other. Just as a Kidney deficiency caused by excessive sexual activity can weaken the Heart (causing palpitations), conversely, a Heart deficiency caused by sadness and anxiety can weaken the Kidneys and cause impotence or inability to achieve an orgasm.

The Liver is responsible for the smooth circulation of Qi and Blood, particularly in the Lower Burner. Stagnation of Liver-Qi and/or Liver-Blood can therefore influence the sexual life and lead to inability to reach an orgasm, frigidity or impotence in men.

CHRONIC ILLNESS

As mentioned before, most chronic diseases eventually affect the Kidneys. In the late stages of a chronic disease a pattern of Kidney-Yin or Kidney-Yang deficiency can nearly always be seen.

OLD AGE

Kidney-Essence declines with age and in fact, Chinese Medicine sees the process of ageing as the result of the decrease of Kidney-Essence throughout our life.

Most of the symptoms and signs associated with old age are due to deficiency of Kidney-Essence. Hearing decreases because Kidney-Essence cannot reach the ears, bones become brittle and weak because Kidney-Essence fails to nourish bones and bone-marrow, the sexual function decreases because the declining Kidney-Essence and the Fire of the Gate of Vitality cannot nourish the sexual organs.

OVERWORK

This is intended both in a physical and mental sense. Physical overwork over a long period of time will weaken Kidney-Yang. Mental overwork under conditions of stress will eventually weaken Kidney-Yin. This is, in fact, the most common cause of Kidney-Yin deficiency in Western industrialized societies. A lifetime of work under conditions of stress, lack of relaxation, long hours of work, hurried meals, irregular eating schedule, eating late at night, discussing business while eating, excessive mental work not balanced with physical exercise, all these factors combine to erode the Yin energies because the body is never given a chance to recuperate. The result is that, instead of using Yang energies which are quickly replenished by the Post-Heaven Qi, the body starts using the Yin essences which are stored in the Kidneys. This eventually causes Kidney-Yin deficiency. If, in addition, there is great stress, worry and anxiety usually associated with overwork, this may also give rise to Empty-Heat.

The patterns discussed are:

- Deficiency patterns
  - Kidney-Yin deficiency
  - Kidney-Yang deficiency
  - Kidney-Qi not Firm
  - Kidney failing to receive Qi
  - Kidney-Essence deficiency
- Deficiency/Excess patterns
  - Kidney-Yang deficient, Water overflowing
  - Kidney-Yin deficient, Empty-Fire blazing
- Combined patterns
  - Kidney- and Liver-Yin deficiency
  - Kidney- and Heart-not harmonized
  - Kidney- and Lung-Yin deficiency
  - Kidney- and Spleen-Yang deficiency.

KIDNEY-YIN DEFICIENCY

Clinical manifestations

Dizziness, tinnitus, vertigo, poor memory, deafness, night sweating, dry mouth at night, 5-palm heat, thirst, sore back, ache in bones, nocturnal emissions, constipation, dark-scanty urine.

Tongue: Red, no coating, cracks.

Pulse: Floating-Empty and Rapid

Key symptoms: dry mouth at night, night sweating, Red-Peeled tongue.

Pathology

This pattern is characterized by deficiency of Yin and also Essence of the Kidneys, as Essence is part of Kidney-Yin.

Kidney-Yin deficient fails to produce enough Marrow to fill the brain resulting in dizziness, tinnitus, vertigo and poor memory. The dizziness would be slight and the tinnitus would be of gradual and slow onset with a sound like rushing water.

The deficiency of Kidney-Yin leads to lack of Body Fluids and ensuing dryness, resulting in a dry mouth at night, thirst, constipation and scanty-dark urine.

The deficiency of Kidney-Yin leads to the arousal of Empty-Heat within the Kidneys, hence the 5-palm heat, night sweating, Red tongue and Rapid pulse. In particular, night sweating is due the Yin being deficient and failing to hold Defensive Qi in the body at night (Defensive Qi retires into the Yin at night), so that the precious Yin nutritive essences come out with the sweat. Also, Empty-Heat causes evaporation of the Yin fluids which come out at night as sweat. Thus night sweating is very different from daytime sweating as with the former, the Yin nutritive essences are lost, whilst with the latter, Yang fluids are lost. Night sweating is also called *"evaporation from the bones"*, whilst daytime sweating is called *"evaporation from the muscles"*. The term for night sweating is *"rob sweating"*, probably to indicate that with it the body is robbed of precious Yin essences.

Kidney-Yin deficiency may cause deficiency of Essence which results in nocturnal emissions.

The sore back and ache in the bones are due to the failure of Kidney-Essence in nourishing bones.

Aetiology

1) A long, chronic illness usually transmitted from the Liver, Heart or Lungs.
2) Overwork over a period of several years.
3) Excessive sexual activity, especially during the teen-age years, which depletes Kidney-Essence.
4) Depletion of Body Fluids which can be consumed by Heat after a febrile disease.
5) Loss of blood over a long period of time (such as from menorrhagia) can cause deficiency of Liver-Blood which, in turn, can lead to deficiency of Kidney-Yin. It is said in Chinese Medicine that Liver and Kidney share the same root.
6) Overdosage of Chinese herbal medicines to strengthen Kidney-Yang or administration of wrong medicine (to strengthen Kidney-Yang when Kidney-Yin should be strengthened). The former situation is very common in China as the habit of taking medicines to strengthen Kidney-Yang as middle-age approaches is ingrained in Chinese culture. If this is overdone and Kidney-Yang is over-stimulated by the administration of too hot herbal medicines, Kidney-Yin will be injured.[3]

Treatment

Principle of treatment: nourish Kidney-Yin.

Points: Guanyuan Ren-4, Taixi KI-3, Zhaohai KI-6, Yingu KI-10, Zhubin KI-9, Sanyinjiao SP-6, Huiyin Ren-1.

Method: reinforcing method, no moxa.

Explanation

Ren-4 without moxa tonifies Kidney-Yin and Kidney Essence (with moxa it can tonify Kidney-Yang).

KI-3 tonifies the Kidneys.

KI-6 is specific to tonify Kidney-Yin and it benefits the throat (particularly indicated for dry mouth at night).

KI-10 is specific to tonify Kidney-Yin.

KI-9 tonifies Kidney-Yin, particularly useful in case of anxiety and emotional tension of Kidney origin.

SP-6 tonifies Liver and Kidney Yin and calms the mind.

Ren-1 tonifies Kidney-Yin and Essence and is used for chronic nocturnal emissions (from Kidney-Yin deficiency) combined with Taixi KI-3 and Shenmen He-7.

Case history

A man of 50 suffered from a severe pain in the left loin, with very dark and scanty urine, dry mouth and night sweating. This pain came in bouts and was caused by a kidney stone lodged in the ureter. The tongue was Deep-Red and nearly completely without coating, the tip was redder, it had an extremely deep crack in the midline with smaller cracks arising out of it and it was dry. The pulse at the time of examination was Deep and Wiry (when a pulse has these two qualities it is also called Firm).

The night sweating, dry mouth and very dark and scanty urine point to Kidney-Yin deficiency. This is confirmed by the tongue which is completely peeled: this always indicates Kidney-Yin deficiency. It is also indicated by its dryness. The deep crack in the midline with smaller cracks also indicates severe Kidney-Yin deficiency. The Deep-Red colour of the tongue indicates that Kidney-Yin deficiency has given rise to Empty-Heat. The pulse in this case is affected by the acute episode and it reflects the internal stagnation of Qi and Blood and intense pain caused by the stone in the ureter.

From interrogation, it transpired that this person had been very worried and anxious about job insecurity for the past years. The anxiety was reflected in the red tip of the tongue indicating Heart Empty-Heat. Presumably, the anxiety, fear and insecurity caused the Kidney deficiency.

KIDNEY-YANG DEFICIENCY

Clinical manifestations

Soreness of the back, cold knees, sensation of cold in the back, aversion to cold, weak legs, bright-white complexion, weak knees, impotence, premature ejaculation, lassitude, abundant-clear urination, scanty-clear urination, apathy, oedema of the legs, infertility in women, poor appetite, loose stools.

Tongue: Pale, Swollen, Wet.

Pulse: Deep-Weak.

Key symptoms: cold in the back, abundant-clear urination, Pale tongue, Deep Pulse.

Pathology

This is the classical pattern of Yang deficiency and it is therefore characterized by interior Cold symptoms.

When Kidney-Yang is deficient, the Fire of the Gate of Vitality fails to warm the body, causing the feeling of cold in the back and knees and the aversion to cold.

When Kidney-Yang is deficient, the Kidneys have not enough Qi to give strength to bones and the back, hence the soreness of the back and weakness of the legs and knees.

Kidney-Yang deficient fails to warm the Essence, hence the sexual energy is deprived of the nourishment of the Essence and warmth of Kidney-Yang. This results in impotence and premature ejaculation in men and infertility or frigidity in women.

When Kidney-Yang is deficient it fails to transform the fluids which therefore accumulate, resulting in abundant and clear urination. In special cases when Kidney-Yang is so deficient that it cannot move the fluids at all, there may be the opposite, i.e. scanty (but clear) urination. If the fluids accumulate under the skin there will be oedema of the legs. The accumulation of fluids in the tongue makes it Swollen and wet.

Kidney-Yang deficient fails to nourish the Blood and the Spleen, hence the muscles lack nourishment: this causes the lassitude and Pale tongue. From a psychological point of view, it is manifested with apathy, lack of will power and unwillingness to undertake any project.

The poor appetite and loose stools are due to the Spleen lacking the nourishment from the Kidneys.

Aetiology

1 A chronic illness can cause Kidney-Yang deficiency after a protracted period of time.

2 Excessive sexual activity can also cause Kidney-Yang deficiency. This happens in par-

ticular if one is exposed to cold immediately after intercourse (see p. 138).

3 Retention of Dampness (resulting from Spleen deficiency) over a long period of time will eventually affect the Kidneys by obstructing the movement of fluids and therefore leading to deficiency of Yang.

4 Old age, in the sense explained above.

Treatment

Principle of treatment: tonify and warm the Kidneys, strengthen the Fire of the Gate of Vitality.

Points: Shenshu BL-23, Mingmen Du-4, Guangyuan Ren-4, Qihai Ren-6, Taixi KI-3, Fuliu KI-7, Zhishi BL-52, extra point Jinggong (0.5 cun lateral to Zhishi BL-52).

Method: reinforcing, moxa should be used.

Explanation

BL-23 tonifies Kidney-Yang.

Du-4 strengthens the Fire of the Gate of Vitality. Moxa is applicable.

Ren-4 (with moxa) tonifies Kidney-Yang and the Original Qi.

Ren-6 (with moxa) tonifies Kidney-Yang.

KI-3 tonifies the Kidneys.

KI-7 is specific to tonify Kidney-Yang.

BL-52 tonifies the Kidneys and in particular their mental aspect, i.e. the will power.

Jinggong tonifies Kidney-Yang and warms the Essence.

KIDNEY-QI NOT FIRM

Clinical manifestations

Soreness and weakness of the back, clear-frequent urination, weak-stream urination, abundant urination, dribbling after urination, incontinence of urine, enuresis, urination at night, nocturnal emissions without dreams, premature ejaculation, spermatorrhoea, in women prolapse of uterus, chronic vaginal discharge.

Tongue: Pale.

Pulse: Deep-Weak especially in the Rear positions.

Key symptoms: dribbling after urination, nocturnal emissions without dreams.

Pathology

This pattern is usually considered as a Cold pattern even if there are no obvious cold symptoms. It is basically a type of Kidney-Yang deficiency pattern and it is to be treated as such.

It is characterized by a weakness of one of the two "lower Yin orifices" (urethra) and the "Sperm Gate", leading to manifestations of "leaking". The symptoms broadly fall into two categories of urinary and sexual manifestations. This pattern is also called "Lower Original Qi not Firm", to indicate that it is also caused by a weakness of the Original Qi and the Fire of the Gate of Vitality. Original Qi is weak in the Lower Burner, Qi cannot hold fluids and sperm, hence the leaking character of most of the manifestations.

When Kidney-Qi and Original Qi are weak, the Kidneys cannot provide enough Qi to the Bladder for its function of Qi transformation, hence the urine cannot be held and this causes frequent urination, incontinence, enuresis, weak-stream urination and dribbling after urination.

When Kidney-Qi is deficient it cannot hold the sperm (or vaginal secretions in women), and this causes spermatorrhoea, premature ejaculation, nocturnal emissions without dreams and chronic vaginal discharge. The nocturnal emissions are without dreams because they are caused by a totally Deficient condition, so that the sperm leaks out because Kidney-Qi cannot hold it in. If nocturnal emissions are accompanied by vivid sexual dreams, this indicates that there is some Empty-Fire within the Kidneys arousing sexual desire.

There is urination at night because Yang Qi is not Firm, Yang cannot control the Yin at night, hence Yin predominates and the person needs to urinate during the night.

When Kidney-Yang is deficient, it fails to nourish the Spleen which, in turn, fails in its function of raising Qi, hence the prolapse of the uterus. The chronic vaginal discharge can also be seen to be a manifestation of the sinking of Qi from chronic Kidney and Spleen deficiency.

Aetiology

1 Excessive sexual activity is the most important and frequent cause of this pattern.
2 In women, too many childbirths too close together can cause this pattern to arise.

Treatment

Principle of treatment: reinforce and stabilize Kidney-Qi.

Points: Shenshu BL-23, Mingmen Du-4, Taixi KI-3, Zhishi BL-52, Guanyuan Ren-4, extra point Jinggong.

Method: reinforcing, moxa is applicable.

Explanation

BL-23 tonifies Kidney-Yang.

Du-4 tonifies Kidney-Yang and the Fire of the Gate of Vitality. It is an important point to stop incontinence, enuresis, excessive urination, etc.

KI-3 tonifies the Kidneys.

BL-52 tonifies Kidney-Yang and strengthens will power.

Ren-4 with moxa, tonifies Kidney-Yang and the Original Qi.

Jinggong tonifies Kidney-Yang and firms the Sperm Gate.

KIDNEYS FAILING TO RECEIVE QI

Clinical manifestations

Shortness of breath on exertion, rapid and weak breathing, difficulty in inhaling, cough, asthma, sweating, cold limbs, cold limbs after sweating, swelling of the face, thin body, mental listlessness, clear urination during asthma attack, soreness of the back.

Tongue: Pale.

Pulse: Weak, Tight, Deep.

Key symptoms: shortness of breath on exertion, sweating, clear urination.

Pathology

This is basically a dysfunction of the Kidney function of reception of Qi, and is also to be considered as a type of Kidney-Yang deficiency pattern.

When the Kidneys are weak and fail to receive and hold Qi down, Qi accumulates above, resulting in Excess above in the chest, and Deficiency below in the abdomen, hence the shortness of breath and asthma. Kidneys control inhalation, hence the asthma is characterized by difficulty in inhalation more than exhalation (the Lungs control exhalation).

When Kidney-Yang is deficient, all the Yang energies of the body are deficient, including Defensive Qi, hence the sweating and cold limbs.

Deficiency of Kidney-Yang also causes the abundant and clear urination, typically during an asthma attack.

This pattern can only appear in long-standing, chronic conditions, hence the general lassitude, thin body and mental exhaustion.

This pattern is also characterized by a failure of communication between Lung and Kidneys. As explained before, Lungs and Kidneys have to communicate with each other and assist each other particularly in the function of respiration (Lung controls exhalation and Kidneys control inhalation) and movement of fluids. When Kidney-Yang is deficient, the fluids cannot be transformed and this can give rise to oedema which, in this case, is localized in the face because of the Lung involvement.

Aetiology

1) Hereditary weakness of Lungs and Kidneys.
2) A long-standing, chronic disease which inevitably reaches the Kidneys, particularly if transmitted from the Lungs.
3) Excessive physical exercise particularly during puberty and excessive lifting and standing.

Treatment

Principle of treatment: tonify and warm the Kidneys, stimulate the Kidney function of reception of Qi, stimulate the Lung descending function.

Points: Taixi KI-3, Lieque LU-7 and Zhaohai KI-6 in combination, Zusanli ST-36, Shenshu BL-23, Mingmen Du-4, Qihai Ren-6, Shanzhong

Ren-17, Shencang KI-25, Shenzhu Du-12, Fuliu KI-7.

Method: reinforcing. Moxa is applicable.

Explanation

KI-3 tonifies the Kidneys.

LU-7 and KI-6 in combination open the Directing Vessel, stimulate the Lung descending function and the Kidney function of reception of Qi and benefit the throat.

ST-36 tonifies Qi in general and is important to use in chronic conditions.

BL-23 and Du-4 tonify Kidney-Yang.

Ren-6 tonifies Kidney-Yang (used with moxa) and draws Qi down to the abdomen.

Ren-17 tonifies Qi and stimulates the Lung descending function.

KI-25 is an important local chest point of the Kidney channel to stimulate the Kidney reception of Qi and improve breathing.

Du-12 tonifies Lung Qi, important in chronic conditions.

KI-7 tonifies Kidney-Yang and is important to use in breathing problems.

KIDNEY-ESSENCE DEFICIENCY

Clinical manifestations

In children: poor bone development, late closure of fontanelle, mental dullness or retardation.

In adults: softening of bones, weakness of knees and legs, poor memory, loose teeth, falling hair or premature greying of hair, weakness of sexual activity, soreness of the back.

Tongue: Red and Peeled.

Pulse: Floating-Empty or Leather.

Key symptoms: children: poor bone development; adults: weak knees, falling hair, weak sexual activity.

Pathology

This pattern can be considered as a type of Kidney-Yin deficiency pattern, as Kidney-Essence is part of Yin. However, there is also a Yang aspect to Kidney-Essence, so that a deficiency of Kidney-Essence can also be seen on a background of Kidney-Yang deficiency. In this case the Tongue would be Pale and the Pulse would be Deep and Weak.

When this pattern is present against a background of Kidney-Yin deficiency, there may be other symptoms of Yin deficiency such as tinnitus and dizziness.

This pattern is characterized by a deficiency of Essence: its manifestations therefore affect growth, reproduction and bones, all of which are under the control of Essence.

When the Kidney-Essence is deficient, it will fail to generate Marrow and nourish the bones, hence the poor bone development, late closure of fontanelle, softening of bones and weakness of knees and legs. Teeth are seen as an extension of bone tissue, hence the looseness of teeth.

The Kidney-Essence generates Marrow which fills the Brain; if the Essence is deficient, not enough Marrow is generated to fill the Brain, hence the poor memory in adults and mental dullness or retardation in children.

The Kidney-Essence also dominates the growth of head-hair, hence the falling of hair or premature greying of hair.

The Kidney-Essence is the material basis for a healthy sexual function, hence the weakness of sexual activity.

Aetiology

1) In children: poor hereditary constitution (which can be due to parents being too old or in poor health at the time of conception).
2) In adults: old age, or excessive sexual activity, especially at puberty time.

Treatment

Principle of treatment: nourish the Essence.

Points: Taixi KI-3, Zhaohai KI-6, Guanyuan Ren-4, Shenshu BL-23, Mingmen Du-4, Xuanzhong GB-39, Baihui Du-20, Dazhui Du-14, Xinshu BL-15, Dashu BL-11.

Method: reinforcing. Moxa is applicable unless there is marked Yin deficiency with Empty-Heat.

Explanation

KI-3 tonifies Kidney-Yin and Essence.

KI-6 tonifies Kidney-Yin.

Ren-4 tonifies the Essence.

BL-23 tonifies the Kidneys.

Du-4 tonifies the Yang aspect of the Essence. This point would only be used if the Kidney-Essence deficiency occurs on a background of Yang deficiency.

GB-39 tonifies the Bone Marrow.

Du-20 stimulates the Marrow to fill the Brain.

Du-14 stimulates the Marrow to reach the Brain.

BL-15 tonifies the Heart to house the Mind, hence it tonifies the brain.

BL-11 nourishes the Bones.

KIDNEY-YANG DEFICIENT,WATER OVERFLOWING

Clinical manifestations

Oedema especially of legs and ankles, cold feeling in legs and back, fullness and distension of abdomen, soreness of lower back, feeling cold, scanty-clear urination.

1) Water overflowing to the Heart: the above symptoms plus palpitations, breathlessness, cold hands.

2) Water overflowing to the Lungs: the above symptoms plus thin-watery-frothy sputum, cough, asthma and breathlessness on exertion.

Tongue: Pale, Swollen, white coating.

Pulse: Deep-Weak-Slow.

Key symptoms: oedema of ankles, Deep-Weak pulse, Pale-Swollen tongue.

a) Water overflowing to the Heart: all the above plus palpitations.

b) Water overflowing to the Lungs: all the above plus thin-watery-frothy sputum.

Pathology

This is a severe case of Kidney-Yang deficiency, when Kidney-Yang fails to transform the fluids which accumulate under the skin and form oedema. From the 8-Principle point of view, this is a Deficiency/Excess pattern since Kidney-Yang deficiency leads to the accumulation of fluids, which, in itself, is an Excess condition.

Besides affecting the Kidney itself, in certain cases, the deficiency of Yang can affect the Heart or the Lungs as well. If it affects the Heart it will be manifested with palpitations and cold hands, which are due to deficiency of Heart-Yang.

If it affects the Lungs, it will be manifested with a thin-watery-frothy sputum which is indicative of Phlegm-Fluid formation. This is due to deficiency of Lung-Qi over a long period of time. In addition, the deficiency of Kidney-Yang implies a failure of the Kidney function of reception of Qi, hence the cough and asthma. This is necessarily a very chronic condition.

Aetiology

1) Chronic, long-standing retention of Dampness which interferes with the Kidney function of transformation of fluids.

2) Transmission from Spleen-Yang deficiency due to excessive consumption of cold-raw foods.

3) In the case of Water overflowing to Heart: transmission from Heart-Yang deficiency due to poor constitution and emotional problems affecting the Mind.

4) In the case of Water overflowing to Lungs: transmission from Lung-Qi deficiency due to retention of exterior cold within the Lungs, not expelled and turned into Phlegm-Fluid in the Interior.

Treatment

Principle of treatment: tonify and warm the Kidneys, transform Water, warm and tonify Spleen-Yang. In case of Water overflowing to Heart or Lungs, warm and tonify Heart-Yang or Lung-Qi respectively.

Points: Mingmen Du-4, Shenshu BL-23, Sanjiaoshu BL-22, Pishu BL-20, Shuifen Ren-9, Shuidao ST-28, Yinlingquan SP-9, Sanyinjiao SP-6, Fuliu KI-7.

1) For Water overflowing to the Heart: Dazhui Du-14 (moxa), Xinshu BL-15.

2) For Water overflowing to the Lungs: Lieque LU-7, Feishu BL-13, Shenzhu Du-12.

Method: reinforcing on points to tonify Kidney-Yang and Spleen-Yang (BL-23, Du-4, BL-

20, KI-7) or Heart-Yang (Du-14, BL-15) or Lung-Qi (BL-13, LU-7, Du-12). Reducing method on all the other points in order to resolve Damp and transform Water. Moxa is applicable. Use thick needles and leave the points open after withdrawal so that a few drops of fluid come out.

Explanation

Du-4 strengthens the Fire of the Gate of Vitality which promotes the transformation of Water.

BL-23 tonifies Kidney-Yang.

BL-22 stimulates the transformation of fluids in the Lower Burner.

BL-20 tonifies Spleen-Yang (with moxa).

ST-28 promotes the transformation of fluids in the Lower Burner.

SP-9 and SP-6 resolve Dampness from the Lower Burner.

KI-7 tonifies Kidney-Yang.

Du-14 with direct moxa tonifies Heart-Yang.

BL-15 with moxa tonifies Heart-Yang.

LU-7 stimulates the Lung function of dominating Water passages and resolves oedema.

BL-13 and Du-12 tonify Lung-Qi.

KIDNEY-YIN DEFICIENT, EMPTY-FIRE BLAZING

Clinical manifestations

Malar flush, mental restlessness, "feeling jagged", night-sweating, low-grade fever, afternoon fever, feeling of heat in the afternoon, insomnia, scanty-dark urine, blood in the urine, dry throat especially at night, soreness of the lower back, nocturnal emissions with dreams, excessive sexual desire, dry stools.

Tongue: Red-Peeled, cracked, red tip.

Pulse: Floating-Empty, Rapid.

Key symptoms: malar flush, mental restlessness, dry throat at night, feeling of heat in the afternoon, Red-Peeled tongue.

Pathology

This pattern corresponds to an advanced stage of Kidney-Yin deficiency which has given rise to Empty-Fire: it therefore is a combined Deficiency/Excess pattern, the Empty-Fire representing the Excess condition.

Most of the symptoms are caused by the flaring of Empty-Fire and dryness from Yin deficiency.

The malar flush is a redness of the face, but only on the small area of the cheek-bones, not the whole cheek. The afternoon fever is typical of Empty-Heat; it can also simply be a feeling of heat in the afternoon, rather than an actual fever.

The Empty-Fire arising from Kidney-Yin deficiency can ascend to disturb the Heart and therefore the Mind, hence the insomnia and "mental restlessness". This is described as "heart feels vexed" in Chinese, and it describes a state of fidget, uneasiness and vague anxiety which is undefinable but very real and distressing to the patient. The insomnia is characterized by falling asleep easily but waking up in the middle of the night several times, or also in the early hours of the morning.

The deficiency of Yin leads to the exhaustion of body fluids and therefore dryness; the Empty-Heat further contributes to drying up the Body Fluids, hence the dry throat at night, concentrated urine and dry stools. In severe cases, the Empty-Heat can also cause Blood to rush out of the blood vessels resulting in blood in the urine.

The deficiency of Yin leads to deficiency of Essence, hence the nocturnal emissions. These are accompanied by vivid sexual dreams because the Empty-Fire agitates the mind and creates a strong sexual desire.

The tongue is Red because of the Empty-Heat and Peeled because of the Yin deficiency. The cracks also reflect deficiency of Yin.

The Floating-Empty and Rapid pulse reflects deficiency of Yin and Empty-Heat.

Aetiology

This is the same as for Kidney-Yin deficiency with the addition of emotional problems such as chronic anxiety and worry.

Treatment

Principle of treatment: nourish Kidney-Yin, clear Empty-Fire, calm the Mind.

Points: Taixi KI-3, Zhaohai KI-6, Rangu KI-2, Zhubin KI-9, Guanyuan Ren-4, Yingu KI-10, Sanyinjiao SP-6, Tongli HE-5, Lieque LU-7, Yuji LU-10.

Method: reinforcing on points to nourish Kidney-Yin (KI-3-6-9-10, Ren-4, SP-6) and reducing method on the others. Positively no moxa.

Explanation

KI-3 tonifies the Kidneys.

KI-6 and KI-10 tonify Kidney-Yin.

KI-9 tonifies Kidney-Yin and calms the Mind.

Ren-4 tonifies Kidney-Yin and calms the Mind.

KI-2 clears Empty-Fire from the Kidneys.

SP-6 tonifies Kidney-Yin and calms the Mind.

HE-5 and LU-7 are used to conduct Heat downwards away from the head (where it disturbs the Mind).

LU-10 clears Lung-Heat and is used if there are symptoms of Heat in the Lungs (dry cough, bloody sputum). It also conducts Heat downwards away from the head.

COMBINED PATTERNS

The Kidneys are the root of the Yin and Yang energies of the whole body. In chronic conditions the Kidneys are nearly always involved so that combined patterns of the Kidneys and other Yin organs appear frequently.

Kidney-Yin, in particular, is the foundation for the Liver and Heart, and Kidney-Yang is the foundation for the Spleen and Lungs:

Heart	Lungs
Liver	Spleen
KIDNEY-YIN	KIDNEY-YANG

The combined patterns discussed will be:

Kidney- and Liver-Yin deficiency

Kidney- and Heart-not harmonized

Kidney- and Lung-Yin deficiency

Kidney- and Spleen-Yang deficiency.

There are other possible combinations besides the above, i.e. Kidney and Lung Yang deficiency, and Kidney and Heart Yang deficiency. These patterns are basically the same as "Kidney-Yang deficient, Water overflowing to Lungs" and "Kidney-Yang deficient, Water overflowing to Heart" respectively.

KIDNEY- AND LIVER-YIN DEFICIENCY

Clinical manifestations

Sallow complexion, dull occipital or vertical headache, insomnia, dream-disturbed sleep, numbness of limbs, malar flush, dizziness, dry eyes, blurred vision, propensity to outburst of anger, soreness of the lower back, dry throat, tinnitus, night sweating, feeling of heat of palms and soles, difficult-dry stools, nocturnal emissions, scanty menstruation or amenorrhoea, delayed cycle, in women infertility.

Tongue: Red-Peeled, cracked.

Pulse: Floating-Empty or Choppy.

Key symptoms: dry eyes, dry throat, night sweating, scanty menstruation, Red-Peeled tongue.

Pathology

This pattern includes symptoms and signs of both Liver- and Kidney-Yin deficiency, bearing in mind that Liver-Yin deficiency embodies Liver-Blood deficiency. The Kidneys correspond to Water and should nourish the Liver, which corresponds to Wood. Thus the Yin and Blood of the Liver are dependent on the nourishment of Kidney-Yin and Kidney-Essence.

Dry eyes are a symptom of Liver-Yin deficiency, due to the Yin of the Liver being unable to moisten the eyes. Sallow complexion, dream-disturbed sleep, insomnia, numbness, blurred vision and scanty menstruation or amenorrhoea, are all symptoms of Liver-Blood deficiency which is part of Liver-Yin deficiency.

The headache is also due to Liver-Blood deficiency and would be either on the occiput (related to the Kidney) or on the vertex of the head (related to the Liver channel). When Liver-Yin is deficient, Liver-Yang may ascend, in which case the headache would be on the temples and be of a throbbing rather than dull character.

All the other symptoms are due to deficiency of Yin of the Kidneys and some Empty-Heat, all of which have already been explained.

The infertility in women would be due both to

deficient Liver-Blood failing to nourish the uterus, and to deficient Kidney-Essence unable to promote conception.

The pulse will be either Floating-Empty reflecting the Yin deficiency, or Choppy reflecting only a Blood deficiency, particularly in the beginning stages of the condition.

Aetiology

This is the same as for Kidney-Yin deficiency and Liver-Blood deficiency, but with the additional component of emotional problems due to anger, frustration and depression.

This pattern may also develop from Liver-Blood and Liver-Yin deficiency.

Treatment

Principle of treatment: nourish Liver and Kidney Yin.

Points: Taixi KI-3, Zhaohai KI-6, Ququan LIV-8, Guanyuan Ren-4, Shenshu BL-23, Pishu BL-20, Geshu BL-17, Ganshu BL-18, Tianzhu BL-10, Baihui Du-20.

Method: reinforcing, moxa could be applied on certain points.

Explanation

KI-3 tonifies the Kidneys.

KI-6 tonifies Kidney-Yin.

LIV-8 tonifies Liver-Blood and Liver-Yin.

Ren-4 tonifies Kidney-Yin and Kidney-Essence.

BL-23 and BL-20 tonify Blood.

BL-17 and BL-18 tonify Liver-Blood (direct moxa can be used on BL-17 to tonify Blood).

BL-10 can be used for occipital headache.

Du-20 can be used for vertical headache (moxa could be used if Liver-Blood deficiency predominates over Liver-Yin deficiency).

KIDNEY AND HEART NOT HARMONIZED

Clinical manifestations

Palpitations, mental restlessness, insomnia, poor memory, dizziness, tinnitus, deafness, soreness of the lower back, nocturnal emissions with dreams, fever or feeling of heat in the afternoon, night sweating, scanty-dark urine.

Tongue: Red-Peeled, tip redder, crack in the midline reaching the tip.

Pulse: Floating-Empty, Rapid.

Key symptoms: palpitations, insomnia, night sweating, Red-Peeled tongue with redder tip and midline crack.

Pathology

This is basically characterized by Kidney-Yin deficiency failing to nourish Heart-Yin which also becomes deficient. This leads to the flaring up of Heart Empty-Fire. In 5-Element terms, it corresponds to Water not flowing upwards to nourish and cool Fire (represented by the Heart). Water and Fire must assist each other: the Fire of the Heart must descend to warm the Kidneys, and the Water of the Kidneys must ascend to cool the Heart.

From a mental point of view, Essence is the foundation for the Mind. If Essence is deficient, the Mind suffers. Thus the relationship of mutual assistance between Kidneys and Heart finds expression also in the relationship between the Essence and the Mind.

When Kidney-Yin is weak and Heart-Yin is deficient, Empty-Fire flares within the Heart, resulting in mental restlessness, insomnia (waking up several times during the night), palpitations and a red tip of the tongue.

Poor memory, dizziness, tinnitus and deafness are all due to deficiency of Kidney-Yin failing to nourish the brain and open into the ear.

The fever or feeling of heat in the afternoon, dark urine, Red tongue and Rapid pulse are all due to the flaring of Empty-Heat within the Kidneys.

Aetiology

1) The same as for Kidney-Yin deficiency, with the additional component of emotional problems such as anxiety, sadness and depression. Emotional shocks and the ensuing sadness from break-

up of relationships are a common cause of Heart-Yin deficiency in this pattern.
2) This pattern can also develop from chronic Heart-Yin deficiency.

Treatment

Principle of treatment: nourish Kidney and Heart Yin, clear Heart Empty-Heat.

Points: Shenmen HE-7, Yinxi HE-6, Tongli HE-5, Yintang extra point, Xinshu BL-15, Jiuwei Ren-15, Benshen GB-13, Shenting Du-24, Taixi KI-3, Yingu KI-10, Zhubin KI-9, Guanyuan Ren-4, Neiguan P-6, Sanyinjiao SP-6.

Method: reinforcing on the points to nourish Kidney-Yin (KI-3-9-10, Ren-4, SP-6), reducing method on the points to clear Heart Empty-Heat (HE-5-6-7, BL-15, P-6), even method on the others (Yintang, Ren-15, GB-13, Du-24).

Explanation

HE-7 calms the Mind.

HE-5 clears Heart Empty-Heat and conducts Heat downwards away from the head.

HE-6 clears Empty-Heat and nourishes Heart-Yin (it is specific for night sweating combined with Fuliu KI-7).

Yintang calms the Mind.

G.B.-13 and Du-24 calm the Mind.

KI-3, KI-9 and KI-10 tonify Kidney-Yin. KI-9, in particular, calms the Mind.

Ren-15 calms the Mind and nourishes Heart-Yin.

P-6 calms the Mind.

Ren-4 nourishes Kidney-Yin and Kidney-Essence and conducts Heat downwards.

SP-6 tonifies Yin and calms the Mind.

KIDNEY- AND LUNG-YIN DEFICIENCY

Clinical manifestations

Dry cough which is worse in the evening, dry mouth, thin body, breathlessness on exertion, soreness of the lower back, weak limbs, fever or feeling of heat in the afternoon, night sweating, nocturnal emissions, 5-palm heat.

Tongue: Red-Peeled with two transversal cracks in the Lung area.

Pulse: Floating-Empty.

Key symptoms: dry cough, feeling of heat in the evening, night sweating, Red-Peeled tongue.

Pathology

This pattern is characterized by both Lung and Kidney Yin deficiency. It is not to be confused with the pattern of "Kidney failing to receive Qi" which is characterized by deficiency of Kidney-Yang and Lung-Qi.

The Yin deficiency leads to exhaustion of body fluids and ensuing dryness, hence the dry cough and dry mouth.

The breathlessness on exertion is caused by the failure of the Kidney in receiving and holding Qi.

This pattern only occurs in very chronic conditions and is therefore characterized by exhaustion of the body's Qi which causes weakness of the limbs and a thin body.

All the other symptoms are typical of Kidney-Yin deficiency (night sweating, nocturnal emissions, afternoon fever, 5-palm heat and Floating-Empty pulse).

Aetiology

1) All the same causes as for Kidney-Yin deficiency, with the additional component of worrying over a long period of time leading to injury of the Lung energy.
2) This pattern can also develop from a chronic condition of Lung-Yin deficiency.

Treatment

Principle of treatment: nourish Lung and Kidney Yin, increase body fluids.

Points: Taixi KI-3, Lieque LU-7 and Zhaohai KI-6 in combination, Gaohuangshu BL-43, Taiyuan LU-9, Zhongfu LU-1, Sanyinjiao SP-6, Guanyuan Ren-4.

Method: reinforcing, no moxa.

Explanation

KI-3 tonifies Kidney-Yin.

LU-7 and KI-6 in combination open the Directing Vessel, benefit the throat, stimulate the Kidney reception of Qi and tonify Lung and Kidney Yin.

BL-43 tonifies Lung-Yin and is specific for chronic conditions.

LU-9 tonifies Lung-Yin.

LU-1 tonifies Lung-Yin and stops cough.

SP-6 tonifies Kidney-Yin and promotes fluids.

Ren-4 tonifies Kidney-Yin and Essence.

KIDNEY- AND SPLEEN-YANG DEFICIENCY

Clinical manifestations

Physical weakness, mental listlessness, phlegm in throat, breathlessness, dislike to speak, desire to lie down, abdominal distension, poor appetite, aversion to cold, cold limbs, abundant-clear or scanty-clear urination, loose stools, diarrhoea at dawn, oedema of the abdomen and legs, feeling of cold in the back, chronic diarrhoea, borborygmi, diarrhoea like water, cold abdomen and legs.

Tongue: Pale, Swollen.

Pulse: Deep, Weak, Slow.

Key symptoms: chronic diarrhoea, chilliness, feeling of cold in the back, Deep-Weak-Slow pulse.

Pathology

This is always a chronic condition. It represents a stage further than Spleen-Yang deficiency, from which it usually develops.

The Spleen is the Root of Post-Heaven Qi and when it is deficient, it fails to nourish the muscles resulting in lack of strength. The general deficiency of Qi causes mental listlessness, dislike to speak and desire to lie down.

When Spleen-Yang is deficient it cannot transport nourishment to the limbs which will feel cold. Furthermore, the deficiency of Kidney-Yang implies a weakness of the Fire of the Gate of Vitality, which further contributes to the various cold symptoms (feeling of cold in back and legs).

Deficient Kidney-Yang cannot transform Water and fluids accumulate, hence the oedema and the abundant urination. In severe cases, the opposite could manifest as well, i.e. scanty urination. This happens when the Yang is so deficient that it cannot move the fluids at all.

Deficient Kidney-Yang fails to transform the fluids in the abdomen and to help the Spleen to transport and transform, resulting in chronic diarrhoea.

Aetiology

1) Same as for Kidney-Yang deficiency, with the additional component of excessive consumption of cold-raw foods.
2) This pattern can also develop from a chronic condition of Spleen-Yang deficiency.

Treatment

Principle of treatment: tonify and warm Spleen and Kidney-Yang.

Points: Taixi KI-3, Fuliu KI-7, Shenshu BL-23, Mingmen Du-4, Pishu BL-20, Weishu BL-21, Zusanli ST-36, Qihai Ren-6, Shangjuxu ST-37, Tianshu ST-25 , Dachangshu BL-25.

Method: reinforcing, moxa must be used.

Explanation

KI-3 tonifies the Kidneys.

KI-7 and BL-23 tonify Kidney-Yang.

Du-4 strengthens the Fire of the Gate of Vitality.

BL-20 and BL-21 tonify Spleen-Yang.

ST-36 tonifies the Spleen.

Ren-6 tonifies Qi in general and Yang if used with direct moxa. It is an important point for chronic diarrhoea.

ST-37 is the Lower-Sea point for the Large Intestine and is specific to stop chronic diarrhoea.

ST-25 stops diarrhoea.

BL-25 is the Back Transporting point for the Large Intestine and it stops diarrhoea.

NOTES

1 Classic of the Simple Girl, p 108.
2 Simple Questions, p 2: *"Nowadays . . . people have sex in a state of drunkenness...hence they barely reach the age of 50"*.
3 Ancient Chinese alchemists of the Daoist school searched for the elixir of immortality or longevity. Most of these prescriptions contained very hot, sometimes toxic, herbs to tonify the Gate of Vitality. These herbal pills became very popular during the Ming dynasty and some emperors actually died from an overdose of such preparations.

Stomach Patterns 26

胃腑病証

The main Stomach function is that of "rotting and ripening" food, i.e. transforming and digesting it so that the Spleen can separate the distilled food essences. It is therefore natural that all Stomach patterns involve some digestive symptoms.

The Stomach, together with the Spleen, occupies a central position in the Middle Burner and is at the centre of all Qi pathways of other organs, some of which are ascending and some descending. Stomach-Qi itself normally descends in order to send the digested food downwards, while Spleen-Qi ascends to direct Food-Qi upwards to the Lungs and Heart. Besides, Lung-Qi descends to communicate with the Kidneys and Bladder, Heart-Qi also descends to communicate with the Small Intestine and Kidneys, Kidney-Qi ascends to communicate with the Lungs and Heart and Liver-Qi flows harmoniously in all directions.

Because of this intricate crossing of Qi pathways in the Middle Burner, the Stomach occupies a strategic position and has a crucial role in ensuring the smooth flow of Qi in the Middle Burner. In disease, the Stomach is often affected by stagnation of Qi or retention of food.

The Stomach, with the Spleen, is the Root of the Post-Heaven Qi: this means that it is the source of all the Qi which is produced by the body after birth. If the Stomach is deficient, not enough Qi is produced by the body, and a person will experience tiredness and weakness which are very common Stomach symptoms.

Finally, it should be remembered that the Stomach is the origin of fluids as all the drink ingested has to be transformed and digested by it. It follows that the Stomach can be affected by Yin deficiency.

GENERAL AETIOLOGY

DIET

Diet is obviously the main cause of disease for the Stomach. This can be approached from many viewpoints concerning the nature of the food eaten, the regularity of eating times and the conditions of eating.

a) The nature of food eaten

This is a very complex subject which cannot be dealt here in depth, as the nature of the food eaten should take into account many variables such as the character of the food, the season, the constitution, state of health and occupation of the person.

Generally speaking, the Stomach prefers foods which are moist and not too dry (the Spleen prefers the opposite, i.e. foods which are dry). If the person eats foods which are too dry (such as baked and broiled foods), the Stomach may become dry and eventually suffer from Yin deficiency.

Besides this, the Stomach may suffer from excessive consumption of either too hot or too cold foods in terms of energy. Excessive consumption of hot foods may cause Heat in the Stomach. Of course, one cannot define in absolute terms what is an "excessive" consumption of these foods, as this is relative to the constitution of the person, the season and the occupation. If a person suffers from a deficiency of Yang, it is appropriate to eat more of the heating foods. These are also more appropriate in wintertime in cold countries. If the person is engaged in heavy physical work, it is also appropriate to eat more of the hot foods.

Excessive consumption of cold foods may cause Cold in the Stomach. Similarly to what was said for the hot foods, a heavier consumption of cold foods could be appropriate for someone suffering from excess of Heat, or living in a very hot country.

b) The regularity of meal times

The Chinese traditionally stress the importance of eating at regular times. This is because the body has a natural rhythm of flow of Qi in different organs at different times, and it would be inappropriate to eat at a time when Stomach-Qi is quiescent. The Stomach would obviously not be able to digest food properly. An advice to eat at regular times may sound very old-fashioned to some patients, but experience shows that irregular eating does produce Stomach disorders. It is therefore important to:

— have meals at regular times
— eat a proper breakfast (in some countries people have just a small cup of very strong coffee)
— not to over- or under-eat
— not to nibble
— not to eat late at night
— not to eat too fast.

Over-eating prevents the Stomach from digesting food properly, so that it stagnates in the Middle Burner and Stomach-Qi cannot descend.

Under-eating or a form of malnourishment due to too strict unsuitable diets leads to Stomach and Spleen deficiency.

Constant nibbling or eating too fast do not give the Stomach time to digest food properly and lead to retention of food.

Eating late at night, a time of Yin, forces the Stomach to use its Yin energy and leads to deficiency of Stomach-Yin.

c) The conditions of eating

Apart from the nature and amount of food eaten and the time at which it is eaten, the accompanying circumstances are also extremely important. One might eat the purest and most balanced food at absolutely regular times, but if this is eaten in a negative frame of mind, such as when one is very sad or worried, it will not do one any good.

The emotional frame of mind at meal times is important. If one eats while worrying about something (such as one's work), it will lead to stagnation of Qi in the Stomach. If meal time is a regular opportunity for family rows (as it sadly is in some cases), even the best of foods will not be digested and will cause retention of food in the Stomach and stagnation of Qi in the Middle Burner. Eating on the run, grabbing a quick bite during a short lunch-hour, also causes stagnation of Qi in the Stomach. Reading while eating leads to deficiency of Stomach-Qi.

EMOTIONS

The Stomach is mostly affected by worry and excessive thinking. Worry will cause stagnation of Qi in the Stomach and will manifest with a niggling, burning pain, belching and nausea.

Excessive mental work over a period of many years leads to deficiency of Stomach-Qi.

Anger also affects the Stomach, though only indirectly via the Liver. Anger, frustration and resentment cause stagnation of Liver-Qi which invades the Stomach resulting in nausea, belching or distending pain.

CLIMATE

The Stomach can be affected by climatic factors directly, in particular by Cold. Cold can invade the Stomach directly (by passing the Exterior layers of the body) and give rise to Interior Cold in the Stomach, with symptoms of sudden acute pain and vomiting.

The patterns discussed are:

- Deficiency patterns
  - Stomach-Qi deficiency
  - Stomach Deficient and Cold
  - Stomach-Yin deficiency
- Excess patterns
  - Stomach Fire (or Phlegm-Fire)
  - Cold invading the Stomach
  - Stomach-Qi rebelling upwards
  - Retention of Food in the Stomach
  - Stagnation of Blood in the Stomach.

STOMACH-QI DEFICIENCY

Clinical manifestations

Uncomfortable feeling in the epigastrium, no appetite, lack of taste sensation, loose stools, tiredness especially in the morning, weak limbs.

Tongue: Pale.

Pulse: Empty, especially on the right Middle position.

Key symptoms: tiredness in the morning, uncomfortable feeling in the epigastrium, Empty pulse on the Stomach position.

Pathology

The Stomach is the Root of Post-Heaven Qi and the beginning stage in the production of Qi from food: if the Stomach is weak, therefore, Qi will be deficient and all other organs will suffer. Tiredness will be the main symptom of Stomach deficiency. It will be worse in the mornings in correspondence with the peak of activity of the Stomach between 7 and 9 am.

Deficient Stomach-Qi will fail to descend, causing a vaguely uncomfortable feeling in the epigastrium, indicative of a Deficiency condition (if it was from an Excess condition, it would be a strong feeling of discomfort or pain).

When Stomach-Qi is deficient, Spleen-Qi is also often deficient as Stomach and Spleen are so closely intertwined. This results in lack of appetite, loose stools, lack of taste and a Pale tongue.

When Stomach-Qi is weak, it cannot transport the food essences to the limbs, resulting in a feeling of weakness of the limbs.

Aetiology

1) The most common cause of Stomach disharmonies is dietary. A diet lacking in nourishment and protein or plain under-eating (due to "dieting") can cause deficiency of Stomach-Qi.
2) Stomach-Qi deficiency can also arise as a consequence of a chronic disease which weakens Qi in general. For example, it is very common to see Stomach-Qi deficiency after a prolonged illness such as mononucleosis (glandular fever).

Treatment

Principle of treatment: tonify Stomach Qi.

Points: Zusanli ST-36, Zhongwan Ren-12, Weishu BL-21, Qihai Ren-6.

Method: reinforcing, moxa is applicable.

Explanation

ST-36 is the main point to tonify Stomach-Qi. Using moxa on the needle is especially effective.

Ren-12 tonifies Stomach and Spleen Qi.

BL-21 tonifies Stomach-Qi. It is an important point in case of extreme tiredness. Moxa is also applicable.

Ren-6 tonifies Qi in general, and is indicated

for chronic cases of Stomach-Qi deficiency, especially with loose stools.

STOMACH DEFICIENT AND COLD

Clinical manifestations

Discomfort or dull pain in the epigastrium which is worse after bowel movements, better after eating and better with pressure or massage, no appetite, preference for warm drinks and foods, vomiting of clear fluid, loose stools, no thirst, cold limbs, tiredness.

Tongue: Pale, Swollen.

Pulse: Deep, Weak, especially on the right Middle position.

Key symptoms: discomfort in the epigastrium which is better after eating, tiredness, cold limbs.

Pathology

This is similar to the previous pattern, with the addition of Empty-Cold. Normally this pattern is associated with Spleen-Yang deficiency which leads to internal Cold, resulting in cold limbs, loose stools, vomiting of clear fluids, no thirst, preference for warm drinks and foods and a Deep Pulse.

When Stomach-Qi is deficient, it may be made worse by the bowel movement (because of the relationship between Stomach and Large Intestine with the Bright Yang), hence the aggravation of the feeling of discomfort in the epigastrium after a bowel movement.

Because the discomfort is caused by a Deficiency condition, it is better with eating and better for pressure or massage.

Aetiology

1) From diet, through insufficient nourishment or protein. It may also be due to excessive consumption of cold foods and drinks, ice-creams, salads, fruit and iced drinks.
2) This pattern can be the consequence of a prolonged illness which damages the Yang of the Spleen and Stomach.
3) Exterior Cold can invade the Stomach, and if it is not expelled, after some time it will interfere with the Stomach function and cause Stomach-Qi deficiency.

Treatment

Principle of treatment: tonify and warm Stomach and Spleen Qi.

Points: Zusanli ST-36, Zhongwan Ren-12, Pishu BL-20, Weishu BL-21, Qihai Ren-6.

Method: reinforcing, moxa must be used.

Explanation

ST-36 tonifies Stomach-Qi.

Ren-12 tonifies Stomach and Spleen Qi.

BL-20 tonifies Spleen-Qi.

BL-21 tonifies Stomach-Qi.

Ren-6 tonifies Qi in general. Moxa on ginger can be used on this point: this is the best method for Empty-Cold in the Stomach.

STOMACH-YIN DEFICIENCY

Clinical manifestations

No appetite, fever or feeling of heat in the afternoon, constipation (dry stools), epigastric pain, dry mouth and throat especially in the afternoon, thirst but with no desire to drink or desire to drink in small sips, feeling of fullness after eating.

Tongue: Peeled in the centre, or with coating "without root" Red in the centre in Empty Heat.

Pulse: Floating-Empty on the right Middle position.

Key symptoms: epigastric pain, dry mouth, tongue Peeled in the centre or with rootless coating in the centre.

Pathology

The Stomach is the origin of fluids and when its Yin is deficient there will be dryness, causing dry stools, dry mouth and throat and thirst. The feeling of thirst in Stomach-Yin deficiency is peculiar in so far as there is "thirst but no desire to drink", as Chinese books usually put it. This apparently contradictory statement indicates that there is a thirst (or, rather than thirst, a dry mouth), but because it is not due to Heat, there is no desire to drink large amounts of cold water. Because the thirst is due to deficiency of Yin, the person likes to drink in small sips or sometimes even likes to drink warm liquids.

The fever or feeling of heat in the afternoon is due to deficiency of Yin.

The most significant sign of deficiency of Stomach-Yin is a tongue that is either Peeled or has a rootless coating in the centre (Stomach area). A coating without root is formed when the Stomach is weak and ceases to send its "dirty dampness" (which is normal by-product of its activity of rotting and ripening) up to the tongue: no new coating is being formed and the old coating therefore loses its root. A coating without root looks patchy, as if it had been sprinkled on top of the tongue, rather than arising out of the tongue surface, as the normal coating does. A coating with root cannot be scraped away while a coating without root can.

Aetiology

The most common cause of Stomach-Yin deficiency is an irregular diet and eating habits, mostly due to eating late at night, skipping meals, "grabbing a quick bite" during a short and hectic lunch-hour, worrying about work while eating, going straight back to work immediately after a meal. All these habits seriously deplete Stomach-Qi and, if they persist over a long period of time, they will begin to weaken Stomach-Yin. In particular, eating late at night depletes Stomach-Yin.

Treatment

Principle of treatment: nourish Stomach-Yin, nourish fluids.

Points: Zhongwan Ren-12, Zusanli ST-36, Sanyingiao SP-6, Taibai SP-3, Neiting ST-44.

Method: reinforcing (except on ST-44 which should be reduced), no moxa.

Explanation

Ren-12 tonifies Stomach-Yin.

ST-36 tonify Stomach-Qi and Stomach-Yin.

SP-6 tonifies Stomach-Yin and nourishes fluids.

SP-3 nourishes fluids.

ST-44 clears Stomach Empty-Heat.

STOMACH-FIRE (OR PHLEGM-FIRE)

Clinical manifestations

Burning sensation and pain in the epigastrium, thirst with desire to drink cold liquids, constant hunger, swelling and pain in the gums, bleeding gums, sour regurgitation, constipation, nausea, vomiting soon after eating and bad breath.

In case of Phlegm-Fire: feeling of oppression of epigastrium, less thirst, mucus in stools, mental derangement and insomnia.

Tongue: Red, thick-yellow-dry coating (in case of Phlegm-Fire: thick-yellow-sticky coating, or yellow prickles inside a midline crack).

Pulse: Full, Deep, Rapid (in case of Phlegm-Fire: Slippery, Full, Rapid).

Key symptoms: burning sensation epigastrium, thirst with desire to drink cold liquids, thick-yellow coating, Red tongue.

Pathology

This is a pattern of Interior Full-Heat in the Stomach. Heat in the Stomach burns the fluids, hence the intense thirst, constipation and dry tongue.

Heat makes the Blood extravasate in the Stomach channel resulting in bleeding from the gums. The swelling and pain in the gums is due to Heat rising in the Stomach channel.

Full-Heat obstructs the Stomach and interferes with the descending of Stomach-Qi, hence the sour regurgitation, nausea and vomiting. The fluid regurgitated is "sour" because the Heat ferments the Stomach fluids.

In case of Phlegm-Fire, Phlegm is more obstructive, causing the feeling of oppression of the epigastrium. There is less thirst because the presence of Phlegm dampens the thirst.

Phlegm and Fire in the Stomach can affect the Mind and cause insomnia or severe mental symptoms such as manic-depression. This is often reflected in the tongue with a large midline crack not reaching the tip with yellow stiff coating (prickles) inside it.

Aetiology

This pattern can be due to excessive consumption of hot foods in the sense described above and to smoking (tobacco has a hot energy). In case of Phlegm-Fire, it is caused by excessive consumption of hot-greasy foods, such as deep-fried foods.

Treatment

Principle of treatment: clear Stomach-Heat, stimulate the Stomach descending function.

Points: Liangmen ST-21, Shangwan Ren-13, Neiting ST-44, Lidui ST-45, Sanyinjiao SP-6, Zhongwan Ren-12, Neiguan P-6.

Method: reducing method, except on Ren-12 and Ren-13 on which even method should be used.

Explanation

ST-21 clears Stomach Heat and stimulates the descending of Stomach-Qi.

Ren-13 subdues rebellious Stomach-Qi.

ST-44 clears Stomach-Heat.

ST-45 clears Stomach Heat and calms the Mind.

SP-6 will nourish the fluids and calm the Mind.

Ren-12 clears Stomach-Heat.

P-6 subdues rebellious Stomach-Qi and calms the Mind.

Case history

A woman of 60 lost her sense of smell and taste two years previously. For the past 10 years, she also suffered from epigastric pain, a sensation of "knot" in the stomach and nausea. She was often very thirsty and drank large amounts of water every day. Occasionally she experienced bleeding of the gums. She also complained of a lack of appetite and loose stools. Her pulse was Full and Wiry especially on the right Middle position, and her tongue was red in the centre and had a dry yellow coating.

This patient suffered from Stomach Full-Heat ("knot" in the stomach, thirst and bleeding gums) and Deficiency of Spleen-Qi (lack of appetite and loose stools). The loss of taste and smell is due to Spleen deficiency, but also to Stomach-Heat "burning" upwards.

COLD INVADING THE STOMACH

Clinical manifestations

Sudden pain in the epigastrium, feeling cold, preference for warmth, vomiting of clear fluid, feeling worse after swallowing cold fluids which are quickly vomited, preference for warm liquids.

Tongue: thick-white coating.

Pulse: Deep, Slow, Tight.

Key symptoms: sudden pain in epigastrium, vomiting, feeling cold, Deep-Tight Pulse.

Pathology

This is a pattern of Interior Full-Cold. It is an acute pattern caused by the invasion of the Stomach by exterior Cold. The Stomach is one of three organs (with Intestines and Uterus) that can be attacked by exterior Cold directly, bypassing the exterior layers of the body.

Exterior Cold blocks the Stomach and prevents Stomach-Qi from descending, hence the vomiting and the pain.

Cold impairs the Yang of the Stomach and Spleen and prevents the food essences from reaching the body, hence the feeling of cold, Slow pulse, preference for warm liquids, and aggravation from cold liquids.

Aetiology

This is caused by invasion of the Stomach by exterior Cold, due to exposure to cold and excessive consumption of cold foods and iced drinks.

Treatment

Principle of treatment: expel Cold, warm the Stomach, stimulate the descending of Stomach-Qi.

Points: Liangmen ST-21, Gongsun SP-4, Shangwan Ren-13, Liangqiu ST-34.

Method: reducing method, moxa can be used in conjunction with needling (not on its own).

Explanation

ST-21 expels Stomach-Cold if used with moxa after needling.

SP-4 expels Stomach-Cold, stimulates the descending of Stomach-Qi, clears obstruction from the Stomach.

Ren-13 stimulates the descending of Stomach-Qi.

ST-34 is the Accumulation point and therefore suitable for acute and painful patterns. It will clear obstructions from the Stomach and stop pain.

STOMACH-QI REBELLING UPWARDS

Clinical manifestations

Nausea, belching, vomiting, hiccup.

Tongue: no changes.

Pulse: Tight on right Middle position.

Pathology

This pattern is an expression of the impairment of the Stomach descending function. It is frequently not a pattern appearing on its own, but accompanying other patterns, such as Stomach-Fire or Cold invading the Stomach.

All the symptoms are caused by the failure of Stomach-Qi to descend and rebelling upwards instead.

Aetiology

This is often due to emotional problems such as anxiety and worry, which interfere with the descending of Stomach-Qi.

Treatment

Principle of treatment: subdue rebellious Qi, stimulate the descending of Stomach-Qi.

Points: Shangwan Ren-13, Xiawan Ren-10, Neiguan P-6, Gongsun SP-4.

Method: reducing.

Explanation

Ren-13 subdues rebellious Stomach-Qi.

Ren-10 stimulates the descending of Stomach-Qi.

P-6 and SP-4 stimulate the descending of Stomach-Qi.

RETENTION OF FOOD IN THE STOMACH

Clinical manifestations

No appetite, fullness and distension of the epigastrium which are relieved by vomiting, nausea, vomiting, foul breath, sour regurgitation, belching, insomnia.

Tongue: thick coating (which could be white or yellow).

Pulse: Full, Slippery.

Key symptoms: epigastric fullness, sour regurgitation, thick coating.

Pathology

This is an Interior Excess pattern. It could be associated either with Cold or Heat, in which case the tongue coating would be white or yellow respectively.

Most of the symptoms are caused by the obstruction of food in the Stomach, preventing Stomach-Qi from descending, hence the nausea, vomiting, feeling of fullness, belching and sour regurgitation.

The foul breath is due to the fermentation of food in the Stomach for too long.

The prolonged retention of food in the stomach creates an obstruction in the Middle Burner and prevents Heart-Qi from descending. This causes the Mind to be disturbed at night resulting in insomnia.

The Slippery pulse indicates the presence of undigested food.

Aetiology

This pattern could be simply due to overeating. It can also be due to eating too quickly, or eating in a hurry or worrying while eating.

Treatment

Principle or treatment: remove retention of food, stimulate the descending of Stomach-Qi.

Points: Shangwan Ren-13, Xiawan Ren-10, Liangmen ST-21, Neiting ST-44, Lidui ST-45, Gongsun SP-4, Neiguan P-6.

Method: reducing.

Explanation

Ren-13 subdues rebellious Stomach-Qi.

Ren-10 stimulates the descending of Stomach-Qi.

ST-21 stimulates the descending of Stomach-Qi and resolves stagnant food.

ST-44 resolves stagnant food and clears Heat.

ST-45 resolves stagnant food and calms the Mind (if there is insomnia).

SP-4 resolves stagnant food.

P-6 stimulates the descending of Stomach-Qi.

STASIS OF BLOOD IN THE STOMACH

Clinical manifestations

Stabbing pain in the epigastrium which is worse with heat and pressure, pain after eating, vomiting of dark blood, blood in the stools.

Tongue: Purple with purple spots. It could be Purple only in the centre.

Pulse: Wiry or Choppy.

Key symptoms: stabbing pain in the epigastrium, vomiting of dark blood.

Pathology

Stasis of Blood always causes pain of a stabbing or boring nature, hence the stabbing epigastric pain. This pain is much more intense than in any of the other Stomach patterns.

Stasis of Blood always manifests with dark-coloured blood, hence the vomiting of dark blood.

Since the Stomach is related to the Large Intestine, the stasis of Blood extends to it and is manifested with blood in the stools.

The Purple tongue reflects the stasis of Blood.

Aetiology

This is always a chronic condition, resulting from various causes. It may be associated with, or be the result of other Stomach patterns, particularly Stomach-Fire, Retention of Food in the Stomach, and Liver-Qi invading the Stomach. Any of the causes indicated for these patterns can therefore cause stasis of Blood in the Stomach.

In addition to this, stasis of Blood is often the result of stagnation of Qi, particularly of the Liver, over a long period of time. This is usually due to long-standing emotional problems such as anger, frustration, resentment and depression.

Treatment

Principle of treatment: remove stasis, revive Blood, stimulate the descending of Stomach-Qi.

Points: Xiawan Ren-10, Liangmen ST-21, Liangqiu ST-34, Xuehai SP-10, Geshu BL-17, Ganshu BL-18.

Method: reducing, no moxa.

Explanation

Ren-10 stimulates the descending of Stomach-Qi.

ST-21 removes obstructions.

ST-34, Accumulation point, moves Qi and Blood in the channel.

SP-10 revives Blood, removes stagnation.

BL-17 (with needle, no moxa) removes stasis and revives Blood.

BL-18 removes stagnation of Liver-Blood.

Small Intestine Patterns 27

小腸腑病証

The main function of the Small Intestine is that of receiving and transforming food by separating a clean from a dirty part. It has an important function in relation to fluids movement as it separates clean from dirty fluids. To explete this function, the Small Intestine is in direct communication with the Bladder, helping the Bladder function of Qi transformation.

The Small Intestine transforms food in coordination with the Spleen, whilst it transforms fluids in coordination with Kidney-Yang. In both cases, the Small Intestine's role is subordinate to that of the Spleen and Kidney-Yang. For this reason, most of the Small Intestine patterns are different manifestations of Spleen or Kidney-Yang patterns.

GENERAL AETIOLOGY

DIET

The Small Intestine is easily and readily affected by the type and "temperature" of food eaten. An excessive consumption of cold and raw foods can create Cold in the Small Intestine, whilst an excessive consumption of hot foods can create Heat.

EMOTIONS

The Small Intestine is affected by sadness which grips a person and destroys the mental clarity and capacity of sound judgement for which this organ is responsible.

The patterns discussed are:

- Excess patterns
  - Full-Heat in the Small Intestine
  - Small Intestine Qi Pain
  - Small Intestine Qi Tied
  - Infestation of worms in the Small Intestine
- Deficiency patterns
  - Small Intestine Deficient and Cold.

FULL-HEAT IN THE SMALL INTESTINE

Clinical manifestations

Mental restlessness, tongue ulcers, pain in the throat, deafness, uncomfortable feeling and heat sensation in the chest, abdominal pain, thirst, scanty and dark urine, painful urination, blood in urine.

Tongue: Red with redder and swollen tip, yellow coating.

Pulse: Rapid, Overflowing, especially in the Front position.

Key symptoms: abdominal pain, tongue ulcers, scanty-dark-painful urination.

Pathology

This pattern is closely associated with blazing of Heart-Fire and from the 8-Principle point of view it is a pattern of Interior Full-Heat.

Fire in the Heart causes the mental restlessness, tongue ulcers, pain in the throat and thirst.

Heart-Fire is transmitted to the Small Intestine with which the Heart is interiorly-exteriorly related, it interferes with the Small Intestine function of separating fluids in the Lower Burner and burns the fluids causing scanty and dark urine and pain on urination. In severe cases of Heat, this may cause the Blood to extravasate resulting in blood in the urine.

Deafness is caused by obstruction of Fire in the Small Intestine channel (which enters the ear).

The tongue reflects Full-Heat as it is Red with a coating; the tip may be redder and swollen reflecting Heart-Fire.

The pulse is Rapid because of the Heat and Overflowing because of the Heart-Fire.

Aetiology

This pattern is caused by emotional problems such as great anxiety over a long period of time, in particular related to the person's life pressures and direction of life. This type of pattern is also seen frequently in manic behaviour, in people who are driven by an unstoppable desire to undertake several different projects and push themselves very hard in many different directions with great dissipation of energy. If this energy can be harnessed with the help of acupuncture treatment, these persons can be very creative, productive, imaginative and usually artistic.

Treatment

Principle of treatment: clear Heart and Small Intestine Fire.

Points: Qiangu S.I.-2, Yanggu S.I.-5, Tongli HE-5, Shaofu HE-8, Xiajuxu ST-39.

Method: reducing, no moxa.

Explanation

S.I.-2 clears Small Intestine Heat.

S.I.-5 also clears Heat in the Small Intestine and it calms the Mind. This point is also very effective in helping the person to gain clarity and a sense of direction in life.

ST-39 is the Lower Sea point for the Small Intestine and it stops abdominal pain.

HE-5 and HE-8 clear Heart-Fire.

SMALL INTESTINE QI PAIN

Clinical manifestations

Lower abdominal twisting pain which may extend to back, abdominal distension, dislike of pressure on abdomen, borborygmi, flatulence, abdominal pain relieved by emission of wind, pain in the testis.

Tongue: white coating.

Pulse: Deep, Wiry, especially on the Rear positions.

Key symptoms: lower abdominal twisting pain, borborygmi, Deep-Wiry pulse.

Pathology

This is due to stagnation of Qi in the Small Intestine, and is usually associated with stagnation of Liver-Qi invading the Spleen. It can be an acute or chronic condition. If it is acute, it is a totally Excess condition, if it is chronic, it is an Excess/Deficiency condition characterized by Excess of Liver-Qi (stagnation) and Deficiency of Spleen-Qi.

All the symptoms and signs are due to stagnation of Qi in the Small Intestine and Liver, preventing the smooth flow of Liver-Qi and the transformation of fluids by the Small Intestine. Stagnation of Qi causes a distending pain, hence the twisting abdominal pain with distension. The person dislikes pressure on the abdomen as this aggravates the obstruction from stagnation of Qi.

The Deep and Wiry pulse reflects the obstruction of Qi in the Interior.

Aetiology

This pattern can be caused by excessive consumption of cold and raw foods which interfere with the Small Intestine transformation function. In addition, it is also caused by any of the factors which induce Liver-Qi stagnation, i.e. anger, frustration and resentment.

Treatment

Principle of treatment: move Qi in the Lower Burner, harmonize the Liver.

Points: Qihai Ren-6, Yanglingquan G.B.-34, Zhangmen LIV-13, Daju ST-27, Guilai ST-29, Sanyinjiao SP-6, Taichong LIV-3, Xiajuxu ST-39.

Method: reducing, moxa can be used if there are some Cold signs.

Explanation

Ren-6 in combination with G.B.-34 moves Qi in the Lower Burner and relieves pain.

LIV-13 harmonizes the Liver and tonifies the Spleen. This point would be used particularly in chronic patterns.

ST-27 and ST-29 move Qi in the lower abdomen, stimulate the Small Intestine functions and stop abdominal pain.

SP-6 stops abdominal pain.

LIV-3 relieves stagnation of Liver-Qi.

ST-39 is the Lower Sea point of the Small Intestine and is specific to stop abdominal pain.

SMALL INTESTINE QI TIED

Clinical manifestations

Violent abdominal pain, dislike of pressure, abdominal distension, constipation, vomiting, borborygmi, flatulence.

Tongue: thick white coating.

Pulse: Deep, Wiry.

Key symptoms: sudden violent abdominal pain, constipation, vomiting, Deep-Wiry pulse.

Pathology

This pattern is very similar to the previous one and it differs in so far as it is always an acute pattern.

It is characterized by great obstruction and stagnation in the Small Intestine, hence the sudden, violent pain and constipation.

The obstruction in the Small Intestine is such that it interferes with the Stomach descending function and causes vomiting.

From a Western point of view, it resembles an acute attack of appendicitis. However, it can occur without appendicitis.

Aetiology

This pattern can be caused by excessive consumption of cold and raw foods which completely block the transformation function of the Small Intestine.

Treatment

Principle of treatment: remove obstruction from the Lower Burner, move Qi of Small Intestine.

Points: Xiajuxu ST-39, Lanweixue extra point, Qihai Ren-6, Yanglingquan G.B.-34, Tianshu ST-25, Sanyinjiao SP-6, Taichong LIV-3.

Method: reducing, electrical stimulation is applicable.

Explanation

ST-39 stops abdominal pain and moves Small Intestine Qi.

Lanweixue is in between Shangjuxu ST-37 and Zusanli ST-36 and corresponds to the appendix.

This point is therefore used if it is tender (one selects the most tender spot between ST-36 and ST-37) and appendicitis is suspected.

Ren-6 and G.B.-34 see above.

ST-25 stops abdominal pain.

SP-6 stops abdominal pain.

LIV-3 stops abdominal pain and spasms and promotes the smooth flow of Liver-Qi.

INFESTATION OF WORMS IN THE SMALL INTESTINE

Clinical manifestations

Abdominal pain and distension, bad taste in mouth, sallow complexion.

Roundworms (ascarid): abdominal pain, vomiting of round worms, cold limbs.

Hookworms: desire to eat strange objects such as soil, wax, uncooked rice or tea leaves.

Pinworms: itchy anus, worse in the evening.

Tapeworms: constant hunger.

Pathology

This obviously consists in obstruction of the Small Intestine by worms, which causes abdominal pain, and in the malnourishment following from worm infestation. According to Chinese Medicine, infestation by worms is thought to be caused by a Cold condition of the Spleen and Intestines which allows the worms to thrive.

Aetiology

A Cold condition of Spleen and Intestines deriving from excessive consumption of cold and raw foods.

Treatment

Acupuncture is not applicable in this case and herbal treatment is the treatment of choice.

SMALL INTESTINE DEFICIENT AND COLD

Clinical manifestations

Abdominal pain, desire for hot drinks and pressure on abdomen, borborygmi, diarrhoea, pale and abundant urination.

Tongue: Pale, white coating.

Pulse: Deep, Slow, Weak.

Key symptoms: abdominal pain, borborygmi, diarrhoea.

Pathology

From the 8-Principle point of view, this is an Interior pattern of Deficiency and Cold. It is usually associated with Deficiency of Spleen-Yang, and it is often hard to distinguish these two patterns. The main symptom of Small Intestine involvement is borborygmi.

All the other symptoms are basically due to an impairment of the Spleen function of transformation and transportation and the Small Intestine function of receiving and transforming resulting in diarrhoea.

The deficiency of Yang of the Spleen results in interior Cold, hence the desire for hot drinks, pale urine, Pale tongue, white coating and Deep and Slow pulse.

The abdominal pain is also caused by the obstruction of Cold in the Intestines.

Aetiology

This pattern is caused by excessive consumption of cold and raw foods.

Treatment

Principle of treatment: warm and tonify Small Intestine and Spleen, expel Interior Cold.

Points: Qihai Ren-6, Tianshu ST-25, Xiajuxu ST-39, Zusanli ST-36, Pishu BL-20, Xiaochangshu BL-27.

Method: reinforcing, moxa should be used.

Explanation

Ren-6 with moxa tonifies Yang and stops diarrhoea.

ST-25 stops diarrhoea and abdominal pain.

ST-39 stops abdominal pain.

ST-36 tonifies Spleen-Yang (with moxa).

BL-20 tonifies Spleen-Qi.

BL-27, Back Transporting point for the Small Intestine, tonifies the Small Intestine.

Large Intestine Patterns 28

大腸腑病証

The main function of the Large Intestine is to receive food from the Small Intestine, absorb fluids and excrete stools.

It is therefore obvious that all the Large Intestine patterns have to do with disturbances of bowel movements.

GENERAL AETIOLOGY

EXTERIOR PATHOGENIC FACTORS

The Large Intestine can be invaded by exterior Cold directly (by passing the exterior layers of the body). This results from exposure to excessive cold over a prolonged period of time, or to normal seasonal cold but without adequate clothing. Cold dampness penetrates from ground level and works its way up to the Lower Burner where it can enter the Large Intestine and cause abdominal pain and diarrhoea.

Many cases of lower abdominal pain are due to interior Cold resulting from the invasion of exterior Cold.

EMOTIONS

The Large Intestine is exteriorly-interiorly related to the Lungs and is equally affected by sadness and worry. Worry depletes Lung-Qi which fails to descend and to help the Large Intestine in its functions. This results in stagnation of Qi in the Large Intestine, with the ensuing symptoms of spastic abdominal pain and constipation with bitty stools alternating with diarrhoea.

DIET

Diet obviously affects the Large Intestine directly. Excessive consumption of cold and raw food can give rise to interior Cold and ensuing diarrhoea.

On the other hand, excessive consumption of greasy and hot foods can give rise to Damp-Heat in the Large Intestine.

The patterns discussed are:
Excess patterns
Damp-Heat in the Large Intestine
Heat in the Large Intestine
Heat obstructing the Large Intestine
Cold invading the Large Intestine
Deficiency patterns
Large Intestine Dry
Collapse of Large Intestine
Large Intestine Cold.

DAMP-HEAT IN THE LARGE INTESTINE

Clinical manifestations

Abdominal pain, diarrhoea, mucus and blood in stools, offensive odour of stools, burning in anus, scanty-dark urine, fever, sweating (which does not decrease the fever), thirst without desire to drink, feeling of heaviness of the body and limbs, stuffiness of chest and epigastrium.

Tongue: Red, sticky-yellow coating.

Pulse: Slippery, Rapid.

Key symptoms: abdominal pain, diarrhoea with mucus and blood in the stools.

Pathology

The retention of Dampness in the Large Intestine interferes with its function of absorbing fluids and excreting stools, hence fluids are not absorbed and diarrhoea results. The mucus in the stools is indicative of Dampness. The blood in the stools is due to Heat in the Large Intestine making the blood come out of the vessels.

Stools with fetid odour, burning in the anus, thirst, dark urine, fever, Red tongue and Rapid pulse are all indicative of Heat.

The feeling of heaviness, stuffiness of chest and epigastrium, sticky tongue coating, and Slippery pulse, are all indicative of Dampness.

Aetiology

This pattern can be caused by excessive consumption of hot and greasy foods, with the additional component of emotional problems such as anxiety and worry over a long period of time, causing interior Heat.

Treatment

Principle of treatment: clear Heat, resolve Damp, stop diarrhoea.

Points: Yinlingquan SP-9, Sanyinjiao SP-6, Zhongji Ren-3, Sanjiaoshu BL-22, Tianshu ST-25, Dachangshu BL-25, Geshu BL-17, Zhongwan Ren-12, Quchi L.I.-11, Shangjuxu ST-37, Pishu BL-20.

Method: reducing, no moxa.

Explanation

SP-9 and SP-6 resolve Dampness from the Lower Burner.

Ren-3 and BL-22 resolve Dampness from the Lower Burner.

ST-25 is the Front Collecting point of the Large Intestine and stops diarrhoea.

BL-17 stops bleeding.

Ren-12 resolves Dampness.

L.I.-11 clears Heat.

ST-37 is the Lower Sea point for the Large Intestine and stops diarrhoea.

BL-20 tonifies the Spleen to resolve Dampness.

BL-25 is the Back-Transporting point of the Large Intestine and it clears Heat.

Case history

A 45-year old man complained of chronic diarrhoea with mucus in the stools, abdominal pain, flatulence and irritability. His pulse was Wiry, Full and slightly Slippery. His tongue was Red with a sticky yellow coating which was thicker on the root. This condition had been diagnosed as Crohn's disease in Western medical terms.

This is a case of Damp-Heat in the Large Intestine with a background of Liver-Fire (as shown by the Wiry pulse, Red tongue and irritability). This shows how the Yang organ patterns are often accompanied or caused by Yin organ patterns. It also worth noting how there is no direct correspondence between Western medical disease entities and the organ patterns of Chinese Medicine. In fact, this condition affected the Small Intestine from a Western medical viewpoint, but the Large Intestine from a Chinese medical viewpoint.

HEAT IN THE LARGE INTESTINE

Clinical manifestations

Constipation with dry stools, burning sensation in the mouth, dry tongue, burning and swelling in anus, scanty-dark urine.

Tongue: thick-yellow (or brown or black) dry coating.

Pulse: Full, Rapid.

Key symptoms: dry stools, burning sensation in anus, thick-yellow-dry coating.

Pathology

This is an Excess pattern with Full-Heat and dryness. The dryness derives not from Deficiency, but is a result of the burning action of Full-Heat on the body fluids.

All the symptoms reflect Full-Heat in the Large Intestine: dry stools, burning and swelling of anus, thick-yellow-dry coating and a Rapid pulse.

The Large Intestine is closely related to the Stomach (within the Bright Yang) and there is also Heat in the Stomach resulting in dry mouth and tongue.

The Heat in the Lower Burner makes the urine more concentrated and scanty, hence its dark colour.

Aetiology

This pattern is caused by the excessive consumption of hot foods (such as lamb, beef and alcohol) and "dry" foods, such as broiled or baked meats.

Treatment

Principle of treatment: clear Heat in the Large Intestine and Stomach, promote Body Fluids.

Points: Guanyuan Ren-4, Quchi L.I.-11, Shangjuxu ST-37, Neiting ST-44, Erjian L.I.-2, Sanyinjiao SP-6, Zhaohai KI-6, Zhongwan Ren-12.

Method: reducing method for points to clear Heat, tonifying method for points to promote fluids (Ren-4, SP-6, Ren-12, KI-6). Positively no moxa.

Explanation

Ren-4 tonifies Yin and therefore fluids.

L.I.-11 clears Heat in the Large Intestine.

ST-37 is the Lower-Sea point for the Large Intestine and is good for chronic conditions of this organ.

ST-44 clears Stomach Heat.

L.I.-2 clears Heat in Large Intestine.

SP-6, KI-6 and Ren-12 promote Body Fluids.

HEAT OBSTRUCTING THE LARGE INTESTINE

Clinical manifestations

Constipation, burning in anus, abdominal distension and pain which is worse with pressure, high fever or tidal fever, sweating especially on limbs, vomiting, thirst, delirium.

Tongue: thick-dry-yellow (or brown-black) coating, Red body

Pulse: Deep, Full, Big.

Key symptoms: constipation, abdominal pain, fever, thick-dry-yellow coating, Big pulse.

Pathology

From the 8-Principle perspective, this pattern is not different from the previous one, as it is also an interior pattern with Full Heat. It differs from the previous one in so far as it is an acute pattern appearing during febrile diseases. It is seen at the Bright Yang stage of the 6-Stage patterns (see App. 1), the Qi level of the 4-Level patterns (see App. 2) and the Middle Burner stage of the 3-Burner patterns (see App. 3).

Heat in the Large Intestine causes constipation, abdominal pain and burning in the anus. Heat in the Large Intestine is transmitted to the Stomach and causes thirst and a thick-dry-yellow coating on the tongue.

Heat in the Stomach and Large Intestine vaporizes the body fluids and causes profuse sweating. Heat in the Stomach interferes with the Stomach descending function and causes vomiting.

Extreme Heat can mist the Mind and cause delirium. A Big and Deep pulse is typical of Interior Heat in Stomach.

Aetiology

This is an acute pattern seen at the middle stage

of febrile diseases caused by exterior Wind-Cold or Wind-Heat.

Treatment

Principle of treatment: clear Heat in Stomach and Large Intestine, promote bowel movement.

Points: Quchi L.I.-11, Hegu L.I.-4, Daheng SP-15, Zhigou T.B.-6, Sanyinjiao SP-6, Erjian L.I.-2, Neiting ST-44, Tianshu ST-25.

Method: reducing, no moxa.

Explanation

L.I.-11 clears Heat in the Large Intestine.

L.I.-4 clears Large Intestine Heat and promotes bowel movement.

SP-15 promotes bowel movement.

T.B.-6 clears Heat in the Intestines and promotes bowel movement.

SP-6 nourishes Yin and stops abdominal pain.

L.I.-2 clears Large Intestine Heat.

ST-44 clears Stomach Heat.

ST-25 clears Large Intestine Heat.

COLD INVADING THE LARGE INTESTINE

Clinical manifestations

Sudden abdominal pain, diarrhoea with pain, feeling of cold, cold sensation in abdomen.

Tongue: thick-white coating.

Pulse: Deep, Wiry.

Key symptoms: sudden abdominal pain, diarrhoea, feeling of cold.

Pathology

This is an acute pattern caused by invasion of exterior Cold in the Large Intestine. Even though the Cold is of exterior origin, it invades the Interior immediately, by-passing the skin outer energetic layers and settling in the Large Intestine. The Large Intestine (together with Uterus and Stomach) is one of three organs which can be invaded by exterior Cold directly.

Cold in the Large Intestine interferes with the movement of Qi in the Lower Burner and causes sudden stagnation of Qi, resulting in the sudden pain which is severe and "twisting" in character.

Cold also interferes with the Large Intestine function of absorption of fluids, hence the diarrhoea.

The thick coating reflects a sudden invasion of a pathogenic factor and the Deep and Wiry pulse suggests that the pathogenic factor is in the Interior.

Aetiology

This is due to invasion of exterior Cold in the Large Intestine which can take place if the person sits on cold and wet surfaces for prolonged periods or is exposed to very cold weather having the abdomen insufficiently covered.

Treatment

Principle of treatment: expel Cold from the Large Intestine, warm the Lower Burner.

Points: Shangjuxu ST-37, Tianshu ST-25, Zusanli ST-36, Sanyinjiao SP-6, Taichong LIV-3, Daju ST-27.

Method: reducing, moxa is applicable after needling.

Explanation

ST-37 is the Lower-Sea point of the Large Intestine and it stops diarrhoea and pain.

ST-25 is the Front Collecting point of the Large Intestine and it stops diarrhoea and pain.

ST-36 can expel Cold from the Large Intestine.

SP-6 calms abdominal pain.

LIV-3 moves Qi in the Lower Burner and calms spasms (in this case of the intestines).

ST-27 expels Cold from the Large Intestine.

LARGE INTESTINE DRY

Clinical manifestations

Dry stools which are difficult to discharge, dry mouth and throat, thin body.

Tongue: dry, either Pale or Red without coating.

Pulse: Fine.

Key symptoms: dry stools which are difficult to discharge, thin body.

Pathology

This pattern is characterized by exhaustion of fluids in the Large Intestine. It seldom arises independently, but it accompanies other patterns, particularly Blood or Yin Deficiency.

All the symptoms are simply due to a state of dryness in Large Intestine and Stomach.

The tongue will be Pale if this condition is due to Blood deficiency, or Red and peeled if due to Yin deficiency (usually of the Kidneys).

This condition is more common in old people and often in those with a thin body, which indicates Yin deficiency. It can also frequently be seen in women after childbirth with heavy loss of blood, as this induces an exhaustion of Body Fluids (of which Blood is part).

Aetiology

This is due either to Blood or Yin deficiency. Therefore any of the causes of these two conditions can cause dryness in the Large Intestine. In some countries with very dry and warm weather, it could arise by itself.

Treatment

Principle of treatment: promote fluids in the Large Intestine.

Points: Zusanli ST-36, Sanyinjiao SP-6, Zhaohai KI-6, Guanyuan Ren-4.

Method: reinforcing.

Explanation

ST-36 can promote fluids in Stomach and Large Intestine.

SP-6 and Ren-4 tonify Yin and promote fluids.

KI-6 tonifies Yin and promotes fluids and is particularly indicated to moisten the stools.

COLLAPSE OF LARGE INTESTINE

Clinical manifestations

Chronic diarrhoea, prolapse ani, haemorrhoids, tiredness after bowel movements, cold limbs, no appetite, mental exhaustion, desire to drink warm liquids, desire to have the abdomen massaged.

Tongue: Pale.

Pulse: Fine, Weak, Deep.

Key symptoms: chronic diarrhoea, prolapse ani.

Pathology

This is due to chronic deficiency of Qi of the Spleen, Stomach and Large Intestine, with sinking of Spleen-Qi.

Sinking of Spleen-Qi causes the prolapse ani and chronic diarrhoea.

The deficiency of Stomach and Spleen Qi and Yang causes lack of appetite, cold limbs and desire to drink warm liquids. The desire to have the abdomen massaged and the tiredness after bowel movements indicate a Deficiency pattern.

Aetiology

This can be caused by any of the causes of Spleen and Stomach deficiency.

Treatment

Principle of treatment: tonify Stomach and Spleen, raise Qi.

Points: Qihai Ren-6, Tianshu ST-25, Zusanli ST-36, Taibai SP-3, Pishu BL-20, Weishu BL-21, Baihui Du-20.

Method: reinforcing, moxa is applicable.

Explanation

Ren-6 tonifies and raises Qi.

ST-25 tonifies Large Intestine and stops diarrhoea. The warm box could be used on Qihai Ren-6 and Tianshu ST-25.

ST-36 tonifies Stomach and Spleen Qi.

SP-3 tonifies Spleen-Qi.

BL-20 and BL-21 tonify Spleen and Stomach.

Du-20 with direct moxa, raises Qi and is used for prolapse ani.

LARGE INTESTINE COLD

Clinical manifestations

Loose stools like duck droppings, dull abdominal pain, borborygmi, pale urine, cold limbs.

Tongue: Pale.

Pulse: Deep, Fine.

Key symptoms: loose stools, cold limbs, Fine pulse.

Pathology

This is an interior pattern with Deficient Cold, and it is basically the same as Spleen-Yang deficiency.

Aetiology

This pattern can be caused by excessive consumption of cold and raw foods and by chronic exposure to cold weather on the abdomen.

Treatment

Principle of treatment: tonify and warm Large Intestine and Spleen.

Points: Tianshu ST-25, Qihai Ren-6, Zusanli ST-36, Shangjuxu ST-37, Dachangshu BL-25, Pishu BL-20.

Method: reinforcing, moxa should be used.

Explanation

ST-25 stops diarrhoea and pain.

Ren-6 tonifies Qi and stops chronic diarrhoea. The warm box can be used on these two points.

ST-36 tonifies Spleen-Qi.

ST-37 stops chronic diarrhoea.

BL-25 is the Back Transporting point and tonifies the Large Intestine.

BL-20 tonifies Spleen-Qi.

Gall-Bladder Patterns 29

胆腑病証

The main Gall-Bladder function is that of storing bile and its patterns are nearly always very closely related to those of the Liver. The Gall-Bladder's job of storing and emptying the bile is dependent on the Liver ensuring the smooth flow of Qi.

The Gall-Bladder is easily affected by Dampness deriving from an impairment of the Spleen function of transformation and transportation.

GENERAL AETIOLOGY

DIET

An excessive consumption of greasy and fatty foods leads to the formation of Dampness which can lodge in the Gall-Bladder.

EMOTIONS

The Gall-Bladder, like the Liver, is affected by anger. Anger, frustration and bottled-up resentment can cause stagnation of Liver-Qi which, in turn, can produce Heat which affects the Gall-Bladder. Pent-up anger over a long period of time implodes to give rise to Fire in Liver and Gall-Bladder with symptoms of irritability, bitter taste, thirst, headaches, etc.

From an emotional point of view, the Gall-Bladder also affects courage and spirit of initiative. A weak Gall-Bladder energy may result in timidity and lack of courage. This is also expressed in certain Chinese language expressions such as "big gall-bladder" for "courage" and "small gall-bladder" for "cowardice or timidity".

CLIMATE

Exterior Dampness and Heat, as it is found in tropical or sub tropical regions, can cause Damp-Heat in the Gall-Bladder.

The patterns discussed are:
Excess pattern
Damp-Heat in the Gall-Bladder
Deficiency pattern
Gall-Bladder Deficient.

DAMP-HEAT IN THE GALL-BLADDER

Clinical manifestations

Hypochondriac pain and distension, nausea, vomiting, inability to digest fats, yellow complexion, scanty and dark yellow urine, fever, thirst without desire to drink, bitter taste.

Tongue: thick-sticky yellow coating, either bilateral or only on one side.

Pulse: Slippery, Wiry.

Key symptoms: hypochondriac pain, bitter taste and thick-sticky yellow coating on the right side.

Pathology

Underlying this pattern there is always a deficiency of Spleen-Qi leading to the formation of Dampness which obstructs the Gall-Bladder. Hence the sticky tongue coating and Slippery pulse.

Dampness in the Gall-Bladder interferes with the smooth flow of Liver-Qi which stagnates and causes hypochondriac pain and a feeling of distension.

Nausea and vomiting are caused both by stagnant Liver-Qi invading the Stomach, and by Dampness preventing Stomach-Qi from descending.

Bitter taste, fever, dark urine, thirst, are all signs of Heat. There is thirst because of the Heat, but no desire to drink (or desire to drink in small sips) because of the presence of Dampness.

From a Western point of view, this pattern is often seen in cholelithiasis (stones in Gall-Bladder). From a Chinese perspective, stones are an extreme form of Dampness in its most substantial state. They are formed over a long period of time from Dampness under the "steaming and brewing" action of Heat. Thus stones are always considered a manifestation of Damp-Heat or Phlegm-Fire.

Aetiology

This pattern is often caused by feelings of anger over a long period of time causing stagnation of Liver-Qi and implosion of stagnant Qi into Fire.

The excessive consumption of greasy and fatty foods leads to the formation of Dampness which combines with the Heat.

In tropical or sub-tropical regions, it can be caused by climatic Damp-Heat.

Treatment

Principle of treatment: resolve Damp, clear Heat in Gall-Bladder, stimulate the smooth flow of Liver-Qi.

Points: Riyue G.B.-24, Qimen LIV-14, Zhongwan Ren-12, Yanglingquan G.B.-34, Dannangxue special point, Zhiyang Du-9, Danshu BL-19, Ganshu BL-18, Pishu BL-20, Quchi L.I.-11, Zhigou T.B.-6.

Method: reducing (except on Ren-12 and BL-20).

Explanation

G.B.-24 and BL-19 (respectively Front Collecting and Back Transporting points) clear Heat in Gall-Bladder.

LIV-14 and BL-18 clear Heat in the Liver.

Ren-12 and BL-20 resolve Dampness.

G.B.-34 stimulates the smooth flow of Liver-Qi, resolves Dampness and clears Heat.

Dannangxue special point (slightly below G.B.-34) has the same functions as G.B.-34 and is only used if it is tender on pressure.

Du-9 clears Heat in Gall-Bladder, stimulates the smooth flow of Liver-Qi and resolves Dampness.

L.I.-11 clears Heat and resolves Damp.

T.B.-6 stimulates the smooth flow of Liver-Qi and clears Heat in the Lesser Yang channels.

GALL-BLADDER DEFICIENT

Clinical manifestations

Dizziness, blurred vision, nervousness, timidity,

propensity to being easily startled, lack of courage and initiative, sighing.

Tongue: Pale or normal.

Pulse: Weak.

Key symptoms: timidity, sighing, lack of courage.

Pathology

The Gall-Bladder is the Yang aspect of the Liver, and it is said in Chinese Medicine that Liver-Yang can only be in excess, never deficient. However, in this case, this pattern describes a state of deficiency of the Gall-Bladder.

More than a "pattern", this is really the description of a certain character or personality. The key feature of this "pattern" is the character of the person, i.e. the lack of courage, timidity and lack of initiative.

As was discussed before, the Liver houses the Ethereal Soul and its weakness can be manifested with timidity and fear.

Aetiology

In this case, there is no "aetiology" as such as the pattern depends on the character of the person. Of course, the timidity and lack of courage could also be the result of certain interrelationships within the family during childhood, such as a younger child always "bullied" by the older brothers or a child who is never encouraged and only reproached.

From a Chinese physiological perspective, severe deficiency of Blood may result in fear and lack of courage (whilst Heat in the Blood may result in anger). As mentioned before, Blood and Yin are the root of the Ethereal Soul. If Blood is deficient, the Ethereal Soul suffers and this manifests with fear (especially on going to bed at night). The "Classic of Categories" (1624) by Zhang Jie Bin says: *"The Liver stores Blood and Blood is the residence of the Ethereal Soul. If the Liver is deficient there is fear, if it is in excess there is anger"*.[1]

Treatment

Principle of treatment: tonify and warm the Gall-Bladder.

Points: Qiuxu G.B.-40.

Method: reinforcing, moxa is applicable.

Explanation

G.B.-40 is the Source point to tonify the Gall-Bladder, and it has a good effect on this particular mental aspect of the Gall-Bladder.

NOTES

1 Zhang Jie Bin, 1982 Classic of Categories (*Lei Jing* 类经). People's Health Publishing House, p 53. This book was first published in 1624.

Bladder Patterns 30

膀胱腑病証

The main Bladder function is that of "Qi transformation", i.e. transforming and excreting fluids by the power of Qi.

Physiologically, the Bladder is directly connected to the Small Intestine from which it receives the "dirty" part of fluids after separation into a dirty and "clean" part.

The Bladder receives the Qi for this function from the Kidneys: in disease, therefore Bladder deficiency often results from Kidney-Yang deficiency. However, the Kidney does not have a pattern of Excess, so all Excess patterns pertaining to the urinary system fall under the category of Bladder patterns. From this point of view, the Bladder patterns are very important, as they fill a gap within the urinary disease patterns.

Accumulation of Dampness is the most common pathological factor in Bladder patterns.

GENERAL AETIOLOGY

CLIMATE

Climate has an important influence on Bladder conditions. Excessive exposure to cold and damp weather, sitting on damp surfaces, or living in damp places, can lead to the accumulation of Dampness in the Bladder. This can be manifested as Damp-Cold or Damp-Heat (even if it derives from exterior Cold).

Excessive exposure to Damp-Heat in tropical countries also leads to the accumulation of Damp-Heat in the Bladder.

EMOTIONS

From an emotional point of view, the Bladder, like the Kidneys, is affected by fear. In particular in children, fear or anxieties or insecurity leads to the sinking of Qi in the Bladder resulting in nocturnal enuresis.

In adults, Bladder disharmonies are often manifested with feelings of suspicion and jealousy over a long period of time.

EXCESS SEX

Excessive sexual activity depletes Kidney-Yang and therefore indirectly also the Bladder, as this derives its energy from Kidney-Yang. This can result in frequent and abundant urination, nocturia or incontinence.

The patterns discussed are:
- Excess patterns
  - Damp-Heat in the Bladder
  - Damp-Cold in the Bladder
- Deficiency patterns
  - Bladder Deficient and Cold.

DAMP-HEAT IN THE BLADDER

Clinical manifestations

Frequent and urgent urination, burning on urination, difficult urination (stopping in the middle of flow), dark-yellow and/or turbid urine, blood in the urine, sand in the urine, fever, thirst.

Tongue: Red, thick-sticky yellow coating on the root with red spots.

Pulse: Rapid, Slippery, slightly Wiry on left Rear position.

Key symptoms: burning on urination, dark urine, difficult urination.

Pathology

This pattern is one of Interior Full-Heat from the 8-Principle point of view. It is characterized by the presence of Dampness and Heat in the Bladder.

Dampness obstructs the smooth flow of fluids in the Lower Burner, giving rise to difficult urination, urgent urination, turbid urine and a sticky tongue coating. In extreme cases, Dampness can materialize into urinary sand or stones.

Heat in the Bladder causes burning on urination, a dark urine, a Red tongue with yellow coating and red spots and a Rapid pulse.

Fever and thirst are manifestations of generalized Heat.

Aetiology

This pattern can be caused by excessive exposure to exterior Damp-Heat or Dampness and Cold. Dampness and Cold penetrate the Bladder from below and, in time, can turn into Damp-Heat. Thus it is important to realize that exterior Cold Dampness can cause a pattern of Damp-Heat in the Bladder. In fact, the pattern of Damp-Heat in the Bladder is very common in most countries, including very cold ones.

From an emotional point of view, this pattern can be caused by feelings of suspicion or jealousy bottled-up over a long period of time.

Treatment

Principle of treatment: resolve Dampness, clear Heat, open the Water passages of the Lower Burner.

Points: Yinlingquan SP-9, Sanyinjiao SP-6, Sanjiaoshu BL-22, Pangguangshu BL-28, Zhongji Ren-3, Jinmen BL-63, Tonggu BL-66.

Method: reducing, no moxa.

Explanation

SP-9 and SP-6 resolve Dampness from the Lower Burner.

BL-22 stimulates the transformation of Water in the Lower Burner and opens its Water passages.

BL-28 is the Back Transporting point of the Bladder and clears Heat from the Bladder.

Ren-3 is the Front Collecting point of the Bladder and clears Heat from the Bladder.

BL-63 is the Accumulation point for the Bladder and stops pain on urination, particularly in acute cases.

BL-66 clears Heat from the Bladder.

Case history

A young woman of 30 had been suffering from recurrent and persistent discomfort on urination for 7 years. The problem started 7 years previously with three acute attacks of burning on urination which were treated with antibiotics even though urine cultures showed no bacterial infections. Ever since then she had been suffering from a constant discomfort in the urethra, sometimes burning on urination and a sensation of constantly needing to urinate. The colour of the urine varied between dark yellow and pale. She always felt cold. Her pulse was very Fine, Weak and Deep. Her tongue was Pale, without "spirit" and with a dirty-yellow coating on the root.

The urinary symptoms themselves were obviously due to Damp-Heat obstructing the Bladder (burning on urination, urine sometimes dark, constant discomfort, dirty-yellow coating on tongue root). However, this occurred on a background of Kidney-Yang deficiency (very Deep and Fine pulse, very Pale tongue without "spirit", sometimes pale urine). In treatment, it would be important to clear the Damp-Heat in the Bladder before tonifying and warming Kidney-Yang as a warming method of treatment might aggravate the Damp-Heat of the Bladder.

Case history

A woman of 73 suffered from persistent burning on urination. The pain was experienced in the urethra and hypogastrium. The urine was dark. Occasionally, there was some hesitancy in urination. Her pulse was Full and Wiry, especially on the Rear position. Her tongue was Deep-Red with a thick-sticky yellow coating on the root with red spots on it.

These manifestations indicate retention of Damp-Heat in the Bladder. This is very clearly reflected on the tongue, having a thick yellow coating (indicating Heat) which was sticky (indicating Dampness). The burning on urination was caused by the Heat and the occasional retention of urine by the Dampness obstructing the water passages in the Lower Burner.

DAMP-COLD IN THE BLADDER

Clinical manifestations

Frequent and urgent urination, difficult urination (stopping in mid-stream), feeling of heaviness in hypogastrium and urethra, pale and turbid urine.

Tongue: white-sticky coating on root.

Pulse: Slippery, Slow, slightly Wiry on Rear position.

Key symptoms: difficult urination, feeling of heaviness, turbid urine.

Pathology

This pattern is characterized by the presence of Dampness and Cold in the Lower Burner. Dampness is heavy, it obstructs the Water passages of the Lower Burner and interferes with the Bladder function of Qi transformation. This causes the urgent and difficult urination and the feeling of heaviness which is typical of Dampness.

The sticky coating and Slippery pulse reflect Dampness.

Aetiology

This pattern is caused by excessive exposure to exterior Dampness and Cold.

Treatment

Principle of treatment: resolve Dampness, expel Cold, remove obstruction from the Lower Burner's Water passages.

Points: Yinlingquan SP-9, Sanyinjiao SP-6, Sanjiaoshu BL-22, Zhongji Ren-3, Shuidao ST-28, Shuifen Ren-9, Pangguangshu BL-28.

Method: reducing, moxa can be used.

Explanation

SP-9 and SP-6 resolve Dampness from the Lower Burner.

BL-22 opens the Lower Burner's Water passages.

Ren-3 and BL-28 resolve Dampness in the Bladder.

ST-28 resolves Damp from the Lower Burner.

Ren-9 resolves Dampness in general.

BLADDER DEFICIENT AND COLD

Clinical manifestations

Frequent-pale-abundant urination, incontinence, enuresis, lower backache.

Tongue: Pale, wet.

Pulse: Weak, Deep.

Key symptoms: frequent-pale-abundant urination.

Pathology

This pattern is basically the same as Kidney-Yang deficiency or Kidney-Qi not Firm.

The Bladder derives its Qi from Kidney-Yang and if this is deficient, the Bladder cannot control the fluids which leak out resulting in frequent abundant and pale urination as well as incontinence or enuresis.

Aetiology

This pattern can be caused by excessive sexual activity that weakens Kidney-Yang.

It can also be caused by excessive exposure to cold or living in cold and damp places. Women are particularly vulnerable to invasion of cold to the Lower Burner, particularly during menstruation.

Treatment

Principle of treatment: tonify and warm Bladder and Kidney-Yang.

Points: Shenshu BL-23, Mingmen Du-4, Pangguangshu BL-28, Guanyuan Ren-4.

Method: reinforcing, moxa is applicable.

Explanation

BL-23 and Du-4 with moxa strongly tonify Kidney-Yang and Bladder.

BL-28 tonifies the Bladder.

Ren-4 with moxa strengthens Qi and Yang in the Lower Burner.

Triple Burner Patterns 31

三焦腑病証

There are no actual Triple Burner patterns as such because the Triple Burner as an organ is not distinct from the other organs. In other words, patterns of the Lung and Heart are patterns of the Upper Burner, patterns of the Stomach and Spleen are patterns of the Middle Burner and patterns of the Bladder, Kidneys, Small and Large Intestine are patterns of the Lower Burner.

Of all the patterns discussed, certain ones are more typical of a disharmony of the Triple Burner functions. These will be briefly discussed below.

UPPER BURNER

The Upper Burner disperses and vaporizes the Body Fluids of the upper part of the body. In this respect, this function falls under the scope of the Lung dispersing function, and for this reason the Upper Burner is compared to a "mist".

In disease, the Upper Burner function of dispersing fluids is blocked, usually by an exterior pathogenic factor (Wind-Cold or Wind-Heat), so that the Defensive Qi circulation is impaired and the skin pores are blocked. This results in sneezing, a runny nose, a sore throat, body aches, a temperature, occipital headache, etc. These are the clinical manifestations occurring in invasion of the Lungs by Wind-Cold or Wind-Heat, already discussed.

In particular, when the Triple Burner channel is directly attacked, which usually happens in invasion of Wind-Heat rather than Wind-Cold, there will be deafness, pain in the outer canthus, earache, pain behind the ears, a swelling of the cheeks and a sore throat. In this case, the tongue would typically have a white or yellow coating on one side only and children would frequently have red points on one side only of the tongue.

MIDDLE BURNER

The Middle Burner digests food and drink and its activity is compared to a process of "rotting and ripening". From this point of view, the Middle Burner function coincides with that of the Stomach.

In disease, the Middle Burner cannot digest food properly, resulting in retention of food in the Stomach, which has already been discussed.

LOWER BURNER

The Lower Burner transforms, separates and excretes fluids, hence the comparison to a "drainage ditch". From this point of view, the function of the Lower Burner coincides with that of the Bladder, Kidneys, and the Intestines.

In disease, the Lower Burner cannot transform, separate and excrete fluids, giving rise to various conditions, such as Damp-Heat in the Bladder or Bladder Deficient and Cold, Kidney-Yang Deficiency, Damp-Heat in Small Intestine. All these conditions affect the Lower Burner causing dysfunctions of urination or defecation.

32 Identification of Patterns According to Pathogenic Factors

六淫辨证

Pathogenic factors invade the body in various forms which are Wind, Cold, Dampness, Heat, Dryness and Fire. Each of these can be of exterior or interior origin. They always correspond to a Full pattern according to the 8 Principles.

Generally speaking, pathogenic factors are more important as patterns of disharmony than as causes of disease. In chapter 15 they were discussed as causes of disease in relation to climate; we will now discuss them simply as patterns of disease, irrespective of climatic influences.

As was explained previously, the diagnosis of a pathogenic factor is made not on the basis of the patient's history, but on the basis of the pattern of symptoms and signs presented. Of course, when considered as causes of disease, climatic factors have a definite, direct influence on the body and they attack it in a way that corresponds to their nature. For example, a person exposed to a hot, dry climate, is likely to develop a pattern of invasion of "Wind-Dryness". However, when considered as pathogenic factors, climatic influences are somewhat irrelevant as the diagnosis is made only on the basis of the clinical manifestations. For example, if a person has a runny nose, aversion to cold, sneezing, a headache, a stiff neck, a cough and a Floating pulse, these clinical manifestations denote a pattern of exterior Wind-Cold. It is irrelevant whether this person was exposed to climatic cold or not and it is not usually necessary to ask.

Some internally-generated pathogenic factors give rise to similar pathological signs and symptoms as the exterior climatic factors. These will be discussed together with the relevant exterior pathogenic factor.

The pathogenic factors are:

Wind
Cold
Summer-Heat
Dampness
Dryness
Fire.

WIND

Wind is Yang in nature and tends to injure Blood and Yin. Wind is often the vehicle through which other climatic factors invade the body. For example, Cold will often enter the body as Wind-Cold and Heat as Wind-Heat.

The clinical manifestations due to Wind mimic the action of wind itself in Nature: it arises quickly and changes rapidly, it moves swiftly, blows intermittently and sways the top of trees.

There is a saying that captures the clinical characteristics of Wind: *"Sudden rigidity is due to Wind"*.[1] This refers to the clinical manifestations resulting from both interior and exterior Wind. In fact, interior Wind can cause paralysis (as in Wind-stroke) and exterior Wind can cause facial paralysis or simply stiffness of the neck.

The main clinical manifestations of Wind are:
— Its onset is rapid
— It causes rapid changes in symptoms and signs
— It causes symptoms and signs to move from place to place in the body
— It can cause tremors, convulsions, but also stiffness or paralysis
— It affects the top part of the body
— It affects the Lungs first
— It affects the skin
— It causes itching.

All the above manifestations apply to both exterior and interior Wind, except for tremors, convulsions and paralysis which only apply to interior Wind. Only facial paralysis (Bell's palsy) can be caused by exterior Wind.

Exterior Wind penetrates via the skin and interferes with the circulation of Defensive Qi in the space between skin and muscles. Since Defensive Qi warms the muscles, the person feels chilly, shivers and has aversion to cold when its circulation is impaired by Wind. "Aversion to cold or wind" is a characteristic and essential symptom of invasion of exterior Wind and consists not only in feeling cold and shivering but also in a reluctance to go outside in the cold. The Lungs control the spreading of Defensive Qi in the Exterior of the body and also the opening and closing of the pores. The presence of Wind in the space between skin and muscles interferes with the Lung dispersing and descending function and causes sneezing and possibly coughing. The impairment of the Lung dispersing and descending function prevents the spreading and descending of Lung fluids, resulting in a runny nose with profuse white discharge.

The fight between the pathogenic Wind and Defensive Qi in the skin and muscles may cause fever. Wind attacks the most superficial channels first which are the Greater Yang channels (Small Intestine and Bladder) and obstructs the circulation of Defensive Qi within them: this causes stiffness and pain along these channels and particularly in the back of the neck.

Wind attacks the top part of the body and often lodges in the throat causing an itchy sensation in the throat.

If Wind combines with Cold with a prevalence of the latter, there will be no sweating because Cold contracts the pores. The pulse will be Tight.

If the Cold is not so prevalent, but Wind predominates, the pores are open, the person sweats slightly and the pulse will be Slow.

If a person has a strong constitution and a tendency to Excess patterns, then the body's Defensive Qi reacts strongly, the pores will be closed and there will be no sweating: this is called Exterior-Excess pattern. If a person has a

Table 18 Comparison between attack of Cold and attack of Wind

	Attack of Cold	Attack of Wind
Sweating	No sweating	Slight sweating
Aches	Pronounced	Slight
Headache	Severe	Less severe
Aversion to cold	Pronounced	Slight
Pulse	Floating-tight	Floating-slow

relatively weak constitution and a tendency to Deficiency patterns, the Defensive Qi reacts less strongly, the pores are open and there will be a slight sweating. This is called Exterior-Deficiency pattern.

With the invasion of exterior Wind, Defensive Qi reacts by rushing to the Exterior of the body, and this is reflected on the pulse which becomes more superficial (Floating pulse).

Thus, to summarize, the symptoms and signs of invasion of Exterior Wind are:
— aversion to cold or wind
— sneezing, cough
— runny nose
— possibly fever
— occipital stiffness and ache
— itchy throat
— sweating or not (depending on whether Wind or Cold is predominant)
— Floating pulse .

Besides this, exterior Wind can invade the channels of the face directly and cause deviation of mouth and eyebrows (facial paralysis).

Exterior Wind can also invade any channel, particularly the Yang channels and settle in the joints, causing stiffness and pain of the joints (Painful Obstruction Syndrome). The pain would typically be "wandering", moving from one joint to the other on different days.

Finally, Wind can also affect some internal organs, principally the Liver. Wind pertains to Wood and the Liver according to the 5-Element system of correspondences. This relationship can often be observed when a person prone to migraine headaches is affected by a period of windy weather (particularly an easterly wind) causing a neck ache and headache.

Wind combines with other pathogenic factors giving rise to the following symptoms and signs:

WIND-COLD

Aversion to cold, shivering, sneezing, cough, runny nose with white-watery mucus, no fever or slight fever, severe occipital stiffness and ache, no sweating, no thirst, Floating-Tight pulse, Tongue body colour unchanged, thin-white coating.

Explanation

This has already been largely explained above. The tongue seldom shows any significant changes in invasion of Wind-Cold as the body colour is unaffected.

WIND-HEAT

Aversion to cold, shivering, sneezing, cough, runny nose with slightly yellow mucus, fever, occipital stiffness and ache, slight sweating, itchy throat, sore throat, swollen tonsils, thirst, Floating-Rapid pulse, Tongue body colour Red on the tip or sides, thin-white coating.

Table 19 Comparison between Wind-Cold and Wind-Heat patterns

	Wind-Cold	Wind-Heat
Aetiology/pathology	Wind-Cold on Exterior obstructing Wei Qi	Wind-Heat preventing descending of Qi
Penetration route	Skin	Nose and mouth
Fever	Light	High
Aversion to cold	Pronounced	Slight
Aches body	Pronounced	Slight
Headache	Deep inside, severe	On occiput
Sweating	No sweating	Slight sweating
Thirst	No	Yes
Urine	Clear	Dark
Tongue	Body colour normal, coating thin-white	Sides or tip slightly Red, coating thin-white
Pulse	Floating-Tight	Floating-Rapid
Treatment	Pungent-warm herbs to cause sweating	Pungent-cool herbs to release the Exterior

Explanation

The pathology here is the same as in Wind-Cold, except that since Wind is combined with Heat, there are some Heat signs such as thirst, yellow mucus, more fever, a rapid pulse and a slightly Red tongue body on the tip or sides.

There is aversion to cold in invasions of Wind-Heat because this interferes with the circulation of Defensive Qi in skin and muscles. Since Defensive Qi warms the muscles, an impairment of its circulation leads to aversion to cold in the beginning stages.

The tongue body is red on the tip or sides because these areas reflect the Exterior of the body, as opposed to the centre of the tongue which reflects the state of the Interior.

WIND-DAMP

Itchy skin, skin rashes, urticaria, fever, aversion to cold, sweating, occipital stiffness, body aches, feeling of heaviness, swollen joints, Floating-Slippery pulse.

Explanation

This consists in invasion of Wind and Damp either on the skin causing skin rashes and itching, or in the channels and joints causing Painful Obstruction Syndrome. The skin rashes would typically appear suddenly and frequently move from place to place around the body.

WIND-WATER

Oedema, especially on the face, swollen face and eyes, cough with profuse white and watery mucus, aversion to cold, sweating, no thirst, Floating pulse.

Explanation

In this case, exterior Wind prevents the Lungs from opening the Water passages and dispersing and lowering fluids. Fluids cannot descend, so they overflow under the skin causing oedema. This would be more prominent in the face as it is caused by a Lung dysfunction which mostly affects the Upper Burner.

The facial oedema that occurs in the beginning stage of acute nephritis would be considered "Wind-Water".

INTERNAL WIND

Although some of the clinical manifestations are the same, internal Wind arises from completely different causes than external Wind. Most of its manifestations are also different.

The main clinical manifestations of interior Wind are: tremors, tics, severe dizziness, vertigo and numbness. In severe cases, they are: convulsions, unconsciousness, opisthotonos, hemiplegia and deviation of mouth.

Interior Wind is always related to a Liver disharmony. It can arise from three different conditions:

1) Extreme Heat can give rise to Liver-Wind. This happens in the late stages of febrile diseases when the Heat enters the Blood portion and generates Wind. This process is like the wind generated by a large forest fire. The clinical manifestations are a high fever, delirium, coma and opisthotonos. These signs are frequently seen in meningitis and are due to Wind in the Liver and Heat in the Pericardium.

2) Liver-Yang can give rise to Liver-Wind in prolonged cases. The clinical manifestations are severe dizziness, vertigo, headache and irritability.

3) Deficiency of Liver-Blood can give rise to Liver-Wind. This is due to the deficiency of Blood creating an empty space within the blood vessels which is taken up by interior Wind. This could be compared to the draughts generated sometimes in certain underground (subway) stations. The clinical manifestations are numbness, dizziness, blurred vision, tics and slight tremors (in Chinese called "chicken feet Wind" as the tremors are like the jerky movements of chicken feet when they scour the ground for food).

COLD

Cold is a Yin pathogenic factor and, as such, it tends to injure Yang. Cold, spearheaded by Wind, can invade the Exterior of the body and give rise to symptoms of Wind-Cold, already described above.

Apart from this, Cold can invade the channels directly and cause Painful Obstruction Syndrome, with pain in one or more joints, chilliness and contraction of the tendons.

Cold contracts tissues and it obstructs the circulation of Yang Qi and Blood causing pain. There is a saying: *"Retention of Cold causes pain"*.[2] Pain is therefore a frequent manifestation of Cold. Other symptoms are stiffness, contraction of tendons and chilliness. Cold can invade any part of the body and any joint, but the most common places it invades are the hands and arms, feet and knees, lower back and shoulders.

Apart from invading muscles, channels and joints, Cold can invade three organs directly. These are the Stomach (causing epigastric pain and vomiting), the Intestines (causing abdominal pain and diarrhoea) and the Uterus (causing acute dysmenorrhoea). In all these three cases the symptoms would be accompanied by chilliness and the pain would be alleviated by application of heat.

Cold is often manifested with thin, watery and clear fluid discharges, such as a clear-white discharge from the nose, very pale urine, watery-loose stools and clear-watery vaginal discharges. Another saying clarifies this characteristic of Cold: *"A disease characterized by thin, clear, watery and cool discharges is due to Cold"*.[3]

INTERNAL COLD

Internal Cold can be Full or Empty (see chapter 18 on the 8 Principles). Interior-Full Cold originates from climatic cold which either invades the channels causing Painful Obstruction Syndrome, or it invades certain organs directly. Both these cases have just been mentioned.

Generally speaking, Interior-Full Cold can only last a relatively short time. After prolonged retention, interior Cold consumes the Yang of the Spleen, giving rise to Empty Cold. Thus a Full-Cold pattern can turn into an Empty-Cold one.

The clinical manifestations of Full and Empty Cold are very similar as they are the same in nature. The main difference is that Full-Cold is characterized by an acute onset, severe pain and a tongue and pulse of the Excess type, e.g. the tongue would have a thick-white coating and the pulse would be Full and Tight. Empty-Cold is characterized by a gradual onset, dull pain and a tongue and pulse of the Deficiency type, e.g. the tongue would have a thin-white coating and be Pale and the pulse would be Empty or Weak.

Internal Cold arises from deficiency of Yang, usually of the Spleen, Lungs or Kidneys. In this case the Cold does not come from the exterior, but is interiorly generated by deficiency of Yang.

The general symptoms are chilliness, dull pain, cold limbs, a desire to drink warm liquids, no thirst, a pale face, a thin-white tongue coating and a Deep, Weak and Slow pulse. Other symptoms vary according to which organ is mostly affected. The Heart, Lungs, Spleen, Kidneys can suffer from deficiency of Yang and Interior Cold.

The symptoms of Heart-Yang deficiency (in addition to the above-mentioned general symptoms) with interior Cold are stuffiness and pain in the chest, purple lips and a Knotted pulse. In Lung-Qi deficiency they are propensity to catch colds, sweating and a cough with white mucus. In Spleen-Yang deficiency they are diarrhoea or loose stools and lack of appetite. In Kidney-Yang deficiency they are frequent, pale and profuse urination, lower back ache, cold feet and knees and impotence in men or white leucorrhoea in women.

The manifestations of Yang deficiency of the various organs have been discussed in much greater detail in the chapter on the Identification of Patterns according to the Internal Organs.

SUMMER-HEAT

Summer-Heat is a Yang pathogenic factor and, as such, it tends to injure Yin. This pathogenic factor is slightly different from the others, in so far as it is definitely related to a specific season since it can only occur in summertime.

The main clinical manifestations are aversion to heat, sweating, headache, scanty-dark urine, dry lips, thirst, a Rapid pulse and a Red tongue on the sides and tip.

In severe cases, Heat can invade the Pericardium and cause clouding of the mind, manifesting with delirium, slurred speech or unconsciousness.

DAMPNESS

Dampness is a Yin pathogenic factor and it tends to injure Yang. Dampness refers not only to damp weather, but also to damp living conditions, such as living in damp houses. Exterior Dampness can also be caught by wearing wet clothes, wading in water, working in damp places or sitting on damp ground.

The characteristics of Dampness are that it is sticky, it is difficult to get rid of, it is heavy, it slows things down, it infuses downwards and it causes repeated attacks. When exterior Dampness invades the body, it tends to invade the lower part first, typically the legs. From the legs, it can flow upwards in the leg channels to settle in any of the pelvic cavity organs. If it settles in the female genital system it causes vaginal discharges, if it settles in the Intestines it will cause loose stools and if it settles in the Bladder it will cause difficulty, frequency and burning of urination.

The clinical manifestations of Dampness are extremely varied according to its location and nature (hot or cold), but the general ones are a feeling of heaviness of body or head, no appetite, a feeling of oppression of chest or epigastrium, a sticky taste, urinary difficulty, a white-sticky vaginal discharge, a sticky tongue coating and a Slippery pulse.

The various clinical manifestations can be correlated to the main characteristics of Dampness:

— Heaviness: this causes a feeling of tiredness, heaviness of limbs or head, or a "muzzy" feeling of the head. Since Dampness is heavy it causes a feeling of fullness and oppression of chest or epigastrium, and it tends to settle in the Lower Burner. However, Dampness often affects the head too causing the above-mentioned symptoms. This happens because it prevents the clear Yang from ascending to the head to brighten the sense orifices and clear the brain.

— Dirtiness: Dampness is dirty and is reflected in dirty discharges, such as cloudy urine, vaginal discharges or skin diseases characterized by thick and dirty fluids oozing out such as in certain types of eczema.

— Stickiness: Dampness is sticky and this is reflected in a sticky tongue coating, sticky taste and Slippery pulse. The sticky nature of Dampness also accounts for its being very difficult to get rid of. It often becomes chronic, manifesting in frequent, recurrent bouts.

External Dampness can be characterized by any of the above symptoms with acute onset, a thick-sticky tongue coating and a Slippery and Full pulse. If it is accompanied by Heat, there would also be fever, the tongue coating would be sticky and yellow and the pulse would be Slippery and Rapid. Damp-Heat is most frequent in summertime and just after the summer.

External Dampness tends to injure Spleen-Yang and impair its function of transformation and transportation. After the initial attack, therefore, the Spleen will become deficient which, in turn, will tend to produce more Dampness. At that point, it will be impossible to distinguish exterior from interior Dampness.

External Dampness can invade the channels and settle in the joints causing a dull ache and swelling of the joints. These are the clinical manifestations of Damp-Painful Obstruction Syndrome.

Case history

A young woman of 32 suffered from pain in the muscles of neck, shoulders and arms and extreme tiredness. This had started 4 months previously when she fell ill with influenza symptoms, a sore throat, ache in the joints and a temperature in May. After two weeks she developed more pain in both joints and muscles, the temperature continued at night, she had a feeling of heaviness and she felt hot and cold. This continued for three months. The appetite was poor, the sleep was disturbed and she experienced epigastric fullness and distension after eating. The tongue was of a normal colour and had a sticky-yellow coating on the root extending towards the centre. The pulse was Weak-Floating (Soft).

The sudden attack of fever with ache in the muscles and joints and a feeling of heaviness indicates the invasion of exterior Damp-Heat. The temperature at night also indicates Damp-Heat, which is also confirmed by the sticky-yellow coating on the tongue. The long duration of the problem and retention of Dampness have weakened Spleen-Qi, hence the extreme tiredness and Soft pulse. Her pains in the muscles are still due to the retention of Damp-Heat in the muscles.

INTERNAL DAMPNESS

Interior Dampness arises from a deficiency of Spleen and sometimes Kidneys. If the Spleen function of transformation and transportation of Body Fluids fails, these will not be transformed and will accumulate to form Dampness.

The clinical manifestations of internal Dampness are the same as those of external Dampness, with the only difference that the onset is gradual rather than sudden. The tongue and pulse are also slightly different. In exterior Dampness the tongue has a thick-sticky coating, whereas in internal Dampness it will be sticky but thinner. The pulse in external Dampness will be Full and Slippery whereas in internal Dampness it is Slippery and Fine, or Weak-Floating.

Dampness and Phlegm are similar in nature. They both originate from a dysfunction of the Spleen in transforming and transporting fluids. There are, however, some differences between Dampness and Phlegm:

1) Dampness can be of exterior or interior origin, whereas Phlegm can only originate from an interior dysfunction.

2) Interior Dampness originates mostly from the impairment of the Spleen in transforming and transporting Body Fluids, whereas the Lungs and Kidneys are also involved in the formation of Phlegm.

3) Although Dampness can settle in the head preventing the clear Yang from ascending, it primarily affects the lower part of the body, while Phlegm primarily affects the middle and upper part of the body. For example, urinary problems are often caused by Dampness in the Lower Burner and Bladder, while intestinal problems manifesting with mucus or blood in the stools are due to Dampness and Heat in the Intestines. Phlegm, on the other hand, mostly affects the chest causing a feeling of oppression in the chest, the throat causing a feeling of obstruction in the throat, or the head causing a feeling of heaviness, muzziness and dizziness.

4) Dampness in the head causes a characteristic feeling of heaviness while Phlegm, contrary to Dampness, also causes dizziness.

5) Phlegm can "mist" the Mind causing mental problems or sometimes mental retardation in children while Dampness has no such effect.

6) Phlegm can be retained in the channels and under the skin causing swellings and lumps, while Dampness mostly affects the Internal Organs or joints.

7) Although there are various different types of Phlegm including Cold or Damp-Phlegm, Phlegm easily combines with Fire, especially in chronic diseases. Dampness has no such characteristic. Phlegm is so frequently associated with Fire that there is a saying in Chinese Medicine: *"Phlegm is a substantial form of Fire and Fire is a non-substantial form of Phlegm"*.

8) Interior Dampness originates only from a Spleen dysfunction, while Phlegm can also originate from the condensing action of Fire on Body Fluids.

9) Dampness affects mostly the Spleen, Gall-Bladder, Bladder, and Intestines (hence, apart from the Spleen, mostly the Yang organs), while Phlegm affects mostly the Lungs, Heart, Kidney and Stomach (hence, apart from the Stomach, mostly the Yin organs).

10) Dampness affects the Spleen, while Phlegm often affects the Stomach.

11) Although Phlegm has the nature of heaviness, it does not have Dampness's characteristics of being sticky, dirty and flowing downwards.

12) Phlegm can associate with various other pathogenic factors giving rise to Cold-Phlegm, Damp-Phlegm, Wind-Phlegm, Dry-Phlegm, Phlegm-Fire and Qi-Phlegm, while Dampness only associates with Cold or Heat.

13) Phlegm can assume a very watery and dilute form called Phlegm-Fluids while Dampness only assumes one form.
14) From the point of view of pulse diagnosis, both Dampness and Phlegm can manifest with a Slippery pulse. However, Dampness can also manifest with a Weak-Floating pulse, while Phlegm can manifest with a Wiry pulse.
15) From the point of view of tongue diagnosis, both Dampness and Phlegm can manifest with a sticky coating but Phlegm can also manifest with a dry and rough coating with prickles. This type of coating is frequently seen inside a central crack in the Stomach area of the tongue indicating the presence of Phlegm-Fire in the Stomach.
16) From the point of view of acupuncture treatment, although there are many similarities in the treatment of Dampness and Phlegm, the Spleen channel is mostly used to eliminate Dampness, while the Stomach channel is mostly used to resolve Phlegm. For example, Yinlingquan SP-9, Sanyinjiao SP-6 and Taibai SP-3 are the main points to eliminate Dampness, while Fenglong ST-40 is the most important point to resolve Phlegm.
17) Finally, from the point of view of herbal treatment, the herbs used to drain Dampness or resolve Phlegm belong to two entirely different categories with different therapeutic effect.

DRYNESS

Dryness is a Yang pathogenic factor and it tends to injure Blood or Yin. It arises in very dry weather, but it can also occur in some artificial conditions such as in very dry, centrally-heated buildings.

The clinical manifestations are simply characterized by dryness and they are a dry throat, dry lips, a dry tongue, a dry mouth, dry skin, dry stools and scanty urination.

INTERNAL DRYNESS

Internal Dryness arises from deficiency of Yin, particularly of the Stomach and/or Kidneys and the symptoms are the same as for exterior Dryness. Interior Dryness is not always the result of Yin deficiency as it is sometimes the stage preceding it. There is a saying: "*Withering and cracking is due to Dryness*".[4] This describes the dry skin and cracked tongue often seen in Dryness.

The Stomach is the origin of fluids and if one has an irregular diet, such as eating late at night, eating in a hurry or going back to work straight after eating, the Stomach fluids are depleted and this leads to a state of dryness which is the precursor of Yin deficiency.

This dryness is manifested with a dry throat and mouth and a dry tongue possibly slightly peeled in the centre, but not yet Red.

FIRE

Fire is an extreme form of Heat which can derive from any of the other exterior pathogenic factors. Strictly speaking, it is not really an exterior pathogenic factor. It either arises from the Interior or derives from other exterior pathogenic factors, but once it manifests in the body, it is an interior pathogenic factor.

Extreme Heat and Fire are not exactly the same in nature, although very similar. Fire is more "solid" than Heat, it tends to move and dry-out more than Heat. Heat can cause pain as well as all the other symptoms of Heat, such as a Red tongue, thirst and a Rapid pulse, but Fire moves upwards (causing mouth ulcers for example) or damages the blood vessels (causing bleeding). Also, Fire tends to affect the mind more than Heat causing anxiety, mental agitation, insomnia or mental illness.

The differentiation between the Bright-Yang channel pattern and Bright-Yang organ pattern of the 6-Stage Pattern Identification, illustrates the difference between Heat and Fire well. The Bright-Yang channel pattern is characterized by Heat manifesting with fever, thirst and sweating, but no constipation or abdominal pain. The organ pattern is characterized by similar manifestations, but in addition, there is constipation and abdominal pain. This is because in the organ pattern the Heat has become "solid" and has been transformed into Fire which dries up the faeces in the intestines and causes constipation. In addition, the organ pattern can be characterized by mental changes, such as delirium, as Fire affects the mind.

To give another example, Heat in the Stomach can cause thirst, but Fire in the Stomach will cause bleeding gums, gum ulcers, and haematemesis as Fire moves upwards more than Heat and it agitates the Blood causing bleeding.

The difference between Liver-Yang ascending and Liver-Fire blazing upwards is another appropriate example of the difference between Heat and Fire. Ascending Liver-Yang results from an imbalance between Yin and Yang within the Liver: when Liver-Yin or Liver-Blood is deficient, Liver-Yang may rise upwards excessively and cause dizziness, headaches, a dry throat, irritability and probably a red face. These are symptoms of Heat, but not of Fire. If the Liver has excessive Fire, in addition to these symptoms and signs, there will be intense thirst, bitter taste, scanty-dark urine and dry stools. All these are symptoms and signs of Fire which dries fluids more than Heat does.

The nature of Fire therefore is to rise to the head, to dry fluids, to injure Blood and Yin, to deplete Qi and to affect the mind.

There are many sayings that describe the nature and clinical manifestations of Heat or Fire. Some of them are:

— *"Diseases manifesting with tympanic sounds are due to Fire"*.[5] This describes the condition of Fire or Heat in the Intestines causing borborygmi and a distended abdomen.

— *"Abnormal changes and dark fluids are manifestations of Heat"*.[6] This describes the tendency of Heat or Fire to produce rapid changes for the worse in an acute condition. For example, when exterior Wind-Heat invades the Lung-Defensive Qi portion, the Heat can in a few cases rapidly penetrate to the Pericardium causing a high temperature and coma. This is called "abnormal transmission". The second part of the saying refers to dark and concentrated fluids often produced by Heat or Fire, such as a dark and scanty urine.

— *"Vomiting of sour fluids and sudden downpouring are manifestations of Heat"*.[7] The first part of this saying describes a condition of Stomach-Heat causing vomiting and sour regurgitation. The second part of the saying describes the sudden diarrhoea with foul-smelling stools which can occur with Heat in the Intestines.

— *"Manic behaviour is a manifestation of Fire"*.[8] Fire can easily affect the Mind causing restlessness, agitation and in severe cases a manic behaviour (laughing uncontrollably, shouting, hitting people, talking incessantly, etc.). This is a specific characteristic of Fire as opposed to Heat.

Fire can be of the Excess or Deficient type. The clinical manifestations of Excess Fire are a high fever, a red face and eyes, a dry mouth, a bitter taste, constipation, scanty-dark urine, thirst, mental agitation, a Red tongue with yellow coating and a Full-Rapid pulse. When Fire enters the Blood, it may give rise to dark purple spots under the skin (macules) and vomiting of blood or other haemorrhages.

Deficient Fire arises from deficiency of Yin and is manifested with night sweating, a feeling of heat in the chest, palms and soles, red cheekbones, a dry mouth, afternoon fever, a Red and peeled tongue and a Floating-Empty and Rapid pulse.

Fire can affect the Heart, Liver, Stomach, Kidneys, Lungs and Intestines and its clinical manifestations related to each of these organs have been described in detail in the chapter on the Identification of Patterns according to the Internal Organs (see p. 199 to 202).

PHLEGM AND STASIS OF BLOOD

Phlegm originates from a dysfunction of the Spleen in transforming and transporting fluids, while Stasis of Blood is usually caused by stagnation of Qi. They are therefore pathogenic factors.

However, in chronic conditions, they become further causes of disease in themselves. For this reason, a discussion of the causes of disease in Chinese books always includes these two pathogenic factors. These will not be discussed here as they have already been discussed in the chapter on the Identification of Patterns according to Qi, Blood and Body Fluids (see page 191).

NOTES

1 Zhai Ming Yi 1979 Clinical Chinese Medicine (*Zhong Yi Lin Chuang Ji Chu* 中医临床基础) Henan Publishing House, p 132.
2 Clinical Chinese Medicine, p 133.
3 Clinical Chinese Medicine, p 133.
4 Clinical Chinese Medicine, p 135.
5 Clinical Chinese Medicine, p 133.
6 Clinical Chinese Medicine, p 133.
7 Clinical Chinese Medicine, p 134.
8 Clinical Chinese Medicine, p 134.

33 Identification of Patterns According to the Five Elements

五行辨证

The Identification of Patterns according to the 5 Elements is based on the pathological changes occurring in dysfunctions of the Generating, Over-acting and Insulting sequences of the 5 Elements.

These patterns are not of primary importance in practice as most of them describe clinical conditions which are better expressed by the Internal-Organ patterns. In certain cases, however, some 5-Element patterns can describe conditions which fall outside the scope of the Internal-Organ patterns. An example of this is the pattern of Deficient Qi of Wood (manifesting with timidity and indecision) which is not included among the Internal Organ patterns.

We can distinguish the 5-Element patterns according to the Generating, Over-acting and Insulting sequences.

GENERATING SEQUENCE PATTERNS

These patterns describe conditions of deficiency of each organ when this is induced by its Mother Element.

WOOD NOT GENERATING FIRE

The clinical manifestations are timidity, a lack of courage, indecision, palpitations and insomnia (in particular, waking up in the early hours of the morning).

This pattern is sometimes also described as a pattern of Deficient Gall-Bladder. It is an unusual pattern in so far as, according to the theory of the Internal Organs, Liver-Qi or the Gall-Bladder can hardly ever be deficient. This pattern describes such a situation. More than a pattern, it really describes a certain character and personality, and its salient feature is the lack of courage and timidity. It corresponds to the Internal-Organ pattern of Deficient Gall-Bladder.

FIRE NOT GENERATING EARTH

The clinical manifestations are loose stools, chilliness and weakness of the limbs.

This pattern basically describes a condition of Spleen-Yang deficiency due to failure of Fire in providing Heat to the Spleen to transform and transport. According to the theory of the Internal Organs, however, the Spleen derives the warmth necessary to its functions not from the Heart, but from Kidney-Yang. This is because, even though the Kidneys pertain to the Water Element, they also are the source of Fire in the body. The relationship between Kidney-Yang and the Spleen is clinically more relevant than that between the Fire of the Heart and the Spleen.

EARTH NOT GENERATING METAL

The clinical manifestations are phlegm in the chest, cough and tiredness.

This pattern describes the situation when a Spleen deficiency (causing the tiredness) leads to the formation of Phlegm which obstructs the Lungs.

METAL NOT GENERATING WATER

The clinical manifestations are cough, breathlessness, loss of voice and asthma.

This pattern corresponds to the Internal-Organ pattern of Kidneys not receiving Qi.

WATER NOT GENERATING WOOD

The clinical manifestations are dizziness, blurred vision, headaches and vertigo.

This pattern is the same as the Internal-Organ pattern of Kidney and Liver Yin deficiency.

OVER-ACTING SEQUENCE PATTERNS

WOOD OVER-ACTING ON EARTH

The clinical manifestations are hypochondriac and epigastric pain, a feeling of distension, irritability, loose stools, poor appetite and a greenish face.

When the clinical manifestations pertain to one Element and the face colour pertains to the Element which over-acts on it, the face colour usually shows the origin of the disharmony. In this case, loose stools and poor appetite are symptoms of deficiency of Earth (Spleen) but the face is greenish: this indicates that the root of the problem is in Wood, i.e. Wood over-acting on Earth. This same principle applies to all the following cases of disharmony of the Over-acting sequence.

The pattern of Wood over-acting on Earth is very common and it is exactly the same as the pattern of "Liver invading the Spleen" already discussed (see page 227).

EARTH OVER-ACTING ON WATER

The main clinical manifestations are oedema, difficult urination and a yellow face.

This pattern occurs when a deficient Spleen fails to transform and transport fluids which accumulate and obstruct the Kidney function of transformation and excretion of fluids.

WATER OVER-ACTING ON FIRE

There is no such pattern as the Kidneys cannot be in Excess.

FIRE OVER-ACTING ON METAL

The clinical manifestations are cough with profuse yellow sputum, a feeling of heat and a red face.

This pattern corresponds to Full-Heat in the Lungs.

METAL OVER-ACTING ON WOOD

The clinical manifestations are tiredness, irritability, a feeling of distension and a white face.

INSULTING SEQUENCE PATTERNS

WOOD INSULTING METAL

The clinical manifestations are cough, asthma and a feeling of distension of chest and hypochondrium.

The Liver channel influences the chest and stagnant Liver-Qi or Liver-Fire can obstruct the chest and prevent Lung-Qi from descending.

METAL INSULTING FIRE

The clinical manifestations are palpitations, insomnia and breathlessness.

This pattern basically describes a condition of both Lung and Heart Qi deficiency.

FIRE INSULTING WATER

The clinical manifestations are a malar flush, dry mouth at night, insomnia, dizziness, lower back ache and night-sweating.

This pattern is identical to the Internal-Organ pattern of "Kidney and Heart not harmonized", i.e. Kidney-Yin deficiency giving rise to Heart Empty-Heat.

WATER INSULTING EARTH

The clinical manifestations are loose stools, oedema, tiredness and weakness of the limbs.

This pattern corresponds to Spleen and Kidney Yang deficiency.

EARTH INSULTING WOOD

The clinical manifestations are jaundice and hypochondriac pain and distension.

This pattern is caused by a failure of the Spleen in transforming fluids leading to Dampness. Dampness accumulates and obstructs the smooth flow of Liver-Qi, impeding the free flow of bile.

Identification of Patterns According to the Channels

34

经络辨証

The Pattern Identification according to the channels is the oldest of the pattern identification methods. It is found in the "Spiritual Axis" in chapter 10.[1]

Basically, this method of pattern identification allows us to distinguish symptoms and signs according to the involved channel: it is therefore concerned with the pathological changes occurring in the channel rather than the organ.

ORGAN VERSUS CHANNEL

The organs and their relevant channels form an indivisible energetic unit: problems of the internal organs can affect the relevant channels, and conversely, problems which start as channel problems can penetrate in the Interior and be transmitted to the organs.

It is important, however, to appreciate both the unity and the separation between the organ and the channel. They form a unity, but they are also energetically separate: the channels pertain to what is called the Exterior, i.e. the superficial energetic layers of the body (including skin and muscles), and the organs pertain to the Interior, i.e. the deep energetic layer of the body including the organs and bones.

In disease, there can be problems of the channels not affecting the organs and vice versa. It is very important to appreciate (and be able to identify) when a problem is situated in the Exterior and affecting the channels only, as there has been a certain tendency in Western acupuncture to overemphasize the role of the Internal Organs.

For example, if a person has a pain in the shoulder along the Large Intestine channel without any Large Intestine-organ symptoms, one can safely conclude that this is a channel problem only, not affecting the Internal Organs. If, on the contrary, a person suffers from chronic diarrhoea over a long period of time with mucus and blood in the stools and, after some years, develops a pain the shoulder along the Large Intestine channel, then this channel problem is possibly caused by its corresponding Internal Organ disease. However, even in this case there could be an overlap of an internal organ problem with a separate invasion of an exterior pathogenic factor in the channel.

Channel problems can arise from four factors.

1) First of all, they arise from invasion of exterior pathogenic factors, such as Cold,

Wind, Dampness or Heat. These invade the superficial channels first, and then the main channels, settling in the joints and causing Painful Obstruction Syndrome. This is an extremely frequent cause of channel problems which affects most people at one time or another.

Channel pathology is, in fact, closely related to joint pathology. Joints in Chinese Medicine are more than just anatomical entities: they have an important function with regard to the circulation of Qi and Blood, with several implications in pathology.

Joints are places where Qi and Blood concentrate or gather, and they are also the places where Qi goes from the Interior to the Exterior or vice versa. As will be remembered from chapter 4, Qi has complex directions of movement, upwards and downwards and in and out. The joints are the places along the channels where Qi enters and exits. It is not by chance that many of the major Transporting points of the limbs below elbows and knees, are situated on joints. As a consequence of this concentration of Qi, the joints are the places where a pathogenic factor easily settles.

When a pathogenic factor invades the joint, it alters the balance of Yin-Yang, it upsets the circulation of Qi in the channel and it causes Qi and Blood to stagnate: this causes pain and in the long run it gives rise to Painful Obstruction Syndrome. If the pathogenic factor is associated with Heat, the joint will feel hot; if it is associated with Cold, it will feel cold.

Besides being affected by exterior pathogenic factors, joints are affected by general deficiency of Qi and Blood which may cause their lack of nourishment and hence weakness.

2) Another frequent cause of channel problem is from over-use of a limb or part of the body, giving rise to local stagnation of Qi. Anyone who, because of their work circumstances, has to constantly repeat the same movements, will be liable to suffer from channel problems, manifesting with local stagnation of Qi.

3) Sports injuries are another frequent cause of channel problems, causing local stagnation of Qi in the channel.

4) Finally, channel problems can of course spring from Internal-Organ disharmonies.

The Channel-Pattern Identification describes the pathological changes occurring in channels.

However, although this is the main aim of this Pattern Identification, it can be slightly confusing as the symptoms and signs described in the "Spiritual Axis" include also some from the relevant organ and sometimes even from other organs.

For example, among the Lung-channel symptoms and signs are:

— congested and sore throat, sensation of fullness in the chest, pain in the clavicle and arm, which are due to the Lung channel;

— cough, asthma, which are due to the Lung organ;

— pain in the shoulders and upper back, which is due to the Large Intestine channel, to which the Lung channel is related.

Thus channel patterns include some symptoms and signs from the organs themselves. These can safely be ignored, as for organ problems, one would much rather use the Internal-Organ Pattern Identification. For example, "cough" and "asthma" are not specific enough to give an indication of the possible pattern involved. In order to do so, it is necessary to use the Internal-Organ Pattern Identification which is more specific about the picture formed by the pattern. For example, if cough is accompanied by profuse white sputum with a feeling of oppression of the chest and the tongue has a sticky white-thick coating, we know that the pattern involved is Damp-Phlegm obstructing the Lungs. If the cough is dry and there is night-sweating with a feeling of heat in the chest, soles and plams, we know that the pattern in question is Deficiency of Lung-Yin.

However, we must also remember that a channel problem can affect the orifices and sense organs. For example, Triple Burner channel symptoms include pain in the ear and deafness. By this is obviously meant a pain in the ear and deafness of acute onset, probably from invasion of exterior Wind-Heat. Liver channel symptoms include blurred vision and tinnitus. Thus, not all sense organ problems are related to Internal-Organ diseases.

The Channel-Pattern Identification is important to identify the affected channel from the symptoms and signs. The clinical manifestations related to the channel itself are therefore more important.

Of course, the Channel-Pattern Identification needs to be based on a thorough knowledge of the main channels and their deep pathways.[2]

Apart from this, one must also distinguish Full from Empty conditions of the channels. Full conditions are characterized by intense pain, stiffness, contractions and cramps. Empty conditions are characterized by dull ache, weakness of the muscles, atrophy of the muscles and numbness.

Fullness and Emptiness of the channels can also be differentiated from the colour appearing along the course of the channel and its temperature to the touch. In Full conditions there may be a Red colour indicating Heat or a Bluish colour indicating Cold. In the case of Heat, it would also feel hot to the touch. In Empty conditions, there may be a pale streak along the course of the channel and this would feel cold to the touch.

To summarize, if we know the pathway of the channels thoroughly and are able to identify Full or Empty conditions of the channels according to the above guidelines, any clinical manifestation appearing along the channel can be correctly identified.[3]

The following is a list of the Channel patterns from chapter 10 of the "Spiritual Axis". For the sake of clarity, I have omitted the symptoms and signs of Internal Organ problems, and limited them only to the channel symptoms and signs. In addition to the following clinical manifestations, any pain, numbness, stiffness, tingling or ache along the course of a channel is obviously a channel symptom.

LUNGS

Fever, aversion to cold, stuffiness of the chest, pain in the clavicle, shoulders and arms.

LARGE INTESTINE

Sore throat, tooth-ache, epistaxis, runny nose, swollen and painful gums, swollen eyes, pain along the course of the channel.

STOMACH

Pain in the eyes, epistaxis, swelling of neck, facial paralysis, cold legs and feet, pain along the course of the channel.

SPLEEN

Vaginal discharge, cold feeling along the channel, weakness of the leg muscles.

HEART

Pain in the eyes, pain on the inner side of the arm, pain along the scapula.

SMALL INTESTINE

Pain in the neck, pain in the elbow, stiff neck, pain along the lateral side of the arm and scapula.

BLADDER

Fever and aversion to cold, headache, stiff neck, pain in the lower back, pain in the eyes, pain behind the leg along the channel.

KIDNEYS

Pain in the lower back, pain in the sole of the foot.

PERICARDIUM

Stiff neck, pain along the course of the channel, contraction of elbow or hand.

TRIPLE BURNER

Pain along the course of the channel, pain in the elbow, alternation of chills and fever, deafness, pain and discharge from the ear, pain at the top of the shoulders.

GALL BLADDER

Alternation of chills and fever, headache, deafness, pain in the hip and lateral side of legs, pain and distention of breasts.

LIVER

Headache, pain and swelling of the eye, cramps in the legs.

As will be realized, some of the symptoms and signs of some of the Yin channels are actually symptoms of the associated Yang channels. For example:
— Lungs: pain in the shoulders (=Large Intestine channel)
— Heart: pain in the scapula (=Small Intestine channel)
— Pericardium: pain in the neck (=Triple Burner channel)

NOTES

1 Spiritual Axis, p 30-38.
2 For a description of the main channels and their deep pathways see Acupuncture, a Comprehensive Text, and also Essentials of Chinese Acupuncture.
3 For a description of the symptoms and signs of the channels, see Acupuncture, a Comprehensive Text.

35 Principles of Treatment

治疗原则

After making a diagnosis and identifying the pattern, the next logical step is that of determining the principle of treatment to be adopted. The practitioner of Chinese Medicine will need to formulate a rational and coherent plan of action as to what should be treated first, what is primary and what is secondary in the patient's condition, what is the relative importance of the acute or chronic condition and what method of treatment should be used.

Over the centuries, Chinese medical theory has answered these questions and provided a coherent system of principles of treatment. In practice, these principles provide a logical framework according to which a practitioner can evaluate the objectives of his or her treatment. A principle of treatment should always be established before treatment commences. This is achieved by a rigorous analysis of the clinical manifestations and a synthesis of the patient's condition and therapeutic needs at that particular time. The principles of treatment follow logically from the establishment of the relevant pattern of disharmony.

A few examples will clarify this.

A patient with chronic bronchitis presents with an acute attack of Wind-Cold or Wind-Heat (a common cold or influenza, for example): should we treat the acute attack first and ignore the chronic condition? Or should we treat both at the same time?

A patient with deficiency of Qi causing great tiredness also has symptoms of Dampness and a thick-greasy tongue coating. Should we concentrate on tonifying Qi or on eliminating Dampness?

A patient has been having a recurrent temperature and flu-like symptoms for weeks; she is completely exhausted, but her pulse is Full and Wiry. Should we tonify her body's Qi or expel the exterior pathogenic factor still lingering in the Interior?

An old man has deficiency of Yin with rising of Liver-Yang causing hypertension. We need to reduce Liver-Yang, but as the patient is old and frail, will reducing Liver-Yang reduce his energy?

These are a few examples of complex situations encountered in everyday clinical practice requiring a clear differentiation of what is primary and what is secondary, an assessment of the patient's condition and a clear principle of treatment and plan of action.

The principles of treatment can be discussed from four points of view:
1) The question of "Root" ("*Ben*") and "Manifestation" ("*Biao*").
2) The question of the relative strength of the Upright Qi and the pathogenic factors and when to support the former or eliminate the latter.
3) The question of when to tonify and when to reduce.
4) The question of assessing the patient's constitution.
Points 2 and 3 will actually be discussed together as they are concerned with the same basic issue.

THE ROOT AND THE MANIFESTATION

The Root is called "*Ben*" in Chinese, which literally means "root", and the Manifestation is called "*Biao*" which literally means "outward sign" or "manifestation", i.e. the outward manifestation of some inner, unseen root.

Root and Manifestation acquire different meanings in different contexts. These are:
a) From the point of view of Upright Qi and pathogenic factor: the Root is the Upright Qi and the Manifestation is the pathogenic factors.
b) From the point of view of aetiology-pathology: the Root is the root of the disease and Manifestation is the clinical manifestations.
c) From the point of view of onset of the disease: the Root is the initial condition while the Manifestation is the later condition.
d) From the point of view of duration of the disease: the Root is a chronic disease while the Manifestation is an acute disease.

Thus when treatment of Root or Manifestation is discussed, we need to be clear about the particular standpoint or context being considered. For example, to say that in a certain case the Root needs to be treated first, could mean that the Upright Qi needs to be treated first, or that the root (or cause) of the disease needs treating, or that the chronic conditions should be treated first.

In clinical practice, however, Root and Manifestation are usually considered in context (b) above, i.e. as root and clinical manifestations of the disease.

When considering the Root and Manifestation, it is important to understand the connection between the two. They are not separate entities, but two aspects of a contradiction, like Yin and Yang. As their names suggest, they are related to one another, just as the roots of a tree are connected to its branches, the former under the ground and invisible, the latter above the ground and visible. The same relation exists between the root of a disease and its clinical manifestations: they are indissolubly related and they form two aspects of the same entity. There is no separation between the two. For this reason, it is not entirely correct to translate "Ben" as "cause" since the relation between the Root and Manifestation is not a causal one. The root is not the "cause" of the branches, but the two together form the entity of a tree. The art of diagnosis consists precisely in identifying the Root (i.e. the root-cause of symptoms and signs) by looking at the Manifestation (i.e. the clinical manifestations).

For example, if a person has diarrhoea, chilliness, tiredness, poor appetite, abdominal distention, a Weak pulse and a Pale tongue, the complex of these clinical manifestations clearly points to its Root, i.e. Spleen-Yang Deficiency. In this simple example, therefore, Spleen-Yang deficiency is the Root and all the symptoms and signs are the Manifestation of the disease. It is only when we master the art of pattern identification that we can identify the Root by looking at the pattern woven by the Manifestation, much like a botanist can identify a tree by looking at its leaves.

Why do we need to identify the Root? In the course of a disease, the clinical manifestations can be very numerous and complicated and sometimes contradictory. Different clinical manifestations will appear and develop in the course of a long chronic illness; they may combine with superseding acute symptoms, interior conditions may overlap with exterior ones, Deficient conditions may co-exist with Excess ones, Cold can co-exist with Heat, and so on.

Identification of the Root (which need not be a single one, but could be a multiple one) allows us to understand and unravel the numerous clinical manifestations to see the underlying pattern and decide on the principle of treatment according to the condition of the patient and the character of the diseases.

There is a saying in Chinese Medicine *"To treat a disease, find the Root"*. This succinctly summarizes the importance of always tracing the clinical manifestations back to their Root in order to treat a disease. This is because, generally speaking, the Root is the primary aspect of the contradiction, i.e. it is generally primary in relation to the clinical manifestations. As the Root is primary, treatment of the clinical manifestations is usually carried out by treating the Root.

For example, if a patient complains of acute occipital headache, a slight temperature, a stiff neck, aversion to cold, a runny nose, sneezing and a Floating-Tight pulse, all these clinical manifestations (the Manifestation) obviously point to their root (the Root) which is invasion of the Lung-Defensive Qi portion by exterior Wind-Cold. This pattern was discussed in detail in the chapter on the Identification of Patterns according to Pathogenic Factors (see ch. 32). In this case treatment is aimed at the Root, i.e. dispersing the Cold, releasing the Exterior and restoring the Lung dispersing and descending function. When this is done, all the clinical manifestations will disappear. This is a simple example as to how the various clinical manifestations form a pattern which, when properly identified using the tools of Chinese diagnosis and pattern identification, lead us to recognize the Root and treat it accordingly. In this example, if the practitioner were not skilled in Chinese diagnosis and pattern identification and unable to identify the Root, he or she might set about treating each of the clinical manifestations individually, which would of course be wrong.

Another example: a patient suffers from a low-grade fever in the afternoon, night sweating, a feeling of heat in the palms and soles, a dry mouth at night and has a Red-Peeled tongue. These are the clinical manifestations that, when properly interpreted, lead us to identify their root, i.e. Yin deficiency. To treat all the various clinical manifestations, it is sufficient to treat the Root, i.e. tonify Yin.

Another example: a patient has an unremitting high fever, irritability, thirst, a Rapid pulse, a Red tongue with yellow coating and very cold limbs. In this case there is a contradiction as the patient has a high fever but cold limbs. However, taking all the clinical manifestations into account, we can identify interior Heat as the Root. The correct treatment is therefore to clear interior Heat, in spite of the cold limbs. These are due to interior Heat obstructing the circulation of Yang Qi to the limbs, so that there can be the apparent paradox that the stronger the Heat, the colder the limbs.

In conclusion, generally speaking, the Root is primary and is treated first. However, under certain circumstances, the Manifestation can become primary and needs to be treated first, even though the ultimate aim is always to treat the Root. The decision to treat the Root or the Manifestation depends on the severity and urgency of the clinical manifestations.

There are three possible courses of action:

Treat the Root only

Treat both the Root and the Manifestation

Treat the Manifestation first, and the Root later.

1 TREAT THE ROOT ONLY

Generally speaking, treating the Root only is sufficient to clear all clinical manifestations in most cases. The method of treating the Root can be used in both interior or exterior as well as chronic or acute diseases. Examples of this approach have been given above: in case of Spleen-Yang deficiency (the Root) causing the previously mentioned clinical manifestations, treating the Root (i.e. tonifying and warming the Spleen) will be the correct approach which, in time, should clear all the clinical manifestations. Similarly for the clinical manifestations caused by Wind-Cold or those caused by Yin deficiency. In both these cases it will be sufficient to treat the Root (i.e. expel Wind-Cold in the former case, and nourish Yin in the latter) to clear all the clinical manifestations.

This approach is applicable in cases when the clinical manifestations are not too severe. If the clinical manifestations are severe or even life-threatening, the approach should be changed, as will be explained below.

2 TREAT BOTH THE ROOT AND THE MANIFESTATION

This approach is widely used in practice. In chronic cases when the clinical manifestations are severe and distressing for the patient, it is necessary to treat both the Root and the Manifestation simultaneously. This approach is also applied when the clinical manifestations themselves are such that they would perpetuate the original problem. For example, in the case of a woman with Qi deficiency leading to excessive menstrual bleeding (Qi not holding Blood), prolonged menstrual bleeding over many years will in itself lead to further deficiency of both Blood and Qi.

To return to the previous example of Spleen-Yang deficiency: if this is causing very severe and debilitating diarrhoea, particularly in an elderly patient, it would be necessary to treat the Root, i.e. tonify and warm the Spleen, but at the same time also take active steps to treat the Manifestation, i.e. stop the diarrhoea. In acupuncture terms this would involve using points which are known to stop diarrhoea (whatever the cause), such as Tianshu ST-25 and Shangjuxu ST-37.

In the case of a patient suffering from Spleen-Yang deficiency causing severe oedema, the correct approach would again be to treat both the Root (i.e. tonify and warm the Spleen) and the Manifestation (i.e. eliminate the oedema). In acupuncture terms, this would involve combining the reinforcing method (to tonify the Spleen) with the reducing method (by reducing points to move fluids, such as Shuifen Ren-9, Shuidao ST-28 and Sanjiaoshu BL-22).

In the case of a child who has severe whooping cough caused by Phlegm-Heat in the Lungs, it would be necessary again to adopt the method of treating both the Root (by clearing Lung-Heat and resolving Phlegm) and the Manifestation (by stopping the cough). This is the correct approach since the cough is very distressing and debilitating to the child, so it would be wrong to simply treat the Root and wait for the symptoms to improve. This example can be compared and contrasted with a case of a chronic slight dry cough caused by Yin deficiency, in which case the cough is not bad or serious enough to warrant treating the Manifestation.

3 TREAT THE MANIFESTATION FIRST AND THE ROOT LATER

Under certain circumstances the Root becomes secondary and the Manifestation needs to be treated first and usually urgently too. This approach is applicable in all cases when the clinical manifestations are very severe or even life-threatening, generally in acute cases.

For example, a patient has a productive cough with profuse watery sputum, breathlessness, chilliness, a thick-sticky coating and a Slippery pulse. The clinical manifestations reflect Spleen-Yang deficiency (the Root) causing retention of Phlegm in the Lungs (the Manifestation). In this case, if the clinical manifestations are severe and acute (particularly in an elderly person), the correct approach is to deal with the Manifestation first, by resolving Phlegm and stimulating the Lung descending function. Later, when the symptoms of phlegm have subsided, one can treat the Root, i.e. tonify and warm the Spleen.

Another example: a woman suffering from dysmenorrhoea caused by stasis of Blood, itself caused by deficiency of Qi. In this case, the correct approach is to concentrate on treating the Manifestation (i.e. move Blood and stop pain) before or during the period, and treating the Root (i.e. tonify Qi) just after and in between periods.

MULTIPLE ROOTS AND MANIFESTATIONS

So far fairly simple examples have been given when only one Root gives rise to one Manifestation. In reality, however, actual clinical cases are often more complex. There can be more than one Root as well as more than one Manifestation.

There are three possible situations:

More than one Root, each giving rise to different Manifestations

One Root giving rise to different Manifestations

The Root coincides with the Manifestation.

1) It is very common to have more than one Root. This is due to the fact that, in the course of one's life, several different causes of disease occurring at different times may overlap. For example, a previous trauma to a joint may predispose someone to subsequent invasion of exterior Cold and Damp in that joint. Or someone may suffer from a Liver disharmony caused by dietary reasons and later on in life develop Liver-Yang rising from repressed anger. Thus there can be different Roots, each reflected in various different Manifestations.

For example, a patient may have Liver-Fire (the Root) caused by certain emotional problems over a long period of time. Later on, he or she may be exposed to Cold, invading the channels of the shoulder and causing pain and stiffness. In this case there are two separate roots, one being Liver-Fire (caused by emotional problems), the other being exterior Cold invading the shoulder channels (caused by exposure to exterior Cold). It would be wrong then in this case to try and interpret all the clinical manifestations in the light of one Root only, such as Liver-Fire. As for the treatment, when there is more than one Root, each one must be treated.

Another example: a patient may suffer from Kidney-Yang deficiency (the Root) caused by excessive sexual activity. Later in life he also suffers from stagnation of Liver-Qi (another Root) caused by emotional problems. In this case there are two separate Roots (Kidney-Yang deficiency and Liver-Qi stagnation) from two different causes, and it would be wrong to try and weave all the clinical manifestations into a common pattern.

Of course the different Roots do not co-exist independently, but may also interact with one another, further complicating the picture. For instance, in the example just given, the stagnant Liver-Qi may invade the Spleen and cause Spleen-Yang deficiency which would further aggravate the Kidney-Yang deficiency.

2) One Root can give rise to several different Manifestations. For example, if a patient (particularly a woman) suffers from Spleen-Qi deficiency, this can give rise to oedema (because Spleen-Qi is unable to transport and transform fluids) and also to deficiency of Blood (because the Spleen is unable to make Blood). There will therefore be two Manifestations (the oedema and the deficiency of Blood) arising from the same Root. The treatment in this case is still simply directed at treating the Root.

3) In certain cases the Root and the Manifestation coincide. This can only happen when the clinical manifestations are caused by external physical trauma, such as in an accident. For example, if a person has an accident to the knee, this will cause stagnation of Qi and/or Blood in the knee channels leading to pain. In this case, the stagnation of Qi (the Root), coincides with the knee pain (the Manifestation).

WHEN TO SUPPORT UPRIGHT QI, WHEN TO EXPEL PATHOGENIC FACTORS

This is the second important question to consider when working out a plan of treatment. This question is closely related to the question of when to tonify and when to reduce, so that the two can be discussed together.

Upright Qi is not a particular type of Qi but simply the sum total of all of the body's Qi mostly in relation to its capacity to fight pathogenic factors. Upright Qi could therefore also be described as the body's resistance to disease. It is a term which is used only in relation and in contrast to pathogenic factors.

Pathogenic factors (in Chinese called "*Xie*" which means "evil") indicate any disease factor, whether exterior (such as Wind, Damp, Cold, Heat) or interior (such as Phlegm, Fire, Interior Wind, Stasis of Blood or Stagnation of Qi).

An Excess condition is characterized by the presence of a pathogenic factor, whether interior or exterior, while the Upright Qi is still relatively intact and fights the pathogenic factors.

A Deficient condition is characterized by weakness of the Upright Qi and the absence of a pathogenic factor.

A mixed Deficient/Excess condition is characterized by weakness of the Upright Qi, but also by the presence of a pathogenic factor. Although there is a pathogenic factor, the Upright Qi is weak and does not react adequately or successfully to the pathogenic factor. This is a very common situation in practice, probably more common than a purely Excess condition.

All the various pathological changes and developments of a disease can be seen as various stages in the struggle between the Upright Qi and pathogenic factors. All the numerous changes, improvements and aggravations are due to fluctuations in the relative strength of the Upright Qi and pathogenic factors.

When planning a treatment it is essential to have a clear idea as to the relative strengths of Upright Qi and pathogenic factors, or whether there is a pathogenic factor at all. This is important in order to adopt the correct strategy of treatment. The main question is whether the condition calls for tonification or sedation or both. If both are required, should they be applied simultaneously or in succession, and if so, which one should be applied first? In order to answer these questions we can consider three possible approaches:

1 To tonify Upright Qi
2 To expel pathogenic factors
3 To tonify Upright Qi and expel the pathogenic factors

In this last case there are still three possible courses of action:

a) First tonify Upright Qi, then expel the pathogenic factors
b) First expel the pathogenic factors, then tonify Upright Qi
c) Tonify Upright Qi and expel the pathogenic factors simultaneously.

TONIFY UPRIGHT QI

This includes any method that strengthens the body condition and increases resistance to disease. This may be achieved with acupuncture, herbal treatment, exercise, diet, *Qi Gong*, meditation or simply rest. More specifically, from the acupuncture point of view, it implies tonification of Qi, Blood and Original Qi, by use of the reinforcing method of needling or moxibustion.

The method of tonifying the Upright Qi is applicable when this is weak, or more specifically, in purely Deficient patterns. This approach can also be used in mixed Deficiency/Excess patterns but only if the pattern is predominantly Deficient. Here tonifying Upright Qi strengthens Qi so that it can eliminate any pathogenic factor that there might be. Hence the saying: "*Support Upright Qi, to eliminate the pathogenic factors*".

It must be stressed, however, that this approach is only applicable if a mixed Deficient/Excess pattern is predominantly Deficient. If, however, there is a strong pathogenic factor, tonifying Upright Qi may not only fail to eliminate it, but actually in certain cases, even reinforce it and make the condition worse.

The approach of tonifying Upright Qi is only applicable in interior conditions, as exterior conditions are by definition of the Excess type, being characterized by the presence of a pathogenic factor. Only in very few cases of exterior conditions is it necessary to combine expelling the pathogenic factor with tonifying Upright Qi. This will be discussed later within this chapter.

Examples of purely Deficient patterns, when the approach of tonifying Upright Qi is applicable, are Spleen-Qi Deficiency (manifesting with lack of appetite, tiredness, loose stools and an Empty pulse) or Blood Deficiency (manifesting with dizziness, blurred vision, poor memory, scanty periods, a Choppy pulse and a Pale tongue).

An example of a mixed Deficiency/Excess pattern, but predominantly Deficient, might be that of Stomach and/or Spleen Deficient allowing themselves to be invaded by Liver-Qi (manifesting with tiredness, no appetite, loose stools, an Empty pulse, a slight dull epigastric pain and slight nausea). The last two symptoms are due to stagnant Liver-Qi invading the Stomach. In this case, however, it is not that Liver-Qi invades the Stomach, but rather that Stomach-Qi is weak and allows itself to be invaded by Liver-Qi. This is borne out by the prevalence of Deficiency symptoms and signs. In this case, the correct course of action is to tonify the Stomach, so that when this is strengthened, Liver-Qi will not be able to invade it.

EXPEL THE PATHOGENIC FACTORS

This includes any method that eliminates the pathogenic factors, whether exterior or interior. This might be acupuncture, herbal treatment, massage or cupping.

From acupuncture's point of view, it involves eliminating the pathogenic factors by using the reducing method, bleeding or cupping.

This approach is applicable only in purely Excess patterns characterized by the presence of an exterior or interior pathogenic factor. Expelling the pathogenic factor will remove any obstruction caused by it and will indirectly contribute to strengthening Upright Qi (because it can circulate unhampered by the obstruction of the pathogenic factors). Hence the saying: *"Eliminate the pathogenic factors to strengthen Upright Qi"*.

It is important to note that the decision to expel a pathogenic factor by using a reducing method must be based purely on the Excess character of the pattern and not on subjective feelings about the patient. We should not "translate subjective emotional feelings into a desire to tonify or sedate".[1] In other words, if the pattern identification is correct and the pattern is definitely of an Excess character, a reducing method is called for, even if the patient might be elderly or apparently weak. If the pattern is of an Excess character and the pathogenic factor is expelled, the patient will feel better and have more energy because the obstruction of the pathogenic factor is removed.

This is especially true in Exterior conditions, when it is necessary to use the reducing method to expel the exterior pathogenic factor. Were the reinforcing method used to tonify Qi, the patient would become worse because tonifying Qi in acute exterior conditions tends also to "tonify" the pathogenic factor, and thus aggravate the situation. For example, if a patient has symptoms of an attack of Wind-Cold (such as an aversion to cold, a runny nose, sneezing, a stiff neck, and a Floating-Tight pulse), this is an Excess condition, even though the person might have suffered from deficiency of Qi or Blood previously to the exterior attack. This condition is therefore treated by expelling the pathogenic factor, in this case Wind-Cold. We can later attend to the underlying deficiency and tonify Qi and Blood, but only after the pathogenic factor has been expelled. Of course, in a few cases, when the patient is extremely weak and debilitated, it might be necessary to combine the reducing method to expel the pathogenic factor, with the reinforcing method to tonify Qi. This is, however, rarely necessary and it will be discussed under the next heading.

Another example of an Excess pattern, in this case interior, which requires treatment by the method of expelling pathogenic factors is that of Liver-Fire with symptoms and signs such as thirst, red eyes, a red face, a bitter taste, constipation, dark urine, headaches, irritability, a Red tongue with yellow coating and a Rapid and Wiry pulse.

TONIFY UPRIGHT QI AND EXPEL THE PATHOGENIC FACTORS

First tonify Upright Qi, then expel the pathogenic factors

This approach is used when there is a pathogenic factor to be expelled, but the Upright Qi is too weak to use a reducing method, as this would weaken it further. This situation is however, rather rare and applies only to exterior patterns, when a very weak and possibly elderly person has been attacked by an exterior pathogenic factor and Upright Qi is extremely weak. In this situation it is not possible to expel the pathogenic factor as the reducing method might further weaken Upright Qi. One can therefore first tonify Upright Qi, and then expel the pathogenic factor.

It must be noted here that tonifying Upright Qi alone is not sufficient to expel the pathogenic factor.

This approach does not apply to interior conditions, as in these cases one can tonify the body's Qi and expel the pathogenic factor at the same time.

For example, if a very weak elderly person with chronic bronchitis has an attack of Wind-Cold, one could tonify Qi first, and then expel Wind-Cold. This approach, however, is seldom necessary and is not widely applied.

First expel the pathogenic factors, then tonify Upright Qi

This approach is suitable when there is a pathogenic factor and Upright Qi is weak, but eliminating the pathogenic factor is called for due to the urgency or severity of the clinical manifestations. This approach is also used because tonifying Upright Qi alone can in certain cases also stimulate the pathogenic factor.

This strategy is widely used in clinical practice both in exterior and interior conditions. In fact, when there is a pathogenic factor and the body's Qi is weak, this is the standard procedure to adopt, apart from a few rare cases already mentioned.

We can expel the pathogenic factor first using the reducing method. Once the pathogenic factor is expelled and the Excess-type clinical manifestations have gone, only then can we tonify Upright Qi. This approach is applicable in both exterior and interior conditions, but particularly in exterior ones. We should pay attention when tonifying the Upright Qi, that there is no pathogenic factor left.

In exterior patterns this is generally the approach adopted. For example, if a patient previously suffering from deficiency of Qi is attacked by exterior Wind-Heat and has symptoms of fever, headache, slight sweating, aversion to cold, body aches and Floating-Rapid pulse, the correct approach would be to expel Wind-Heat and release the Exterior (by reducing such points as Hegu L.I.-4, Quchi L.I.-11 or Waiguan T.B.-5). When the exterior symptoms have totally gone (no fever, body aches, aversion to cold, Floating pulse), only then can one tonify the Upright Qi. Tonifying the Upright Qi before the Wind-Heat has been expelled can somehow stimulate the Wind-Heat too and lead to a worsening of the condition. For example, the fever might rise.

It is also important to pay attention to this point even when a fairly long time has elapsed after an exterior attack. In certain cases, if the exterior pathogenic factor is not expelled properly, it can penetrate the Interior and lurk there for a long time after the initial attack. To continue with the previous example of attack of Wind-Heat, the person would find it difficult to recover from the attack, experience great tiredness and become prone to strange recurrent sore throats: these would be due to some remaining Heat "lurking" in the Interior. In Chinese this is called "left-over pathogenic factor". In these cases it is important to be able to recognize it and clear the remaining Heat before tonifying the Upright Qi, as normally one would tend to tonify the Upright Qi straight away since the person would complain of great tiredness. Symptoms and signs of "left-over pathogenic factor" after an exterior attack would be tiredness, a feeling of heat, recurrent sore throats, a Red tongue with a thin yellow coating in the area between the tip and the centre (Lung area) and a slightly Wiry pulse. In this case we could use points to clear interior Heat such as Chize LU-5, Quchi L.I.-11 or Dazhui Du-14.

In interior patterns this approach is used whenever the symptoms caused by the pathogenic factors are so severe or urgent that they need to be dealt with without delay.

For example, a patient with a chronic Kidney and Heart Yang deficiency suffers an acute episode of total retention of urine leading to hypertension and oedema. In this case the pathogenic factor is "Water overflowing" causing oedema and retention of urine. Since this needs to be dealt with without delay, one must first expel the pathogenic factor, in this case "Water overflowing", by using a reducing method (on points such as Yinlingquan SP-9, Shuidao ST-28, Shuifen Ren-9, Weiyang BL-39 or Sanjiaoshu BL-22) as the Lower Burner is in an Excess condition. After the oedema is resolved and the urinary function restored, one can tonify Kidney and Heart Yang.

Another example: a patient with a chronic condition of Liver Blood deficiency has an acute episode of Liver-Wind causing a temporary spasm of a cerebral vessel and a small stroke, with temporary giddiness, numbness, paralysis of mouth and slurred speech. In this case, it is essential to eliminate the pathogenic factor first, i.e. the Liver Wind, by using the reducing method (on points such as Taichong LIV-3 and Xingjian LIV-2). Only when Liver Wind has been eliminated and the symptoms of it gone, can we tonify Liver-Blood.

This approach is not only applicable in acute and urgent cases such as those mentioned above, but also in chronic cases where the symptoms do not have a character of urgency but are nevertheless, very distressing and painful.

For example, a patient may suffer from a chronic deficiency of Liver and Kidney Yin leading to the rising of Liver-Yang. This would cause severe headaches as well as dizziness, irritability, and so on. Although the symptoms are not acute or urgent, the headaches may nevertheless be extremely painful and distressing. It is therefore necessary to subdue Liver-Yang first, and then tonify Liver and Kidney Yin.

Tonify the Upright Qi and expel the pathogenic factors simultaneously

This is a widely used approach in cases when there is a pathogenic factor and the Upright Qi is relatively weak, but not so weak as to need to be tonified first (as in case 1, p. 317).

This approach can only be used in interior conditions, as in exterior conditions it is usually necessary to expel the pathogenic factor first and then tonify the Upright Qi.

Thus this method is used in cases of mixed Deficiency/Excess interior patterns. Many examples could be given. If there is a condition of Liver-Yin deficiency with rising of Liver-Yang, one can simultaneously tonify Liver-Yin and subdue Liver-Yang. In case of Spleen-Qi deficiency leading to the formation of Dampness, one can tonify Spleen-Qi and resolve Dampness at the same time.

From the acupuncture point of view, this involves using the reinforcing method on some points and the reducing method on others. In the two above examples, one could tonify Taixi KI-3, Sanyinjiao SP-6 and Ququan LIV-8 to nourish Liver-Yin and reduce Xingjian LIV-2 and Xiaxi G.B.-43 to subdue Liver-Yang. In case of Spleen deficiency with Dampness, one could tonify Pishu BL-20 and Zusanli ST-36 to tonify Spleen-Qi and reduce Yinlingquan SP-9 and Sanyinjiao SP-6 to eliminate Dampness.

THE CONSTITUTION

When planning a treatment, besides considering the Root and the Manifestation, one must also take into account the constitution of a person.

ESSENCE-QI-MIND

By constitution we mean the fundamental physical and mental make-up of an individual. According to Chinese Medicine, the constitution is made up of three factors, i.e. Essence, Qi and Mind (in Chinese *Jing-Qi-Shen*). Of these three elements, Essence is the foundation for the other two. If the inherited Essence is strong, this will constitute a basis for a healthy life from the physical and mental point of view. Obviously this does not mean a totally disease-free life as many other causes of disease can undermine a person's health, but it does mean that the person will have a strong resistance to disease.

Essence, Qi and Mind are called in Chinese the "Three Treasures" (*San Bao*). Health, strength, vitality, happiness, volition, mental stability and clarity, all depend on a good supply of these three vital substances and their harmonious interaction. Essence is related to the Kidneys, Qi to the Lungs, and Mind to the Heart.

These three substances also represent three different states of "rarefaction", Essence being the coarsest and densest constituent is the foundation. Qi is the refined energy that nourishes the body and mind, and the Mind is the most refined and immaterial of the three substances. Thus the three Treasures represent an interaction between two poles of matter and energy, substantial and non-substantial, physical and mental, which is typical of Chinese Medicine and philosophy.

The interaction of Essence and Qi determines the state of the Mind: if Essence and Qi are strong, the Mind will be healthy and if the Essence and Qi are weak, the Mind will suffer.

The state of the Essence gives an indication of the congenital, hereditary Qi and the inherited constitution, while the state of Qi gives an indication of the acquired Qi. The two together determine the state of the Mind.

The state of the Essence can be gauged by the general vitality, symptomatology, pulse and eyes.

Vitality and resistance to disease is indicative of a strong Essence. If this is weak, a person may feel extremely tired and lethargic and be prone to attacks of exterior pathogenic factors.

Essence generates bones and nourishes the brain, so that when it is strong, the bones develop normally and do not degenerate too rapidly with age. In addition, the mental faculties are clear and memory good. If Essence is weak, there may be poor bone development in children, or early bone degeneration in adults, poor mental development in children or poor memory and loss of hair or premature greying of the hair in adults.

The so-called Leather pulse (a pulse that feels stretched like a drum on the superficial level and empty on the deep level) is indicative of a deficient Essence.

In some cases, a very Deep pulse which is nearly non-existent on both Rear positions also indicates a deficiency of Essence.

The state of the Essence is also reflected in the eyes: eyes with "glitter" show a good state of the Essence and Mind, while eyes which are dull and opaque show a depleted state of the Essence and a Mind disturbed by deep emotional problems.

The state of Qi can of course be gauged by normal Chinese diagnosis based on the symptomatology and observation particularly of the tongue and palpation of the pulse.

The state of the Mind is primarily a result of the interaction of Essence and Qi, and is also reflected in the eyes in the way mentioned above. The state of the Mind is also reflected in the Heart pulse: if the Mind is strong the Heart pulse is strong but not overflowing. If the Mind is weak, the Heart pulse may be very deep and "without wave", i.e. it gives the impression of not flowing smoothly up towards the wrist. On the other hand, if the Mind is disturbed, and the person has mental problems, the Heart pulse may be Full, Hard and Overflowing.

Chinese language shows how these concepts are rooted in Chinese culture. The word *"Jing-Shen"* (i.e. Essence-Mind) means "mind" or "consciousness", showing the interaction and integration of body and mind typical of Chinese philosophy. *"Jing-Shen"* can also mean "vigour", "vitality", "drive", all qualities which are present when both Essence and Mind are healthy and strong. *"Jing-Shen-bing"* means "mental illness".

THE FIVE ELEMENTS AND THE CONSTITUTION

Five constitutional types can be identified each referring to one of the Five Elements. Identifying a particular type can be useful in determining the character and prognosis of any disease.

Wood

Wood types have a darkish face, a tall, slender body, and fairly broad shoulders. They are typified by their strong bones and sinews and they should have a strong and straight back. Wood types are hard workers and have a tendency to worry (Fig. 62).

Fire

The Fire type has a reddish face, a small pointed head or pointed chin, curly hair or not much hair, small hands and he or she walks fast. The Fire type is quick and energetic and active. People of this type tend to be unconcerned about material wealth, and fond of beauty. They often have a short life (Fig. 63).

Their strong point is their blood vessels and Blood.

Metal

The Metal type has broad and square shoulders, a triangular white face, a strongly-built body and he or she walks slowly and deliberately.

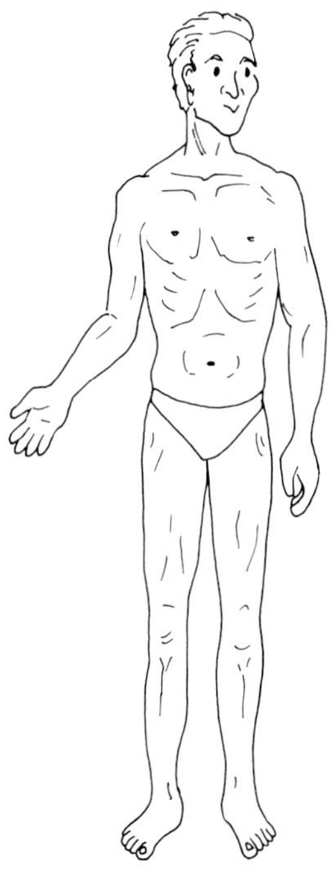

Fig. 62 Wood type

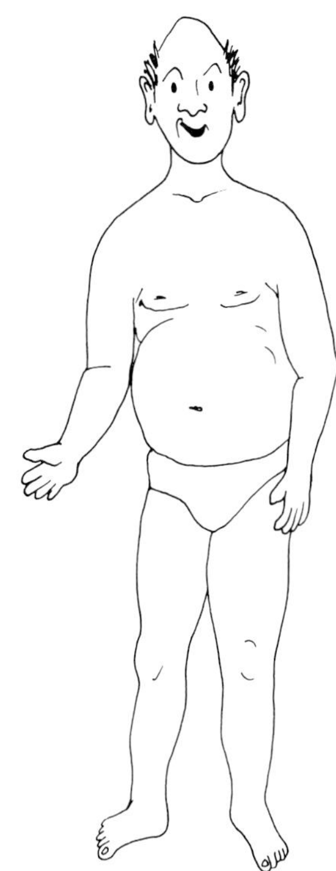

Fig. 63 Fire type

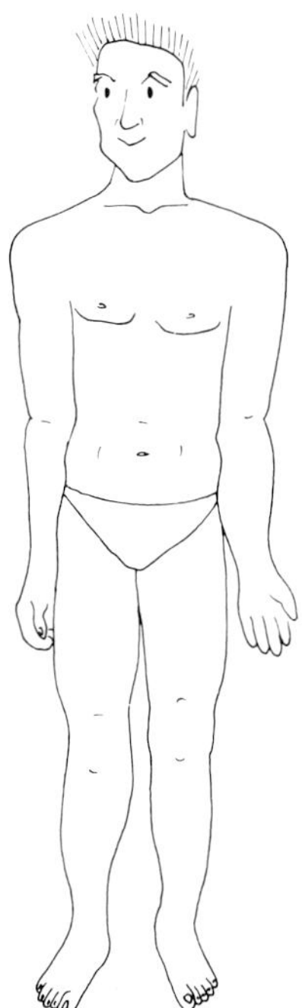

Fig. 64 Metal type

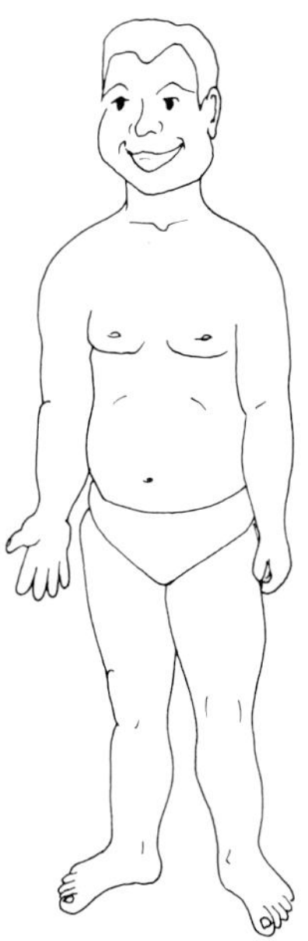

Fig. 65 Earth type

They are meticulous, rational, independent and strong-willed. Their strong point should be their Lungs and they should have a strong voice (Fig. 64).

Earth

Earth types have a darkish complexion and somewhat fat body, a large head, a large belly, strong thighs and wide jaws. They are calm and generous and they are not ambitious. They walk without lifting their feet very high and their strong point are the muscles (Fig. 65).

Water

Water types have a round face and body and soft-white skin. They love movement and their spine is longer than normal (Fig. 66). They are sympathetic and slightly lazy and they do not always tell the truth. They are good negotiators and loyal to their work colleagues. They are aware, sensitive and sometimes psychic. Their strong point should be the digestive system.[2]

This typology can be used in diagnosis and prognosis. These portraits describe an archetype but in reality, due to the way people live their lives and other factors, there can be considerable variations. For example, although a Wood type typically has a tall and slender body, if there is a tendency to over-eat, he or she may obviously become fat and deviate from their type.

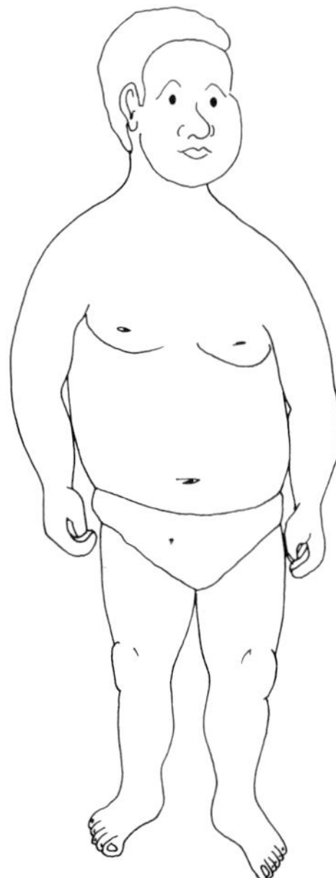

Fig. 66 Water type

Moreover, a person may be a mixture of two or more types; one can have a mixed Earth-Wood type for example.

As far as diagnosis and prognosis are concerned, it is the deviations from the ideal types that are important.

If a Wood type does not have a tall and slender body, it may indicate health problems. If they lose too much hair, it may indicate that there is too much Fire within Wood, burning the hair on top of the head.

The Fire type should walk fast: if they do not, it indicates disease. Their strong point should be the Blood and blood vessels, but if it is not, they are then prone to high blood pressure and heart disease. A poor Fire constitution may be indicated by a very weak and deep heart pulse and a central midline crack on the tongue running to the tip.

Metal types should walk slowly and deliberately: if they habitually walk fast, it may indicate a health problem. Their voice should be strong: if it is weak, it indicates a problem with their Lungs. A poor Metal constitution may be indicated by two small transversal cracks on the tongue in the Lung area and by a pulse that runs from the Front position up towards the base of the thumb medially (see p. 135).

The Earth type should have strong muscles. If they do not, it indicates problems, and they become prone to arthritis and rheumatism.

Water types tend to overindulge in sexual activity, and this may cause Kidney-Essence problems which would be reflected in the eyes with a lack of lustre.

To sum up, each person must be observed carefully and the type assessed so that deviations from the type can be noted. If a person has a certain trait which is unrelated to that particular type, the prognosis is better than if that trait represents a deviation from the type. For example, the Fire type should walk fast. If they walk too fast, it is not so bad as a Metal type walking fast (as the Metal type should walk slowly). Or if a Metal type has a weak voice, it is worse than if another type has a weak voice.

In conclusion, when assessing a person's constitution, we must weigh up the relative strength or power of the "Three Treasures" (Essence, Qi and Mind) and the 5-Element types.

There is often a correspondence between the prevailing Root and the constitution. For example, if a person has a constitutional weakness of the Lungs, he will tend to suffer from a Lung pattern. However, a constitutional weakness may not cause any symptoms or signs, and yet still be visible to an experienced practitioner. In these cases, the question arises whether one should treat according to the constitution even if there are no clinical manifestations.

Generally speaking, it is usually better to treat according to the constitution only towards the end of the treatment in order to consolidate the results. On the other hand, one must pay attention not to exceed in treating the constitution and stir up problems unnecessarily. For example, concentrating on treating according to the constitution ignoring the present pattern of disharmony may disturb the body's Qi unnecessarily and in some cases conflict with the therapeutic needs of the patient. For example, a weak constitution of a Fire-type person may manifest with a slow walk (instead of rapid, as would be normal for a Fire-type), a midline crack on the tongue and a Weak Heart pulse. If this person, through various disease-factors during his or her life, has developed a Kidney-Yang deficiency giving rise to chilliness, weak knees, frequent and pale urination, a lower back ache and slight mental depression, it would probably be wrong to concentrate on treating the constitution, i.e. the Heart. This might stir up the Mind unnecessarily and lead to a further imbalance between Fire and Water perhaps causing anxiety and insomnia. The correct approach would be to attend to the presenting pattern of Kidney-Yang deficiency first. Owing to the relationship among Essence, Qi and Mind, this will also indirectly invigorate the Mind and the Heart and therefore strengthen the constitution. Only at a late stage of the treatment, it might be useful to treat the constitution by tonifying the Heart, thus consolidating the therapeutic results.

It is thus important to strike a balance between treating according to the findings from a presenting pattern, and according to a person's constitution.

CASE HISTORIES

MAN, AGE 44

Clinical manifestations

Headaches over a long period, on either temple. The ache was intense and of a stabbing character; there was occasionally vomiting, numbness of the right arm and thirst. He also suffered from tinnitus of the left ear for 3 years with a low-pitch sound. His sleep was not good as he often woke up, unable to fall asleep again.

Pulse: Wiry, especially on the left side.

Tongue: body colour normal, sides slightly pale.

Diagnosis

Liver-Blood deficiency with Liver-Yang rising.

Explanation

The symptoms of Liver-Blood deficiency are numbness of the right arm, Pale tongue-sides and insomnia. The symptoms of Liver-Yang rising are intense temporal headache, vomiting, tinnitus and a Wiry pulse.

Treatment principle

This is a Deficient Interior pattern. Deficiency of Liver-Blood is the Root as it is the primary aspect of the condition, and Liver-Yang rising is the Manifestation.

In this case we need simultaneously to tonify Upright Qi (in this case Liver-Blood) and to subdue the pathogenic factor (Liver-Yang rising). Here we simultaneously treat the Root and the Manifestation as the symptoms are severe and distressing. Had the patient had more symptoms of Liver-Blood deficiency and only slight occasional headaches, treating only the Root (i.e. tonifying Liver-Blood) might have been sufficient.

WOMAN, AGE 35

Clinical manifestations

Prior to the initial consultation this lady had had a very heavy cold with a congested chest, an occipital headache and alternating feelings of heat and cold. When she came for the consultation she complained of a feeling of exhaustion, slight depression, a slight hypochondriac pain and loose stools.

Pulse: Wiry.

Tongue: body colour normal, thin white coating in the Lung area.

Diagnosis

This was originally an attack of exterior Wind-Cold at the Lesser Yang stage; now it is still at the Lesser Yang stage, but combined with the Greater Yin stage (see App. 1).

Explanation

The symptoms of the Lesser Yang pattern are alternating feeling of heat and cold, hypochondriac pain, slight depression and a Wiry pulse.

The symptoms of the Greater Yin pattern are exhaustion and loose stools.

Although this patient was seen three weeks after the onset, the pattern was still partially at the Lesser Yang stage, and the pulse was all important in the diagnosis. Since this was Wiry and Full, it indicated that the pattern was still primarily of an Excess character, even though the patient felt very tired, which is a Deficiency symptom.

Treatment principle

Since the pattern is still primarily of an Excess nature and is characterized by the presence of a pathogenic factor (Wind-Cold turned into Heat at the Lesser Yang stage), the correct approach is to concentrate on expelling the pathogenic factor, even though the patient feels tired. When the pathogenic factor has been expelled, one can tonify the Upright Qi, in this case Spleen and Lung Qi.

This was the plan of treatment adopted and in the first treatment Waiguan T.B.-5, Zhigou T.B.-6 and Dazhui Du-14 were needled with reducing method, to clear Heat and regulate the Lesser Yang (Triple Burner). Reducing these points produced a nearly immediate and dramatic improvement including the return of her energy. After reducing similar points again in the second treatment and the disappearance of the Lesser Yang symptoms (hypochondriac pain and Wiry pulse), attention was diverted to tonifying the body's Qi, reinforcing Taiyuan LU-9, Sanyinjiao SP-6, Zusanli ST-36 and Neiguan P-6.

This is an example of the principle of expelling the pathogenic factor first and tonifying the Upright Qi later. From the point of view of Root and Manifestation, the Root is represented by the Heat which is half in the Interior and half in the Exterior (Lesser Yang stage) producing the various clinical manifestations. In this case, only the Root was treated, clearing all the clinical manifestations.

WOMAN, AGE 38

Clinical manifestations

This woman had suffered from hypochondriac pain on the right side and a feeling of "lump" in the right abdominal region for a long time. In addition, she also suffered from diarrhoea if she ate too many cold-raw foods. For the last year she sweated slightly at night. Her urination was frequent and pale, she felt very cold all the time and the menstrual blood had clots but was not dark.

Pulse: Deep-Weak and Minute.

Tongue: Pale on the sides, Bluish-Purple on the root and centre.

Diagnosis

Long-standing Liver-Blood deficiency giving rise to slight Yin deficiency (just starting) and causing stasis of Blood.

There is also a Kidney-Yang deficiency causing interior Cold and stasis of Blood in the Lower Burner.

Explanation

This is a complicated situation. There are two Roots, each of them giving rise to two Manifestations.

The first Root is the chronic deficiency of Liver-Blood as manifested in the pale sides of the tongue. This gives rise to a slight deficiency of Yin (night sweating) and also to stasis of Blood (feeling of a lump in the abdomen, clots in the menstrual blood and Purple colour of the tongue on the root and centre).

The second Root is Kidney-Yang deficiency (feeling cold, diarrhoea from cold-raw foods, frequent-pale urination and Deep-Minute pulse), causing interior Cold and stasis of Blood in the Lower Burner (tongue body Purple). In this case, therefore, the stasis of Blood can be attributed both to the chronic deficiency of Liver-Blood and to the obstruction from interior Cold. For this reason, the tongue is Bluish-Purple. The bluish colour indicates Cold while the Purple colour indicates stasis.

As for the relative strength of Upright Qi and pathogenic factors, this is an interior condition characterized by extreme weakness of the Upright Qi and by the presence of pathogenic factors, which are the stasis of Blood and the interior Cold. It is therefore a mixed Deficiency/Excess pattern. The Deficiency patterns are the Liver-Blood and Kidney-Yang deficiency, the Excess factors are the interior Cold and the stasis of Blood.

Treatment principle

In this case treatment must be aimed primarily at tonifying the body's Qi, hence concentrating on treating the Root. This can be achieved by tonifying Ququan LIV-8, Sanyinjiao SP-6, Ganshu BL-18 and Geshu BL-17 to tonify Liver-Blood and Taixi KI-3 and Shenshu BL-23 to tonify Kidney-Yang.

The clinical manifestations can be treated simultaneously to relieve the symptoms caused by the stasis of Blood with such points as Neiguan P-6 and Xuehai SP-10 to move Blood.

WOMAN, AGE 24

Clinical manifestations

This patient had an exterior condition overlapping a chronic interior one, and only came for treatment after the exterior condition had set in and penetrated to the Interior.

As this is a complicated case, I shall give the clinical manifestations in three groups: the underlying chronic condition, the acute exterior attack and the sequelae of such an attack (when she came for treatment)

1 *Chronic condition*: propensity to catching colds, giddiness, Deep-Fine Pulse, both Rear positions very Weak.

Tongue: Pale-Purple, dry.

2 *Acute, exterior attack*: temperature of 101°F (38.5°C), feeling of heaviness, body aches, headache, "buzzing in ears", giddiness.

3 *Sequelae*: constant temperature of 99.5°F (37.5°C), lack of balance and coordination, tinnitus, nystagmus, extreme tiredness, poor sleep, lethargy, feeling of heaviness of the legs, numbness of limbs, occipital headache. In particular, the lack of balance and coordination was very pronounced and led Western doctors to suspect a neurological lesion.

Diagnosis and explanation

1 *Chronic condition*: severe Kidney-Yang deficiency. In this case the tongue is dry from deficient Yang-Qi unable to transport fluids to it. It is also Purple as the deficiency of Kidney-Yang has caused interior Cold which, in turn, causes stasis of Blood.

2 *Acute, exterior attack*: this was an attack of exterior Wind-Damp-Heat.

3 *Sequelae*: these are caused by the exterior pathogenic factors penetrating in the Interior. The Heat and Dampness have become interior and caused the constant low-grade temperature. Once in the Interior, they disturb the circulation of Qi and Blood and, overlapping with the pre-existing condition of Kidney-Yang deficiency,

they cause the rising of Liver-Wind (nystagmus, lack of balance and coordination). These are caused by interior Wind arising from the deficiency of Blood and Kidney-Yang. In addition, Damp-Heat is steaming in the Interior causing the constant low-grade temperature, numbness, extreme tiredness, feeling of heaviness and lethargy.

Treatment principle

The patient only came at the sequelae stage, when the condition was an interior one. It was characterized by an extreme deficiency of Upright Qi and by the presence of formerly exterior pathogenic factors, now become interior (Damp-Heat).

In addition, the exterior attack had also given rise to another interior pathogenic factor, i.e. Liver-Wind. This is a good example of a situation when the Manifestation becomes primary. The Root is represented by the chronic condition of Kidney-Yang deficiency, which must eventually be treated as it also predisposes to Liver-Wind. However, the Manifestation in this case assumes primary importance as it causes symptoms which require urgent treatment. The Manifestation in this case is represented partly by the Damp-Heat and partly by Liver-Wind. Both these, particularly the Liver-Wind, need to be treated without delay.

Treatment in this case was aimed at treating the Manifestation first, or expelling the pathogenic factors first, and later tonifying the Upright Qi. The treatment was aimed at clearing interior Heat, resolving Dampness, subduing Wind and pacifying the Liver. Various groups of points were used at different times to achieve these aims. Quchi L.I.-11 and Dazhui Du-14 were used to clear interior Heat. Points on the Governing Vessel are particularly important to clear latent interior Heat resulting from invasion of previously exterior Heat. Points such as Yinlingquan SP-9, Sanyinjiao SP-6, Shuifen Ren-9 and Sanjiaoshu BL-22 were used to resolve Dampness; Taichong LIV-3, Fengchi G.B.-20 and Fengfu Du-16 were used to subdue Liver-Wind. Only after the symptoms of Damp-Heat and Liver-Wind had gone, was the treatment aimed at tonifying Kidney-Yang by tonifying and warming (with moxa) Shenshu BL-23, Guanyuan Ren-4 and Fuliu KI-7.

WOMAN, AGE 72

Clinical manifestations

Chronic bronchitis and emphysema for a very long time. She caught colds easily, was breathless and coughed up a lot of yellow-sticky sputum.

Pulse: Slippery, both Front positions Weak.

Tongue: Red, sticky-yellow coating.

During the course of treatment she caught a heavy cold and had the following symptoms: aversion to cold, a headache, cough, runny nose, sneezing, breathlessness and a Floating pulse.

Diagnosis

Retention of Phlegm-Heat in the Lungs and Spleen-Qi deficiency. During the acute exterior attack: invasion of Lung-Defensive Qi portion by exterior Wind-Cold.

Explanation

This condition is chronic and, as often happens in chronic conditions, there is interior Heat. There is also Phlegm, which is caused by deficient Spleen-Qi being unable to transform fluids which accumulate into Phlegm.

The Spleen-Qi deficiency is the Root and the retention of Phlegm in the Lungs is the Manifestation.

The Upright Qi is weak and there is a pathogenic factor in the form of Phlegm-Heat, hence the condition is a mixed Deficient/Excess one.

The acute attack of Wind-Cold represents another Root, causing the various clinical manifestations.

Treatment principle

Treatment must primarily be aimed at the Root, i.e. tonifying Spleen-Qi because, as long as the Spleen is weak, new Phlegm will always be formed. However, the clinical manifestations are in this case severe and distressing and also need treatment. So in this case both the Root and the Manifestation need to be treated simultaneously and the treatment must combine tonifying the Upright Qi (in this case Spleen-Qi) with resolving the pathogenic factor (in this case Phlegm-Heat).

During the acute attack of common cold, the treatment principle is entirely different. In this case, treatment of the acute condition takes precedence over the chronic one for several reasons. First of all, the acute condition is exterior, and one cannot simultaneously tonify the Upright Qi and expel an exterior pathogenic factor with acupuncture. Secondly, this patient has emphysema and chronic bronchitis, and therefore an exterior attack of Wind-Cold can have very serious consequences if not treated promptly. The Wind-Cold attack, for instance, could very easily turn into pneumonia, considering the tendency to Lung trouble and the retention of Phlegm-Heat in the Lung.

During the acute attack of Wind-Cold, the primary aim of treatment is to expel the pathogenic factor first and tonify the Upright Qi later. Points used to expel Wind-Cold were Lieque LU-7 and Fengmen BL-12 with cupping.

NOTES

1 1982 Report on Dr T Kaptchuk Seminar. Journal of Oriental Medicine (Australia) no.1: 18.
2 These types are taken from chapter 64 of the Spiritual Axis, p 115, and from a seminar given by Dr JHF Shen in London in 1979.

Principles of Combination of Points 36

配穴法

After identifying the patterns and formulating a plan of treatment, the next step for an acupuncturist is that of the selection of points to use. There are two different considerations:

— the selection of points according to their action
— the combination of points according to channel dynamics.

In other words, in order to give an effective acupuncture treatment, it is not enough to select the points according to their individual characteristics and energetic action. We must also be able to combine points harmoniously according to their action within the channel system.

Acupuncture works via the channels, not just via isolated points so that each point should not only be considered for its individual action but also for its place within the channel system. Even if we master the action of each individual point, this is still not enough to give an effective acupuncture treatment, as each point must be seen not in isolation but within the dynamics of the channel system so as to attain a harmonious combination of points.

For example, one might treat Spleen-Qi deficiency and Liver-Qi stagnation by tonifying Pishu BL-20 and Weishu BL-21 and reducing Ganshu BL-18 and Danshu BL-19. Although technically correct from the point of view of energetic action of the individual points, it would be an unbalanced point prescription as all the points selected are on the back.

To give another example, one might treat Liver and Kidney Yin deficiency by tonifying Taixi KI-3, Taichong LIV-3, Sanyinjiao SP-6 and Zhaohai KI-6. Again, this would be correct according to the functions of the individual points, but also rather unbalanced as all the points are on the distal part of the legs.

Let us then look at the principles regulating the combination of points according to the channel-system dynamics.

BALANCE OF POINTS

TOP AND BOTTOM

The channel system forms a closed circuit of energy circulation with a maximum potential of energy on the head, minimum on the chest and average on the hands and feet. In order to maintain the balance between the upper and lower part of the body, it is important to balance the chosen points between these two areas.

After a needle is inserted in a point, it tends to cause a rush of energy towards the top of the body, particularly for the points at the opposite end, i.e. the lower part of the body. This movement of Qi is irrespective of the channel direction of flow.

Keeping this in mind, it is important to balance the points on the upper part of the body with those of the lower part.

An example of point prescription balancing upper and lower part of the body might be Hegu L.I.-4 and Taichong LIV-3 (called the *"Four Gates"*). This combination clears Wind from the head and has a powerful calming effect.

Another example might be the combination of Neiguan P-6 with Zusanli ST-36. P-6 harmonizes the upper and middle part of the Stomach and subdues rebellious Qi (which causes nausea and vomiting) while ST-36 tonifies Stomach-Qi. The combination of these two points provides a balanced tonification of Stomach and Spleen and can be used in many cases of epigastric problems.

Another example might be the combination of Zhigou T.B.-6 with Fengshi G.B.-31. These two points clear Wind-Heat from the Blood and can be used for herpes zoster or any skin disease manifesting with a red and itchy rash that changes position rapidly. This combination would be particularly effective if the flanks are affected.

Of course, there are numerous examples of achieving a balance by using upper and lower points together; such combinations are frequently used.

However, this does not mean that one should always balance upper with lower part. In some cases, one might deliberately want to choose an unbalanced point prescription to obtain a specific effect.

For example, if there is an imbalance of energy between the upper and lower part of the body, with a very red face, hypertension, dizziness, anxiety and insomnia caused by a deficiency of Kidney-Yin (Deficiency below) and the flaring up of Liver-Fire (Excess above), one might choose to needle only Yongquan KI-1 in order to draw the excess energy on the top downwards.

On the other hand, if a woman suffers from prolapse of the uterus caused by the sinking of Spleen-Qi, one might deliberately use a point on the upper part of the body in order to draw the energy upwards, e.g. moxibustion on Baihui Du-20.

In both cases, the channel-system dynamics is exploited to draw the energy to the upper or the lower part of the body.

There is another case in which the principles of balancing top with bottom is not applied: this is when a distal point is reduced in acute cases of sprain of the back or a joint. For example, one can strongly reduce the point Renzhong Du-26 for acute sprain of the lower back on the midline over the sacrum.

DISTAL AND LOCAL POINTS

Distal points are those on the limbs, local points are those on the trunk and head. The combination of local and distal points is the most widely used technique of balancing of points.

In channel problems, the use of local points only might sometimes be sufficient, but it is much more common to balance the local points with distal ones. The distal points actually play an important role in clearing the channel from obstructions (which may be from exterior Cold, Damp or Wind, or only from stagnation of Qi and/or Blood in cases of sprain). When choosing a distal point, we should keep in mind that distal points on the feet are more powerful than those on the hands. If we want to moderate the effect of the treatment because the patient is rather weak or old, we can then choose a distal point on the hands. For example, both Hegu L.I.-4 and Neiting ST-44 have an effect on the face and teeth and both can be used to clear Heat in the Stomach channel affecting the face and they are somewhat interchangeable. To give another example, both Waiguan T.B.-5 and Xiaxi G.B.-43 affect the temple area and can be used as distal points for the treatment of migraine headaches on the temple. The Yang channels (Greater Yang, Lesser Yang and Yang Ming) are more closely connected than the Yin channels (Greater Yin, Lesser Yin and Terminal Yin). This is because the Yang channels all end or start on the face and actually merge into one another, so that we could look upon the Large Intestine and Stomach channel for example, as one channel from this point of view. The same applies to Triple Burner-Gall Bladder and Small Intestine-Bladder. Thus, in the case of the Yang channels, we have a choice of distal points to use, either on the hands or feet, as the points are quite interchangeable. For the Yin channels, it is somewhat different. The Yin channels all end or start in the chest or abdominal cavity and they do merge into one another, but only internally, whereas the Yang channels merge into each other directly and superficially on the face. Thus, in the case of the Yin channels, we do not have the same free choice of distal points as for the Yang channels. For example, Neiguan P-6 and Taichong LIV-3 have some common properties is so far as they both move Liver-Qi, but, besides that, they have quite different actions and there is not really a question of choice between them as a distal point.

In acute cases, the distal point is used first on its own with a reducing method in order to clear the obstruction of the pathogenic factors and open the channel to make it ready for the use of the local points. A few examples will clarify this technique.

In acute sprain of the lower back on the midline, just above the sacrum, one can reduce Renzhong Du-26 first while the patient gently bends forwards and backwards. This helps to clear the obstruction in the channel (the Governing Vessel in this case). After the manipulation of the distal point, the patient lies down and local points are used according to tenderness. These may also be cupped after insertion of the needle.

In acute sprain of the shoulder joint affecting the Large Intestine channel one can strongly reduce Tiaokou ST-38, while the patient gently moves and rotates the arm, perhaps with the help of a third person if possible. After manipulation of the distal point, local points are used according to tenderness and according to the channel involved. If the affected channel is the Small Intestine, Feiyang BL-58 is used as a distal point instead.

In acute sprain of the wrist one would use a distal point on the feet, choosing the channel on the foot related to the involved channel of the wrist. For example, supposing the main tenderness is on the point Yangchi T.B.-4, one can choose the leg channel related to the Triple Burner channel with an upper-lower relation, i.e. the Gall Bladder channel. On the Gall Bladder channel one would choose the point with a corresponding location to the wrist point, i.e. on the ankle joint: this would be Qiuxu G.B.-40.

This is based on the principle of correspondence between shoulder and hip, elbow and knee, wrist and ankle, and on the relationship of leg and arm channels of the same polarity, e.g.

Table 20 Correspondence of points on joints of the upper and lower part of the body

Joint	Arm	Leg
Shoulder		
Large Intestine	Jianyu L.I.-15	Biguan ST-31
Triple Burner	Jianliao T.B.-14	Huantiao G.B.-30
Small Intestine	Naoshu S.I.-10	Chengfu BL-36
Elbow		
Large Intestine	Quchi L.I.-11	Zusanli ST-36
Triple Burner	Tianjing T.B.-10	Yanglingquan G.B.-34
Small Intestine	Xiaohai S.I.-8	Weizhong BL-40
Wrist		
Large Intestine	Yangxi L.I.-5	Jiexi ST-41
Triple Burner	Yangchi T.B.-4	Qiuxu G.B.-40
Small Intestine	Yanggu S.I.-5	Kunlun BL -60

Lung-Spleen, Heart-Kidney, Pericardium-Liver, Large Intestine-Stomach, Triple Burner-Gall Bladder and Small Intestine-Bladder. Supposing the main tender point had been on Lieque LU-7, the point used on the foot would have been Shangqiu SP-5. If the sprain had been on the elbow and the main tenderness on Quchi L.I.-11, the point of the foot chosen would have been Zusanli ST-36.

Bearing in mind the above correspondences between joints and related leg and arm channels, we can make a table of related distal points to use for each joint according to the two above correspondences (Table 20).

In interior organ problems, the method of combining distal with local points is always used. One cannot treat the internal organs without using distal points, and the local points are often not necessary, except in chronic conditions.

Of course, countless examples could be given of the use of distal points to treat internal organ diseases, such as Taichong LIV-3 to treat Liver diseases, Zusanli ST-36 to treat Stomach diseases, and so on.

In chronic conditions it is essential to use local points in combination with distal ones. The local points used are mainly the Back Transporting points and Front Collecting points for the relevant internal organs. For example, in chronic deficiency of Spleen-Qi, it would be essential to use Pishu BL-20 and possibly Weishu BL-21.

When treating chronic headaches some local points on the head are added to the point prescription to treat the Manifestation while the distal points treat the Root.

For example, in a chronic case of headaches due to deficiency of Kidney-Yin with rising of Liver-Yang, one can use Taixi KI-3, Sanyinjiao SP-6, Xiaxi G.B.-43 and Taichong LIV-3 to treat the Root (i.e. tonify Kidney-Yin and subdue Liver-Yang). To treat the Manifestation, it would be necessary to add local points according to the channel involved such as Tianchong G.B.-9 and Xuanli G.B.-6 for the Gall Bladder channel or Tongtian BL-7 for the Bladder channel. The use of local points on the head is important to remove the local stagnation of Qi or Blood in the head which results from chronic headaches especially if they always occur on the same spot.

LEFT AND RIGHT

The balancing of points on the left and right side of the body is very useful in clinical practice.

Generally speaking, in the majority of cases, bilateral needling is the rule. Such a technique is adopted when a strong effect is needed; however, there are cases when unilateral needling is just as effective.

Sometimes points can be needled unilaterally in order to balance the left and right side. This technique obtains the same therapeutic effect using fewer needles, which is always a bonus, especially for nervous patients, those who are being treated for the first time or those who have a severe deficiency of Qi and Blood. Even in other normal cases, reducing the number of needles used to the minimum without compromising the therapeutic effect is a desirable goal.

Unilateral needling balancing a point on the left with another on the right side can sometimes give even better results than bilateral needling. In particular, if the points balanced between left and right are also at opposite ends, i.e. one on the arm and the other on the leg, the effect is particularly dynamic. It is as if a pressure was applied along the tangent of a circle at opposite ends making it spin (Fig. 67).

The use of the opening and coupled points of the extraordinary vessels is, of course a good example of the use of unilateral needling and balancing of left and right. The same technique can be applied to other points.

An example of unilateral needling could be the needling of Neiguan P-6 on the right side

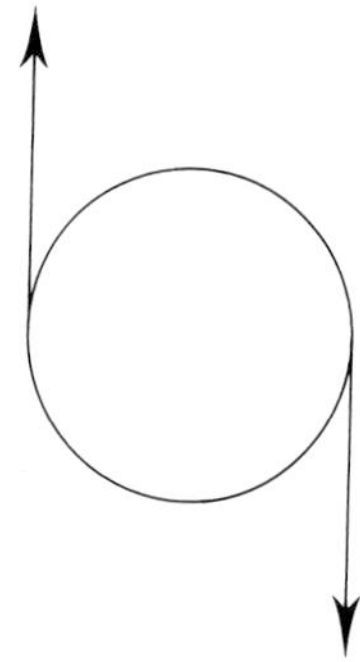

Fig. 67 Left-right unilateral needling

and Taichong LIV-3 on the left. LIV-3 eliminates stagnation of Liver Qi or Blood and P-6 moves Blood and calms the Mind. The combination of these two points can therefore eliminate stagnation of Liver Qi or Blood particularly if it derives from bottling-up of emotional problems. Very often this situation is also accompanied by a deficiency of Stomach and Spleen which may arise independently or as a result of invasion of stagnant Liver-Qi to Stomach and Spleen. In such cases, one could combine the needling of P-6 on one side, LIV-3 on the other and Zusanli ST-36 and Sanyinjiao SP-6 bilaterally. The combination of these four points (with 6 needles instead of 8) can tonify the Stomach and Spleen, calm the Mind and eliminate stagnation of Liver Qi or Blood.

Another example could be the combination of Neiguan P-6 on one side and Fenglong ST-40 on the other. P-6 harmonizes the Stomach and ST-40 calms the Stomach in Excess patterns: this combination has a good effect in treating Stomach problems of Excess nature. Besides its effect on the Stomach, this particular combination is also used for acute bruising of the rib-cage.

Unilateral needling is particularly effective when using two channels of the same polarity, one of the arm the other of the leg, e.g. Triple Burner and Gall-Bladder (Lesser Yang), Pericardium and Liver (Terminal Yin), and so on. For example, one can use Waiguan T.B.-5 on one side and Zulinqi G.B.-41 on the other for Lesser Yang type of headaches or Hegu L.I.-4 and Zusanli ST-36 for Bright Yang headaches.

The method of using unilateral needling of points on arm and leg channels of the same polarity can be used in the treatment of sprains as illustrated above and be combined with the method of using the opposite side. For example, in sprain of the right wrist with tenderness on Yangchi T.B.-4, one would use G.B.-40 on the left side, so using a point on the related leg channel of the same polarity on the opposite side to the sprained side.

Another case when balancing of left and right is used is simply to balance the two sides when several points are used on one side. If several points are used on one side to treat a specific problem of that side, these can be balanced with a few points on the opposite side according to a presenting pattern. For example, if one is treating a pain in the shoulder using Jianyu L.I.-15, Quchi L.I.-11 and Hegu L.I.-4 on one side, it might be desirable to balance these points with one or two on the opposite side according to a presenting pattern: this could be for example Zusanli ST-36 (in case of Spleen-Qi deficiency) or Taichong LIV-3 (in case of stagnation of Liver-Qi). Of course, one would not choose a point on the other side simply to balance the others, but also to treat a specific pattern.

Sometimes unilateral needling is used with the Connecting points. These are often used on the opposite side to the diseased side, in chronic conditions when the channel is in a deficient state. The use of the Connecting point of the exteriorly-interiorly related channel (either with reducing or even method) will achieve the effect of rebalancing the left and right side of the channel. For example, if we are treating a chronic pain of the arm along the Large Intestine channel and the channel on the diseased side is in an Empty condition (manifested by dull ache and slight wasting of the muscles), we could use Lieque LU-7 on the healthy side with reducing or even method to rebalance left and right and shift energy from the healthy to the diseased side.

YIN AND YANG

Balancing the Yin and Yang character of the point used is also important. The nature of the acupuncture points gives us a great choice in the use of points, and we should not think that in order to treat a Yin organ a Yin channel should be used as it is possible to use a Yang channel to treat a Yin organ or vice versa. For example, Zusanli ST-36 tonifies the Spleen.

This makes it possible to have a wide choice in the balancing of Yin and Yang points.

Generally speaking, it is better to balance Yin and Yang points within one treatment. The excessive use of Yang points may make a person slightly uneasy or edgy, while the excessive use of Yin points may make a person tired. Especially when several points of one polarity are used, it is a good idea to balance them with one or more points of the opposite polarity.

To use the same example as above, if one is treating a shoulder problem with several points on the Large Intestine channel, it would be good to balance them with a single Yin point such as Taichong LIV-3. This balancing technique could be combined with balancing of left and right and top and bottom. Thus one might use Jianyu L.I.-15, Quchi L.I.-11 and Hegu L.I.-4 on the left side and Taichong LIV-3 on the right, i.e. balancing Yin and Yang, left and right and top and bottom.

Of course, balancing points should not be chosen just for the sake of balance, but preferably according to a presenting pattern. In other words, it is always better if there is more than one reason for using a certain point.

In balancing Yin and Yang, it is particularly advisable to pay attention to balancing Yang channels with the Yin channel of the Yin organ across the Over-acting cycle of the 5 Elements, as follows:

Gall-Bladder — Spleen
Small Intestine — Lungs
Stomach — Kidneys
Large Intestine — Liver
Bladder — Heart.

The example of balancing a series of points on the Large Intestine channels with a point on the Liver channel has been given above. Another example of the balancing of points of Yang channels with points of Yin channels across the Over-acting sequence might be the use of Sanyinjiao SP-6 or Taibai SP-3 to balance a series of points on the Gall-Bladder channel such as Huantiao G.B.-30, Fengshi G.B.-31 and Yanglingquan G.B.-34 treating a sciatica for example.

The "Simple Questions" deals with the effects of over-action across the Over-acting cycle in chapter 69.[1]

FRONT AND BACK

Generally speaking it is not necessary to balance front and back within one treatment. The front points are usually used in acute cases, while the back ones are used in chronic cases. However, this distinction is by no means absolute and both sets of points could be used for acute or chronic cases.

In chronic cases it is often necessary to treat both front and back points. In particular, in very chronic conditions, it is nearly always necessary to use the Back Transporting points at some time during the course of treatment. If treatments are given frequently, i.e. two or three times a week, one can alternate points on the front with those on the back within each treatment: this is a good way to balance the front and back. If treatment is given at more infrequent intervals, points on both the front and back can be used during one treatment. If both back and front points are used in the same treatment, it is better to start with the back points.

Balancing the front and back points can be useful to correct an excessively strong reaction to a treatment. Supposing one has used several back points during one treatment and the patient experiences a fairly strong reaction (whether the treatment was the right one or not), one could correct this by using points on the front in a successive treatment. This method applies to all other categories of balancing mentioned. If a patient experiences a strong reaction, one can analyse the point prescription used and see if it was unbalanced in any way, e.g. too many Yin (or Yang) points, too many front (or back) points, too many points on the top (or bottom), too many points on the left (or right) or too many distal (or local) points. If the point prescription appears to be unbalanced, one can balance it appropriately using the opposite type of points.

NOTES

1 Simple Questions, p 403 – 407.

The Five Transporting Points 37 输穴

These are the points that lie between the fingers and elbows or between the toes and knees. They are also assigned to the 5 Elements so that they are mostly known in the West as "Element points" or sometimes "command points".

The Chinese name for these points is *"Shu"* 输 which is nearly the same character as for the Back Transporting points, meaning "transporting".

In order to illustrate the nature of these points, the ancient Chinese compared the section of channel between fingers/toes and elbows/knees to a river, starting from a "well"-point at the tips of the fingers or toes, getting gradually larger and deeper and ending in "sea"-point at the elbows or knees. Thus from fingers/toes to elbows/knees there is a progression in the size and depth of the channel: it is narrowest and most superficial at the fingers/toes and widest and deepest at the elbows/knees.

This progression of size and depth of the channel is irrespective of the direction of flow of the channel, i.e. it applies equally to Yin or Yang channels of both arms and legs. Even though the Yin channels of the hand flow downwards towards the fingers, and the Yang channels of the hand flow upwards towards the chest, the comparison of the channel to a river, with its springhead at the fingers and its delta at the elbows applies equally to both. Exactly the same applies to the leg channels (Fig. 68).

The implication of this is that the section of channel between fingers/toes and elbows/knees is more superficial than the rest, and this is one of the reasons for the importance of the points lying along its path. The energetic action of the points situated along this section of a channel is much more dynamic than other points and this explains their frequent use in clinical practice. One could conceivably practice acupuncture using only these points. As one may have experienced many times, the effect of, say, Taichong LIV-3 is far more dynamic than, say, LIV-10 or LIV-11 (situated on the thigh).

The other implication of the fact that the section of channel between fingers/toes and elbows/knees is more superficial is that this section represents the connection between the body and the environment. It is the section of channel which is influenced most promptly and directly by climate and exterior pathogenic factors. For this reason the points along this section of channel are more directly related to the seasons and can be used according to their cycle. For the same reason, the points along this section of channel are the points of entry of exterior pathogenic factors such as Cold, Dampness and Wind.

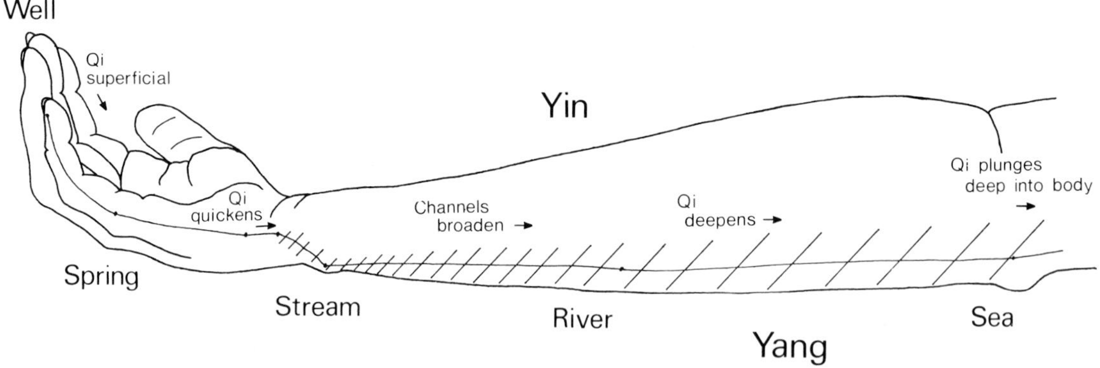

Fig. 68 Flow of Qi in the 5 Transporting points

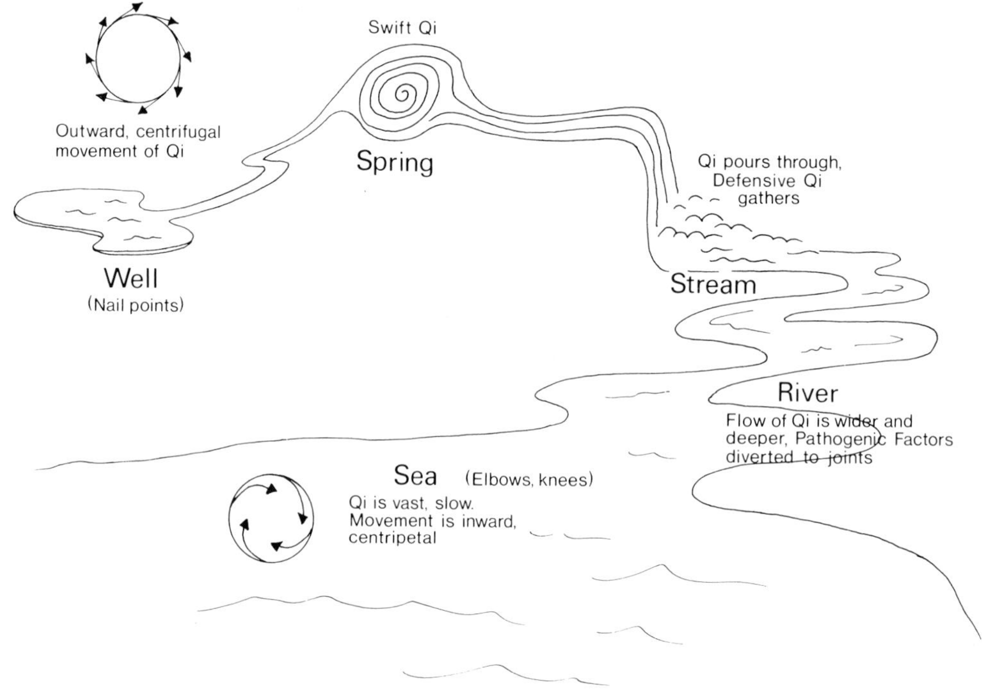

Fig. 69 The channel as a river

Another reason for the dynamism of the points in this section of the channel is that at the fingertips and toes the energy changes polarity from Yin to Yang or vice versa. Due to this change of polarity, the Qi of the channel is more unstable and therefore more easily influenced. (Fig. 69)

Even though we normally say that this change of polarity takes place at the fingers and toes, it cannot take place immediately at one single point and the inertia from one channel at its end carries on to a certain extent through the next channel up to the elbow or knee. For example, the Lung channel ends at the tip of the thumb where the polarity changes to Yang and the energy flows into the Large Intestine channel. However, this change from Yin to Yang polarity cannot take place instantly in one point at the fingertips, but the inertia from the Lung channel is, to a certain extent, carried through to the initial section of the Large Intestine channel. This can be compared to the meeting of two rivers: when two wide rivers meet, they do not just merge at the point of junction, but often the current from one river carries on flowing independently within the second river for some time. The progression of the 5-Element points along the channel is probably in relation to this change of polarity, as the second point belongs to Fire in Yin channels and Water in Yang channels. This might be because the second point represents the point at which the inertia of the incoming channel is felt most and manifests itself. For example, the Lung channel inertial movement continues into the Large Intestine channel particularly at the second point along the channel which therefore belongs to Water, reflecting the Yin character of the Lung channel. Similarly, the second point of Yin channels belongs to Fire reflecting the inertia of the incoming Yang channels. Thus, the second points along the channel represent the points of maximum inertia from the previous channel, after which the inertia becomes less and less to disappear totally at the fifth point along the channel. This explains the particularly unstable state of the energy in this section of channel. This instability also accounts for the dynamism of the points along it and is made use of in practice.

Five of the points situated along this section of channel are particularly important, and they are called the 5 Transporting points: they also coincide with what we call the Element points. However, the dynamics of these points is irrespective of their 5-Element character.

Each of the five points occupying the same location along the channel has a name. The names I will use are:

WELL point	The point at the tips of fingers or toes
SPRING point	The second point of the five: in all cases it is the second point along the channel
STREAM point	The third point of the five: in all cases it is the third point along the channel (except for the Gall Bladder channel where it is the fourth)
RIVER point	The fourth point of the five, not always the fourth point along the channel
SEA point	The fifth point of the five: in all cases it is the point at the elbows and knees

These names do not represent a literal translation of the Chinese names, but I have preferred them to the literal translation as this might have created some confusion. The use of the above names is also justified by the analogy of these points with stages in the course of a river found in chapter 1 of the "Spiritual Axis", where it says that *"... at the Well points Qi flows out, at the Spring points it slips and glides, at the Stream points it pours, at the River points it moves, at the Sea points it enters ..."*.[1]

The "Classic of Difficulties" gives the same description in chapter 69.[2]

The actual meanings of their names are:

JING = WELL
YING = SPRING (of water), POOL (of water)
SHU = TO TRANSPORT
JING = TO PASS THROUGH
HE = TO UNITE, JOIN.

Each of the five Transporting points has a specific energetic action within the channel dynamics which explains the meaning of these points names. These are as follows:

1. WELL point: it is the point of departure of Qi (in the sense outlined above and therefore applying to both Yin and Yang channels of arm and leg). At this point the channel is at its most superficial and thinnest and the energy changes polarity from Yin to Yang or vice versa. Because the energy is more superficial and changes polarity, the Well point has a particularly dynamic effect when needled. The energy is at its most unstable state here, so that it can be easily and readily influenced and changed. This explains the use of these points in acute situations, as the Well points tend to be used to eliminate pathogenic factors quickly. According to the "Classic of Difficulties" these points have an "outward" movement, i.e. the energy of the channel tends to go outwards in a centrifugal movement at these points.[3] The outward, centrifugal tendency of the Well points is exploited to eliminate pathogenic factors quickly as they pass through these points. Several

examples can be cited, such as the use of Shaoshang LU-11 for fainting, Zhongchong P-9 for fainting and heat-stroke, Shaochong HE-9 and Shaoze S.I.-1 for loss of consciousness, Yinbai SP-1 for convulsions, Yongchuan KI-1 for loss of consciousness and infantile convulsions and Shangyang L.I.-1 for loss of consciousness.

2 SPRING point: at this point the Qi of the channel is very powerful and full of potential energy ready to manifest, like the swirling movement of water in a mountain spring. Hence the "Spiritual Axis" says that at this point the Qi "slips" or "glides", i.e. it is swift. Because of this nature, the Spring points are also very dynamic and powerful points which can quickly change situations: they all have a particularly strong action and are generally used to eliminate pathogenic factors (whether interior or exterior) and in particular to clear Heat.

Because of their dynamism, these points are to be used sparingly. As mentioned in the previous chapter (see p. 330), the Spring points of the feet are more powerful than those of the hands and, if there is a choice, those of the hands are to be chosen first. For example, in deciding on a distal point to affect the temples in migraine headaches due to rising of Liver-Yang, one might have a choice between using the Gall-Bladder or Triple Burner channel Spring point: the Triple Burner Spring point is slightly less powerful and dynamic than that of the Gall-Bladder channel and therefore it might be preferred, especially in case of first treatment. Of course, this does not mean that the Spring point of a hand channel is always to be preferred to that of a foot channel as, in many cases, one does not have a choice, or one might deliberately want to have a particularly strong effect.

3. STREAM point: at this point the Qi of the channel "pours" through, it swirls and the flow starts to be bigger and slightly deeper within the channel. At this point, the flow of Qi is rapid and large enough to carry other things with it, hence its name "transporting".[4] At these points, exterior pathogenic factors can be "transported" into the Interior and penetrate deeper in the channels. On the other hand, at these points Defensive Qi gathers.

4. RIVER point: at this point the Qi of the channel is much bigger, wider and also deeper. The Qi flows like a large current after coming a long distance from its source. At these points, exterior pathogenic factors are deviated towards joints, bones and tendons.

5. SEA point: at this point the Qi of the channel is vast and deep, it collects, comes together and joins the general circulation of the body, like a large river flowing into the sea. According to chapter 65 of the "Classic of Difficulties" at this point, the Qi has an inward, centripetal movement (as opposed to the outward, centrifugal movement of the Well point).[5] Compared and contrasted to the Well points, the Sea points are much less dynamic and their effect is less quick and dramatic. This is due to the fact that at the Sea points, Qi flows much slower and it flows inwards and deeper so that it is not so unstable and cannot be quickly and easily affected.

We can discuss the clinical use of the five Transporting points from four different viewpoints:

According to chapter 68 of the "Classic of Difficulties"

According to the "Spiritual Axis", chapters 4, 6 and 44

According to the seasons as in "Simple Questions", chapter 61

According to the 5-Element character of the points as in chapter 64 and 69 of the "Classic of Difficulties".

ACCORDING TO THE "CLASSIC OF DIFFICULTIES"

Chapter 68 of the "Classic of Difficulties" deals with the use of the 5 Transporting points and gives guidelines which are still valid and widely followed today. These are:

WELL points: used for "fullness under the heart"

SPRING points: used for "hot sensations of the body"

STREAM points: used for "feeling of heaviness and joint pain"

RIVER points: used for "cough and hot and cold sensations"

SEA points: used for "rebellious Qi and diarrhoea".[6]

We can expand on the clinical use of these points as follows:

WELL points: used for irritability, mental restlessness, anxiety. This applies to both Yin and Yang channels. The Well points have a particularly strong effect on the mental state and quickly change the mood. Examples of Well points used in this way are Zhongchong P-9 (irritability, insomnia), Shaochong HE-9 (mental disorders, anxiety, manic-depression), Yinbai SP-1 (hysteria, insomnia), Lidui ST-45 (insomnia, mental confusion) and Yongquan KI-1 (anxiety).

SPRING points: used for febrile diseases or to clear Heat. The Spring points are very widely used to clear Heat and practically all of them do. It is important to note that their Heat-clearing action is irrespective of their 5-Element character. For example, Shaofu HE-8 is a Fire point and Neiting ST-44 is a Water point, but they both clear Heat by virtue of being the Spring points. Virtually all Spring points clear Heat in their respective channel and organ. Examples of widely used points are Shaofu HE-8 and Laogong P-8 to clear Heart-Fire, Xingjian LIV-2 to clear Liver-Fire, Neiting ST-44 to clear Stomach-Heat, Rangu KI-2 to clear Kidney Empty-Heat, Shaoshang LU-10 to clear Lung-Heat or Wind-Heat.

STREAM points: used for Painful Obstruction Syndrome, especially if from Dampness. This applies to Yang channels more than Yin ones. Examples are: Sanjian L.I.-3, Zhongzhu T.B.-3 and Houxi S.I.-3 for Painful Obstruction Syndrome of the fingers and Xiangu ST-43 for the toes.

These points can be used not only as local points for Painful Obstruction Syndrome of fingers and toes, but also as distal points to clear Wind and Dampness from the channels. For example, Xiangu ST-43 is an important distal point to clear Wind-Damp and Heat from the channels; Houxi S.I.-3, Zhongzhu T.B.-3 and Sanjian L.I.-3 can all be used as distal points to clear obstructions from Dampness and Cold from the respective channels.

RIVER points: used for cough, asthma and upper respiratory diseases. This applies more to Yin than Yang channels, and among the Yang channels it applies more to the Bright Yang channels. Examples are: Jingqu LU-8 for cough and asthma, Shangqiu SP-5 for dry cough, Jiexi ST-41 and Yangxi L.I.-5 for sore throat of an Excess nature. The River point Jianshi P-5 is used for hot and cold sensations.

SEA points: used for all stomach and intestinal diseases. This applies mostly to Yang channels, but also to Yin ones. Obvious examples of Sea points of Yang channels treating stomach and intestinal problems are Zusanli ST-36 and Yanglingquan G.B.-34. The Sea points of the Yin channels of the leg also treat problems of the Yang organs as Yinlingquan SP-9, Yingu KI-10 and Ququan LIV-8 can all clear Damp-Heat in Bladder or Intestines. Finally, the Sea points of the Pericardium channel Quze P-3 can also clear Heat in the Intestines.

In addition to these Sea points, the Yang channels of the arm have also a so-called Lower-Sea point. These are:

Shangjuxu ST-37 for the Large Intestine
Xiajuxu ST-39 for the Small Intestine
Weiyang BL-39 for the Triple Burner.

These three points are directly connected to their respective organs and function like Sea points, i.e. they treat problems of the Yang organs. In particular, Shangjuxu ST-37 is used for chronic diarrhoea and Damp-Heat of the Large Intestine, Xiajuxu ST-39 for intestinal pain and Weiyang BL-39 for enuresis (if tonified when the Lower Burner is deficient) or retention of urine and oedema (if reduced when the Lower Burner is in Excess).

The "Spiritual Axis" deals with the use of Weiyang BL-39 in chapter 2: *"Weiyang [BL-39] receives the Lower Burner, if it is in Excess there is retention of urine, if it is deficient there is enuresis or incontinence. The point is to be reduced in the former case and tonified in the latter"*.[7]

The "Spiritual Axis" lists all the Sea points in chapter 4 and it gives Shangjuxu ST-37 for the Large Intestine, Xiajuxu ST-39 for the Small Intestine and Weiyang BL-39 for the Triple Burner.[8]

These three points therefore function as Sea points for the Large Intestine, Small Intestine and Triple Burner and their upper Sea points

(Quchi L.I.-11, Xiaohai S.I.-8 and Tianjing T.B.-10) mostly treat channel problems of the neck, shoulders and face.

ACCORDING TO THE "SPIRITUAL AXIS"

A) CHAPTER 44

The "Spiritual Axis" says in chapter 44: *"When the Yin organs are affected use the Well points; when the disease affects a change in the complexion colour, use the Spring points; when the disease manifests intermittently, use the Stream points; when the disease affects the voice and there is stagnation of Qi and Blood in the channels, use the River points; when the Stomach is affected and the person lacks appetite, use the Sea points".*[9]

These rules are fairly straightforward and have some points in common with those from chapter 68 of the "Classic of Difficulties". The "Spiritual Axis" recommends the use of the Well points in Yin organs diseases: this is similar to the "Classic of Difficulties" recommendation of these points in mental restlessness and irritability, particularly if deriving from a Heart pattern. The "Spiritual Axis" use of the River points for problems of the voice coincides with the "Classic of Difficulties" use for problems of the throat. The use of the Sea points is also practically the same in the two classics.

However, the "Spiritual Axis" recommendations are much less followed in clinical practice than those from the "Classic of Difficulties" as they are of lesser practical significance.

B) CHAPTER 4

The "Spiritual Axis" gives other guidelines to the use of the 5 Transporting points, some of them in contradiction with each other. It says in chapter 4: *"The divergent branches of the Yang channels reach into the Interior and connect with the Yang organs ... the Spring and Stream points [together, Tr.] treat channel problems, the Sea points treat organ problems".*[10] It then goes on to list the Sea points of the Yang channels, listing only the Lower-Sea points for the Yang channels of the arm, Large Intestine, Small Intestine and Triple Burner.

The Spring and Stream points of the Yang channels are frequently used in the treatment of Painful Obstruction Syndrome as the Stream point is a point of concentration of Defensive Qi and the Spring point is a powerful point which can be used to move the Qi of the channel.

The use of the Yang Sea points is in agreement with the use of these points according to the "Classic of Difficulties" and to chapter 44 of the "Spiritual Axis" itself, i.e. to treat problems of the Yang organ themselves. This method is frequently applied in clinical practice.

C) CHAPTER 6

Chapter 6 of the "Spiritual Axis" gives yet different recommendations for the clinical use of the five Transporting points.

It says: *"In the Interior there are 5 Yin and 6 Yang organs, in the Exterior there are bones, sinews and skin. Both in the Interior and Exterior there is Yin and Yang. Within the Interior, the 5 Yin organs pertain to Yin and the 6 Yang organs pertain to Yang; within the Exterior sinews and bones pertain to Yin and the skin pertains to Yang. For diseases of Yin within Yin [i.e. Yin organs, Tr.], use the Spring and Stream points of the Yin channels together. For diseases of Yang within Yang [i.e. the skin, Tr.], use the Sea points of the Yang channels. For diseases of Yin within Yang [i.e. sinews and bones, Tr.], use the River points of the Yin channels. For diseases of Yang within Yin [i.e. the Yang organs, Tr.], use the Connecting points".*[11]

To summarize:
YIN WITHIN YIN = Yin Organs = Use Spring and Stream points of Yin channels in combination
YANG WITHIN YANG = Skin = Use the Sea points of Yang channels
YIN WITHIN YANG = Sinews and bones = Use the River points of Yin channels
YANG WITHIN YIN = Yang organs = Use the Connecting points.

These recommendations are only partially applied in clinical practice. The Spring and Stream points are frequently used together to clear Heat from the Yin organs; sometimes the Spring point can be reduced to clear Heat, and the Stream point tonified to nourish the Yin of the channel. A good example is the use of Xingjian LIV-2 (reduced to clear Liver-Fire) and Taichong LIV-3 (reinforced to nourish Liver-Yin). This technique can be used to nourish Liver-Yin and subdue Liver-Yang in headaches, or to nourish Liver-Yin and clear Liver-Fire in urinary diseases caused by Liver-Fire and Bladder-Heat.

The Sea points of the Yang channels, especially the upper Sea points (such as Quchi L.I.-11, Xiaohai S.I.-8 and Tianjing T.B.-10) are frequently used to treat the "skin", i.e. release the Exterior in invasions of exterior pathogenic factors. In particular, L.I.-11 and T.B.-10 are used to release the Exterior and expel Wind-Heat.

The River points of the Yin channels are frequently used to treat problems of sinews and bones, i.e. in Painful Obstruction Syndrome. This is also because the Qi at these points is diverted to sinews, bones and joints.

The rule of using the Connecting points to treat problems of the Yang organs, is not widely followed as the Lower Sea points would be preferred in this case.

ACCORDING TO THE SEASONS

Chapter 44 of the "Spiritual Axis" gives guidelines as to the use of the 5 Transporting points according to the seasons. It says: *"In winter use the Well points, in Spring use the Spring points, in Summer use the Stream points, in Late Summer use the River points, in Autumn use the Sea points"*.[12]

These rules find only limited application in clinical practice as it is not always possible to choose points according to the cycle of seasons, as this choice might conflict with the requirements of treatment according to the actual condition of the patient. However, these guidelines may be followed more when giving preventive seasonal treatments to patients who seek treatment to keep well rather than for specific conditions.

ACCORDING TO THE 5 ELEMENTS

The 5 Transporting points are also used according to their 5-Element character. This was established in the "Classic of Difficulties" for the first time. In chapter 64 it says that the Yin channels' Well point belongs to Wood and the Yang channels' Well point belongs to Metal.[13]

The use of the 5 Transporting points according to their 5-Element character was discussed in chapter 69. It tersely says: *"In case of Deficiency tonify the Mother, in case of Excess sedate the Child"*.[14]

Following this principle and keeping in mind the Generating cycle of the 5 Elements, in case of Deficiency of a channel we can choose the point corresponding to the "Mother" Element in order to tonify it. In case of Excess, we would choose the point corresponding to the "Child" Element in order to sedate it. For example, if the Liver is deficient, the Liver belongs to Wood, Water is the Mother of Wood, we therefore select (and tonify) the point Ququan LIV-8 which corresponds to Water. If the Liver were in Excess, we would choose (and reduce) the point Xingjian LIV-2 corresponding to Fire, as Fire is the Child of Wood.

In accordance with this theory, therefore, every channel has a tonification and sedation point corresponding to its Mother and Child Element respectively. It must be stressed, however, that the needle technique is all important when tonifying or sedating; in other words we cannot rely only on the tonification or sedation character of a point, in order to tonify or sedate.

Furthermore, the tonification or sedation character of a point is very often overridden by its other characteristics, so that the rule of tonifying and sedating according to tonification and sedation points suffers many exceptions.

For example, Shaochong HE-9 and Zhongchong P-9 are tonification points but are more often used for sedation instead in acute cases, by virtue of their being the Well points. Shenmen HE-7 is the sedation point but is more often used to tonify Heart Blood to nourish the Mind and similarly for Daling P-7. Quchi L.I.-11 is the tonification point, but it also cools Blood and releases the Exterior and is by its very nature a reducing point. Dadun SP-2 is the tonification point, but would not be the most indicated point to tonify the Spleen, as either Taibai SP-3, Zusanli ST-36 or Pishu BL-20 would be much better for this purpose. SP-2, on the contrary, is often used in febrile diseases to clear Heat and promote sweating. Zhiyin BL-67 is the tonification point but again, owing to its being a Well point, is often used to sedate in acute cases, or also to subdue rising Qi which is causing headaches.

Apart from being applied in the theory of tonification and sedation points, the 5-Element points are also used in another very common way to eliminate pathogenic factors.

There is a correspondence between the 5 Elements and pathogenic factors:

WOOD corresponds to Wind
FIRE corresponds to Heat or Fire
EARTH corresponds to Dampness
METAL corresponds to Dryness
WATER corresponds to Cold.

In accordance with this correspondence, the 5-Element points can be used to expel the relevant pathogenic factors (whether exterior or interior). The only exception is the Metal point which is not used to eliminate Dryness. The reason for this lies in the very nature of Dryness. While Heat, Fire, Wind, Dampness and Cold are pathogenic factors that manifest as an Excess pattern, Dryness manifests as a deficiency of Body Fluids, and the way to correct this is by nourishing fluids.

The application of this correspondence between the 5 Elements and pathogenic factors is mostly used in Excess patterns to eliminate the relevant pathogenic factor (Table 21). It also applies more to Yin rather than Yang channels.

Table 21 lists all the Yin channel Transporting points with their clinical use in the elimination of the pathogenic factors related to the 5 Elements .

This method of using the Element points to expel the relevant pathogenic factors can be applied to some of the points of Yang channels too. In particular, some of the Wood points are used to subdue Interior Wind, such as Houxi S.I.-3, and some of the Fire points are used to clear Heat, such as Yangxi L.I.-5 and Jiexi ST-41.

Table 21 Correlation between Element points and pathogenic factors

Element	Point	Pathogenic factor	Use
WOOD	All Yin channels Wood points	Wind	Expel Internal Wind (acute stage of Wind stroke)
FIRE	Shaofu HE-8	Heat or Fire	**Expels Summer-Heat or Heart-Fire**
	Yuji LU-10		**Expels Wind-Heat or Lung-Heat**
	Laogong P-8		**Expels Summer-Heat or Heart-Fire**
	Xingjian LIV-2		**Subdues Liver-Fire**
	Dadu SP-2		**Clears Heat in febrile diseases**
	Rangu KI-2		**Subdues Empty-Heat, cools Blood**
EARTH	Shenmen HE-7	Dampness	Not used to resolve Phlegm
	Daling P-7	Phlegm	Resolves Phlegm from Heart
	Taiyuan LU-9		Resolves Phlegm from Lung
	Taibai SP-3		Resolves Dampness
	Taichong LIV-3		Resolves Dampness
	Taixi KI-3		Not used to resolve Phlegm
WATER	Shaohai HE-3	Cold	Not used to expel Cold
	Quze P-3		Not used to expel Cold
	Chize LU-5		Expels Cold from Lungs
	Ququan LIV-8		Expels Damp-Cold from Lower Burner
	Yinlingquan SP-9		Expels Damp-Cold from Lower Burner
	Yingu KI-10		Expels Damp-Cold from Lower Burner

Table 22 Characteristics and functions of the 5 Transporting points

	Well	Spring	Stream	River	Sea
Description "Spiritual Axis" ch.1	Qi goes out	Qi is swift, slips	Qi pours	Qi moves, goes	Qi enters
Other descriptions	Like spring-head, Qi of channel comes out, Qi is small, superficial	Minute trickle from a spring Qi begins to flow Qi is bigger	Like water flowing from surface to depth, Qi irrigates the body	Like water freely flowing in a river Qi flowing in the channels, Qi flows swiftly	Like many streams returning to the sea, Qi of channel comes to an end, Qi is vast and deep, it comes together
"Spiritual Axis" ch.2 and ch.6	Point of departure of Qi	Point of convergence	Point of entry of pathogenic factors	Concentration point	Qi joins body circulation
Use from "Classic of Difficulties" ch. 68	Fullness under heart Mental irritation	Hot sensation, Heat diseases	Heaviness of body, painful joints, Painful Obstruction Syndrome	Wheezing, cough feeling hot and cold. Lung diseases	Rebellious Qi, Diarrhoea, Diseases of Yang organs
Use from "Spiritual Axis" ch. 44	When Yin organs are affected	When illness manifests on complexion	When illness is characterized by amelioration and and aggravation	When illness reflects in the voice	For Stomach diseases
Use from "Spiritual Axis" ch.4		Exterior diseases (Yang channels)	Exterior diseases (Yang channels)		Interior diseases
Use from "Spiritual Axis" ch.6		For Yin organs (Yin channels)	For Yin organs (Yin channels)	For tendons and bones	For skin and muscles

NOTES

1 Spiritual Axis, p 3.
2 Classic of Difficulties, p 148.
3 Classic of Difficulties, p 142.
4 Acupuncture, A Comprehensive Text, p 126.
5 Classic of Difficulties, p 142.
6 Classic of Difficulties, p 148.
7 Spiritual Axis, p 7.
8 Spiritual Axis, p 14.
9 Spiritual Axis, p 86.
10 Spiritual Axis, p 14.
11 Spiritual Axis, p 18–19.
12 Spiritual Axis, p 86.
13 Classic of Difficulties, p 139.
14 Classic of Difficulties, p 151.

38 The Functions of Specific Points

穴位学

SOURCE POINTS

The nature and use of the Source points is dealt with in the first chapter of the "Spiritual Axis" and chapter 66 of the "Classic of Difficulties". In order to understand the use of the Source points, it is worth looking at these two chapters closely.

CHAPTER 1 OF THE "SPIRITUAL AXIS"

This chapter makes two statements in connection with the Source points, one regarding their use in diagnosis, the other in treatment.

The first statement says: *"Select the Source points when the 5 Yin organs are diseased"*.[1] This clearly indicates that the Source points directly affect the Yin organs.

The other statement says: *"If the 5 Yin organs are diseased, abnormal reactions will appear at the 12 Source points. If we know the correspondence of Source points to the relevant Yin organ, we can diagnose when a Yin organ is diseased."*[2] This statement clearly indicates that the Source points are in relation with the Original Qi and that changes on the skin over the Source points indicate abnormalities in the Yin organs function and can therefore be used for diagnosis.

Abnormalities which can be observed on the Source points include swellings, redness, congested blood vessels (common on Taixi KI-3), varicose veins, a deep sunken dip around the point (also commonly seen on KI-3), whiteness, a bluish colour or very flaccid skin.

When the "Spiritual Axis" proceeds to list the Source points, however, it gives different points from the ones we usually consider. The "Spiritual Axis" lists the Source points as:

Taiyuan LU-9 for the Lungs	2 points
Daling P-7 for the Heart	2 points
Taibai SP-3 for the Spleen	2 points
Taichong LIV-3 for the Liver	2 points
Taixi KI-3 for the Kidneys	2 points
Total	10 points
Jiuwei Ren-15, Source point for Fat tissue	1 point
Qihai Ren-6, Source point for Membranes	1 point
Grand total	12 points

Regarding these last two points, the "Spiritual Axis" says: *"The Original Qi of Fat tissues [Gao] gathers at Jiuwei [Ren-15], the Original Qi of Membranes [Huang] gathers at Qihai [Ren-6]"*.[3] Although the book uses a different name for Ren-6 (Boyang), this is the old name for Qihai i.e. Ren-6.

Ren-15 and Ren-6 are also considered the Original points for the chest and abdomen respectively, as well as the Original points for all the Yin and all the Yang organs respectively. Ren-15 is used for neurosis, anxiety or psychosis and is an extremely useful point to calm the Mind. Ren-6 is used in Deficiency conditions of the Yang organs as it strongly tonifies Yang Qi.

The surprising element in this chapter is that the "Spiritual Axis" only mentions Source points for the Yin organs. This is because the Source points energy stems from the Original Qi which is related to the Yin organs and the Kidneys in particular. The Source points are therefore used mostly to tonify the Yin organs.

In contrast, the Source points of the Yang organs do not have a similar function and do not tonify the Yang organs in the same way the Yin Source points tonify the Yin organs. The Yang Source points are mostly used in Excess patterns to expel pathogenic factors. For example, Hegu L.I.-4 is used to release the Exterior and expel Wind-Heat, Yanggu S.I.-4 can be used to move stagnant Liver-Qi and stop pain in the costal region, Jinggu BL-64 can be used to expel Damp-Heat from the Lower Burner, Qiuxu G.B.-40 can be used for stagnation of Liver-Qi, Chongyang ST-42 can be used to expel Wind-Cold from the face in facial paralysis and Yangchi T.B.-4 can be used to clear Gall-Bladder Heat causing deafness or to regulate the Lesser Yang. Of course, the Source points of the Yang channels can also be used to tonify the relevant Yang organs, but this is not their main use, and they would not be the best points to do that. To tonify the Yang organs, the best points would be the Lower Sea points.

The other surprising statement in this chapter is the mention of Daling P-7 as the Source point of the Heart. This is because in the times when the "Spiritual Axis" was written the Heart and Pericardium were considered as a single organ, hence the constant reference to "5 Yin and 6 Yang organs". It was only later that the Pericardium and Heart were split into two separate organs to preserve the symmetry of 12 organs and 12 channels.

To summarize, the functions of the Source points as from the "Spiritual Axis" are:

1) The Source points are in relation with the Original Qi.
2) They can be used in diagnosis as they reflect the state of the Original Qi of each Yin organ.
3) They are used in treatment mostly to tonify the Yin organs.
4) The Source points of the Yin organs are more important than those of the Yang organs.

CHAPTER 66 OF THE "CLASSIC OF DIFFICULTIES

This chapter of the "Classic of Difficulties" lists the 12 Source points as we know them, i.e. one for each of the Yin and Yang organs. The only difference with the Source points as normally known nowadays is that it lists both P-7 and HE-7 as Source points for the Heart.[4] This is due again to the fact that in those times the Heart and Pericardium were considered as one organ, and the Pericardium could not therefore have a Source point.

The rest of this short chapter clarifies the relation between Original Qi, Triple Burner and Source points.

It says: *"The Original Qi is the motive force situated between the two kidneys, it is life-giving and is the root of the 12 channels. The Triple Burner acts as the ambassador for the Original Qi, which passes through the three Burners and it then spreads to the 5 Yin and 6 Yang organs [and their channels].*

The places where the Original Qi stays are the Source points." [5]

This chapter therefore confirms that the Source points are in relation with the Original Qi. In contrast with chapter 1 of the "Spiritual Axis", the "Classic of Difficulties" says that the Source points can be used to tonify both Yin and Yang organs.

In particular, the role of the Triple Burner as the "ambassador" or "avenue" through which the Original Qi arises from in between the two Kidneys to spread to the 5 Yin and 6 Yang organs, explains a particular use of the Source point of the Triple Burner channel, Yangchi T.B.-4. This point can be used to tonify Original Qi directly and activate its circulation in the channels. Combined with the Source point of the Stomach, Chongyang ST-42, T.B.-4 strongly tonifies Qi and the Original Qi.

CONNECTING POINTS

To understand the use of the Connecting (Luo 络) points, we must know the pathway and nature of the Connecting channels. These are described in chapter 10 of the "Spiritual Axis".

There are 16 Connecting channels, one for each of the 12 main channels, one each for the Directing and Governing Vessels, one "Great Connecting" channel for the Spleen and one "Great Channel" for the Stomach. [6]

Each of the 12 Connecting channels related to the main channels departs from its relevant Connecting point and branches out in two directions: one branch connects with its interiorly-exteriorly related channel and the other departing from its Connecting point travels upwards along a separate trajectory.

Although there are two branches for each Connecting channel, it must be realized that these are not entirely separate and still form part of the same channel.

There are two ways of using the Connecting points according to the functions of each of the two branches.

The Connecting point can be used in conjunction with the Source point of its interiorly-exteriorly related channel; or it can be used on its own, according to the symptomatology of the Connecting channels themselves. In the latter case we must distinguish between Empty and Full conditions of the Connecting channel.

Let us now discuss these two ways of using the Connecting points.

USE IN CONJUNCTION WITH THE SOURCE POINTS

Since each Connecting channel joins with its interiorly-exteriorly related channel (e.g. Lungs-Large Intestine), the Connecting point can treat not only the channel to which it belongs, but also its interiorly-exteriorly related channel.

When a Source point is used to tonify a given channel/organ, the Connecting point of its interiorly-exteriorly related channel can be used to strengthen the treatment. The Connecting point is thus chosen as a secondary point to reinforce the action of the Source point, chosen as the main point to treat the primarily affected channel.

For example, in case of Lung-Qi deficiency we may choose to use the Lung channel Source point, i.e. Taiyuan LU-9 and reinforce its action by using the Connecting point of its interiorly-exteriorly related channel, i.e. Pianli L.I.-6.

This technique finds its rationale in the pathway of the Connecting channels as these join-up with their interiorly-exteriorly related channels. This is also reflected in the fact that the symptomatology of each Connecting channel often includes symptoms of its interiorly-exteriorly related channel.

USE ON THEIR OWN

The use of the Connecting points by themselves is based on the Full or Empty symptomatology of each Connecting channel. The Full and Empty symptoms of the Connecting channels are described in chapter 10 of the "Spiritual Axis". [7]

These are listed in Table 23.

The "Spiritual Axis" also says in the same chapter that *"When the Connecting channels are*

Table 23 Full and Empty symptoms and signs of the Connecting channels

Connecting Channel	Empty	Full
Lungs	Shortness-of breath, frequent urination, enuresis	Hot palms
Large Intestine	Sensation of cold in teeth, feeling of tightness in diaphragm	Toothache, deafness
Stomach	Flaccidity or atrophy of leg muscles	Epilepsy, insanity, sore throat, aphasia
Spleen	Abdominal distension	Abdominal pain
Heart	Aphasia	Congested diaphragm
Small Intestine	Scabies	Loose joints, stiff elbow
Bladder	Runny nose, nose bleed	Stuffy nose, headache backache
Kidney	Lower back ache	Mental restlessness depression
Pericardium	Stiffness of head	Pain in chest
Triple Burner	Loosening of elbow joint	Spasm of elbow
Gall Bladder	Weakness and flaccidity of foot muscles	Fainting
Liver	Itching of pubis	Swelling of testicle, colic, abnormal erection
Directing Vessel	Itching of abdomen	Pain on skin of abdomen
Governing Vessel	Heaviness and shaking of head	Stiffness of spine
Great Connecting Channel of Spleen	Weakness of all joints	Aches all round the body
Great Connecting Channel of Stomach	Palpitations	Feeling of congestion in chest

Full they can be seen, when they are Empty they cannot be seen".[8]

This is due to the fact that the Connecting channels are more superficial than the main channels and branch out into smaller branches of which there are three types: Superficial channels, Blood channels and Minute channels. For example, when congested venules can be seen under the skin, those are the Blood channels of the Connecting channels.

In Full patterns, the Connecting channels and their smaller branches are congested and can therefore be seen. A greenish coloration suggests Cold in these channels, while a reddish coloration suggests Heat. The channel pathway areas can also be cold or hot to the touch. This, together with the coloration, indicates retention of Cold or Heat in the Connecting channels and their branches, i.e. an Excess condition.

In Deficiency patterns, the Connecting channels and their branches are void of Qi, so nothing can be observed outwardly in terms of colour, but in chronic severe cases, a flaccidity of the muscles can be observed.

In Excess conditions of the Connecting channels the Connecting point must be reduced, and in Deficiency conditions it must be tonified.

Since the Connecting channels and their branches are more superficial than the main channels, the Connecting points are often used for superficial channel problems as opposed to internal problems, although they can treat the latter too.

When they are used for channel problems, the Connecting points are often chosen on the opposite side to where the problem is, and on the interiorly-exteriorly related channel. For example, if there is a pain in the right shoulder along the Large Intestine channel and some local points on the Large Intestine are used on the right side, Lieque LU-7 on the left side can be added to reinforce the treatment.

Apart from the above uses of the Connecting points, they are also often used in practice according to their specific action, irrespective of their being Connecting points. For example, Fenglong ST-40 is very much used to resolve Phlegm, irrespective of it being the Connecting point of the Stomach channel. Waiguan T.B.-5 is often used to expel Wind-Heat, Neiguan P-6 is very much used for chest problems and emotional problems, Lieque LU-7 can be used to affect the head, and so on.

In conclusion, the Connecting points can basically be used in four different ways:

a) In conjunction with the Source point of the primarily affected channel to reinforce its action.

b) According to the symptomatology from chapter 10 of the "Spiritual Axis". They are not often used in this way.

c) According to their range of action in terms of energetic layers, i.e. to affect the superficial layers in channel problems. They are very much used in this way.

d) According to their specific energic action, irrespective of their being Connecting points (e.g. Fenglong ST-40 to resolve Phlegm).

BACK TRANSPORTING POINTS

The importance of the Back Transporting points in treatment cannot be over-emphasised. They are particularly important for the treatment of chronic diseases and, indeed, one may go so far as to say that a chronic disease cannot be treated without using these points at some time during the course of treatment.

The Chinese character (Shu 俞) denoting these points means "to transport" indicating that they transport Qi to the inner organs. Each point takes its name from the corresponding organ. For example, "*Xin*" means "Heart" and "*Xinshu*" is the Back Transporting for the Heart.

There is a Back Transporting point for each of the Yin and Yang organs. They are:

Lungs	Feishu BL-13
Pericardium	Jueyinshu BL-14
Heart	Xinshu BL-15
Liver	Ganshu BL-18
Gall Bladder	Danshu BL-19
Spleen	Pishu BL-20
Stomach	Weishu BL-21
Triple Burner	Sanjiaoshu BL-22
Kidneys	Shenshu BL-23
Large Intestine	Dachangshu BL-25
Small Intestine	Xiaochangshu BL-27
Bladder	Pangguangshu BL-28

In addition to these points, there are a few others which are situated on the Bladder channel very close to the Back Transporting points but are not related to organs. They are related to parts of the body or channels. These are:

Governing Vessel	Dushu BL-16
Diaphragm	Geshu BL-17
Sacrum	Zhonglushu BL-29
Anus	Baihuanshu BL-30

The Back Transporting points affect the organs directly and are therefore used in Interior diseases of the Yin or Yang organs. They can be used in both acute or chronic conditions, but are more frequently used in chronic ones.

The Back Transporting points are Yang in character and are especially used to tonify the Yang. However, they can be used for deficiency of Yin as well.

Another characteristic of these points is that they are used to affect the sense organ of the corresponding organ. For example, Ganshu BL-18 is the Back Transporting point of the Liver and can be used for eye diseases.

In practice, these points tend to produce a stronger and more rapid effect than the Front Collecting points (see p. 351). They are therefore very useful when the patient feels very tired, exhausted or depressed. In these cases, if the Stomach and Spleen are deficient, the use of Pishu BL-20 and Weishu BL-21 will produce a strong tonifying effect.

The use of Geshu BL-17 and Danshu BL-19 (in Chinese called the "Four Flowers"), also has a strong tonifying effect on Qi and Blood. The point Shenshu BL-23 should be used in any deficiency of the Kidneys, particularly Kidney-Yang, as it strongly tonifies the Kidneys.

Although the Back Transporting points are mostly used to tonify the organs, they can also be used in Excess patterns to sedate Qi. In particular, they can be used to subdue rebellious Qi. For example, the point Weishu BL-21 can be used to subdue rebellious Stomach-Qi in case of belching, nausea or vomiting. The point Ganshu BL-18 can be used to move stagnant Liver-Qi. Xinshu BL-15 can be used to clear Heart-Fire and Feishu BL-13 to stimulate the dispersing and descending of Lung-Qi and release the Exterior.

The Back Transporting points can also be used for diagnostic purposes as they become tender on pressure or even spontaneously tender when the corresponding organ is diseased. The "Spiritual Axis" discusses this and other aspects of the Back Transporting points in chapter 51: *"The Back Transporting point for the centre of the thorax is below the tip of the big vertebra (Dazhui Du-14), that for the Lungs is below the 3rd vertebra, that for the Heart below the 5th vertebra, that for the diaphragm below the 7th vertebra, that for the Liver below the 9th vertebra, that for the Spleen below the 11th vertebra, that for the Kidneys below the 14th vertebra, all of them are situated 3 inches from the spine. Soreness is relieved on pressing on these points. Moxa is applied on these points, never needling. In order to tonify them one lets the moxa cones burn out on the skin slowly, in order to sedate them one blows on the moxa cones and then puts them out quickly."* [9]

This passage establishes the use of the Back Transporting points in diagnosis when they become tender on pressure. The last statement could seem surprising as it forbids the needling of these points, which are needled so frequently in practice. The prevalent view is that prohibiting the needling of these points was an over-cautious attitude so that they would not be needled too deeply. In fact, these points, and especially those on the upper part, should not be needled deeply because of possible injury to the lungs. **They should be needled quite superficially (but not just under the skin) and obliquely towards the midline.**

Another point of interest in this passage is the mention of a method of moxibustion for sedation, contrary to the prevalent idea that moxibustion is generally used for tonification only.

In addition to the above line of Back Transporting points along the Bladder channel, there are also six other points on the outer line of the Bladder channel on the back which are particularly important.

These are:

Pohu BL-42	Door of the Corporeal Soul
Gaohuangshu BL-43	The Transporting point of *"Gaohuang"*
Shentang BL-44	Hall of the Mind
Hunmen BL-47	Door of the Ethereal Soul
Yishe BL-49	House of the Mind
Zhishi BL-52	Room of the Will Power

With the exception of Gaohuangshu BL-43, the other five points exert a special effect on the corresponding mental aspect of each of the five Yin organs, i.e. the Corporeal Soul (Lungs), Mind (Heart), Ethereal Soul (Liver), Mind (Spleen) and Will Power (Kidneys). These points can therefore be used in emotional and psychological problems of the relevant Yin organs.

For example, Pohu BL-42 can be used for deep emotional problems related to sadness or grief affecting the Lungs. Shentang BL-44 can be used for emotional problems related to the Heart causing anxiety and insomnia, in particular if due to Heart-Fire or Heart Empty-Heat. Hunmen BL-47 can be used to help a person find a sense of direction in life. It is very useful in certain cases of depression when the person feels confused and unable to plan his or her life. This point is also effective to treat other emotional problems related to the Liver manifesting with mood swings, a feeling of frustration, resentment and anger. Yishe BL-49 can be used in patients who exceed in mental work. Zhishi BL-52 can be used for Kidney deficiency manifesting with great exhaustion, depression, lack of will power and a feeling of powerlessness and hopelessness.

The action of these points is stronger if they are combined with the relevant Back Transporting points of the corresponding Yin organ, e.g. Shenshu BL-23 and Zhishi BL-52 for the Kidneys.

The point Gaohuangshu BL-43 is the Back Transporting point for the area below the diaphragm (which is called "Gaohuang"). However, its use can only be understood by referring to the other meaning of "Gaohuang". "Gaohuang" also indicates the site of any disease which is chronic and very difficult, if not impossible, to treat. This point is therefore used in very chronic diseases, particularly of the Lungs, and especially Lung-Yin deficiency. Historically, it was used for tuberculosis of the Lungs (see also p. 420).

FRONT COLLECTING POINTS

The Front Collecting points are all located on the chest or abdomen (with the exception of one). The Chinese character *Mu* (募) literally means "to raise, collect, enlist, recruit". In this context it has the meaning of "collecting", i.e. the points where the energy of the relevant organs collects or gathers.

These points are used both in diagnosis and treatment. They are used in diagnosis because they become tender, either on pressure or spontaneously, when their relevant organ becomes diseased.

In treatment, they are used to regulate the internal organs either by tonification or sedation.

The Front-Collecting points are Yin in character and are more often used in acute diseases; however, they can also be used in chronic ones.

The combination of the Front Collecting points with the Back Transporting points enhances the therapeutic results and provides a particularly strong treatment. If a patient is seen at rather infrequent intervals (two weeks or more), the combination of Front Collecting and Back Transporting points is effective in providing more lasting therapeutic results. If a patient is seen at frequent intervals (twice a week or more), it is better to alternate the use of the Front Collecting points with that of the Back Transporting points in each treatment session.

The Front-Collecting points are:

Lungs	Zhongfu LU-1
Pericardium	Shanzhong Ren-17
Heart	Juque Ren-14
Liver	Qimen LIV-14
Gall-Bladder	Riyue G.B.-24
Spleen	Zhangmen LIV-13
Stomach	Zhongwan Ren-12
Triple Burner	Shimen Ren-5
Kidney	Jingmen G.B.-25
Large Intestine	Tianshu ST-25
Small Intestine	Guanyuan Ren-4
Bladder	Zhongji Ren-3

The main therapeutic uses of these points are as follows:

— Zhongfu LU-1: used in acute Excess patterns of the Lungs, to clear Lung-Heat.

— Shanzhong Ren-17: used to tonify and/or move Qi in the chest.

— Juque Ren-14: used in Heart patterns with anxiety to calm the Mind.

— Qimen LIV-14: used to move Liver-Qi when it stagnates in the hypochondrium. It harmonizes Liver and Stomach.

— Riyue G.B.-24: used to clear Gall-Bladder Damp-Heat in acute Excess patterns of Liver and Gall Bladder.

— Zhangmen LIV-13: used to move Liver-Qi when it stagnates in the epigastrium or lower abdomen causing Spleen deficiency. It harmonizes Liver and Spleen.

— Zhongwan Ren-12: widely used to tonify Stomach-Qi or Stomach-Yin and Spleen-Qi to resolve Phlegm.

— Shimen Ren-5: used in Excess patterns of the Lower Burner, such as Damp-Heat accumulating in the Lower Burner.

— Jingmen G.B.-25: used in acute Excess patterns of the Bladder, to clear Heat and Damp.

— Tianshu ST-25: used to regulate the Intestines and stop diarrhoea and pain.

— Guanyuan Ren-4: used to regulate the Small Intestine.

However, this point is not much used in this capacity as it has many other important functions such as tonifying the Kidneys and Original Qi.

— Zhongji Ren-3: used in acute Excess patterns of the Bladder, such as Damp-Heat.

A more detailed account of the actions of these points will be given in the chapter on the functions of points (see page 367).

The Front-Collecting points are mentioned in chapter 47 of the "Simple Questions".[10]

ACCUMULATION POINTS

The Accumulation points are all located between the fingers/toes and elbows/knees, with the exception of Liangqiu ST-34.

They are points where the Qi of the channel gathers and are used mostly in acute patterns, especially when there is pain. They are therefore primarily indicated for channel problems and are usually reduced, as they are mostly used for Excess patterns.

The Accumulation points are:

Kongzui LU-6
Wenliu L.I.-7
Liangqiu ST-34
Diji SP-8
Yinxi HE-6
Yanglao S.I.-6
Jinmen BL-63
Shuiquan KI-5
Ximen P-4
Huizong T.B.-7
Waiqiu G.B.-36
Zhongdu LIV-6.

For example, Kongzui LU-6 is frequently used for an acute attack of asthma, Liangqiu ST-34 can be used for acute epigastric pain, Diji SP-8 for acute dysmenorrhoea, Jinmen BL-63 and Zhongdu LIV-6 for acute cystitits.

In addition, there are four Accumulation points for four of the extraordinary vessels, i.e. the Yang and Yin Heel Vessel and the Yang and Yin Linking Vessel. These are:

Fuyang BL-59 for the Yang Heel Vessel
Jiaoxin KI-8 for the Yin Heel Vessel
Yangjiao G.B.-35 for the Yang Linking Vessel
Zhubin KI-9 for the Yin Linking Vessel.

The Qi of the extraordinary vessels accumulates at these points which makes them particularly powerful points to activate the Qi of these vessels. They can be used in combination with the opening points of the extraordinary vessels.

GATHERING POINTS

The Gathering points are points that have a special influence on certain tissues, organs, energy or Blood. The Chinese character (*Hui* 会) denoting these points means "to gather" or "to meet".

The Gathering points are:

Zhangmen LIV-13 for the Yin organs
Zhongwan Ren-12 for the Yang organs
Shanzhong Ren-17 for Qi
Geshu BL-17 for Blood
Yanglingquan G.B.-34 for sinews
Taiyuan LU-9 for arteries
Dashu BL-11 for bones
Xuanzhong G.B.-39 for Marrow.

Each of these points has a special influence on the above tissues, organs, energy or Blood.

— Zhangmen LIV-13 is used to affect all the Yin organs, but in particular the Spleen and is used for Spleen deficiency especially if accompanied by stagnation of Liver-Qi.

— Zhongwan Ren-12 is very frequently used to tonify Stomach and Spleen thus influencing all the Yang organs.

— Shanzhong Ren-17 is used to tonify the Lungs and Heart and is often combined with other points to tonify Qi. It can also be used to move Qi in the chest especially in emotional problems, particularly worry and anxiety.

— Geshu BL-17 is used to either tonify Blood if used only with moxa, or to move Blood if used only with needle. It is also useful to move Blood locally to relieve upper back ache.

— Yanglingquan G.B.-34 is used for weakness or stiffness of joints and arthritis.

— Taiyuan LU-9 is used to tonify Lung-Qi particularly when all the pulses are deep and thin. It also stimulates the circulation as it influences the arteries.

— Dashu BL-11 can be used for chronic arthritis to affect the bones, and for all bone diseases.

— Xuanzhong G.B.-39 is used to nourish Marrow and Yin in case of Wind-stroke. It is also used with moxa to prevent Wind-stroke.

The above-mentioned functions of these points are only those related to their particular characteristic as Gathering points. Each of them has several other actions which may be unrelated to this particular characteristic. Other actions of these points are discussed in the chapter "Functions of the Points".

NOTES

1 Spiritual Axis, p 3.
2 Spiritual Axis, p 3.
3 Spiritual Axis, p 4.
4 Classic of Difficulties, p 143.
5 Classic of Difficulties, p 144.
6 For a detailed description of the Connecting channels pathways, see Acupuncture, A Comprehensive Text, p 83–90.
7 Spiritual Axis, p 37–39.
8 Spiritual Axis, p 39.
9 Spiritual Axis, p 100.
10 Simple Questions, p 262.

The Extraordinary Vessel Points

39

奇経八脉交会穴

In order to discuss the function and clinical use of the extraordinary vessel points, it is necessary to discuss the nature and functions of the vessels themselves.

The main source of knowledge for the extraordinary vessels derives from the following classics:

— the "Spiritual Axis", chapters 17, 21 and 62
— the "Classic of Difficulties", chapters 27, 28 and 29
— the "Study of the 8 Extraordinary Vessels" (*Qi Jing Ba Mai Kao*) by Li Shi Zhen, 1578
— the "Compendium of Acupuncture" (*Zhen Jiu Da Cheng*) by Yang Ji Zhou, 1601.

The 8 extraordinary vessels and their opening points are:

Directing Vessel (*Ren Mai*) LU-7
Governing Vessel (*Du Mai*) S.I.-3
Penetrating Vessel (*Chong Mai*) SP-4
Girdle Vessel (*Dai Mai*) G.B.-41
Yin Linking Vessel (*Yin Wei Mai*) P-6
Yang Linking Vessel (*Yang Wei Mai*) T.B.-5
Yin Heel Vessel (*Yin Qiao Mai*) KI-6
Yang Heel Vessel (*Yang Qiao Mai*) BL-62.

The main functions of the extraordinary vessels can be summarized as follows:

1) They act as reservoirs of energy in relation to the main channels which are compared to rivers. This idea comes from the "Classic of Difficulties" in chapter 27. It says: "*When there are heavy rains, canals and ditches are full to the brim . . . similarly, the extraordinary vessels are left out of the channel-system so that they can take the overflow from the main channels*"[1]

This means that the extraordinary vessels can both absorb energy from the main channels and transfer energy to them when needed. This happens in cases of shock, for example.

2) The extraordinary vessels all derive their energy from the Kidneys and all contain the Essence which is stored in the Kidneys. They circulate the Essence around the body, thus contributing to integrating the circulation of Nutritive Qi with that of the Essence.

For this reason, the extraordinary vessels are the link between the Pre-Heaven and the Post-Heaven Qi in so far as they are connected to the main channels and circulate the Essence all over the body. The extraordinary vessels therefore represent a deeper level of treatment related to the Pre-Heaven Qi and the basic constitution of an individual.

3) The extraordinary vessels circulate Defensive Qi over the thorax, abdomen and back. This is a function which is performed by the Penetrating, Directing and Governing Vessels only. Since they circulate Defensive Qi, which protects the body from exterior pathogenic factors, the extraordinary vessels also play a role in the body's resistance to pathogenic factors. This also explains the important role played by the Kidneys in the resistance to pathogenic factors since all extraordinary vessels derive from the Kidneys.

4) The Directing and Penetrating vessels regulate the 7 and 8 year cycles of women's lives and men's respectively. These life cycles are described in the "Simple Questions" in chapter 1.[2]

Beyond the above functions, it is impossible to generalize as each of the extraordinary vessels has special characteristics and functions of its own.

CLINICAL USE OF THE EXTRAORDINARY VESSELS

The extraordinary vessels can be grouped in two different ways. First of all they can be arranged into 4 pairs of vessels of the same polarity (both Yin or both Yang) sharing similar pathways, i.e.

Directing Vessel and Yin Heel Vessel
Governing Vessel and Yang Heel Vessel
Penetrating Vessel and Yin Linking Vessel
Girdle Vessel and Yang Linking Vessel

Because of this arrangement in pairs, the opening point of one vessel is usually used in conjunction with the opening point of the paired vessel. For example, when using the Directing Vessel, one would needle Lieque LU-7 and Zhaohai KI-6. These two points are needled on opposite sides according to sex: the opening point of the vessel being treated is needled on the left side for men and right side for women, and the opening point of the coupled vessel on the opposite side. For example, if one were to use the Directing Vessel in a man, one would needle LU-7 on the left and KI-6 on the right; in a woman, one would needle LU-7 on the right and KI-6 on the left. The opening point of the vessel being used (in our example the Directing Vessel) is needled first (in this example, LU-7 first).

When paired in this way, the extraordinary vessels within a pair have a common range of action in terms of body areas.

These are:

— Directing Vessel and Yin Heel Vessel: abdomen, chest, lungs, throat, face.
— Governing Vessel and Yang Heel Vessel: back of legs, back, spine, neck, head, eyes, brain.
— Penetrating Vessel and Yin Linking Vessel: inner aspect of leg, abdomen, chest, heart, stomach.
— Girdle Vessel and Yang Linking Vessel: outer aspect of leg, sides of body, shoulders, side of neck.

Another way in which the extraordinary vessels can be coupled is according to their functions. From this point of view, they can be grouped as follows:

Directing, Governing and Penetrating Vessels
Yin and Yang Heel Vessels
Yin and Yang Linking Vessels
Girdle Vessel.

DIRECTING, GOVERNING AND PENETRATING VESSELS

All these three vessels originate directly from the Kidneys and flow down to the perineum (at Huiyin Ren-1) from where they take different pathways: the Directing vessel flows up the abdomen along the midline, the Governing vessel up the back and the Penetrating vessel up the abdomen along the Kidney channel. These three vessels can be seen as the source of all the other extraordinary vessels as they originate directly from the Kidneys and are therefore connected to the Essence. They, more than the other extraordinary vessels, can be used in clinical practice to affect the patient's energy at a deep constitutional level.

YIN AND YANG HEEL VESSELS

These two vessels are directly complementary: the Yin Heel vessel starts at Zhaohai KI-6 and flows up to the eye carrying Yin energy to it, the Yang Heel vessel starts at Shenmai BL-62 and flows up to the eye carrying Yang energy to it. Thus, when the energy is in excess in the Yin Heel vessel, the person will be constantly sleepy and the eyes will want to close, while when the energy is in excess in the Yang Heel vessel, the person is awake and the eyes are open.[3]

The two Heel vessels also control the state of the muscles of the legs. When the Yin Heel vessel is diseased the Yin is tight and the Yang is relaxed (i.e. the muscles of the inner aspect of the leg are tight and those of the outer aspect too relaxed). When the Yang Heel vessel is diseased the Yang is tight and the Yin relaxed (i.e. the muscles of the inner aspect of the leg are relaxed and those of the outer aspect tight).[4]

YIN AND YANG LINKING VESSELS

These two vessels complement each other in so far as they link the Yin and Yang channels. In addition, their opening points belong to the Lesser Yang and Terminal Yin (Triple Burner and Pericardium) respectively which are externally-internally related.

GIRDLE VESSEL

The Girdle Vessel stands on its own as it is the only horizontal channel in the body. It encircles the main channels and because of this, it exerts an influence on the circulation of energy to the legs.

Thus the extraordinary vessels form an energetic pattern of the whole body which develops from the Kidneys, in much the same way as the embryo develops along a central axis. The Penetrating Vessel is at the centre of this energetic vortex as it is also the "Sea of the 5 Yin and 6 Yang organs", the "Sea of Blood" and "Sea of the channels" (the meaning of which will be explained later) and it starts from the Kidney itself. The energy of the Penetrating vessel is then distributed all over the body in small channels at the Defensive Qi energetic level. When its energy reaches Zhaohai KI-6, Zhubin KI-9, Shenmai BL-62, Jinmen BL-63 and Daimai GB-26 it gives rise to the Yin Heel Vessel, Yin Linking Vessel, Yang Heel Vessel, Yang Linking Vessel and Girdle Vessel respectively. Thus, the Penetrating Vessel can be seen as the origin of these five extraordinary vessels.

The Directing and Governing Vessel determine and define the coronal plane of the body, the Girdle Vessel defines the transverse plane, while the Yang Heel and Linking Vessels define the sagittal plane (see Fig. 70).

We can now discuss the function and clinical use of each extraordinary vessel and their opening points individually.

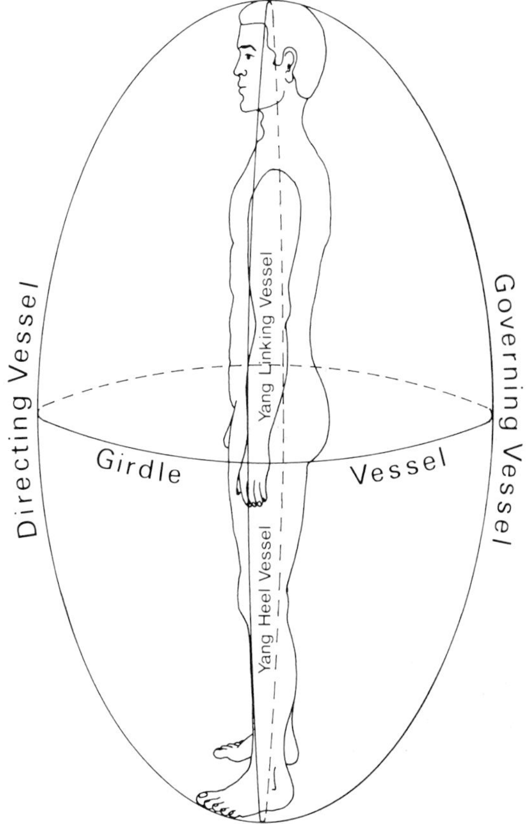

Fig. 70 Planes defined by the extraordinary vessels

GOVERNING VESSEL

Opening point: Houxi S.I.-3
Coupled point: Shenmai BL-62
Starting point: Changqiang Du-1
Area of body influenced: back, spine, back of neck and head.

The Governing vessel is called the "Sea of Yang channels" as it exerts an influence on all the Yang channels and it can be used to strengthen the Yang of the body. It can strengthen the spine and tonify Kidney-Yang.

The Governing vessel also nourishes the spine and brain as the inner pathway of the vessel enters the brain. In this sense, it can be used to strengthen the Kidney function of nourishing Marrow and Brain, for such symptoms as dizziness and poor memory. To summarize, the opening and coupled points can be used for the following cases:

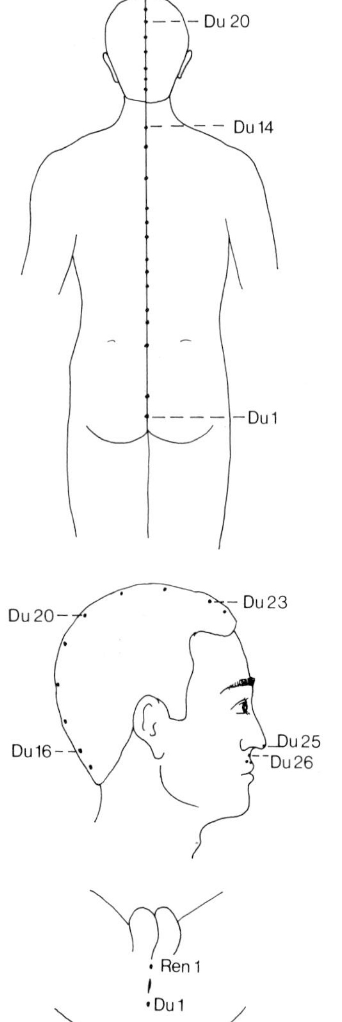

Fig. 71 The Governing Vessel

1) To tonify Kidney-Yang and strengthen the back. The Governing vessel is extremely useful in all cases of chronic lower back ache due to Kidney deficiency, especially (but not exclusively) when the pain is on the midline of the back. The use of the opening and coupled points can strengthen the back and actually straighten the spine. In men the Governing Vessel can be used on its own, and in women it is best combined with the Directing Vessel, crossing over the opening and coupled points. Thus in a woman, one would use Houxi S.I.-3 on the right, Shenmai BL-62 on the left, Lieque LU-7 on the left and Zhaohai KI-6 on the right, the needles being inserted in this order and taken out in the reverse order.

When used for lower back ache, the Governing Vessel opening and coupled points are used first and left in about 10-15 minutes. This has the effect of opening the Governing Vessel, making it more receptive to further treatment with local points. It also has the effect of actually straightening the spine. After withdrawal of the opening and coupled point needles, local points can be used, particularly Yaoyangguan Du-3 or the extra point Shiqizhuixia situated on the midline below the tip of L-5 lumbar vertebra.

2) To expel Wind: this can be either internal or external Wind. In exterior attacks, the Governing vessel can be used to release the Exterior and expel Wind at the Greater Yang stage of the 6 Stages (see App. 1). It is therefore used for such symptoms as fever, runny nose, headache, stiff neck and a Floating pulse.

In interior conditions, the Governing Vessel can be used to subdue interior Wind, for such symptoms as dizziness, tremors, convulsions, epilepsy, or for the sequelae of Wind-stroke.

3) To nourish the spine and the brain. Using the opening and coupled points of the Governing Vessel can strengthen the Kidney function of nourishing Marrow and Brain, for such symptoms as dizziness, tinnitus and poor memory.

Case history

A man suffered from chronic back ache on the midline in the lumbar area. This was caused by a Kidney deficiency and the Governing Vessel opening and coupled points (Houxi S.I.-3 and Shenmai BL-62) were used, together with Taixi KI-3 and Shenshu BL-23, producing an immediate marked improvement.

DIRECTING VESSEL

Opening point: Lieque LU-7
Coupled point: Zhaohai KI-6
Starting point: Huiyin Ren-1
Area of body influenced: abdomen, thorax, lungs, throat, face.

The Directing vessel is called the "Sea of the Yin channels" as it exerts an influence on all the Yin channels of the body. It originates from the Kidneys and flows through the uterus down to Huiyin Ren-1 where the superficial pathway starts. The Directing Vessel is of paramount importance for the reproductive system of both men and women, but particularly women, as it regulates menstruation, fertility, conception, pregnancy, childbirth and menopause. Its functions and clinical use can be summarized as follows:

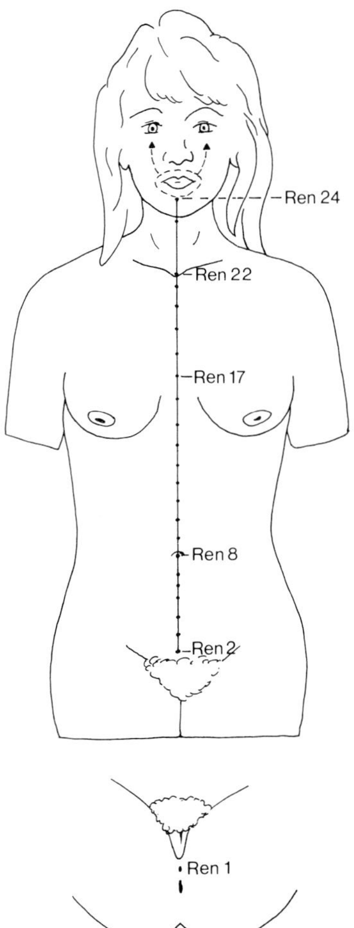

Fig. 72 The Directing Vessel

1) It can be used to nourish the Yin energy of the body. In this context, it is particularly useful to nourish Yin in women after menopause as the Directing channel controls the uterus and determines the 7-year life cycles of women. It can therefore regulate the energy of the reproductive system and, after the menopause, tonify Blood and Yin to reduce the effects of Empty-Heat symptoms deriving from Yin deficiency.

It can therefore be used for such symptoms as night sweating, hot flushes, feeling of heat, mental irritability, anxiety, dry mouth at night, dizziness, tinnitus or insomnia, all symptoms of Kidney-Yin deficiency and Heart Empty-Heat. When used in this way, the opening and coupled points are best combined with Guanyuan Ren-4.

2) It regulates the uterus and Blood in women, so that it is responsible for menstruation, fertility, conception, pregnancy, childbirth and menopause. It can be used for infertility to promote the supply of Blood to the uterus and in many menstrual disorders such as dysmenorrhoea, amenorrhoea, menorrhagia and metrorrhagia.

3) It moves Qi in the Lower Burner and uterus, so that it can be used for lumps, fibroids and carcinoma of the uterus. In men, it is used for hernia.

4) The sphere of action of the Directing Vessel extends not only to the Lower Burner, but also the Middle and Upper Burner. It can in fact be used also to stimulate the Lung descending function and the Kidney function of reception of Qi. For this reason, it is used for chronic asthma, for which it is excellent.

Case history

A man of 37 suffered from chronic asthma characterized by difficulty in inhalation. There was no sputum and he felt very tired generally. His voice was low and his complexion Pale. He also had a lower back ache and felt cold. His pulse was Deep and Weak and his tongue was Pale. These manifestations clearly point to deficient Kidney-Yang unable to hold Qi resulting in asthma. Besides this there was also a Lung-Qi deficiency as evidenced by the low voice and pale complexion.

The opening and coupled points of the Directing Vessel (Lieque LU-7 on the left and Zhaohai KI-6 on the right) were used to tonify the Lungs, stimulate the descending of Lung-Qi and stimulate the Kidney function of reception of Qi.

Case history

A woman of 41 had a large fibroid in the uterus for several years. Her periods were very heavy and painful and the menstrual blood was dark. Her lower abdomen was extremely hard and the fibroid was clearly felt on palpation.

She was treated several times using the opening and coupled points of the Directing Vessel producing a complete normalization of her periods and a very marked softening of her lower abdomen. The size of the abdominal swelling was also markedly reduced. Obviously a fibroid of that size cannot be dissolved but the use of the Directing Vessel at least normalized her periods, took the menstrual pain away and made her lower abdomen much more comfortable.

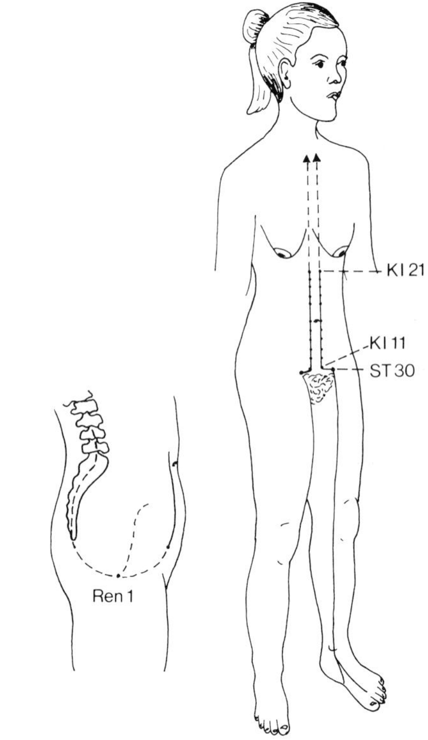

Fig. 73 The Penetrating Vessel

PENETRATING VESSEL

Opening point: Gongsun SP-4
Coupled point: Neiguan P-6
Starting point: Huiyin Ren-1
Area of body influenced: abdomen, uterus, chest, heart.

The Penetrating Vessel is very complex as it has many different functions at different levels. In a way, it could be considered to be the origin of the other extraordinary vessels (excluding Governing and Directing Vessels) as it originates in the Kidneys and spreads its Qi all over the body at the Defensive Qi level. When this energy arrives at the relevant starting points, it gives rise to the Yin and Yang Linking Vessels, the Yin and Yang Heel Vessels and the Girdle Vessel.

The Penetrating Vessel is described as the "Sea of the 5 Yin and 6 Yang organs" [5] and also as the "Sea of the 12 channels".[6] It is described as the Sea of the 5 Yin and 6 Yang organs as it is a fundamental vessel which connects the Pre-Heaven and the Post-Heaven Qi, due to its connection with Kidneys and Stomach. It is connected to the Kidneys as it originates in them and it distributes Essence all over the body, and it is connected to the Stomach as it passes through the point Qichong ST-30 which is a point for the Sea of Food. Furthermore, the Penetrating Vessel is connected to the Spleen channel along which it flows on the inner aspect of the thigh, down to the big toe.

It is called the "Sea of the 12 channels" because it branches out in many small capillary-like vessels that circulate Defensive Qi over the abdomen and chest.

The functions and clinical use of the Penetrating vessel can be summarized as follows:

1) The Penetrating Vessel is excellent in cases of rebellious Qi[7] and is therefore often used to move Qi and Blood when they stagnate in the abdomen and chest, for such cases as dysmenorrhoea, flatulence, borborygmi, abdominal distension or abdominal masses. In this respect, it is used mostly for Excess patterns charac-

terized by stagnation and obstruction with a characteristic feeling of fullness of the chest or epigastrium.

2) The Penetrating Vessel, together with the Directing vessel, regulates the uterus and menstruation and it nourishes Blood. It can be used for such conditions as dysmenorrhoea, amenorrhoea and menorrhagia. The main difference between the Directing vessel and the Penetrating vessel in relation to menstruation is that the former controls Qi and can be used to tonify and nourish, whereas the latter controls Blood and is mostly used to move Qi and Blood and remove obstructions.

3) Since the Penetrating vessel provides the link between the Pre-Heaven and Post-Heaven Qi, it can be used in all cases of weak constitution with digestive symptoms, such as poor appetite, abdominal distension and poor assimilation of food.

4) The Penetrating Vessel exerts an influence on the heart, as it flows through it, and it can be used to move the Blood of the Heart in cases of pain in the chest, feeling of stuffiness of the chest and palpitations.

Case history

A man of 45 suffered from chronic indigestion with a sensation of fullness of the epigastrium, belching and nausea. His pulse was Full and Tight especially in the Middle position, and his tongue had a thick white coating. The clinical manifestations point to retention of food in the Middle Burner. The opening and coupled points of the Penetrating Vessel (Gongsun SP-4 and Neiguan P-6) were used producing a complete recovery after several treatments.

GIRDLE VESSEL

Opening point: Zulinqi G.B.-41
Coupled point: Waiguan T.B.-5
Starting point: Daimai G.B.-26
Area of body influenced: genitals, waist, hips.

The Girdle Vessel is the only horizontal vessel of the body. It divides the body in two halves and flows through Zhangmen LIV-13, Daimai G.B.-26, Wushu G.B.-27 and Weidao G.B.-28. It is closely related to the Liver and Gall-Bladder and it connects with the Kidney divergent channel.

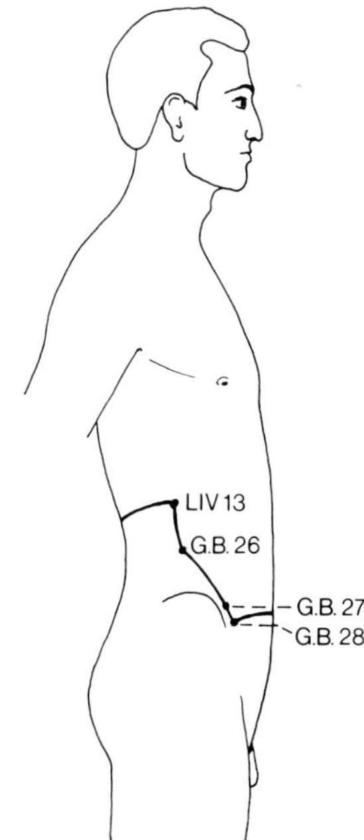

Fig. 74 The Girdle Vessel

The functions and clinical use of the Girdle Vessel can be summarized as follows:

1) It can be used to harmonize the Liver and Gall-Bladder, particularly in Excess patterns of the Liver, when the Gall-Bladder pulse is Full and Wiry, for such symptoms as temporal headaches.

2) The Girdle Vessel can be used to disperse Damp-Heat in the genitals, causing such symptoms as burning on urination and difficulty in urination.

3) The Girdle Vessel encircles the leg channels and it affects their circulation. Disorders of this channel can therefore impair the circulation of Qi in the leg channels, resulting in such symptoms as cold legs and feet, purple feet or tense outer leg muscles (due to Liver-Blood not moistening the sinews).

4) The Girdle Vessel particularly affects the circulation of Qi in the Stomach channel and can cause weakness of the leg muscles, and in severe cases, atrophy. In these cases the opening and coupled point of the Girdle Vessel can be used to ease the vessel and tonify the Stomach and Spleen channels.

5) The Girdle Vessel flows through the waist and

influences the hip. It can therefore be used for hip pain, particularly when there is a condition of deficiency of Liver-Blood and excess of Liver-Yang, with Liver-Blood deficiency leading to malnourishment of sinews and joints.

Case history

A woman of 45 suffered from chronic migraine headaches characterized by a severe throbbing ache on the temple. Her pulse was Wiry and Full and her tongue was Red with a yellow coating. The headaches were clearly due to the rising of Liver-Yang and the Girdle Vessel opening and coupled points (Zulinqi G.B.-41 and Waiguan T.B.-5) were used several times in successive treatments producing a complete cure.

Case history

A woman of 72 suffered from chronic cystitis characterized by severe burning on urination and dark-scanty urine. She also experienced a severe distending sensation in the hypogastrium. Her pulse was Full, Rapid and very Wiry particularly in the Middle position. Her tongue was Deep-Red and had a yellow coating which was thicker on the root. The root of the tongue also had red spots. This problem was caused by the downward infusion of Liver-Fire affecting the Bladder. The opening and coupled points of the Girdle Vessel were used several times in succession, together with other points to clear Liver and Bladder Heat, producing a nearly complete cure.

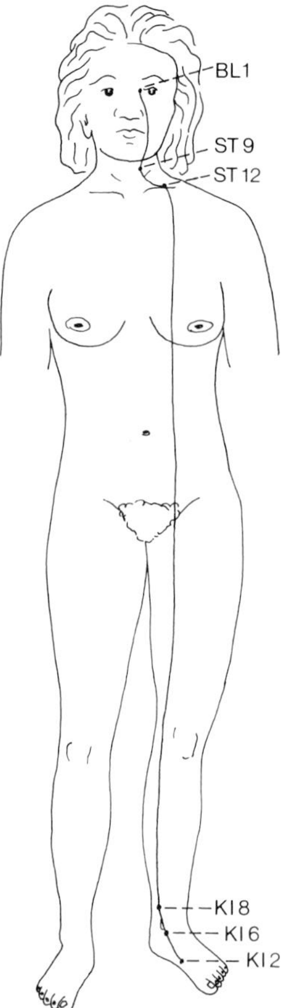

Fig. 75 The Yin Heel Vessel

YIN HEEL VESSEL

Opening point: Zhaohai KI-6
Coupled point: Lieque LU-7
Starting point: Zhaohai KI-6
Accumulation point:Jiaoxin KI-8
Area of body influenced: inner side of legs, abdomen, eyes.

The Yin and Yang Heel Vessels are closely related, especially in their relation with the eyes. They both flow up to the eyes, the Yin Heel Vessel bringing Yin energy to them, the Yang Heel Vessel bringing Yang energy to them. When the Yin Heel Vessel is diseased, the eyes cannot stay open and tend to close all the time, i.e. the person feels always sleepy. When the Yang Heel Vessel is diseased, the eyes cannot close and tend to stay open all the time, i.e. the person cannot sleep.[8]

The Yin and Yang Heel Vessels also exert an influence on the tone of the leg muscles. When the Yin Heel Vessel is in Excess the inner leg muscles are tight, and the outer leg muscles loose; when the Yang Heel Vessel is in Excess, the inner leg muscles are loose and the outer ones tight.[9]

The Yin Heel Vessel is an offshoot of the Kidney channel, while the Yang Heel Vessel is an offshoot of the Bladder channel.

The clinical uses of the Yin Heel Vessel can be summarized as follows:

1) Because of its relation with the eyes, it can be used in disturbances of sleep, either insomnia or somnolence. In this context, it is often used in conjunction with the Yang Heel Vessel. In case of insomnia, the Yin Heel Vessel is tonified (by tonifying Zhaohai KI-6) and the Yang Heel Vessel sedated (by reducing Shenmai BL-62). In case of somnolence, the Yin Heel Vessel is

sedated (by reducing KI-6) and the Yang Heel Vessel tonified (by reinforcing BL-62). In both cases, the point Jingming BL-1 can be added to establish a connection between the Yin and Yang Heel Vessels, so that Yin and Yang energy in the eyes can be balanced.

2) The Yin Heel Vessel can be used in certain cases of Atrophy Syndrome, when the muscles of the inner aspect of the legs are loose and the foot turns inwards, partly pulled by the tight outer leg muscles: this makes walking very difficult and a person prone to tripping. The Yin Heel Vessel opening and coupled points can be used to balance the tension of the inner and outer leg muscles.

3) The Yin Heel Vessel extends its range of action to the abdomen, and can be used in Excess patterns of the Lower Burner in women, for such symptoms as abdominal distension, abdominal masses, lumps, fibroids, difficult delivery or retention of placenta.

4) Finally, the Yin and Yang Heel Vessels can harmonize left and right, and can therefore be used in structural imbalances between left and right side of the body.

Case history

A man of 28 suffered from continuous somnolence. This followed a car accident during which he suffered a fracture of the skull. He came for treatment as he was studying hard for an exam and could not keep awake.

The point Shenmai BL-62 on the left side was reinforced to stimulate the Yang Heel Vessel, Zhaohai KI-6 on the right side was reduced to sedate the Yin Heel Vessel, and the point Jingming BL-1 was used bilaterally with even method. After only one treatment the somnolence completely disappeared and he could not actually sleep for two days!

YANG HEEL VESSEL

Opening point: Shenmai BL-62
Coupled point: Houxi S.I.-3
Starting point: Shenmai BL-62
Accumulation point: Fuyang BL-59

Area of body influenced: lateral aspect of leg, back, neck, head, eyes.

The Yang Heel Vessel is an offshoot of the

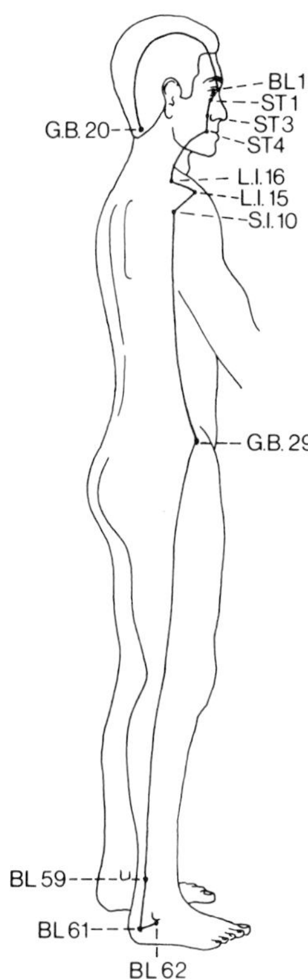

Fig. 76 The Yang Heel Vessel

Bladder channel and it brings Yang energy up to the eyes. Its influence on the eyes and the muscle tone of the lateral side of the legs, has already been mentioned in the discussion of the Yin Heel vessel.

Although the Yin and Yang Heel Vessels are somewhat symmetrical in their functions, there are some differences in their practical use.

Whilst the Yin Heel Vessel's sphere of influence is mostly in the lower abdomen and genitals (apart from its action on the eyes), the Yang Heel Vessel's sphere of action is mostly in the head, absorbing excess Yang energy or stagnation in the head area. For this reason, it is used for Wind-stroke, hemiplegia, aphasia and facial paralysis.

The functions and clinical use of the Yang Heel Vessel can be summarized as follows:

1) It absorbs excess Yang energy from the head, and it is therefore used to subdue internal or external Wind from the head (Wind is a Yang pathogenic factor), in such conditions as facial

paralysis (exterior Wind), Wind-stroke, severe dizziness and aphasia (interior Wind).

2) It is used to expel exterior Wind and release the Exterior in invasions of exterior Wind-Heat or Wind-Cold, causing such symptoms as sneezing, headache, stiff neck, runny nose and Floating pulse. It is particularly indicated if the exterior attack is accompanied by severe headache and stiff neck.

3) It is extremely effective for lower back ache with pain along the Bladder channel of the leg, but only if this pain is of Excess nature, i.e. acute in character and due to sprain or invasion of Cold. It is only used if the pain is unilateral.

4) The Yang Heel Vessel is also very useful in cases of extreme nervous tension, particularly in young men, when the pulse is very Wiry and the face is red (showing excess Yang energy in the head).

5) As the Yang Heel Vessel flows through the point Juliao G.B.-29, its opening and coupled points can be used as distal points for the treatment of pain in the hip.

Case history

A man of 43 suffered from giddiness and an ache on the lateral side of the legs. His blood pressure was high. His face was red and the muscles on the lateral side of the legs were very tight. He appeared very tense. His pulse was Full, Rapid and Wiry and his tongue was Red.

The Yang Heel Vessel was chosen to calm the Yang, relax the muscles on the lateral side of the legs, subdue interior Wind (manifested by the giddiness) and calm the Mind. The successive use of its opening and coupled points (Shenmai BL-62 on the left and Houxi S.I.-3 on the right) produced a marked improvement.

YIN LINKING VESSEL

Opening point: Neiguan P-6
Coupled point: Gongsun SP-4
Starting point: Zhubin KI-9
Accumulation point: Zhubin KI-9
Area of body influenced: chest, heart.

The Yin Linking vessel connects all the Yin channels. This is partly due to the fact that its opening point is P-6 pertaining to the Terminal Yin which is the "hinge" of the Yin channels.

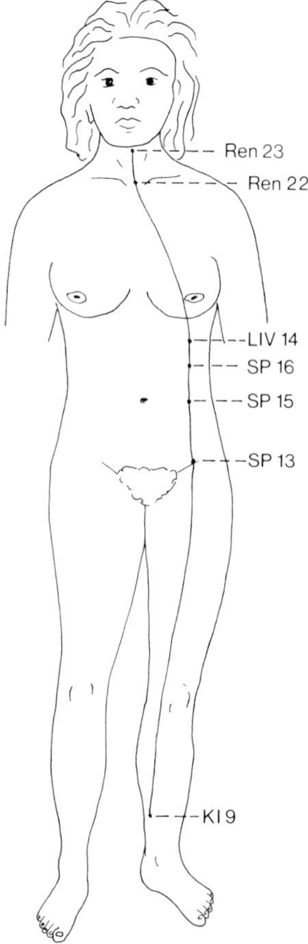

Fig. 77 The Yin Linking Vessel

Its functions and clinical use can be summarized as follows:

1) Since it connects all the Yin channels, it can be used for deficiency of Blood and/or Yin, especially if accompanied by psychological symptoms such as insomnia, anxiety and mental restlessness. In this context, it has a remarkable effect in calming the mind, especially in women.

2) Since it tonifies Blood, it has a tonifying action on the Heart and can be used for such symptoms as chest pain or a feeling of stuffiness of the chest, a feeling of oppression or tightness of the chest, anxiety, apprehension, depression or nightmares.

3) The Yin Linking Vessel is effective in treating headaches from deficiency of Blood, especially if they are at the back of the neck. This is due to the fact that it nourishes Blood and its opening

point P-6, being also the Connecting point of the Pericardium channel, affects the Triple Burner channel area on the neck.

Case history

A woman of 54 suffered from severe anxiety and claustrophobia. She was afraid to go to the theatre, church or in the underground. She was anxious when alone at home and felt a tight, gripping sensation in the chest. Her pulse was Choppy and her tongue Pale, but with a red tip. The clinical manifestations are due to deficiency of Blood, depriving the Mind of its residence resulting in severe anxiety.

Due to the deficiency of Blood and the typical sensation of tightness of the chest, the Yin Linking Vessel was used (Neiguan P-6 on the right and Gongsun SP-4 on the left) producing excellent results.

YANG LINKING VESSEL

Opening point: Waiguan T.B.-5
Coupled point: Zulinqi G.B.-41
Starting point: Jinmen BL-63
Accumulation point: Yangjiao G.B.-35
Area of body influenced: lateral aspect of leg, sides of body, lateral aspect of neck and head, ears.

The Yang Linking Vessel connects all the Yang channels. Its functions and clinical use can be summarized as follows:

1) It is used for intermittent fevers and alternation of chills and fever. These are symptoms of affection of the Lesser Yang stage in the 6-Stage patterns of penetration of exterior pathogenic factor (see App. 1). The chief symptom at this stage is alternation of chills and fever because the pathogenic factor is lodged half in the Interior and half in the Exterior.

2) The Yang Linking Vessel exerts its influence on the sides of the body and is used for such symptoms as hypochondriac pain, pain in the lateral aspect of the leg (such as sciatica along the Gall Bladder channel) and pain in the lateral side of the neck.

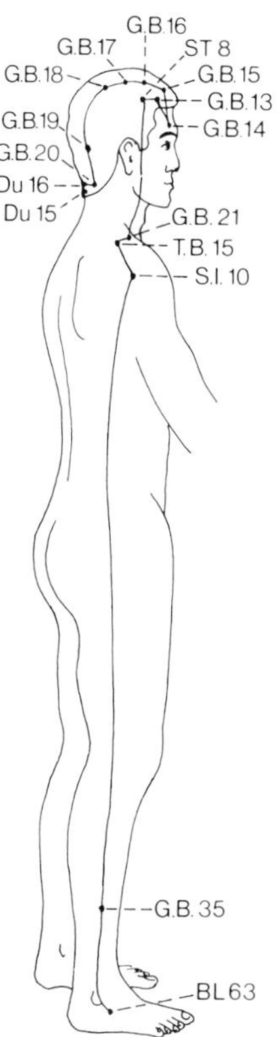

Fig. 78 The Yang Linking Vessel

3) The Yang Linking Vessel affects the ears and can be used for ear problems due to the rising of Liver-Fire, such as tinnitus and deafness. It can also be used in any ear diseases manifesting caused by a Gall-Bladder disharmony.

Case history

A boy of 12 had a middle-ear infection and the Yang Linking Vessel was used (Waiguan T.B.-5 on the left and Zulinqi G.B.-41 on the right), producing a complete cure.

NOTES

1 Classic of Difficulties, p 68–69.
2 Simple Questions, p 4–6.
3 Spiritual Axis, ch 17, p 50.
4 Classic of Difficulties, ch 29, p 73.
5 Spiritual Axis, ch 38, p 79.
6 Spiritual Axis, ch 62, p 112–113.
7 Simple Questions, ch 61, p 320.
8 Spiritual Axis, ch 21, p. 56. Also ch 17, p 50.
9 Classic of Difficulties, ch 29, p 73.

The Functions of the Points 40

穴位作用

Acupuncture points can be classified in various ways according to their common energetic actions. For example, all Accumulation points can be said to have an action on the Qi of the channel and be able to treat acute and painful conditions. Likewise, all Back Transporting points can treat chronic problems while all Source points tonify the Yin organs directly.

The problem with any classification of points is that it always suffers from many exceptions because not all points within a given category have necessarily the same function. This is due to the fact that most theories of Chinese Medicine, and the theory of the function of points in particular, resulted from a combination of the inductive with the deductive method. For example, if a point such as Xingjian LIV-2 was found from experience to eliminate Liver-Fire, after a process of further experimentation, the theory might have been formulated that all Fire points eliminate Heat. Thus, one might say that LIV-2 eliminates Liver-Fire not because it is the Fire point, but it is the Fire point because, according to many centuries'experience, it clears Liver-Fire. The practical experience of LIV-2 clearing Liver-Fire preceded the generalization according to which Fire-points clear Fire.

The implication of this is that each point has certain energetic functions, discovered over centuries of accumulated clinical experience, which may or may not be related to their "classification".

Having discussed the energetic action of the various classes of points, we can now add the energetic action of each point as it was discovered empirically over many centuries by countless doctors.

I will discuss not all the points, but the most commonly used ones.

This information has been drawn from various different sources, some ancient and some modern. The main sources are:

"The Spiritual Axis" (c. 200 BC)[1]

"The Simple Questions" (c. 200 BC)[2]

"The Classic of Difficulties" (c. 200 BC)[3]

"The Compendium of Acupuncture" (1601)[4]

"Clinical Application of Frequently Used Acupuncture Points"[5]

"Selection of Acupuncture Point Combinations from the 'Discussion on Cold-induced Diseases"[6]

"Clinical Records of *Tai Yi Shen* Acupuncture"[7]

Notes from the First Advanced International Acupuncture Course at the Nanjing College of Traditional Chinese Medicine, 1981

Notes from Dr J.H.F. Shen Seminars, 1978, 1979 and 1981

Personal communications from Dr Su Xin Ming of the Nanjing College of Traditional Chinese Medicine

Personal communications from Dr Chen Jing Hua of the Beijing Friendship Hospital

Personal communications from Dr J. H. F. Shen.

In addition to the above sources, the function of certain points has also been drawn from the author's own experience. Whenever this is so, this is made clear in the text.

When discussing the energetic action of each point it is usually implied that different actions require different needle manipulations. For example, if a certain point "eliminates exterior Wind", it is implied that in order to do that it should be needled with reducing method. Likewise, if a certain point "nourishes Blood", it is implied that it should be reinforced.

For the sake of clarity, the following is a list of the main energetic actions mentioned together with their corresponding manipulation method.

Reinforcing method	*Reducing method*
Tonify Qi or Yang	Eliminate Wind (interior or exterior)
Nourish Blood, Yin or Essence	Clear Fire or Heat
Tonify Original Qi	Resolve Dampness
Moisten Dryness	Eliminate interior Cold
Warm	Resolve Phlegm
Lift the Mind	Open the orifices
	Promote resuscitation
	Stop pain
	Regulate Qi
	Regulate Blood
	Remove obstructions from the channels

In some cases, either the reinforcing or reducing method is applicable, according to the nature of the pattern, i.e. whether it is a Deficiency or Excess pattern. These are:

Benefit the sinews

Benefit the eyes or ears

Calm the Mind.

The usual condition applies whereby in certain cases the reducing method, although indicated, should not be applied. These are:

1) When the condition is chronic (over 6-months duration).

2) When the patient is very old.

3) When the patient is very weak.

In all these cases the reducing method should be replaced by the even method.[8]

Finally, in giving the actions of each point I have tried to tread a middle way between giving as detailed information as possible, and giving the essential actions for each point. Giving too little information on a point may miss some important function, but giving too much information may make it impossible for the reader to form an idea of the essential nature and functions of the point. For example, the point Shangwan Ren-13 besides subduing rebellious Stomach-Qi (which is its most essential function), may also tonify Stomach-Qi. I have omitted the latter function as it is not frequently used in this way since the point Zhongwan Ren-12 is much better to tonify Stomach-Qi. There would be no point in using Ren-13 instead of Ren-12 to tonify Stomach-Qi. I have therefore tried to capture the essential nature and functions of each point.

LUNG CHANNEL

肺经

MAIN CHANNEL PATHWAY

The Lung channel originates from the Middle Burner and runs down to connect with the large intestine. It then ascends to the stomach, passes the diaphragm and enters the lung. From here it ascends to the throat and then emerges at Zhongfu LU-1. From here, it descends along the medial aspect of the arm and reaches the styloid process of the radius. It then goes to the thenar eminence and ends at the medial side of the tip of the thumb (Fig. 79).

CONNECTING CHANNEL PATHWAY

After separating from the main channel at Lieque LU-7, the Lung Connecting channel

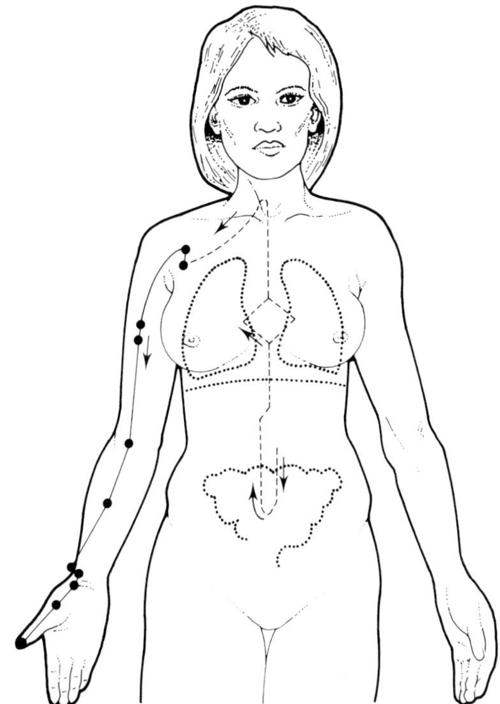

Fig. 79 Lung channel

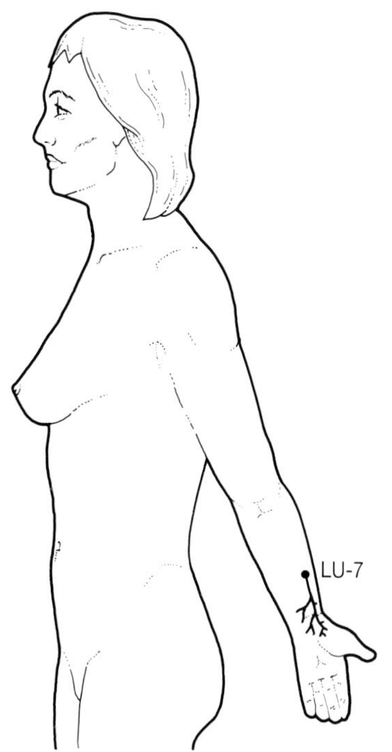

Fig. 79A Lung Connecting channel

connects with the Large Intestine channel. From Lieque LU-7 a branch flows to the thenar eminence where it scatters (Fig. 79A).

ZHONGFU LU-1 *Central Residence*

Nature

Front Collecting point of the Lungs
Meeting point of Greater Yin (Lungs-Spleen).

Action

Regulates Lung-Qi and stops cough
Stimulates the descending of Lung-Qi
Disperses fullness from the chest and stops pain.

Comments

This point is mostly used in acute Excess patterns of the Lungs to disperse fullness from the chest and to clear Lung-Heat. Thus it would be commonly used in the later stages of invasion of the Lungs by an exterior pathogenic factor, when this has penetrated into the Interior. In particular, it is very well indicated for cough caused by retention of Phlegm in the Lungs. This point is not usually used when the pathogenic factor is still on the Exterior. This explains why this point is not indicated for sore throat from invasion of exterior Wind-Heat. However, since it has a good effect on making Lung-Qi descend and stopping cough, it can be used in the beginning stages of invasion from an exterior pathogenic factor if cough is a prominent symptom. In these cases, LU-1 would be needled as a secondary point together with points to release the Exterior, such as Lieque LU-7 and Hegu L.I.-4.

It is an important point for the treatment of whooping cough during its second stage (i.e. Lung-Heat stage).

It is also effective in treating chest pain deriving from stagnation of Heart-Blood or retention of Phlegm in the chest. In the first case, LU-1 can move Lung-Qi and therefore help to move Blood in the chest, particularly if combined with Neiguan P-6. Combined with Fenglong ST-40 it can resolve Phlegm retained in the chest by moving Qi in the chest.

LU-1 is effective in treating shoulder or upper back pain deriving from a Lung channel dysfunction, such as in Lung-Heat, Damp-Phlegm or Phlegm-Heat obstructing the Lungs. The "Simple Questions" in chapter 22 says: *"When the Lungs are diseased, Qi rebels upwards causing breathlessness and there is pain in the shoulders or [upper] back"*.[9]

LU-1 can be combined with Feishu BL-13 both to tonify the Lungs, or to eliminate pathogenic factors in both acute and chronic cases. However, the combination of both front and back points is rather powerful and, in most cases, not necessary. Generally speaking, the Front Collecting point LU-1 would be chosen more for Excess and acute conditions, and the Back Transporting point Feishu BL-13 more for Deficiency and chronic conditions.

Combined with Zusanli ST-36 and Taibai SP-3, LU-1 can be used to tonify the Spleen and Lungs. This combination of points is based on the nature of LU-1 as meeting point of the Lung and Spleen channel. In 5-Element terms, this combination is called "Filling Earth to generate Metal".

It is useful to compare the functions of the Front Collecting point of the Lungs Zhongfu LU-1 with those of the Back Transporting point Feishu BL-13:

LU-1 (Front Collecting point)	*BL-13 (Back Transporting point)*
Mostly for Excess patterns	Mostly for Deficiency patterns
Mostly to treat the Manifestation	Mostly to treat the Root
Better for acute cases	Better for chronic cases
Treats pain in the chest	Treats pain in the upper back

YUNMEN LU-2 *Cloud door*

Action

Disperses fullness from the chest
Stimulates the descending of Lung-Qi
Stops cough.

Comments

The energetic actions of this point are the same as Zhongfu LU-1, but less strong. In addition to these, it can be used for local channel problems such as Painful Obstruction Syndrome of the shoulder, when the person cannot adduct the arm (i.e. bring the arm over close to the body towards the opposite side).

TIANFU LU-3 *Heavenly Residence*

Comments

This point has a powerful psychological effect on all emotional problems deriving from a Lung disharmony, such as depression, claustrophobia, agarophobia, mental confusion and forgetfulness.

CHIZE LU-5 *Foot Marsh*

Nature

Sea point
Water point
Sedation point.

Action

Clears Lung-Heat
Stimulates the descending of Lung-Qi
Expels Phlegm from the Lungs
Benefits the Bladder
Relaxes the sinews.

Comments

This point is used for interior patterns of an Excess nature characterized by Heat in the Lungs with such symptoms as cough, fever, yellow sputum and thirst. This point would be applicable at the Qi level (2nd stage) of the 4-Level Pattern Identification characterized by Full-Interior-Heat in the Lungs. It can also be used in chronic conditions characterized by retention of Phlegm and Heat in the Lungs, such as may happen in chronic bronchitis. In this case it would be combined with Fenglong ST-40.

In cases when Lung-Heat has injured the Body Fluids, LU-5 can be combined with Fuliu KI-7 to clear the Lungs and nourish Yin.

It is also an important point to use in the

second stage of whooping cough usually characterized by Phlegm and Heat in the Lung combined with Yuji LU-10 and Fenglong ST-40.

It can also be used for interior patterns of an Excess-Cold nature, with retention of Cold Phlegm in the Lungs, manifesting with such symptoms as cough with profuse white-sticky sputum and chilliness. In all these cases, this point would be needled with reducing method.

LU-5 also has an effect on the Bladder in opening the Water passages and facilitating urination. It is therefore used for retention of urine caused by obstruction of the Lungs by Damp-Phlegm preventing Lung-Qi from descending and opening the Water passages in the Lower Burner. Also in this case, LU-5 would be reduced and would be combined with such points as Yinlingquan SP-9 and Zhongji Ren-3.

Finally, LU-5 relaxes the tendons of the arm along the Lung channel and can be used in Painful Obstruction Syndrome or paralysis of the arm when the patient is unable to raise the arm. The "ABC of Acupuncture" (AD 259) states: "*When the arm cannot be raised to the head, or there is pain in the elbow, use LU-5*".[10]

The "Illustrated Manual of Acupuncture Points as Shown on the Bronze Man" (AD 1026) says: "*LU-5 can treat Wind-Painful Obstruction Syndrome of the elbow and inability to raise the arm*".[11]

KONGZUI LU-6 *Biggest Hole*

Nature

Accumulation point.

Action

Regulates Lung-Qi and causes Lung-Qi to descend
Clears Heat
Stops bleeding.

Comments

This point is mostly used in acute Excess patterns of the Lungs, especially for an acute attack of asthma. It also stops bleeding, which is a property of all Accumulation points.

LIEQUE LU-7 *Broken Sequence*

Nature

Connecting point
Opening point of the Directing Vessel.

Action

Stimulates the descending and dispersing of Lung-Qi
Circulates the Defensive Qi and releases the Exterior
Expels exterior Wind
Opens the Directing Vessel
Benefits the Bladder and opens Water passages
Opens the nose
Communicates with the Large Intestine.

Comments

This is an extremely important point. It is a major point to release the Exterior in invasions of exterior Wind-Cold or Wind-Heat. This point contributes to the elimination of the pathogenic factor by stimulating the descending and dispersing of Lung-Qi, thus releasing the Lung-Defensive Qi portion and stimulating sweating. The Lungs control the skin where Defensive Qi circulates, and spread fluids all over the skin. The use of this point (with reducing method) will stimulate the circulation of the Defensive Qi and open the pores to cause sweating. It is better for Wind-Cold than Wind-Heat.

It is therefore used in the beginning stages of common cold or influenza, with sneezing, stiff neck, headache, aversion to cold and a Floating pulse. In treating exterior invasions of Wind-Cold or Wind-Heat it is often combined with Hegu L.I.-4, as they both release the Exterior. This combination is called "Guest-Host" as the Connecting channel of the Lungs (the "Guest") joins with the Large Intestine channel (the "Host").

Because of the Lung connection with the nose, LU-7 is used to treat sneezing, nasal obstruction, runny nose and loss of the sense of smell. In all these cases, it would be combined with Yingxiang L.I.-20.

Far from being used only in exterior patterns, Lieque LU-7 has a very wide-ranging energetic action in interior patterns too. It is the best point on the Lung channel to stimulate the Lung descending function and it is therefore a very important point to use in all types of cough or asthma, whether acute or chronic.

LU-7 is also one of the best points to affect the face and head and can be used in combination with other points to direct the effect of the treatment to face and head. Because of this, it is very frequently used in headaches.

In my experience, LU-7 is a very important point from the psychological and emotional point of view, and can be used in emotional problems caused by worry, grief or sadness. LU-7 is particularly indicated in cases in which the person bears his or her problems in silence and keeps them inside. LU-7 tends to stimulate a beneficial outpouring of repressed emotions. Weeping is the sound associated with the Lungs according to the 5 Elements, and those who have been suppressing their emotions may burst out crying when this point is used or shortly after.

The Lungs are the residence of the Corporeal Soul and this point will release the emotional tensions of the Corporeal Soul manifesting at the physical level with tense shoulders, shallow breathing and a feeling of oppression in the chest. These symptoms are often due to excessive worrying over a long period of time preventing the free breathing of the Corporeal Soul and constraining the Lung energy. LU-7 will calm the Mind, settle the Corporeal Soul, open the chest and release tension.

Being the Connecting point, it is very useful and effective in channel problems of the Large Intestine and Lung channels. It is often used as a distal point for Painful Obstruction Syndrome of the shoulder, if the problem is along the Large Intestine channel. In these cases, LU-7 is often used on the opposite side to where the problem is.

In conjunction with Zhaohai KI-6, it opens the Directing Vessel, stimulates the descending of Lung-Qi and the Kidney function of grasping Qi. Because of this, it is beneficial in chronic asthma from Lung and Kidney deficiency and oedema of the face. The combination of LU-7 and KI-6 tonifies Yin, regulates the uterus and the menstrual function, benefits the throat and moistens the eyes. It is excellent for a dry and sore throat deriving from Yin deficiency.

The Lungs are indirectly related to the Bladder and control the Water passages. LU-7 is the main point on the Lung channel to affect the Lung function of opening the Water passages. It is therefore used in oedema and urinary retention in Excess patterns, when an exterior pathogenic factor obstructs the descending of Lung-Qi: this results in Lung-Qi being unable to open the Water passages and connect with the Bladder. In this case, it is needled with reducing method. It is also effective in urinary retention of the Empty type, when deficient Lung-Qi fails to descend and communicate with the Bladder. This gives rise to urinary retention of the Deficient type and is particularly common in the elderly. In this case it is needled with reinforcing method.

Lung-Qi also communicates with the Large Intestine and it provides the Qi necessary for the act of defecation. When Lung-Qi is weak, it may fail to communicate with the Large Intestine and constipation ensues. This constipation is of the Deficient type and is common in old people. It is characterized by difficulty in passing stools, or passing them with great strain and feeling exhausted afterwards. In these cases, LU-7 will tonify Lung-Qi and help it to reach the Large Intestine to give it strength for the act of defecation.

To summarize, the areas controlled by LU-7 are: lungs, throat, nose and head. Because of its connection with the Large Intestine, it also influences the shoulders.

JINGQU LU-8 *Channel canal*

Nature

River point
Metal point.

Comment

This point is effective in treating problems of the throat and lungs, and such symptoms as cough and asthma, fitting into the category of River point indications. It is often added to other points to treat chronic throat problems.

TAIYUAN LU-9 *Greater Abyss*

Nature

Source and Stream point
Earth point
Gathering point for arteries and veins
Tonification point.

Action

Resolves Phlegm
Regulates Lung-Qi, stops cough
Tonifies Lung-Qi and Lung-Yin
Tonifies Gathering Qi
Promotes the circulation of blood and influences the pulse
Clears Lungs and Liver Heat.

Comments

This is another major point of the Lung channel. It is the main point to tonify Lung-Qi and Lung-Yin, especially in chronic conditions.

It is more frequently used in Deficiency rather than Excess patterns, and it treats interior more than exterior conditions.

It is also used to resolve Phlegm obstructing the Lungs with such symptoms as chronic cough with yellow-sticky sputum.

The chest is the seat of Gathering Qi which is closely related to Lungs and Heart. LU-9 tonifies Gathering Qi of the chest and can be used in patients who are particularly Qi-deficient, suffer from cold hands and have a weak voice. These last two are signs of deficiency of Gathering Qi. When tonifying Gathering Qi, LU-9 is often combined with Ren-17.

LU-9 is also indicated when all the pulses are extremely Weak and Deep and nearly impossible to feel.

LU-9 is the Gathering point of all the blood vessels. The "Classic of Difficulties" in chapter 1 says: *"The Inch Mouth [the Front position of the pulse corresponding to LU-9] is the great meeting place of all the blood vessels, and the Lungs give impetus to the pulse"*.[12] The Front position of the pulse is considered the convergence point of all the blood vessels of the body and for this reason the acupuncture point on its site, LU-9, is said to influence all the blood vessels and the pulse.

It is not by chance that this position was chosen as the best place to feel the pulse. It is because the Lungs govern Qi and one can therefore feel the movement of Qi within the Blood at this position. LU-9 can therefore influence all blood vessels and can be used for poor circulation, cold hands and feet, chilblains and varicose veins. The Lungs' influence on the blood vessels is a further expression of the close relationship existing between the Lungs and Heart. The Lungs govern Qi, the Heart controls Blood and they mutually affect each other. LU-9 tonifies Lung-Qi and stimulates the circulation of Heart Qi and Blood in the chest: it is therefore also used to tonify Heart Qi and Blood indirectly, in such symptoms as breathlessness on exertion, listlessness and palpitations.

Finally, LU-9 can be used to clear Lung and Liver Heat in cases when Liver-Fire overflows towards the chest obstructing the descending of Lung-Qi.

It is useful to compare the actions of LU-9 with those of LU-7:

LU-7	*LU-9*
For Exterior problems	For Interior problems
For Excess patterns	For Deficiency patterns
Has an outward movement	Has an inward movement
Affects Qi	Affects Qi and Blood
For channel problems	Not for channel problems
Better for emotional problems	Not so much for emotional problems
Does not resolve Phlegm	Resolves Phlegm
Opens Water passages	Does not open Water passages

YUJI LU-10 *Fish Border*

Nature

Spring point
Fire point.

Action

Clears Lung-Heat
Benefits the throat.

Comments

This is the main point to clear Lung Full-Heat. Chize LU-5 also clears Lung-Heat, but more when Heat is combined with Phlegm obstructing the chest. LU-10, on the contrary, clears Lung-Heat especially in acute situations, e.g. at the Qi level of the 4-Level Pattern Identification.

It also clears Heat from the throat, and is therefore used in sore throat from Heat or from Wind-Heat. It is not used for sore throat from Yin deficiency, except when combined with other points such as Zhaohai KI-6.

SHAOSHANG LU-11 *Lesser Metal*

Nature

Well point
Wood point.

Action

Expels Wind (both exterior and interior).
Stimulates the dispersing and descending of Lung-Qi
Benefits the throat
Opens the orifices and promotes resuscitation.

Comments

This point expels Exterior Wind-Heat and is often used for sore-throat from attack of Wind-Heat: in this case it is bled. It is usually used only for acute sore throat from exterior Wind-Heat.

It is also effective for interior Wind, and is used in conjunction with the other Well points of the hand in apoplexy and loss of consciousness from Wind-stroke to open the orifices and promote resuscitation.

I have translated the name of this point as "Lesser Metal" instead of the usual "Lesser Merchant", as the word *"Shang"*, in this context indicates "Gold" or "Metal", as one of the traditional 5 sounds. This particular sound is the sound of metal when struck.[13] The Lungs pertain to Metal and the Well point is where the channel is at its smallest and most superficial, hence "Lesser Metal".

It is useful to compare the functions of five major points of the Lung channel:

— LU-5 clears Lung-Heat, resolves Phlegm.
— LU-7 releases the Exterior, circulates Defensive Qi, stimulates the dispersing and descending of Lung-Qi.
— LU-9 tonifies the Lungs.
— LU-10 clears Lung-Heat, benefits the throat.
— LU-11 expels Wind-Heat, stimulates the dispersing and descending of Lung-Qi, benefits the throat.

LARGE INTESTINE CHANNEL
大腸经

MAIN CHANNEL PATHWAY

The Large Intestine channel starts from the tip of the index finger. It then runs along the radial side of the index finger and up the lateral-anterior aspect of the arm. It then reaches the shoulder at the point Jianyu L.I.-15. From here, it connects with Dazhui Du-14 and descends to the supraclavicular fossa to enter the lung. From the supraclavicular fossa it ascends along the sternocleidomastoid muscle to the cheek and enters the gums of the lower teeth. It then curves around the philtrum and crosses over to end at the side of the nose where it links with the Stomach channel (Fig. 80).

CONNECTING CHANNEL PATHWAY

The Connecting Channel starts at Pianli L.I.-6 from where a branch connects with the Lung channel. From L.I.-6 a branch runs along the main channel on the arm to the shoulder, jaw and teeth. From the jaw, another branch enters the ear (Fig. 80A).

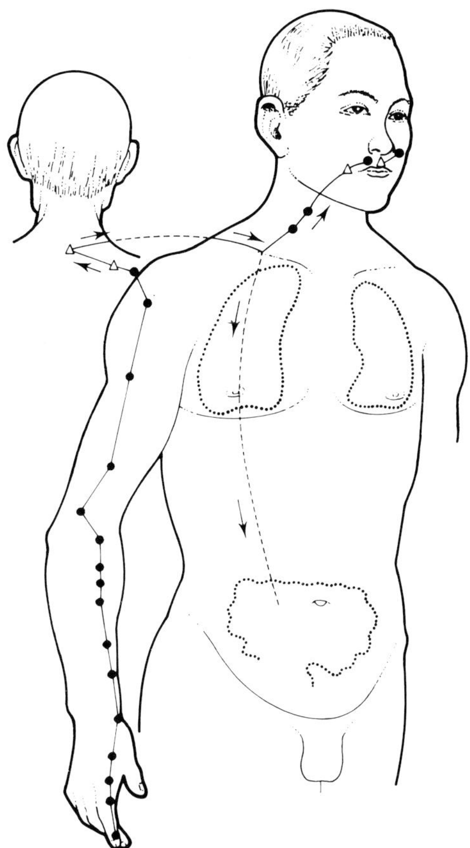

Fig. 80 Large Intestine channel

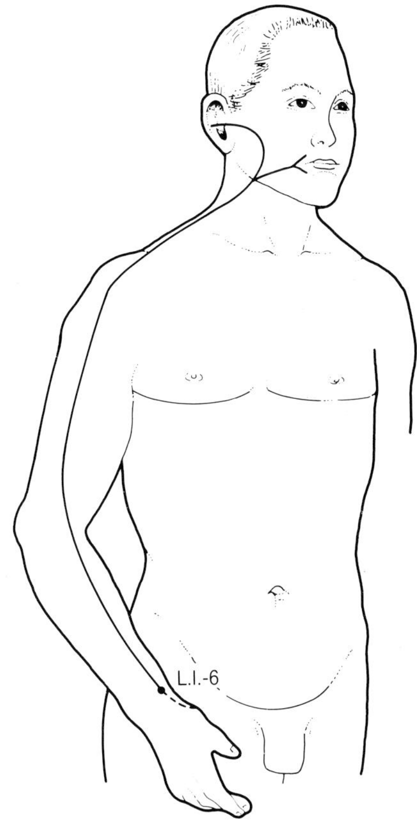

Fig. 80A Large Intestine connecting channel

SHANGYANG L.I.-1 *Metal Yang*

Nature

Well point
Metal point.

Action

Clears Heat
Brightens the eyes
Benefits the throat
Calms the Mind.
Expels Wind and scatters Cold.

Comments

As a Well point this point is effective in Excess patterns to remove obstructions quickly. Hence its use in the acute stage of Wind-stroke, combined with all the other Well points of the hands, to subdue interior Wind.

This point clears both interior and exterior Heat, so that it can be used in exterior attacks of Wind-Heat invading the Lung-Defensive Qi portion especially with sore throat, as well as in case of interior Heat in the Large Intestine.

Its action on the eyes is limited to cases of exterior Wind-Heat invading the eyes, such as in acute conjunctivitis.

Besides clearing Heat, this point can also expel Wind and Cold from the channel for the treatment of Painful Obstruction Syndrome of the shoulder. It can be used in this way as a distal point to clear the channel. If the problem is caused by Wind and Cold, moxa cones can be used instead of needling.

As for LU-11, and for the same reasons, I have translated the word *"Shang"* as "Metal". The

Large Intestine also pertains to Metal, L.I.-1 is the first point of the Metal Yang channel, hence the name "Metal Yang".[14]

ERJIAN L.I.-2 *Second Interval*

Nature

Spring point
Water point
Sedation point.

Action

Clears Heat

Comments

As a Spring point this point clears Heat in the Large Intestine and is used in cases of interior Heat, with symptoms of constipation, dry stools, fever and abdominal pain.

SANJIAN L.I.-3 *Third Interval*

Nature

Stream point
Wood point.

Action

Dispels exterior Wind
Clears Heat
Brightens the eyes
Benefits the throat.

Comments

This point dispels exterior Wind, particularly in Painful Obstruction Syndrome of the hand, for which it is a widely used point. This action is partly due to its being the Stream point as these points are indicated in aches of the joints.

L.I.-3 can also be used to expel Wind-Heat in exterior invasions and it is in this context that it brightens the eyes and benefits the throat.

This point also clears interior Heat of the Large Intestine, but in such a case, Erjian L.I.-2 would be preferred as it has a stronger cooling effect.

HEGU L.I.-4 *Joining Valley*

Nature

Source point.

Action

Dispels exterior Wind
Releases the Exterior
Stimulates the dispersing function of the Lungs
Stops pain
Removes obstructions from the channel
Tonifies Qi and consolidates the Exterior
Harmonizes ascending and descending.

Comments

Hegu L.I.-4 is the main point to expel Wind-Heat and to release the Exterior. L.I.-4 also has a strong direct sphere of influence on the face, so that, in exterior invasions, it is used to relieve nasal congestion, sneezing, burning eyes, etc. It is used in a similar way to relieve the symptoms of allergic rhinitis ("hay fever").

It also stimulates the Lung dispersing function, which explains its strong action in releasing the Exterior and expelling exterior Wind, so that it would be used for such symptoms and signs as nasal congestion, sneezing, cough, stiff neck, aversion to cold and a Floating pulse, i.e. the beginning stages of a common cold, influenza or many other infectious diseases.

L.I.-4 has a powerful calming and anti-spasmodic action, so that it can be used in many painful conditions, with pain originating from the intestines or uterus.

It is also widely used as a distal point in Painful Obstruction Syndrome of the arm or shoulder, since it removes obstructions from the channel.

Since it has a strong direct influence on face and eyes, it is often used as a distal point when treating problems of the face, including mouth, nose and eyes (not so much ears), e.g. allergic rhinitis, conjunctivitis, mouth ulcers, styes, sinusitis, epistaxis, toothache, trigeminal neuralgia, facial paralysis and frontal headaches. There is a saying in Chinese Medicine: *"The face and mouth are reached by L.I.-4"* (this rhymes in Chinese *"Mian kou Hegu shou"*).

It is sometimes combined with Taichong LIV-3 (this combination is called the "Four Gates"), to expel interior or exterior Wind from the head, stop pain and calm the Mind.

In my experience, L.I.-4 has a strong influence on the mind and can be used to soothe the mind and allay anxiety, particularly if combined with Taichong LIV-3 or with Shenting Du-24 and Benshen G.B.-13.

It can also combine with Fuliu KI-7 to regulate sweating, i.e. it can both reduce sweating in case of excessive sweating, or promote sweating to expel Wind-Cold.

L.I.-4 can also be used as a tonifying point rather than in its more common use as a reducing one. Combined with other points, it can tonify Qi and consolidate the Exterior, i.e. strengthen the Defensive Qi. In order to do this, it would be combined with Zusanli ST-36 and Qihai Ren-6. This treatment could be used for chronic allergic rhinitis owing to deficiency of Lung-Qi and weakness of the Exterior energetic layers (i.e. Defensive Qi), which make the person prone to chronic attacks of Wind. This treatment would only be suitable in between the attacks to strengthen Qi and the Exterior in order to reinforce the Defensive Qi to repel Wind. The use of L.I.-4 to tonify Qi is less common than its use to release the Exterior and expel Wind.

L.I.-4 can harmonize the ascending of Yang and descending of Yin. This means that it can be used to subdue ascending rebellious Qi (such as ascending Stomach-Qi, Lung-Qi or Liver-Qi) or to raise Qi when it is sinking (such as sinking Spleen-Qi). Thus, in the former case, it can be used to subdue Stomach-Qi in epigastric pain, Liver-Yang rising in migraine (especially combined with Taichong LIV-3) or Lung-Qi in asthma. In the latter case, it could be used to raise Spleen-Qi, especially in combination with Qihai Ren-6. However, this last use is not common.

Finally, L.I.-4 is an empirical point to promote delivery during labour, hence its contra-indication in pregnancy.

YANGXI L.I.-5 *Yang Stream*

Nature

River point
Fire point.

Action

Expels Wind
Releases the Exterior
Benefits the throat
Stops pain.

Comments

This point has similar functions to Hegu L.I.-4 in releasing the Exterior and expelling Wind-Heat in the beginning stages of exterior invasions. However, in these situations, L.I.-4 would be preferred as it is stronger in its action of releasing the Exterior.

L.I.-5 is frequently used for Painful Obstruction Syndrome of hand and wrist.

PIANLI L.I.-6 *Slanting Passage*

Nature

Connecting point.

Action

Opens the Lung Water passages.

Comments

This point is mostly used to open the Lung Water passages, i.e. whenever the Lung function of controlling Water passages is impaired. This can happen when an exterior pathogenic factor obstructs the circulation of Defensive Qi in the skin, giving rise to oedema of the face and hands. This can also happen in chronic conditions of Lung-Qi deficiency.

L.I.6 also has a marked mental effect, especially in manic depression.

WENLIU L.I.-7 *Warm Flow*

Nature

Accumulation point.

Action

Clears Heat
Stops pain
Expels Wind
Benefits the throat.

Comments

Wenliu L.I.-7, like most Accumulation points, stops pain and removes obstruction from the channel and is mostly used in acute situations. It is widely used in Painful Obstruction Syndrome of the channel and also in invasions of exterior Wind-Heat causing a painful and sore throat or swollen tonsils.

SHOUSANLI L.I.-10 *Arm Three Miles*

Action

Removes obstructions from the channel
Tonifies Qi.

Comments

This is a very important and widely used point for all channel problems of the Large Intestine channel. It also has some tonifying property and is considered by some as a "Zusanli ST-36" of the arm, i.e. a powerful Qi and Blood tonic.

It is a very important point in the treatment of Painful Obstruction Syndrome, Atrophy Syndrome[13] and sequelae of Wind-stroke affecting the arm. It is also a major point for the treatment of any muscular problem affecting the forearm and hands.

QUCHI L.I.-11 *Crooked Pond*

Nature

Sea point
Earth point
Tonification point.

Action

Expels exterior Wind
Clears Heat
Cools Blood
Resolves Dampness
Regulates Nutritive Qi and Blood
Benefits the sinews and joints.

Comments

This point has an extremely wide-ranging action, influencing the Exterior as well as the Interior, in many different types of conditions.

Firstly, it expels exterior Wind-Heat and can therefore be used in the same way as Hegu L.I.-4 in invasions of exterior Wind-Heat with fever, chills, stiff neck, sweating, runny nose and aches in the body. The main difference between these two points is that L.I.-4 has a specific action on the face, which L.I.-11 does not have.

L.I.-11 also clears Heat in general and can be used in interior Heat patterns of virtually any organ and with any fever of internal origin. It is very frequently used in Liver-Fire patterns with hypertension.

It also cools the Blood and is therefore widely used in skin diseases due to Heat in the Blood, such as urticaria, psoriasis and eczema.

L.I.-11 resolves Dampness, particularly Damp-Heat and can therefore be used in such patterns occurring in any part of the body. For example, Damp-Heat causing skin eruptions or acne, Damp-Heat in the Spleen with digestive symptoms, or Damp-Heat in the urinary system causing cystitis or urethritis. It can also be used in invasions of exterior Damp-Heat causing fever, feeling of heaviness, loose stools, abdominal distention, and so on.

L.I.-11 is also used for goitre as a swelling of the thyroid is considered a form of Phlegm.

Finally, L.I.-11 benefits the sinews and joints, which means that it can be used in Painful Obstruction Syndrome, Atrophy syndrome and sequelae of Wind-stroke paralysis, particularly of the arms and shoulders.

ZHOULIAO L.I.-12 *Elbow Seam*

Comments

This is a secondary point, but it is worth mentioning here because it is very useful to treat "tennis elbow" (provided the main problem is along the Large Intestine channel).

BINAO L.I.-14 *Arm and Scapula*

Action

Removes obstructions from the channel
Brightens the eyes
Resolves Phlegm and disperses masses.

Comments

This is not a major point, but still rather important and frequently used.

Firstly, it is very much used in Painful Obstruction Syndrome of the arm and shoulder to remove obstructions from the channel, i.e. obstructions caused by Wind, Cold and Dampness.

It also has an action on the eyes in so far as it clears and enhances vision. In this case the needle should be slanted upwards.

L.I.-14 also resolves Phlegm and disperses Phlegm masses, and is therefore used for goitre.

JIANYU L.I.-15 *Shoulder Transporting Point*

Nature

Point of the Yang Heel Vessel.

Action

Benefits sinews
Promotes circulation of Qi in the channels
Stops pain
Expels Wind.

Comments

This is a major point for the treatment of Painful Obstruction Syndrome of the shoulder as it benefits sinews and stimulates the circulation of Qi in the channel. It is also a major and frequently used point for Atrophy Syndrome and paralysis of the arm.

JUGU L.I.-16 *Great Bone*

Nature

Point of the Yang Heel Vessel.

Action

Moves Blood locally
Removes obstructions from the channel
Opens the chest
Subdues ascending rebellious Qi
Stimulates the descending of Lung-Qi
Benefits the joints.

Comments

This point is frequently used in conjunction with L.I.-15 for channel problems of the shoulder.

Besides this, it has an effect on the Lungs as it stimulates the descending of Lung-Qi and opens the chest: this means that it can be used for breathlessness, cough or asthma caused by impairment of the Lung descending function.

FUTU L.I.-18 *Support the Prominence*

Action

Benefits the throat
Relieves cough
Resolves Phlegm and disperses masses.

Comments

This point is widely used as a local point for throat problems, such as tonsillitis, mumps, laryngitis, nodules on the vocal cords, aphasia, hoarse voice and goitre.

YINGXIANG L.I.-20 *Welcome Fragrance*

Nature

Meeting point of Stomach and Large Intestine.

Action

Dispels exterior Wind

Comments

This is the local point for nose problems of any kind such as sneezing, loss of the sense of smell, epistaxis, sinusitis, runny nose, stuffed nose, allergic rhinitis and nasal polyps.

It also expels exterior Wind and is used as a local point in invasions of Wind-Cold or Wind-Heat when there is sneezing, stuffed nose and runny nose. As it expels exterior Wind, it is also widely used as a local point in facial paralysis, trigeminal neuralgia and tic.

NOTES

1 1981 Spiritual Axis. People's Health Publishing House, Beijing.
2 1979 Simple Questions. People's Health Publishing House, Beijing.
3 1979 Classic of Difficulties. People's Health Publishing House, Beijing.
4 1980 Compendium of Acupuncture. People's Health Publishing House, Beijing.
5 Li Shi Zhen, 1985 Clinical Application of Frequently Used Acupuncture Points (*Chang Yong Shu Xue Lin Chuang Fa Hui* 常用腧穴临床发挥), Beijing.
6 Shan Yu Dang. 1984 Selection of Acupuncture Point Combinations from the Discussion of Cold-induced Diseases (*Shang Han Lun Zhen Jiu Pei Xue Xuan Zhu* 伤寒论针灸配穴选注), Beijing.
7 Ji Jie Yin. 1984 Clinical Records of *Tai Yi Shen* Acupuncture (*Tai Yin Shen Zhen Jiu Lin Zheng Lu* 太乙神针灸临证录). Shanxi Province Scientific Publishing House.
8 There are many different reducing needling techniques. The two main ones are according to rotation or lift and thrust. According to rotation, the needle is rotated back and forth rapidly and with large amplitude; according to lift and thrust, the needle is lifted rapidly and vigorously and thrust slowly and gently. In both cases the manipulation may be repeated a few times during the time of retention of the needle. The even needling method consists in rotating the needle back and forth fairly vigorously for a few rotations and then leaving it in without further manipulation.
9 Simple Questions, p 145.
10 Huang Fu Mi, AD 259. The ABC of Acupuncture In: Clinical Application of Frequently Used Acupuncture Points, p 41.
11 Wang Wei Yi, 1026 Illustrated Manual of Acupuncture Points as Shown on the Bronze Man (*Tong Ren Shu Xue Zhen Jiu Tu Jing* 铜人腧穴针灸图经) In: Clinical Application of Frequently Used Acupuncture Points, p 41.
12 Classic of Difficulties, p 2.
13 Zhang Cheng Xing-Qi Jin 1984 An Explanation of the Meaning of Acupuncture Point Names (*Jing Xue Shi Yi Hui Jie* 经穴释义汇解) Shanghai Translations Publishing Company, Shanghai, p 24.
14 An Explanation of the Meaning of Acupuncture Point Names, p 27.

Stomach and Spleen Channels

41

胃经脾经

STOMACH CHANNEL

胃经

MAIN CHANNEL PATHWAY

The Stomach channel starts from the lateral side of ala nasi (at Yingxiang L.I.-20). It ascends along the nose and meets the Bladder channel at Jingming BL-1. It then enters the upper gums. It curves around the lips and links with the Directing Vessel at Chengjiang Ren-24. It then runs along the lower jaw and ascends in front of the ear to reach the forehead.

From Daying ST-5 a branch goes down to the throat and the supraclavicular fossa. It then passes through the diaphragm, enters the stomach and the spleen.

From the supraclavicular fossa, a branch follows the superficial channel down to the breast and abdomen to pass through Qichong ST-30. Another branch from the stomach connects with the point ST-30. From this point it follows the superficial channel to run along the anterior aspect of the upper leg and the anterior border of the tibia to end at the 2nd toe. A branch from Chongyang ST-42 links with the Spleen channel (Fig. 81).

CONNECTING CHANNEL PATHWAY

The Connecting channel starts at Fenglong ST-40 and connects with the Spleen channel. Another branch runs along the anterior border of the tibia up to the thigh and abdomen to the top of the head where it converges with the other Yang channels. A branch separates from the neck and goes forward to the throat (Fig. 81A).

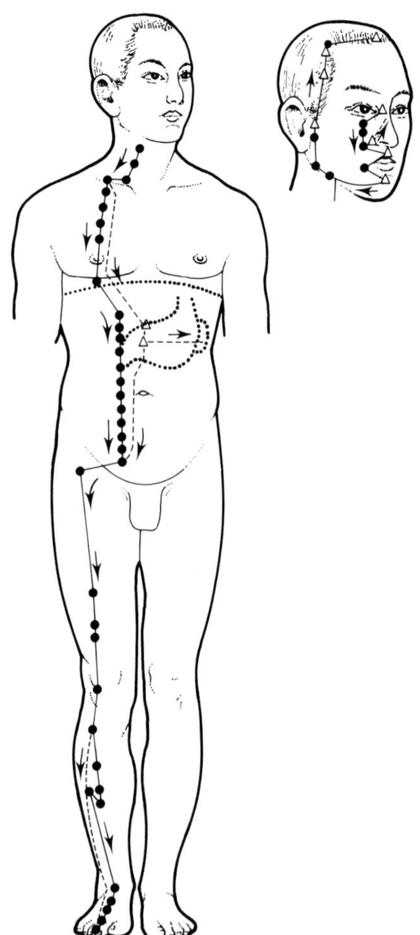

Fig. 81 Stomach channel

CHENGQI ST-1 *Containing Tears*

Nature

Point of the Yang Heel Vessel.

Action

Expels Wind
Brightens the eyes
Stops lacrymation.

Comments

This point is used mostly for eye problems and has a very wide range of indications such as acute and chronic conjunctivitis, myopia, astigmatism, squint, colour blindness, night blindness, glaucoma, atrophy of the optic nerve, cataract, keratitis and retinitis.

As it expels Wind (both interior and exterior) it is used for eye problems deriving from exterior Wind-Heat or Wind-Cold (such as swelling, pain and lacrymation and paralysis of the eyelid), as well as those deriving from interior Wind (such as tic of the eyelid).

SIBAI ST-2 *Four Whites*

Nature

Point of Yang Heel Vessel.

Action

Expels Wind
Brightens the eyes.

Comments

This point is also used mostly for eye problems with the same range of indications as Chengqi ST-1. It is similarly used to expel exterior Wind (swelling of eyes, allergic rhinitis or facial paralysis) and interior Wind (twitch of the eyelid). In particular, it is frequently used as a local point for the treatment of facial paralysis and trigeminal neuralgia.

A curious and seemingly inexplicable empirical use of this point is for biliary ascariasis.

JULIAO ST-3 *Big Bone*

Nature

Point of Yang Heel Vessel.

Action

Expels Wind
Removes obstructions from the channel
Relieves swellings.

Comments

This point is used to expel exterior and interior

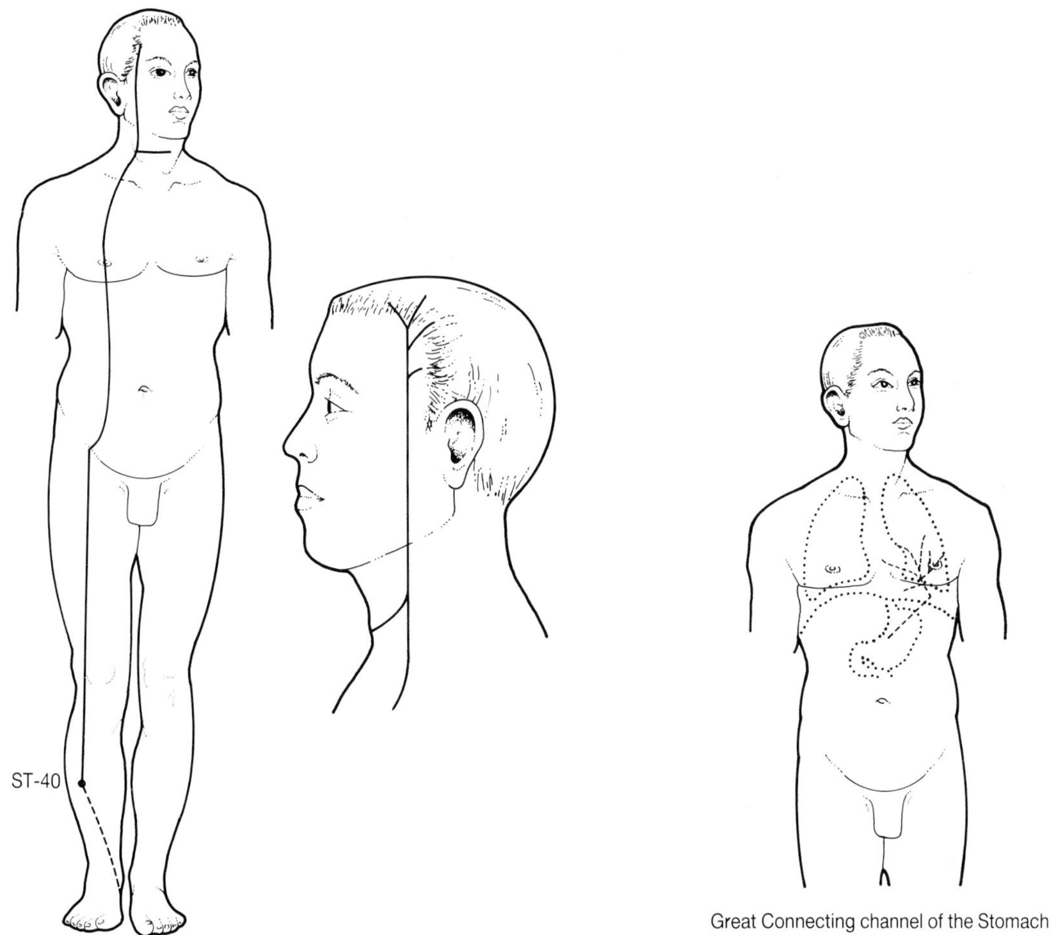

Fig. 81A Stomach Connecting channel and Great Connecting channel.

Wind in exactly the same as manner as Chengqi ST-1 and Sibai ST-2. In particular, it is frequently used for facial paralysis and trigeminal neuralgia.

This point differs from Chengqi ST-1 and Sibai ST-2 in so far as its range of action extends not only to the eye but also to the nose, hence its use in the treatment of epistaxis and nasal obstruction.

DICANG ST-4 *Earth Granary*

Nature

Meeting point of Stomach and Large Intestine
Point of Yang Heel Vessel.

Action

Expels Wind
Removes obstructions from the channel
Benefits tendons and muscles.

Comments

This point eliminates exterior Wind and is a major local point for the treatment of facial paralysis for which it is nearly always used if the mouth is deviated. It also has an effect on the muscles of the face and is therefore used in aphasia.

JIACHE ST-6 *Jaw Chariot*

Action

Expels Wind
Removes obstructions from the channel.

Comments

This is another major point to expel exterior Wind affecting the face and it is nearly always used as a local point in facial paralysis combined with Hegu L.I.-4. It is also used for mumps and spasm of the masseter muscle.

It is combined with Hegu L.I.-4 for problems of the lower jaw including toothache.

XIAGUAN ST-7 *Lower Gate*

Nature

Meeting point of Stomach and Gall Bladder.

Action

Removes obstruction from the channel
Benefits the ear.

Comments

This point is also frequently used in facial paralysis and trigeminal neuralgia but it extends its influence to the ear too, hence its use also for otitis, deafness and earache.

It is combined with Neiting ST-44 for problems of the upper jaw and toothache.

TOUWEI ST-8 *Head Support*

Nature

Point of Yang Linking Vessel
Meeting point of Stomach and Gall Bladder.

Action

Expels Wind
Relieves pain
Brightens the eyes
Clears Heat
Stops lacrymation
Relieves dizziness.

Comments

This is a major local point for dizziness deriving from Dampness and Phlegm retained in the head and preventing the clear Yang from rising upwards to brighten the orifices. It is therefore frequently used for dizziness (only if deriving from Phlegm), "muzziness" of the head and a feeling of cloudiness or heaviness of the head.

It is also an important local point for frontal headaches deriving from Dampness of Phlegm preventing the clear Yang from reaching the head.

It can also be used for eye problems and excessive lacrymation deriving from invasions of exterior Wind-Heat.

RENYING ST-9 *Person's Welcome*

Nature

Point of the Sea of Qi.

Action

Regulates Qi
Removes masses
Benefits the throat
Relieves swellings.

Comments

This is a point which is used to remove obstructions from the head and to send Qi downwards. It is therefore often used in Excess patterns characterized by excess energy on the top part of the body.

It regulates Stomach-Qi in the sense that it subdues Stomach-Qi rebelling upwards and causing hiccup, belching and nausea. Its action in subduing rebellious Stomach-Qi can also be used in certain cases of asthma due to the Stomach channel.

It also removes masses and resolves swellings and "Fire-Poison", i.e. Heat and swelling affecting the Stomach channel, with such symptoms as tonsillitis, swollen and sore throat, adenitis, pharyngitis and swelling of the thyroid.

According to the "Spiritual Axis" (ch. 33), this point is a point of the Sea of Qi (together with Shanzhong Ren-17, Yamen Du-15 and Dazhui Du-14).[1] It can therefore be used to tonify Qi, although it is more often used to regulate Qi and eliminate imbalances in the distribution of Qi resulting in excess above and deficiency below.

QUEPEN ST-12 *Empty Basin*

Action

Subdues rebellious Qi.

Comments

This point is useful in Excess patterns characterized by rebellious Stomach-Qi going upwards causing such symptoms as breathlessness and asthma.

It also has a calming effect on the Mind, by virtue of its sending Qi downwards. It is therefore used for anxiety, nervousness and insomnia due to a Stomach disharmony.

RUGEN ST-18 *Breast Root*

Action

Regulates Stomach-Qi
Regulates the breast and lactation
Dispels stagnation.

Comments

This point is mostly used as a local point for breast problems, especially in women. First of all, it regulates Stomach-Qi in relation to the breast and can be used in mastitis, pre-menstrual swelling of breast and lumps in the breast.

It regulates lactation in nursing mothers, i.e. it will either promote or reduce it as the situation demands.

LIANGMEN ST-21 *Beam Door*

Action

Regulates the Stomach
Subdues rebellious Qi
Stops vomiting
Relieves pain.

Comments

This is an important local point for Stomach problems, particularly of an Excess nature. As a rule of thumb, the epigastric points on the Directing Vessel (such as Ren-12) are used more in Deficiency patterns, whereas the points on the Stomach channel (such as ST-21) are used more in Excess patterns. ST-21, in particular is very frequently used for Excess patterns of the Stomach, with Stomach-Qi rebelling upwards and causing nausea or vomiting.

It also clears Stomach-Heat and is used for thirst and a burning sensation in the epigastrium, especially combined with Neiting ST-44.

It is also used in acute painful patterns with epigastric pain, especially in combination with Liangqiu ST-34.

TIANSHU ST-25 *Heavenly Pillar*

Nature

Front Collecting point of the Large Intestine channel.

Action

Promotes the function of the Intestines
Clears Heat
Regulates Qi
Relieves retention of food.

Comments

This is a very frequently used point. It can be used in all Excess patterns of the Stomach giving rise to abdominal (rather than epigastric) problems. It is particularly indicated to stop diarrhoea and pain.

It clears Heat in the Stomach and Intestines and is therefore used for such symptoms and signs as burning sensation of the epigastrium, thirst, constipation, or foul-smelling loose stools and yellow tongue coating.

As a Front Collecting point, it is especially indicated in acute patterns of the Stomach.

When used with direct moxibustion, it tonifies and warms the Spleen and the Intestines, and is a special point for chronic diarrhoea arising from Spleen-Yang Deficiency. In this case, it is combined with Qihai Ren-6 and Shangjuxu ST-37.

In the context of diseases from invasion of exterior Wind-Heat, it is an important point to use in the Bright Yang stage of the 6-Channel Pattern Identification, or the Qi level of the 4-Level Pattern Identification. In these cases, it is combined with Quchi L.I.-11 and Hegu L.I.-4.

From a psychological point of view, it is effective in mental irritation, anxiety, schizophrenia and mania, when these are due a Stomach disharmony, particularly Excess patterns of the Stomach such as Phlegm-Fire in the Stomach.

DAJU ST-27 *Big Great*

Action

Regulates Stomach-Qi.

Comments

This point is frequently used in Excess patterns of the Stomach giving rise to lateral abdominal pain. It moves Qi in cases of stagnant Qi in the lower abdomen.

It is also used in men's genital problems and hernia.

SHUIDAO ST-28 *Water Passage*

Action

Benefits urination
Opens the Water passages
Benefits Difficult Urination Syndrome[2]
Regulates menstruation
Stops pain.

Comments

This point has several different actions. Firstly, it opens the Water passages of the Lower Burner and stimulates its excretion of fluids. It is therefore used in oedema, difficult urination and retention of urine, if caused by an Excess pattern.

ST-28 also regulates Qi in the lower abdomen, and can be used to regulate the menses in any menstrual problem caused by stagnation of Qi and Blood.

GUILAI ST-29 *Returning*

Action

Relieves stagnation of Blood.

Comments

This is an important point to eliminate stagnation of Blood in the Uterus and regulate the menses. It is very much used in all menstrual problems related to stasis of Blood, particularly for dysmenorrhoea with dark-clotted blood. It can also be used to treat amenorrhorea, but only if caused by stasis of Blood. Some think that its name is due to its action in bringing on the "return" of the menses.

Although this point is used primarily in Excess patterns with stasis of Blood, it can also be used to tonify and raise Qi in case of prolapse of the uterus. In this case, ST-29 is tonified in combination with Hegu L.I.-4, Zusanli ST-36 and Baihui Du-20 (this last point with direct moxibustion).

QICHONG ST-30 *Penetrating Qi*

Nature

Point of the Penetrating Vessel
Point of the Sea of Food.

Action

Regulates Stomach-Qi
Regulates the Penetrating Vessel
Promotes Essence

Tonifies the Sea of Food
Regulates Blood.

Comments

This is a powerful point with many different actions. First of all, it regulates Qi and Blood in the lower abdomen and genitals and is therefore indicated in many abdominal and genital problems of an Excess nature, such as abdominal pain, abdominal masses, hernia, swelling of penis, retention of placenta and swelling of prostate.

Being a major point on the Penetrating Vessel, it can be combined with its opening and coupled points to enhance its action and direct the therapeutic effect to the lower abdomen and genitals.

It also promotes Kidney-Essence due to its connection with the Penetrating vessel. Thanks to its Essence-nourishing effect, it can be used to treat impotence.

Being the point of the Sea of Food means that it stimulates the Stomach function of rotting and ripening and the Spleen function of transformation, thus generally revitalizing the digestive system and tonifying Qi.

Finally, since it is simultaneously a major point of the Penetrating Vessel and the Sea of Food, it is like the link between the Root of the Pre-Heaven Qi (Kidneys) and the Root of the Post-Heaven Qi (Stomach). Because of this connection, it can be used to tonify strongly Pre- and Post-Heaven Qi.

BIGUAN ST-31 *Thigh Gate*

Action

Removes obstruction from the channel.

Comments

This point is frequently used as a local point in Atrophy Syndrome, Painful Obstruction Syndrome and sequelae of Wind-stroke. It strengthens the leg, facilitates its movement and in particular, it facilitates the raising of the leg, an important factor, especially in Atrophy Syndrome, when the leg is often dragged.

When needling this point to affect the whole leg, it is desirable to obtain the needling sensation to propagate all the way down the leg, or at least past the knee.

FUTU ST-32 *Hidden Rabbit*

Action

Removes obstructions from the channel
Expels Wind-Heat.

Comments

This is another local point for leg problems similar in effect to Biguan ST-31, but not with such a strong action in lifting the leg.

In addition, it also has a mild action in expelling Wind-Heat affecting the Blood and can be used to treat certain skin diseases characterized by Wind-Heat in the Blood such as acute urticaria.

LIANGQIU ST-34 *Beam Mound*

Nature

Accumulation point.

Action

Subdues rebellious Stomach-Qi
Removes obstructions from the channel
Expels Dampness and Wind.

Comments

As an Accumulation point, this point is used for acute, Excess and painful patterns of the Stomach. It subdues rising Stomach-Qi causing such symptoms as hiccup, nausea, vomiting and belching.

It is frequently used in the treatment of Painful Obstruction Syndrome of the knee to expel exterior Dampness, Wind and Cold from the knee joint.

DUBI ST-35 *Calf Nose*

Action

Invigorates the channel
Relieves swelling
Stops pain.

Comments

This is an important point for the treatment of Painful Obstruction Syndrome of the knee for which it is nearly always used to expel Dampness and Cold. It is particularly effective when moxa is burned on the needle. This method of treatment should obviously not be used for Hot-Painful Obstruction Syndrome.

This point, together with the corresponding point on the medial side of the knee, is also known as XIYAN *Knee Eye*, an extra point.

ZUSANLI ST-36 *Three Miles of the Foot*

Nature

Sea point
Earth point
Point of the Sea of Food.

Action

Benefits Stomach and Spleen
Tonifies Qi and Blood
Dispels Cold
Strengthens the body
Brightens the eyes
Regulates Nutritive and Defensive Qi
Regulates the Intestines
Raises Yang
Expels Wind and Damp
Resolves oedema.

Comments

This is of course a major point to tonify Qi and Blood in Deficiency patterns. It is the main point to tonify the Root of Post-Heaven Qi, i.e. Stomach and Spleen. Although it is on the Stomach channel, Zusanli ST-36 strongly tonifies Spleen-Qi as well as Stomach-Qi.

It is used in all cases of Deficiency of Stomach and Spleen, and to strengthen the body and mind in very debilitated persons, or after a chronic disease. Since it tonifies Upright Qi, it also strengthens the resistance to attack from exterior pathogenic factors. It can therefore be used for prevention of attacks from exterior climatic factors. When used for prevention, moxa only is applied to this point. Some doctors recommend the use of this point with direct moxibustion every 5 to 7 days for about 10 minutes each time, to strengthen the Upright Qi and the resistance to disease. However, this use of ST-36 is not considered suitable for those under 30 years of age.

Li Dong Yuan (1180-1251), author of the celebrated "Discussion on Stomach and Spleen", said: *"For old people with deficiency of Qi, use St-36 and Ren-6 frequently with 50-60 moxa cones each time"*.[3]

ST-36 is also indicated in all Deficiency patterns of the Stomach, with dull epigastric pain, no appetite, and so on.

It also brightens the eyes and can be used for blurred vision and declining eyesight in old age.

It is also used in attacks of exterior Wind-Cold, with prevalence of Wind (Greater-Yang Wind pattern of the 6-Stage Pattern Identification), to regulate Nutritive and Defensive Qi. In this case, the exterior Wind-Cold invades the skin and interferes with the circulation of Defensive Qi: the pores are open and the person sweats slightly. This situation is characterized by a weakness of Nutritive Qi which causes the person to sweat. Needling ST-36 regulates and harmonizes Nutritive and Defensive Qi so that tonifying the former stops sweating and moving the latter expels the pathogenic factors. When used in this way, ST-36 is needled not with reinforcing, but even method. The "Discussion on Cold-induced Diseases" in clause 8 says: *"At the Greater-Yang stage, if a headache persists for more than seven days, it is because the pathogenic factor has circulated through the Greater Yang channel. If the pathogenic factor tends to be transmitted to the next channel [Bright-Yang channel], needling points on the Stomach channel will stop this transmission"*.[4]

Since it regulates Nutritive and Defensive Qi,

it is also used in all cases of oedema, when the Defensive Qi is weak in the skin layers and fluids overflow from the channels to invade the space under the skin.[5]

Zusanli ST-36 can be used to regulate the Intestines and in particular for constipation of a Deficient nature.

Used with direct moxibustion, it raises Yang and is used for prolapses in combination with Qihai Ren-6 and Baihui Du-20.

ST-36 is not only used as a tonifying point, but it can also be used with even or reducing method to eliminate Dampness or Cold.

ST-36 can also expel Wind and Damp from the channels in Painful Obstruction Syndrome. In my experience, besides its obvious action on Painful Obstruction Syndrome of the knee for which it acts also as a local point, it also has an influence as a distal point for Painful Obstruction Syndrome of the wrist.

SHANGJUXU ST-37 *Upper Great Emptiness*

Nature

Lower Sea point of the Large Intestine channel
Point of the Sea of Blood.

Action

Regulates the function of Stomach and Intestines
Eliminates Damp-Heat
Dispels retention of food.
Calms asthma.

Comments

The most important aspect of this point is related to its character as Lower Sea point for the Large Intestine channel. As such, it serves the same function to the Large Intestine channel as Zusanli ST-36 does to the Stomach channel. It can therefore be used to affect the Large Intestine directly. It is especially indicated for chronic diarrhoea, and for Damp-Heat patterns of the Large Intestine with loose, offensive stools with mucus and blood.

ST-37 opens the chest and can be used to calm asthma and breathlessness.

According to the "Spiritual Axis" (ch. 33), this point, together with Xiajuxu ST-39 and Dashu BL-11 is a point of the Sea of Blood and it can therefore be used to tonify Blood.[5]

TIAOKOU ST-38 *Narrow Opening*

Action

Removes obstruction from the channel.

Comments

This point is mostly used as an empirical distal point for pain and stiffness of the shoulder joint. It is usually needled first with reducing method while the patient gently rotates the shoulder, and then local points are used.

XIAJUXU ST-39 *Lower Great Emptiness*

Nature

Lower-Sea point of the Small Intestine channel.
Point of the Sea of Blood.

Action

Regulates the function of Stomach and Intestines
Eliminates Damp-Heat
Eliminates Wind-Damp
Stops pain.

Comments

Being the Lower-Sea point for the Small Intestine, this point is used for all patterns of this Yang organ. In particular, it is used for lower abdominal pain with borborygmi and flatulence.

It is also used to resolve Damp-Heat in the Small Intestine with such symptoms as cloudy-dark urine.

In combination with Shangjuxu ST-37, it is used for pain in the legs caused by Wind and Dampness.

As a point for the Sea of Blood, it can be used to tonify Blood together with Shangjuxu ST-37 and Dashu BL-11.

FENGLONG ST-40 *Abundant Bulge*

Nature

Connecting point.

Action

Resolves Phlegm and Damp
Calms asthma
Clears Heat
Calms and clears the mind.
Opens the chest.

Comments

This is a very important point since it is the point to resolve Phlegm in all its manifestations and in all parts of the body. It eliminates the Phlegm "that can be seen", such as profuse expectoration from the chest, Phlegm in the form of lumps, such as lumps under the skin, thyroid lumps and uterus lumps, and Phlegm "that cannot be seen" such as when it "mists the mind" causing mental disturbances or simply dizziness and muzziness of the head. In all these cases this point should be needled with reducing method to eliminate Phlegm.

Owing to its Phlegm-eliminating action, it is very much used in the treatment of asthma as it also has the effect of opening the chest and soothing breathing.

Another action of this point is to calm the mind, on which it has a profound effect. It can be used in all cases of anxiety, fears and phobias, if they are caused by misting of the Mind by Phlegm.

Apart from its use to resolve Phlegm, Fenglong ST-40 can also be used to clear Stomach-Heat or simply to calm the Stomach when the person is very anxious, and the anxiety reflects on the Stomach function, with such symptoms as tightness of the epigastrium, a feeling of knot in the Stomach or, as some people say, a feeling of "butterflies in the stomach".

Finally, this point also has an action on the chest and it is used to open and relax the chest when it is painful, or after bruising of the chest and rib-cage. In these cases, it is used in combination with Neiguan P-6, and normally one point can be used on one side, and the other point on the opposite side.

JIEXI ST-41 *Dispersing Stream*

Nature

River point
Fire point
Tonification point.

Action

Removes obstructions from the channel
Eliminates Wind
Clears Heat
Clears the mind
Brightens the eyes.

Comments

This point is frequently used in Painful Obstruction Syndrome of the foot to remove Cold and Damp. As a River point it particularly affects joints and is frequently used for problems of the ankle.

It clears Stomach-Heat and is used for burning epigastric pain and thirst. It is also effective for headache or sore throat due to Stomach-Heat.

It also clears the mind and conducts Heat downwards away from the head.

CHONGYANG ST-42 *Rushing Yang*

Nature

Source point.

Action

Tonifies Stomach and Spleen
Calms the Mind
Removes obstructions from the channel.

Comments

This point can tonify the Stomach and the Spleen as it is the Source point. Combined with Yangchi T.B.-4, it powerfully tonifies the Middle

Burner and dispels Cold from the joints and is used for Painful Obstruction Syndrome from Cold.

This point also calms the Mind and is used for mental illness.

XIANGU ST-43 *Sinking Valley*

Nature

Stream point
Wood point.

Action

Eliminates Wind and Heat
Removes obstruction from the channel.

Comments

This point is mostly used as a general point to expel Wind and Heat from the joints in Painful Obstruction Syndrome.

NEITING ST-44 *Inner courtyard*

Nature

Spring point
Water point.

Action

Clears Heat
Eliminates fullness
Regulates Qi
Stops pain
Promotes digestion
Eliminates Wind from the face.

Comments

This is a very important point of the Stomach channel. First of all, it clears Heat from the Stomach channel, and can be used for bleeding gums and any Stomach complaint with Heat. It is mostly used for Excess patterns.

In the context of diseases from exterior pathogenic factors, it is used at the Bright Yang stage of the 6 Channels, or the Qi level of the 4 Levels.

It is very effective to stop pain along the Stomach channel, particularly the lower jaw.

Combined with Hegu L.I.-4, it eliminates Wind from the face, and is therefore used in facial paralysis and trigeminal neuralgia.

LIDUI ST-45 *Sick mouth*

Nature

Well point
Metal point
Sedation point.

Action

Calms the Mind
Brightens the eyes
Clears the Heart
Relieves retention of food.

Comments

This point is mostly used to calm the Mind, when this is disturbed in the context of a Stomach pattern, usually from an Excess pattern, such as Stomach-Fire being transmitted to the Heart and giving rise to Heart-Fire. The use of this point can, at the same time, sedate the Stomach and calm the Mind. It is often used for insomnia in this context.

It also brightens the eyes particularly when Stomach-Heat is affecting the eyesight.

One particular use of this point is to clear Heart-Fire, in which case it is used with direct moxa cones.

SPLEEN CHANNEL

脾经

MAIN CHANNEL PATHWAY

The Spleen channel starts from the tip of the big toe and runs along the medial aspect of the foot to ascend the medial malleolus. It then follows

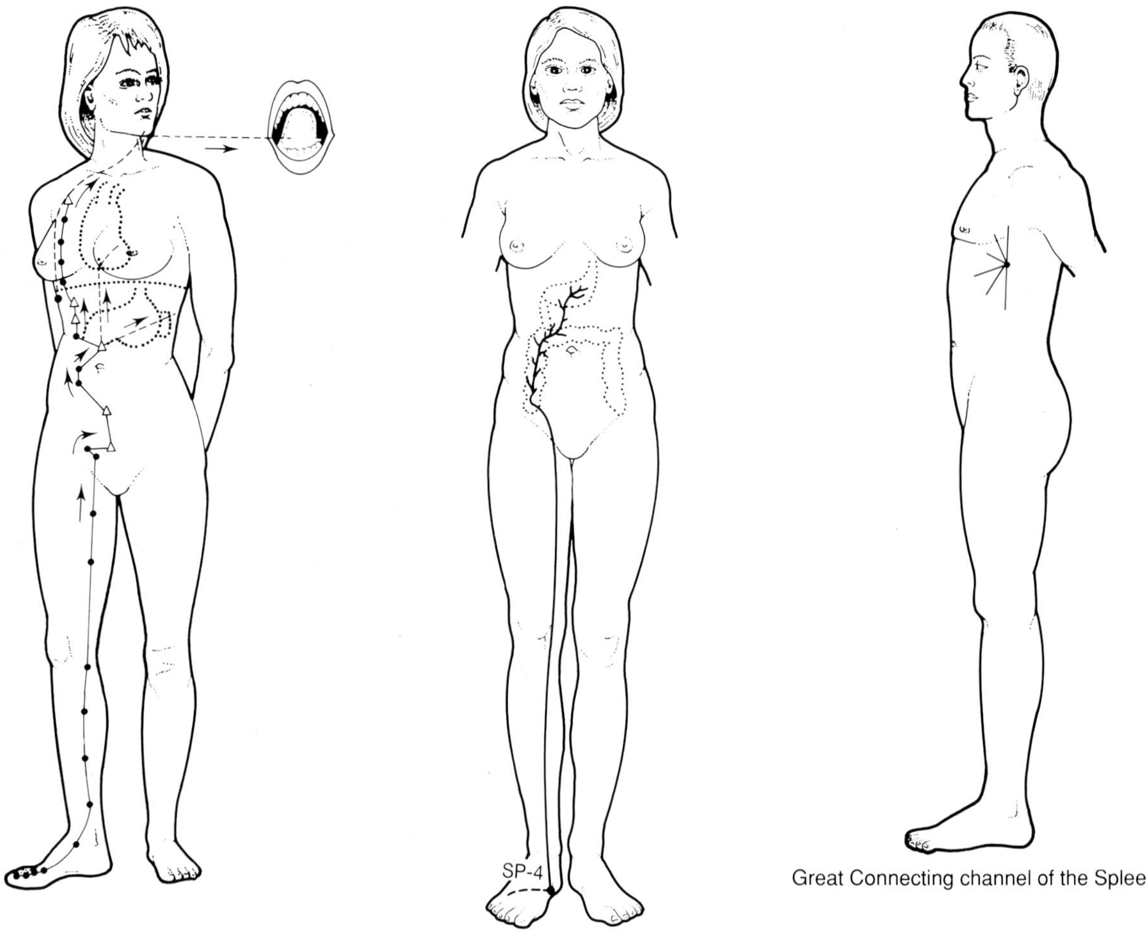

Fig. 82 Spleen channel

Fig. 82A Spleen Connecting channel and Great Connecting channel.

the posterior aspect of the tibia, passes the knee and thigh to enter the abdomen. It then enters the spleen and stomach from where it ascends traversing the diaphragm and reaching the oesophagus. It ends at the centre of the tongue.

From the stomach, a branch goes through the diaphragm and links with the heart (Fig. 82).

CONNECTING CHANNEL PATHWAY

From the point Gongsun SP-4, the Connecting channel links with the Stomach channel. Another branch enters the abdomen and connects with the large intestine and stomach (Fig. 82A).

YINBAI SP-1 *Hidden White*

Nature

Well point
Wood point.

Action

Strengthens the Spleen
Regulates Blood
Calms the Mind.

Comments

This point is normally used in Excess patterns of

the Spleen and Stomach. In particular, it is used to regulate Blood in cases of stasis of Blood in the uterus.

A special use of this point is with direct moxa to stop bleeding from any part of the body and particularly from the uterus. It stops bleeding by strengthening the Spleen's function of holding Blood. It can therefore also be used for bleeding from the nose, stomach, bladder or intestines.

Another use of this point is in cases of mental restlessness and depression in Excess patterns resulting from stasis of Blood. In such conditions it calms the Mind and stops excessive dreaming.

DADU SP-2 *Big Capital*

Nature

Spring point
Fire point
Tonification point.

Action

Strengthens the Spleen
Promotes digestion
Clears Heat.

Comments

Although this is the "tonification" point of the Spleen according to the 5 Elements, it is seldom used to tonify the Spleen, as it is more frequently used to clear Heat in Excess patterns. In particular, it is used in the course of a febrile disease from exterior Heat, at its beginning stage to cause sweating and clear Heat.

TAIBAI SP-3 *Greater White*

Nature

Earth point
Stream and Source point.

Action

Strengthens the Spleen
Resolves Damp
Strengthens the spine.

Comments

This is a major point to tonify the Spleen, as it is the Source point of the channel and also the Earth point of an Earth channel. It is very frequently used to tonify the Spleen in any of its Deficiency patterns. In particular, it stimulates the mental faculties which are associated with the Spleen function in Chinese Medicine, and can be used in cases when Spleen-Qi has been weakened by excessive mental work. The use of Taibai SP-3 can then stimulate the brain, promote memory and induce mental clarity.

Another important function of this point is to resolve Dampness, for which it is a major point. It is used in any Dampness pattern in the Upper, Middle or Lower Burner. When used to resolve Dampness, it should be needled with reducing method. Examples of symptoms and signs of Dampness are: confused thinking, muzziness of the head, feeling of oppression of the chest (Upper Burner), fullness and feeling of oppression of the epigastrium, no appetite (Middle Burner), difficult urination with cloudy urine and vaginal discharge (Lower Burner). In addition, in all these cases there would be a feeling of heaviness and the tongue coating would be sticky.

SP-3 is also frequently used in chronic retention of Phlegm in the Lungs. Phlegm is retained in the Lungs, but it originates from the Spleen due to the impairment of its function of transportation and transformation. Reinforcing SP-3 can at the same time tonify the Spleen to strengthen the Lungs (strengthening the Earth to nourish Metal) and resolve Phlegm.

A more unusual use of this point is to strengthen the spine. According to the "Yellow Emperor's Classic of Internal Medicine", the Spleen controls the spine. In my experience, SP-3 is a very useful point to strengthen and straighten the spine in cases of chronic backache.

GONGSUN SP-4 *Minute Connecting Channels*

Nature

Connecting point
Opening point of Penetrating Vessel.

Action

Tonifies Stomach and Spleen
Regulates the Penetrating Vessel
Stops bleeding
Dispels fullness
Pacifies the Stomach
Removes obstructions
Regulates menstruation.

Comments

This is a complex point with a very wide sphere of action. First of all, it tonifies the Spleen and Stomach (being the Connecting point). However, it is more apt to be used in Excess patterns of the Stomach and Spleen such as retention of Dampness in the epigastrium, stasis of Blood in the Stomach, Stomach-Heat and Stomach-Qi rebelling upwards. It is therefore much used to remove obstructions in these cases, to dispel fullness of the epigastrium and to stop epigastric or abdominal pain.

Its other functions derive from its relation with the Penetrating Vessel. This vessel is the "Sea of the 12 channels" as well as the "Sea of Blood" and it enters the uterus and regulates menstruation. SP-4, by activating and regulating the Penetrating Vessel, regulates menstruation and stops excessive bleeding, also by reinforcing the Spleen function of holding Blood.

The Chinese name of this point is usually translated as "Grandfather Grandson", which is what the two characters can mean, but they can also have the entirely different meaning of "General Minute Connecting Channels". In fact, the character "*gong*" means "general" and "*sun*" is the same character as that indicating the Minute Connecting channels. This name would be quite plausible as the Spleen controls the network of Minute Connecting channels through its point Dabao SP-21. The Minute Connecting channels are capillary-like channels distributed superficially throughout the body. Furthermore, Gongsun SP-4 is the opening point of the Penetrating Vessel which is the "Sea of the 12 channels". This point can affect the circulation in the 12 channels and also the numerous small capillary-like vessels pertaining to the Penetrating Vessel and spreading over chest and abdomen.

SHANGQIU SP-5 *Gold (or Metal) Mound*

Nature

River point
Metal point
Sedation point.

Action

Strengthens Stomach and Spleen
Resolves Damp.

Comments

This point is mostly used to resolve Dampness. Being the River point, it is a point where the Qi of the channel is diverted to bones and joints. This point is in fact very much used for Painful Obstruction Syndrome from Dampness, especially of the knee or ankle. In fact, it can also be used as a general River point for every channel's Painful Obstruction Syndrome from Dampness.

I have translated this point's name as "*Metal (or Gold) Mound*" instead of the usual "*Merchant Mound*", as the first character, in this context, can mean "Metal" or "Gold", in a 5-Element sense.[6]

SANYINJIAO SP-6 *Three Yin Meeting*

Nature

Meeting point of three Yin of the leg.

Action

Strengthens the Spleen
Resolves Damp
Promotes the function of the Liver and the smooth flow of Liver-Qi
Tonifies the Kidneys
Nourishes Blood and Yin
Benefits urination
Regulates the uterus and menstruation
Moves Blood and eliminates stasis
Cools Blood
Stops pain
Calms the Mind.

Comments

This is one of the most important points of all, with a very wide range of action.

First of all, it tonifies the Spleen and can be used in all Spleen Deficiency patterns, with poor appetite, loose stools and tiredness. In particular, combined with Zusanli ST-36, it strongly tonifies the Middle Burner Qi and is extremely effective in tonifying Qi and Blood to relieve chronic tiredness.

Besides tonifying Qi, SP-6 is one of the main points to resolve Dampness, whether it is associated with Cold or Heat, particularly in the Lower Burner. In this context it is a major point to use in all Lower Burner patterns caused by Damp-Cold or Damp-Heat, with symptoms of vaginal discharge, mucus in the stools, cloudy urine and itchiness of the scrotum or vagina.

SP-6 also has a specific action on the urinary function in connection with obstruction of Dampness in the Lower Burner. It is therefore indicated in urinary symptoms caused by Dampness in the Lower Burner, such as difficult urination, painful urination with cloudy urine or retention of urine. This point has a marvellous action in "smoothing out" obstructions and relieving pain.

SP-6 is the crossing point of the Spleen, Liver and Kidney channel, and it therefore has an action on those two channels also. In particular, it can be used to promote the smooth flow of Liver-Qi, when this is stagnant, particularly in the Lower Burner, with such symptoms as abdominal pain, constipation with small-bitty stools and painful periods.

From the emotional point of view, it helps to smooth Liver-Qi to calm the mind and allay irritability.

Being the meeting point of the Kidney channel as well, it tonifies the Kidneys, in particular Kidney-Yin, and is therefore used in cases of dizziness, tinnitus, night sweating, feeling of heat, dry mouth and other Kidney-Yin deficiency symptoms.

SP-6 has a deep influence on Blood. First of all, it can nourish Blood and Yin, and is very frequently used in both Blood or Yin Deficiency.

It can also remove stasis of Blood, especially in relation to the uterus, and is therefore used to move Blood in the Lower Burner, for such symptoms as dysmenorrhoea with clotted blood or bleeding in the stools with dark blood.

It can also cool the Blood and is therefore used in cases of Blood Heat, either in the context of exterior Heat diseases at the Blood stage, or simply in chronic cases of Blood Heat, such as in certain types of skin diseases.

SP-6 also has the function of stopping pain, particularly in the lower abdomen, and it can be used to stop lower abdominal pain, whatever its cause. This function in stopping pain is obviously related to its action in smoothing out Liver-Qi, eliminating Damp and tonifying the Spleen, all of which would help to regulate the energy in the lower abdomen.

SP-6 is also a major point to use in any gynaecological complaint, as it regulates the uterus and menstruation, stops pain and resolves Damp from the genital system. It is used to regulate the period if the cycle is irregular, for leucorrhoea, menorrhagia and dysmenorrhoea. It is an essential point to use in most gynaecological conditions.

Finally, SP-6 has a strong calming action on the Mind, and is often used for insomnia, particularly if from Blood or Yin deficiency. In particular, it is used for Spleen and Heart Blood deficiency, when the Spleen is not making enough Blood, the Heart is not supplied with enough Blood and the Mind lacks residence and floats at night, so that insomnia ensues. SP-6 is the point to use in this case as it will simultaneously tonify the Spleen, nourish Blood and calm the Mind.

DIJI SP-8 *Earth Pivot*

Nature

Accumulation point.

Action

Removes obstructions from the channel
Regulates Qi and Blood
Regulates the uterus
Stops pain.

Comments

Like all Accumulation points, this point removes obstructions and stops pain, particularly in acute Excess patterns. It is very much used in acute cases of dysmenorrhoea to stop pain. It is also used as part of a treatment strategy for chronic dysmenorrhoea, when this point would be used just before the period to move Qi and enliven Blood (usually with reducing method), and other points would be used (usually with reinforcing method) to treat the root of the condition.

Diji SP-8 regulates the uterus and stops pain by enlivening Blood, i.e. removing stasis of Blood.

YINLINGQUAN SP-9 *Yin Mound Spring*

Nature

Sea point
Water point.

Action

Resolves Dampness
Benefits the Lower Burner
Benefits urination
Removes obstructions from the channel.

Comments

This is the point on the Spleen channel to resolve Dampness from the Lower Burner. It is very much used in all conditions caused by obstruction of Dampness in the Lower Burner, whether it is Damp-Cold or Damp-Heat. It is therefore used for such symptoms as difficult urination, retention of urine, painful urination, cloudy urine, vaginal discharge, diarrhoea with foul-smelling stools, mucus in the stools and oedema of the legs or abdomen. In all these cases the point should be reduced to eliminate Dampness.

Yinlingquan SP-9 is also much used for Painful Obstruction Syndrome of the knee, particularly if from Dampness (in which case the knee is swollen), as it removes obstructions and resolves Damp.

XUEHAI SP-10 *Sea of Blood*

Action

Cools the Blood
Removes stasis of Blood
Regulates menstruation
Tonifies Blood.

Comments

This point is also very frequently used. It is an important point to eliminate stasis of Blood, especially in the uterus. It is therefore indicated in a large number of cases when stagnant Blood causes painful or irregular periods. It can be used for both acute and chronic dysmenorrhoea.

It also cools the Blood and is therefore used for Blood Heat patterns causing such skin diseases as eczema, urticaria and rashes. It is also used for menorrhagia or metrorrhagia if they are due to Heat in the Blood. This point is said to make Blood re-enter the Sea of Blood.

Needled with reinforcing method, it can also nourish the Blood, but it is not frequently used in this way, as Sanyinjiao SP-6 would be better.

CHONGMEN SP-12 *Rushing Door*

Nature

Meeting point of Spleen and Liver.

Action

Removes obstructions from the channel
Tonifies Yin.

Comments

This point nourishes Yin and can be used for Kidney-Yin deficiency. It is also useful as a local point for Painful Obstruction Syndrome of the hip, when the pain extends to the groin.

DAHENG SP-15 *Big Horizontal Stroke*

Nature

Point of Yin Linking Vessel.

Action

Strengthens the Spleen
Strengthens the limbs
Resolves Damp
Regulates Qi
Stop pain
Promotes the function of the Large Intestine.

Comments

This is quite an important point for abdominal complaints. First of all, it strengthens the function of the Spleen and promotes the Spleen transformation and transportation, especially in relation to bowel movements. This point is therefore often used in chronic constipation of the Deficiency type, i.e. when Spleen-Qi is deficient and fails to promote the function of the Large Intestine in moving the stools.

By strengthening the Spleen, it particularly strengthens the limbs as it stimulates the Spleen to transport food essences to the limbs. It can be used for cold and weak limbs.

This point can also resolve Dampness in the intestines and is therefore used in chronic diarrhoea with mucus in the stools.

Daheng SP-15 also regulates Qi in the abdomen and promotes its smooth flow of Liver-Qi, so that it can be used to stop abdominal pain from stagnation of Liver-Qi.

This point's name requires an explanation: "*Heng*" means "horizontal", but it also is the horizontal stroke in Chinese writing. The "stroke" in this case is the line drawn across the umbilicus encompassing Shenque Ren-8, Huangshu KI-16, Tianshu ST-25 and Daheng SP-15.

DABAO SP-21 *General Control*

Nature

General Connecting point.

Action

Moves Blood in the Blood Connecting channels.

Comments

This point controls all the minute Blood Connecting channels throughout the body. It is used in generalized pains due to stasis of Blood in the Connecting channels, the main symptoms being muscular pain moving throughout the body.

This point's name is translated as "General Control", as the word "*Bao*" (which normally would mean "envelop") here has the meaning of "controlling", "taking upon oneself". The name therefore refers to the general controlling action of this point on all the Blood Connecting channels.[7]

NOTES

1 Spiritual Axis, p 73.
2 Difficult Urination Syndrome is called "*Lin*" disease in Chinese Medicine. *Lin* literally means "to drip, dribble" and it indicates a series of urinary symptoms and signs characterized by pain and difficulty in urination.
3 Li Dong Yuan 1249 Discussion on Stomach and Spleen In: Clinical Application of Frequently Used Acupuncture Points, p 195.
4 Zhang Zhong Jing c. AD 220 Discussion on Cold-induced Diseases, p 369.
5 Spiritual Axis, p 73.
6 An Explanation of the Meaning of Acupuncture Points' Names, p 89.
7 An Explanation of the Meaning of Acupuncture Points' Names, p 102.

Heart and Small Intestine Channels 42

心经小腸经

HEART CHANNEL

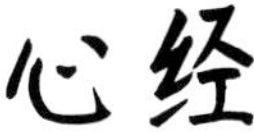

MAIN CHANNEL PATHWAY

The Heart channel originates from the heart. It then emerges, passes through the diaphragm and connects with the small intestine. A branch from the heart ascends to the throat and eye.

Another branch from the heart enters the lung and emerges at the axilla, from where it joins the superficial channel running along the medial aspects of the arm to end at the medial side of the tip of the little finger (Fig. 83).

CONNECTING CHANNEL PATHWAY

From Tongli HE-5, the Connecting channel links with the Small Intestine channel. Another branch follows the main channel, enters the heart and ascends to the tip of the tongue and eye (Fig. 83A).

JIQUAN HE-1 *Supreme Spring*

Action

Nourishes Heart-Yin
Clears Empty-Heat.

Comments

This point is used mostly to nourish Heart-Yin and subdue Heart Empty-Heat with such symptoms as dry mouth, night sweating, mental restlessness and insomnia.

It is also used in the sequelae of Wind-stroke for paralysis of the arm.

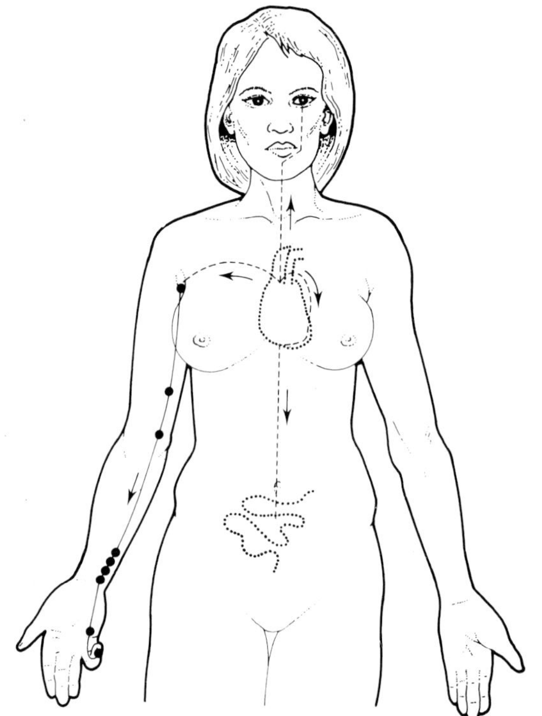

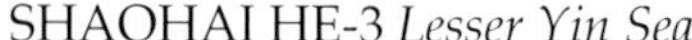

Fig. 83 Heart channel

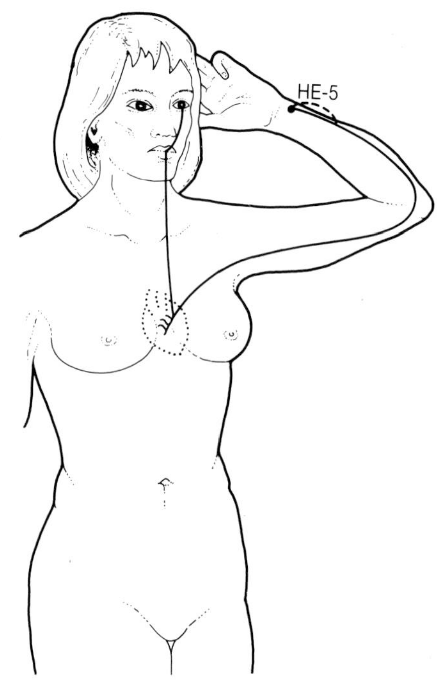

Fig. 83A Heart Connecting channel

SHAOHAI HE-3 *Lesser Yin Sea*

Nature

Sea point
Water point.

Action

Removes obstructions from the channel
Calms the Mind
Clears Heat.

Comments

This point is used mostly to clear Heart-Fire or Heart Empty-Heat, in which case it is sedated.

It has an important calming action on the mental level (by clearing Heart-Fire), and is indicated for epilepsy, depression, mental retardation or hypomania.

Finally, it is also used as a local point to remove obstructions from the Heart channel in Painful Obstruction Syndrome, Atrophy Syndrome or sequelae of Wind-stroke.

I have translated its name as "Lesser Yin Sea" instead of "Lesser Sea", as the "*Shao*" here clearly refers to "*Shao Yin*", i.e. Lesser Yin to which the Heart belongs. It is for this reason that the character "*Shao*" recurs in the points Shaofu HE-8 and Shaochong HE-9.

LINGDAO HE-4 *Mind Path*

Nature

River point
Metal point.

Action

Removes obstructions from the channel.

Comments

This point is mostly used in channel problems, also because, as a River point, it has a special action on joints and bones. It is therefore used for spasm and neuralgia or the forearm and arthritis of elbow and wrist, if the obstruction is along the Heart and Small Intestine channels.

TONGLI HE-5 *Inner Communication*

Nature

Connecting point.

Action

Calms the Mind
Tonifies Heart-Qi
Opens into the tongue
Benefits the Bladder.

Comments

This is one of the main points to tonify Heart-Qi, and is the point of choice out of all the Heart channel points for this purpose. It is indicated in all symptoms of Heart-Qi deficiency and, in particular, it has a marked effect on the tongue, and is the point of choice for aphasia.

Being the Connecting point, Tongli HE-5 connects with the Small Intestine channel; this, in turn, connects with the Bladder channel within the Greater Yang. It is through this route that the Heart channel can influence the Bladder and urination. This connection manifests itself when Heart-Fire is transmitted to the Small Intestine and from this to the Bladder, giving rise to Bladder-Heat. The main manifestations are thirst, bitter taste, insomnia, tongue ulcers, burning on urination and haematuria.

YINXI HE-6 *Yin Accumulation*

Nature

Accumulation point.

Action

Nourishes Heart-Yin
Clears Heat
Stops sweating
Calms the Mind.

Comments

This point is frequently used to nourish Heart-Yin with symptoms of night sweating, dry mouth, insomnia, etc. In particular, in combination with Fuliu KI-7, it is the point of choice to stop night sweating from Heart-Yin deficiency.

It also clears Heart-Fire and in particular Heart Empty-Heat and is therefore useful for mental restlessness and a feeling of heat deriving from Empty Heat.

SHENMEN HE-7 *Mind Door*

Nature

Source point
Stream point
Sedation point.

Action

Calms the Mind
Nourishes Heart-Blood
Opens the orifices.

Comments

This is the most important point on the Heart channel and one of the major points of the body. It can be used in virtually any Heart pattern in order to calm the Mind, which is its main action. However, it primarily nourishes Heart-Blood and is the point of choice for Heart-Blood deficiency causing anxiety, insomnia, poor memory, palpitations and a Pale tongue.

In my experience, it is a "gentle" point and therefore not the choice point in Excess patterns of the Heart, characterized by Heart-Fire or Heart Phlegm-Fire, for which other points would be better indicated (such as Jianshi P-5, or Shaofu HE-8). But it is the best point to calm the Mind when there is great anxiety, and worrying under stressful situations.

As the Heart is the residence for the Mind, which in Chinese Medicine includes mental activity, thinking, memory and consciousness, this point has an effect not only on emotional problems such as anxiety, but also on memory and mental capacity. In fact, this point can be used for mental retardation in children.[1] Interestingly, the ancient classics do not always stress the use of this point for emotional or mental problems. For example, the "ABC of Acupuncture" (AD 282) by Huang Fu Mi says only that this point is used for cold hands, vomiting of blood and rebellious Qi.[2] The "Thousand Ducat Prescriptions" (AD 652) by Sun Si Miao says that this point can be used for contraction of the arm.[3]

A comparison between the functions of HE-7 and Daling P-7 is given under the latter point on page 436.

SHAOFU HE-8 *Lesser Yin Mansion*

Nature

Spring point
Fire point.

Action

Clears Heart-Fire, Heart Empty-Heat and Heart Phlegm-Fire
Calms the Mind.

Comments

This is a "harsh" point, quite different than Shenmen HE-7. Its main action is to clear Heat in the Heart, whether it is Full-Heat, Empty-Heat or Heat with Phlegm. Its main range of action is therefore in Excess patterns of the Heart. The main symptoms would be insomnia with vivid dreams, thirst, bitter taste, mental restlessness or hypomania, dark urine, tongue ulcers, and a Red tongue with redder tip and yellow coating.

It also calms the mind, but only in the context of Excess patterns with Heat in the Heart, and its indications are different from those of HE-7, as they include more serious mental problems such as hypomania, schizophrenia and psychosis. Of course, this does not limit the function of HE-8 to the problems just mentioned.

SHAOCHONG HE-9 *Lesser Yin Rushing*

Nature

Well point
Wood point
Tonification point.

Action

Clears Heat
Subdues Wind
Opens the Heart orifices
Relieves fullness
Restores consciousness.

Comments

This point is mostly used in Excess patterns with Heat in the Heart. It is similar in action to Shaofu HE-8 in so far as it clears Heat, but it also subdues internal Wind and can therefore be used for Wind-stroke. In this context, it is used to restore consciousness as it opens the Heart orifices when these are obstructed by internal Wind.

Table 24 Comparison of Heart channel points

Point	Action	Action on Mind
HE-3	Clears Full-Heat	For severe mental symptoms such as hypomania and severe depression
HE-5	Tonifies Heart-Qi	To lift the Mind, in mild depression and sadness
HE-6	Tonifies Heart-Yin	For the typical mental restlessness of Yin deficiency, i.e. vague and indefinable restlessness and anxiety, fidgeting, with feeling of heat in the face
HE-7	Tonifies Heart-Blood	The main point for anxiety and worry deriving from a stressful life and insomnia
HE-8	Clears Heart-Fire	For severe mental disturbances in Excess patterns with Full Heat, such as hypomania, excessive dreaming and psychosis
HE-9	Clears Heat, subdues internal Wind	To open the "Heart orifices" and restore consciousness. Also for severe anxiety, hysteria and hypomania

In accordance with the general action of Well points indicated in the "Classic of Difficulties" (see p. 339), this point relieves a feeling of fullness in the heart region.

As all Heart channel points "calm the Mind", it might be useful to illustrate the differences among the various points in a tabular form (Table 24).

SMALL INTESTINE CHANNEL

小腸经

MAIN CHANNEL PATHWAY

The Small Intestine channel starts at the ulnar side of the tip of the little finger. Following the ulnar side of the dorsum of the hand it reaches the wrist and ascends along the posterior aspect of the arm to the shoulder joint. Circling around the scapula, it connects with Dazhui Du-14 and goes forward to the supraclavicular fossa to connect with the heart. From here it descends to the oesophagus and connects with the small intestine.

The superficial pathway of the channel from the supraclavicular fossa ascends to the neck and the cheek to enter the ear. From the cheek, a branch goes to the infra-orbital region to link with the Bladder channel at the inner canthus (Jingming BL-1) (Fig. 84).

CONNECTING CHANNEL PATHWAY

From Zhizheng S.I.-7 the Small Intestine Connecting channel links with the Heart channel. Another branch goes up the arm and elbow and joins with the shoulder (Fig. 84A).

SHAOZE S.I.-1 *Lesser Marsh*

Nature

Well point
Metal point.

Action

Expels Wind-Heat
Subdues Wind

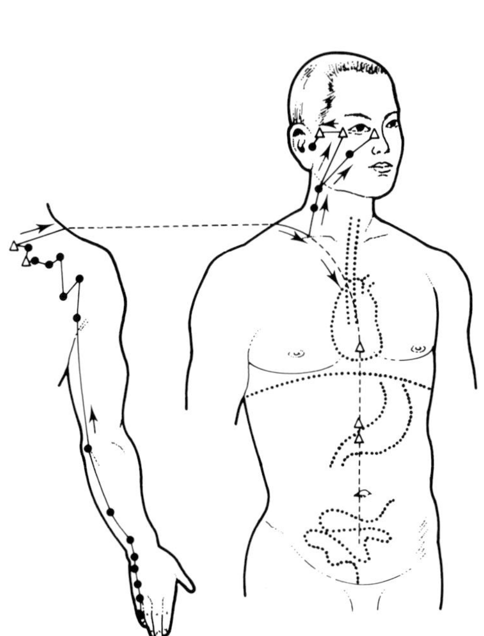

Fig. 84 Small Intestine channel

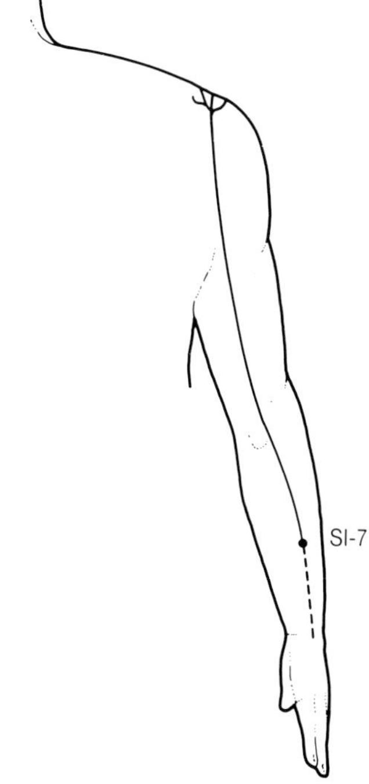

Fig. 84A Small Intestine Connecting channel

Opens the orifices
Removes obstructions from the channel
Promotes lactation.

Comments

Like most of the Well points, this point is used for Excess patterns to eliminate pathogenic factors. Shaoze S.I.-1 mostly eliminates Wind-Heat in exterior attacks, especially when the symptoms affect the head and neck, causing stiff neck and headache. It is also good to treat acute tonsillitis from invasion of exterior Wind-Heat.

It also eliminates internal Wind which is a property of all Well points.

It can also be used to open the orifices and promote resuscitation in cases of internal Wind and Phlegm blocking the orifices and causing sudden unconsciousness, as in Wind-stroke.

Apart from its role in exterior patterns, it can also be used as a distal point for channel problems of the neck, such as chronic stiff neck or acute torticollis.

Finally, it is an empirical point to promote lactation after childbirth, mostly in Excess patterns, i.e. when lactation is inhibited by the presence of some pathogenic factor or stagnation (such as stagnant Liver-Qi).

QIANGU S.I.-2 *Front Valley*

Nature

Spring point
Water point.

Action

Clears Heat.

Comments

Like all Spring points, Qiangu S.I.-2 clears Heat, both interior and exterior. It can therefore be used to expel exterior Wind-Heat, especially if it affects neck and eyes, and also to clear interior Heat from the Small Intestine, but mostly in acute febrile diseases.

Owing to its relationship with the Bladder within the Greater Yang, it can also be used to clear Bladder-Heat when this causes burning on urination.

HOUXI S.I.-3 *Back Stream*

Nature

Stream point
Wood point
Opening point of Governing Vessel
Tonification point.

Action

Eliminates interior Wind from the Governing Vessel
Expels exterior Wind
Benefits sinews
Resolves Dampness
Resolves jaundice
Clears the mind.

Comments

This point has a wide range of action. Firstly, it is the opening point of the Governing Vessel, and is therefore needled for all symptoms of this extraordinary vessel. In particular, it eliminates interior Wind from the Governing Vessel. Symptoms and signs of interior Wind in this vessel include convulsions, tremors, epilepsy, stiff neck, giddiness and headache.

Houxi S.I.-3 also eliminates exterior Wind and is widely used in attacks of exterior Wind-Cold or Wind-Heat whenever there are pronounced symptoms affecting neck and head, such as stiff neck, occipital headache, aches down the spine and back, and chills and fever.

This point has also a deep effect on the muscles and tendons along the course of the Governing Vessel, Small Intestine and Bladder channel (because the Small Intestine and Bladder channels are closely connected within the Greater Yang area). It is therefore widely used for any channel problem along these three channels. In particular, it affects the upper more than lower back area along the Small Intestine and Bladder channel. It is more effective in acute rather than chronic cases.

In combination with Shenmai BL-62, it activates the Governing Vessel and can be used to affect the whole spine and back (upper and lower) in both acute and chronic cases.

This combination is only indicated if the backache is either on the spine itself or across the lower back on both sides, but not if the pain is only on one side of the lower back. The treatment is also different according to sex. In men, it is sufficient to treat only the Governing Vessel by using S.I.-3 and BL-62. In women, it is better to treat the Governing and Directing Vessels simultaneously by using S.I.-3, BL-62, Lieque LU-7 and Zhaohai KI-6. The order and laterality of needling in a woman would be as follows: S.I.-3 on the right, BL-62 on the left, LU-7 on the left and KI-6 on the right. The needles should be withdrawn in the reverse order. This combination of distal points is extremely effective for chronic lower backache in women. These points would be used first to remove obstructions from the Governing Vessel, and the local points would be used afterwards.

Also in combination with BL-62, S.I.-3 activates the Governing Vessel and it tonifies the Kidneys as this extraordinary vessel emerges from the Kidneys. The use of S.I.-3 and BL-62 to tonify the Kidneys is more appropriate in men rather than women.

S.I.-3 also resolves Dampness affecting the chest and the Gall Bladder resulting in jaundice and a feeling of stuffiness of the chest.

Finally, in my experience S.I.-3 has an effect on the mind, in so far as it affects the brain, via the Governing Vessel. It "clears the mind" in the sense that it helps the person to gain strength to face up to choices and difficult decisions in life and to gain clarity of mind and judgement. Just as S.I.-3 strengthens the spine on a physical level, it can strengthen the mind and gives the person strength of character to face difficulties.

WANGU S.I.-4 *Wrist Bone*

Nature

Source point.

Action

Removes obstructions from the channel
Eliminates Damp-Heat.

Comments

This point is mostly used for channel problems of the Small Intestine, extending its influence to the wrist, elbow and neck. It is therefore used for Painful Obstruction Syndrome of the wrist or elbow.

In spite of its being the Source point, this point is not much used for internal problems of the Small Intestine, for which the Lower-Sea, Front Collecting or Back Transporting points would be preferred.

An empirical use of this point is for jaundice from Damp-Heat obstructing the Gall-Bladder, hypochondriac pain and cholecystitis.

YANGGU S.I.-5 *Yang Valley*

Nature

River point
Fire point.

Action

Clears the mind
Removes obstructions from the channel
Expels exterior Damp-Heat.

Comments

This point is very useful for its mental effect: it "clears the mind" in the sense that it helps the person to gain mental clarity and distinguish the right path to take among several. It can help a person at difficult times to distinguish what is right to do at a particular moment in life.

Yanggu S.I.-5 can be used in a similar way to Wangu S.I.-4 for channel problems, and in my experience, it also helps to eliminate Dampness from the knees when they are swollen and hot.

YANGLAO S.I.-6 *Nourishing the Old*

Nature

Accumulation point.

Action

Benefits sinews
Brightens the eyes
Removes obstructions from the channel.

Comments

This point is used for any channel problems of the Small Intestine, particularly when there is tightness of the tendons and ligaments causing stiff neck and shoulders.

Yanglao S.I.-6 also benefits the eyesight but only in patterns related to Heart or Small Intestine.

ZHIZHENG S.I.-7 *Branch to Heart Channel*

Nature

Connecting point.

Action

Removes obstructions from the channel
Calms the Mind.

Comments

This point can treat any channel problem, as all Connecting points do. It is particularly good for elbow problems.

Being the Connecting point, a branch from it departs to connect with the Heart channel, and because of this connection, it can be used to calm the mind in severe anxiety.

In my experience, this point helps to resolve thyroid Phlegm swellings when combined with Pianli L.I.-6.

I have translated this point's name as "Branch to Heart Channel", because "Zheng" in this case means "chief" or "ruler", i.e. the Heart (which is the "Monarch" of all the other organs).

XIAOHAI S.I.-8 *Small Intestine Sea*

Nature

Sea point
Earth point
Sedation point.

Action

Resolves Damp-Heat
Removes obstructions from the channel
Calms the Mind.

Comments

This point resolves Damp-Heat (as all the Sea points of the three arm Yang channels do) and is therefore effective in treating acute swelling of the glands of the neck and parotitis.

It also removes obstructions from the channel and is used in Painful Obstruction Syndrome of the elbow and neck.

Finally, it calms the Mind and can be used in addition to Heart channel points in the treatment of anxiety associated with a Heart pattern.

I have translated this point's name as "Small Intestine Sea" rather than "Small Sea", as the character "*Xiao*" here indicates "*Xiao Chang*", i.e. the Chinese name for "Small Intestine".

JIANZHEN S.I.-9 *Upright Shoulder*

Comments

This is not a major point, but it is worth remembering as it is one of several important local points for shoulder problems. Jianzhen S.I.-9 is one of the points which should always be checked for tenderness when selecting local points for Painful Obstruction Syndrome of the shoulder.

NAOSHU S.I.-10 *Humerus Transporting Point*

Nature

Point of Yang Heel Vessel
Point of Yang Linking Vessel.

Comments

This is another important point for Painful Obstruction Syndrome of the shoulder, and one always to be checked for tenderness when selecting local points. In particular, this point is situated both on the Yang Heel and Yang Linking Vessels trajectory and it especially increases the mobility of the shoulder whenever its joint movement is limited (as in "frozen shoulder").

TIANZONG S.I.-11 *Heavenly Attribution*

Comments

The indications of this point are the same as for Jianzhen S.I.-9. It is more frequently used than S.I.-9 as it is nearly always tender on pressure in Painful Obstruction Syndrome of the shoulder. In my experience, it gives particularly good results in this condition when chosen as one of the local points. After obtaining the needling sensation, a reducing technique should be applied, which should then be followed by application of moxa to the needle. It is best to needle this point with the patient sitting up.

BINGFENG S.I.-12 *Watching Wind*

Nature

Meeting point of Small Intestine, Gall Bladder, Triple Burner and Large Intestine.

Comments

Same as for Jianzhen S.I.-9.

QUYUAN S.I.-13 *Bend Wall*

Comments

The indications for this point are the same as for the previous four points. However, this is a particularly important local point for Painful Obstruction Syndrome of the shoulder and neck, and should always be checked for tenderness when selecting local points.

Similarly to Tianzong S.I.-11, this point should also be reduced and moxa applied to the needle afterwards. It is best to needle this point with the patient sitting up.

JIANWAISHU S.I.-14 *Transporting Point of the Outside of the Shoulder*

Comments

Same as for Quyuan S.I.-13.

JIANZHONGSHU S.I.-15 *Transporting Point of the Centre of the Shoulder*

Comments

The indications for this point are the same as for the previous two points. However, this point is slightly less important as a local point and is less often tender on pressure.

TIANRONG S.I.-17 *Heaven Appearance*

Action

Resolves Damp-Heat
Expels Fire-Poison
Removes obstructions from the channel.

Comments

This point resolves exterior or interior Damp-Heat and is indicated in the treatment of swelling of the cervical glands, parotitis and tonsillitis.

QUANLIAO S.I.-18 *Zygoma Crevice*

Nature

Meeting point of Small Intestine and Triple Burner.

Action

Expels Wind
Relieves pain.

Comments

This is an important local point in the treatment of facial paralysis, tic or trigeminal neuralgia and all manifestations of Wind in the face.

TINGGONG S.I.-19 *Listening Palace*

Nature

Meeting point of Small Intestine, Gall Bladder and Triple Burner.

Action

Benefits the ears.

Comments

This is an important and frequently used local point for tinnitus and deafness. It is particularly indicated for Deficiency types of tinnitus and deafness, especially if associated with a Lung and Heart-Qi Deficiency.

NOTES

1 Tai Yi Shen Acupuncture, p 23.
2 Zhang Shan Chen 1982 Essential Collection of Acupuncture Points from the ABC of Acupuncture (*Zhen Jiu Jia Yi Jing Shu Xue Zhong Ji* 针灸甲乙经腧穴重辑). Shandong Scientific Publishing House, Shandong, p 112 (first published AD 282).
3 Sun Si Miao AD 652 . Thousand Ducat Prescriptions. In: Anwei College of Traditional Chinese Medicine-Shanghai College of Traditional Chinese Medicine 1987 Dictionary of Acupuncture, Shanghai Scientific Publishing House, p 477.

43 Bladder and Kidney Channels 膀胱经肾经

BLADDER CHANNEL
膀胱经

MAIN CHANNEL PATHWAY

The Bladder channel starts at the inner canthus of the eye. It ascends the forehead and joins the Governing Vessel at the point Baihui (Du-20). From here a branch goes to the temple. From the vertex, the channel enters the brain to re-emerge at the nape of the neck. From here, it flows down the occiput and all the way down the back. From the lumbar area, it enters the kidney and bladder.

Another branch from the occiput runs down the back along the medial aspect of the scapula, down the back to the gluteus and the popliteal fossa. Here it meets the previous branch and runs along the posterior aspect of the leg to end at the lateral aspect of the 5th toe where it links with the Kidney channel (Fig. 85).

CONNECTING CHANNEL PATHWAY

The Bladder Connecting channel separates at Feiyang BL-58 on the leg and flows down to connect with the Kidney channel (Fig. 85A).

JINGMING BL-1 *Eye Brightness*

Nature

Point of Yin and Yang Heel Vessels
Meeting point of Bladder, Small Intestine and Stomach.

Action

Expels Wind
Clears Heat
Brightens the eyes
Stops pain
Stops itching
Stops lacrymation.

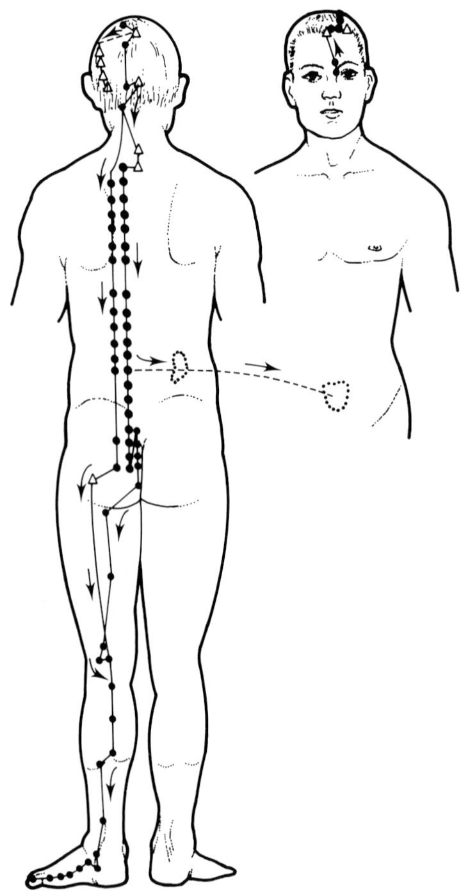

Fig. 85 Bladder channel

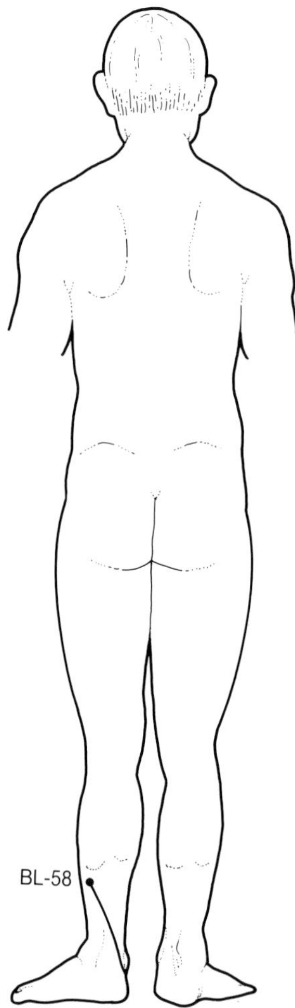

Fig. 85A Bladder Connecting channel

Comments

This point is obviously used mostly for eye diseases, of both interior and exterior character.

It can expel exterior Wind and clear Heat, which means that it can treat eye problems from Wind-Heat, such as conjunctivitis and runny eyes. It can also clear interior Heat and therefore help eye problems deriving from Liver-Fire, such as red, painful, swollen and dry eyes. It stops pain and itching of the eyes deriving from Heat.

One particular use of this point is in conjunction with the opening points of both the Yin and Yang Heel Vessels for the treatment of insomnia. As explained in the chapter "The Extraordinary Vessel Points" (see p. 355), the Yin Heel Vessel transports Yin Qi to the eye, whilst the Yang Heel Vessel transports Yang Qi to it. If Yang is in excess, the eyes will stay open and the person finds it difficult to fall asleep. In this case one can tonify Zhaohai KI-6 to stimulate the Yin Heel Vessel, reduce Shenmai BL-62 to sedate the Yang Heel Vessel and needle BL-1 with even method. The needling of BL-1 closes the circle between the Yin and Yang Heel Vessels and allows the balance of Yin and Yang Qi in the eyes to be re-established.

This combination of points can also be used to treat chronic somnolence simply by reversing the type of needle technique used. In this case we can tonify Shenmai BL-62 to stimulate the Yang Heel Vessel to carry Yang Qi to the eyes, reduce Zhaohai KI-6 to sedate the Yin Heel Vessel and needle BL-1 with even method.

ZANZHU (or CUANZHU) BL-2 *Collecting Bamboo*

Action

Expels Wind
Brightens the eyes
Soothes the Liver
Removes obstructions from the channel
Stops pain.

Comments

This is an important local point for the eye. First of all, it expels exterior Wind from the face and removes obstructions from the channel: this means that it can be used to treat facial paralysis, facial tics and trigeminal neuralgia, all problems caused by Wind affecting the channels of the face.

It brightens the eyes and soothes the Liver, but only locally in relation to the Liver function of nourishing the eyes. It can therefore be used in any Liver pattern affecting the eyes, such as "floaters" in the eyes, red eyes, blurred vision and persistent headaches around or "behind" the eyes.

WUCHU BL-5 *Five Places*

Action

Subdues interior Wind
Restores consciousness.

Comments

This is a local point to subdue interior Wind affecting the Governing Vessel. It is used for the treatment of epilepsy, convulsions or rigidity of the spine in children during a febrile disease.

It is also used in acute sudden attacks of interior Wind (as in Wind-stroke) to restore consciousness.

TONGTIAN BL-7 *Reaching Heaven*

Action

Subdues Wind
Clears the nose
Brightens the eyes
Stops convulsions
Opens the orifices.

Comments

This is an important local point that dispels both exterior and interior Wind from the head. It can be used for attacks of exterior Wind-Cold or Wind-Heat which cause severe headache or facial paralysis, as well as for interior Wind patterns causing dizziness, headache and vertigo. It is particularly important as a local point for headaches on the vertex deriving from Liver-Yang or Liver-Wind rising, as well as from Liver-Blood Deficiency.

It is also used as a local point to subdue interior Wind which may result in convulsions and unconsciousness.

This point also has an effect on both the nose and the eyes, and can be used in rhinitis to clear the nose or in eye diseases to increase vision.

TIANZHU BL-10 *Heaven Pillar*

Nature

Point of the Sea of Qi.

Action

Expels Wind
Clears the brain
Opens the orifices
Soothes the sinews
Removes obstructions from the channel
Brightens the eyes
Invigorates the lower back.

Comments

This is an important point to expel both interior and exterior Wind from the head and is a major local point for occipital or vertical headache from any origin. It can be used to expel exterior Wind in case of stiff neck and headache deriving from invasions of Wind-Cold.

It can subdue interior Wind and is used in this way mostly for occipital headaches deriving from Liver-Wind rising. However, it can be used for virtually any type of occipital headache.

As it is a point of the Sea of Qi and is situated at the point where the Bladder channel emerges from the brain, this point can be used to clear the brain and stimulate memory and concentration.

It has a special effect on the eyes and is used to increase vision, especially if the eyesight is diminished from Kidney deficiency.

Finally, it can be used as a distal point for bilateral acute lower back ache. This point is usually needled first with reducing method while the patient (in a standing position) gently bends forwards and backwards. After a few minutes of this, the patient is made to lie down and local points are used on the lower back.

DAZHU BL-11 *Big Reed*

Nature

Point of the Sea of Blood
Gathering point for Bones
Meeting point of Bladder and Small Intestine.

Action

Nourishes Blood
Expels Wind
Strengthens bones
Soothes the sinews
Releases the Exterior.

Comments

This point has three main areas of influence. Firstly, it is a point of the Sea of Blood and it can be used to nourish Blood. In this case it should be needled with reinforcing method. Another use of this particular function is for generalized muscular ache (Painful Obstruction Syndrome from Wind). This point helps by nourishing Blood and therefore strengthening the Nutritive Qi to throw off the pathogenic factor.

Secondly, it releases the Exterior and expels exterior Wind, in a similar way to Fengmen BL-12, and can be used in the beginning stages of attacks of exterior Wind-Cold or Wind-Heat. In this case it should be needled with reducing method or cupped.

Thirdly, it is a Gathering point for Bones, and it can nourish the bones. It is therefore used either to promote bone formation in children and prevent bone degeneration in the elderly, or to treat bone deformities in chronic arthritis.

Finally, it also strengthens the sinews and can be used for contractions of the tendons.

FENGMEN BL-12 *Wind Door*

Action

Expels and prevents exterior Wind
Releases the Exterior
Stimulates the Lung dispersing function
Regulates Nutritive and Defensive Qi.

Comments

This is the point to use in the very beginning stages of invasions of exterior Wind-Cold or Wind-Heat; reducing this point will release the Exterior, relieve all the exterior symptoms (stuffy nose, sneezing, chills, aversion to cold and headache) and expel Wind. It is extremely effective especially if it is cupped. When reduced or cupped in these cases, it acts by stimulating the Lung dispersing function, i.e. spreading the Defensive Qi all over the skin to fight off the pathogenic factor.

It can also be used with even needling to regulate Nutritive and Defensive Qi, i.e. in invasions of exterior Wind-Cold with the prevalence of Wind resulting in slight sweating (see p. 294).

FEISHU BL-13 *Lung Back Transporting Point*

Nature

Back Transporting point of the Lungs.

Action

Stimulates the Lung dispersing and descending function
Regulates Lung-Qi
Regulates Nutritive and Defensive Qi
Tonifies Lung-Qi
Stops cough
Clears Heat.

Comments

This point can be used in both exterior and interior patterns of the Lungs. In exterior patterns, it releases the Exterior by stimulating the Lung dispersing and descending function, and thus helps to expel Wind-Cold or Wind-Heat. In particular, it is indicated if the exterior attack is accompanied by cough.

In invasions of exterior Wind-Cold with the prevalence of Wind, it can regulate Nutritive and Defensive Qi in the same way as Fengmen BL-12.

In interior patterns, it restores the Lung descending function and is therefore used for cough, asthma or breathlessness.

It also clears interior Heat from the Lungs, and is therefore used in acute conditions of the Lungs characterized by Heat at the Qi level (of the 4-Level Pattern Identification), as may happen in acute bronchitis or pneumonia. The symptoms at this stage are a high fever, thirst, a cough with sticky-yellow sputum, breathlessness, restlessness, a Rapid pulse and a Red tongue body with a thick yellow dry coating.

Needled with reinforcing method, or direct moxa, it tonifies Lung-Qi and is effective for chronic deficiency of Lung-Qi, especially if combined with Shenzhu Du-12. It can also be combined with Gaohuanshu BL-43 to tonify Lung-Yin.

JUEYINSHU BL-14 *Terminal Yin Back Transporting Point*

Nature

Back Transporting point for the Pericardium.

Action

Regulates the Heart.

Comments

This point is frequently used in heart conditions, such as arrhythmia, tachycardia, angina pectoris and coronary heart disease.

XINSHU BL-15 *Heart Back Transporting Point*

Nature

Back Transporting point for the Heart.

Action

Calms the Mind
Clears Heat
Stimulates the brain
Invigorates Blood
Nourishes the Heart.

Comments

This is a very important point for many Heart patterns. Firstly, it calms the Mind and can be used for nervous anxiety and insomnia mostly deriving from Excess conditions of the Heart, such as Heart-Fire or Heart Empty-Heat. In these cases it is needled with reducing method.

It is not indicated for anxiety and insomnia deriving from an Empty condition, such as Heart-Blood or Heart-Yin Deficiency. This is because it mostly calms the Mind by clearing Heat in the Heart.

At the same time as calming the Mind, it also stimulates the brain if used with reinforcing method or with direct moxibustion. In particular, used with direct moxibustion, it has a good effect in stimulating the brain and is effective for depression in adults.

BL-15 also invigorates Blood and is therefore used for pain in the chest deriving from stasis of Blood.

DUSHU BL-16 *Governing Vessel Back Transporting Point*

Nature

Back Transporting point for the Governing Vessel.

Action

Regulates the Heart
Invigorates Blood.

Comments

This point is mostly used for stasis of Blood of the Heart causing heart and chest pain.

GESHU BL-17 *Diaphragm Back Transporting Point*

Nature

Back Transporting Point for the diaphragm
Gathering point for Blood.

Action

Nourishes Blood
Invigorates Blood
Opens the chest
Removes obstructions from diaphragm
Pacifies Stomach-Qi
Tonifies Qi and Blood
Clears Heat
Calms the Mind.

Comments

This is an important point with many functions. Firstly, it can nourish Blood if used with direct moxibustion: it is therefore used for Deficiency of Blood of any organ. It is usually combined with the Back Transporting points to nourish the Blood of the relevant organs. For example, it is combined with Ganshu BL-18 to nourish Liver-Blood, with Xinshu BL-15 to nourish Heart-Blood and with Pishu BL-20 to promote the Spleen function of producing Blood.

Secondly, it invigorates Blood, i.e. removes stasis of Blood from any organ, but only if needled (no moxa) with either reducing or even method. It is used as a general point to remove stasis of Blood in any organ and from any part of the body. Again, it is combined with the Back Transporting points to move stasis of Blood of the relevant organs. For example, combined with Ganshu BL-18 it removes stasis of Liver-Blood whilst combined with Xinshu BL-15 it removes stasis of Heart-Blood.

Thirdly, it moves Qi in the diaphragm and chest and is used for feeling of stuffiness and pain of the chest, fullness in the epigastrium, belching and hiccup.

Fourth, it pacifies Stomach-Qi and it subdues rebellious Stomach-Qi, i.e. Stomach-Qi going upwards instead of downwards. It therefore treats such symptoms as hiccup, belching, nausea and vomiting.

Fifth, it has a general tonification effect on all Qi and Blood of the whole body, if used with direct moxibustion. To this effect, it is usually combined with Danshu BL-19, and the combination of these two points is called the "Four Flowers".[1]

Another combination to tonify Qi and Blood in general is with Ganshu BL-18 and Pishu BL-20, with direct moxibustion. This combination is called the "Magnificent Six" (counting each point bilaterally).

GANSHU BL-18 *Liver Back Transporting Point*

Nature

Back Transporting point for the Liver.

Action

Benefits Liver and Gall Bladder
Resolves Damp-Heat
Moves stagnant Qi
Benefits the eyes
Eliminates Wind.

Comments

This point can be used in most Liver patterns, but it is mostly used either for stagnation of

Liver-Qi or retention of Damp-Heat in Liver and Gall-Bladder. It is frequently used to move stagnant Liver-Qi causing distension of the epigastrium and hypochondrium, sour regurgitation, nausea, etc. In clearing Damp-Heat it can be used for jaundice and cholecystitis.

However, it can also be used for Liver Deficiency patterns, such as Deficiency of Liver-Blood; in this case it should be needled with reinforcing method, or only direct moxibustion should be applied. When used to nourish Liver-Blood, it can be combined with Geshu BL-17.

When needled with reducing method, BL-18 can be used to subdue interior Wind.

Finally, BL-18 can be used to promote vision in all eye disorders related to a Liver disharmony, such as poor night vision, blurred vision, floaters in the eyes, red and painful and swollen eyes.

DANSHU BL-19 *Gall Bladder Back Transporting Point*

Nature

Back Transporting point for the Gall-Bladder.

Action

Resolves Damp-Heat in Liver and Gall-Bladder
Pacifies the Stomach
Relaxes the diaphragm.

Comments

This point also resolves Damp-Heat from the Liver and Gall-Bladder and is therefore used in cholecystitis and jaundice.

It pacifies the Stomach and stimulates the descending of Stomach-Qi, which makes it useful to treat belching, nausea and vomiting.

Similarly to Geshu BL-17, it relaxes the diaphragm, and is used for hiccup and a feeling of fullness under the diaphragm, usually caused by stagnation of Liver-Qi.

PISHU BL-20 *Spleen Back Transporting Point*

Nature

Back Transporting point for the Spleen.

Action

Tonifies Spleen and Stomach
Resolves Damp
Nourishes Blood.

Comments

This is a very important point among all the Back Transporting points. It is a major point to tonify the Spleen and Stomach and invigorate the Spleen function of transformation and transportation. It is used in any Spleen-Qi deficiency pattern with symptoms of tiredness, loose stools, no appetite, abdominal distention and possibly prolapse of stomach or uterus. Combined with Weishu BL-21, it provides a powerful tonification of the Root of Post-Heaven Qi, i.e. Stomach and Spleen and is used to tonify Qi and Blood when a person is physically and mentally exhausted over a long period of time.

By tonifying Spleen-Qi, this point also resolves Dampness and Phlegm, which derive from the dysfunction of the Spleen activity of transformation and transportation of fluids. BL-20 is therefore used in practically every condition with chronic Dampness or Phlegm.

By tonifying Spleen-Qi, BL-20 also nourishes Blood as the Spleen is the origin of Blood. This point is therefore very much used to nourish Blood, often in combination with Shenshu BL-23. In this case the point should be tonified or direct moxa applied.

In conclusion, BL-20 is a very important point to be reinforced in nearly all chronic diseases when the person is very depleted in energy.

WEISHU BL-21 *Stomach Back Transporting Point*

Nature

Back Transporting point for the Stomach.

Action

Regulates and tonifies Stomach Qi
Resolves Damp
Pacifies the Stomach
Relieves retention of food.

Comments

This, like Pishu BL-20, is also a major point to tonify Stomach and Spleen Qi. It tonifies both Stomach-Qi and Spleen-Qi, and is often combined with Pishu BL-20 to tonify Qi and Blood in general. The main difference with BL-20 is in the direction of Qi stimulated by the point: BL-21 stimulates the descending of Stomach-Qi, whereas BL-20 stimulates the ascending of Spleen-Qi. Hence the use of BL-21 to subdue ascending Stomach-Qi when this causes belching, hiccup, nausea and vomiting.

BL-21 also resolves Damp, by tonifying Spleen-Qi and promoting the Spleen function of transformation and transportation of fluids.

Finally, when needled with reducing method, BL-21 stimulates the descending of Stomach-Qi and relieves retention of food in the Stomach, the cause of fullness of the epigastrium, sour regurgitation and belching.

SANJIAOSHU BL-22 *Triple Burner Back Transporting Point*

Nature

Back Transporting point for the Triple Burner.

Action

Resolves Dampness
Opens the Water passages
Regulates the transformation of fluids in the Lower Burner.

Comments

This is a major point to stimulate the transformation and transportation of fluids in the Lower Burner. The Lower Burner keeps the Water passages open so that "dirty" fluids may be excreted. This point regulates this particular function of the Lower Burner and thus ensures that the Water passages are open, fluids are properly transformed and dirty fluids excreted.

By stimulating the transformation and excretion of fluids, it resolves Dampness in the Lower Burner and treats such symptoms as urinary retention, painful urination, oedema of the legs, and any other manifestation of Dampness in the Lower Burner.

SHENSHU BL-23 *Kidney Back Transporting Point*

Nature

Back Transporting point for the Kidneys.

Action

Tonifies the Kidneys and nourishes the Kidney-Essence
Strengthens the lower back
Nourishes Blood
Benefits bones and Marrow
Resolves Dampness
Strengthens the Kidney function of reception of Qi
Brightens the eyes
Benefits the ears.

Comments

This is one of the major points and the main point to tonify the Kidneys. This point must be used (obviously with reinforcing method) in any chronic Kidney deficiency. Being on the back (a Yang surface) it is slightly better to tonify Kidney-Yang, but it can also be used to nourish Kidney-Yin. The main difference between its use for tonifying Kidney-Yang or Kidney-Yin is in the use of moxa: this would be used to tonify Kidney-Yang, but not to tonify Kidney-Yin. This point can therefore be used in the treatment of any Kidney deficiency whether Yin or Yang.

It is also one of the main points to nourish the Kidney-Essence (the other is Guanyuan Ren-4) and is used for impotence, nocturnal emissions, infertility, spermatorrhoea and lack of sexual desire. It is also very frequently used for chronic asthma with Kidney deficiency to stimulate the Kidney function of receiving Qi.

The Kidneys store Essence and are the foundation of life. Essence is the material foundation for the Mind. If Essence is strong and flourishing, the Mind will be happy and positive. If Essence is weak, the body is always weak and exhausted, and the Mind also will suffer, with a lack of will power, negativity, a lack of initiative and depression. In all these cases, BL-23 is a powerful tonic for the Kidneys and their mental aspect: it will stimulate the Mind, strengthen the will power, stimulate the spirit of initiative and lift depression. This effect is particularly strong if BL-23 is combined with Zhishi BL-52.

As the Kidneys rule the lower back, this point is very frequently used to strengthen the lower back in chronic backache. Indeed, it is a point which should be always employed for the treatment of chronic lower backache.

As the Kidneys play a role in the formation of Blood, this point is frequently used in combination with Pishu BL-20 to promote the formation of Blood in Blood deficiency.

As the Kidneys control the bones and produce Marrow, this point is also used in any bone pathology (such as arthritic bone deformities, osteoporosis and osteomalacia) and to nourish Marrow in a Chinese Medicine sense. It is therefore used in symptoms of deficiency of the Sea of Marrow, i.e. dizziness, poor memory, tinnitus, weak legs, blurred vision, fatigue and a constant desire to sleep.[2]

This point also resolves Dampness from the Lower Burner. It is commonly said that the Kidney cannot have Excess patterns: this is not entirely true, as they can suffer from retention of Dampness in conjunction with the Bladder. In these cases, BL-23 can be needled with reducing method together with Pangguangshu BL-28 and Yinlingquan SP-9 to resolve Damp-Heat from the Lower Burner. In this connection, it is used for the treatment of acute urinary stones.

The Kidney opens into the ears, and this point can treat all chronic ear problems related to Kidney deficiency, mostly tinnitus and deafness. It is not indicated for the treatment of acute ear problems (such as otitis or ear infections) as these would be treated more via the Triple Burner and Gall-Bladder channels.

Finally, the Kidneys also influence the eyes and vision. Kidney-Yin nourishes and moistens the eyes and promotes good sight. Many chronic eye disorders, such as poor vision and dry eyes in the elderly, are the result of a deficiency of Kidney-Yin failing to nourish and moisten the eyes. BL-23 is the main point to affect the eyes in these cases.

QIHAISHU BL-24 *Sea of Qi Back Transporting Point*

Action

Strengthens the lower back
Removes obstructions from the channel
Regulates Qi and Blood.

Comments

This is not a major point in terms of its energetic action, but it is frequently used as a local point in chronic or acute lower back ache.

Apart from this, it also regulates Qi and Blood and removes Blood stasis in the Lower Burner, and is therefore used for uterine bleeding and irregular menstruation.

DACHANGSHU BL-25 *Large Intestine Back Transporting Point*

Nature

Back Transporting point for the Large Intestine.

Action

Promotes the function of the Large Intestine
Strengthens the lower back
Removes obstructions from the channel
Relieves fullness and swelling.

Comments

First of all, this point promotes the excreting function of the Large Intestine and can be used to treat both constipation and diarrhoea in combination with Pishu BL-20. Being the Back Transporting point, it is especially indicated for any chronic disease of the Large Intestine.

It is also indicated in Excess patterns of the Large Intestine to relieve abdominal fullness and distension.

It is also frequently used as a local point for both chronic or acute lower back ache. In acute backache, this point is often tender on pressure and, if so, it should be needled with reducing method.

GUANYUANSHU BL-26 *Origin Gate Back Transporting Point*

Action

Strengthens the lower back
Removes obstructions from the channel.

Comments

This point is very frequently used as a local point in chronic lower back ache and should always be used if tender on pressure.

XIAOCHANGSHU BL-27 *Small Intestine Back Transporting Point*

Nature

Back Transporting Point for the Small Intestine.

Action

Promotes the function of the Small Intestine
Resolves Dampness
Clears Heat
Benefits urination.

Comments

This point stimulates the Small Intestine function of receiving and separating, and can be used in any Small Intestine pattern, with such symptoms as borborygmi, abdominal pain and mucus in the stools. BL-27 also eliminates Damp-Heat from the Lower Burner and benefits urination, so that it can be used to treat such symptoms as cloudy urine, difficult urination and burning on urination.

PANGGUANGSHU BL-28 *Bladder Back Transporting Point*

Nature

Back Transporting point for the Bladder.

Action

Regulates the Bladder
Resolves Dampness
Clears Heat
Stops pain
Eliminates stagnation
Opens the Water passages in the Lower Burner
Strengthens the loins.

Comments

This point is very much used in urinary disorders. Firstly, it expels Dampness from the Bladder and the Lower Burner and it can therefore treat retention of urine, difficult urination and cloudy urine. It also clears Heat from the Bladder and can be used for painful and burning urination. Combined with Shenshu BL-23 and Yinlingquan SP-9, it is used to expel renal stones.

BL-28 also generally opens the Water passages of the Lower Burner and makes sure that the dirty fluids are transformed and excreted. It is a point that is often combined with Pishu BL-20 to transform fluids in the Lower Burner and promote diuresis.

Combined with Shenshu BL-23, it strengthens the lower back.

BAIHUANSHU BL-30 *White Ring Transporting Point*

Comments

This point has an effect on the anus, and is mostly used for anal problems, such as haemorrhoids, prolapse of anus, spasm of anus and incontinence of faeces.

SHANGLIAO BL-31 *Upper Crevice*

Action

Regulates the Lower Burner
Tonifies the lumbar region and knees
Nourishes the Kidneys.

Comments

The next four points located in the four sacral

foramina (BL-31-32-33-34) have similar properties. They are important points to treat genital disorders in men and women. In women they can treat leucorrhoea, prolapse of the uterus and sterility. In men they can treat impotence, orchitis and prostatitis.

All these points tonify the Kidneys and benefit Essence, so that, apart from having a specific effect on genital disorders, they also have a tonifying effect on the whole body.

As they tonify the Kidneys, these points are also used to strengthen the lower back and knees.

CILIAO BL-32 *Second Crevice*

Action

The same as for Shangliao BL-31.

Comments

These have already been discussed under the point BL-31. However, BL-32 is the most important of these four points, and the one which is most tonifying to the Kidneys and Essence. BL-32 is an important point to use for the treatment of infertility in women.

In addition, this point is also used to stimulate the ascending of Qi in prolapse of the anus or uterus.

ZHONGLIAO BL-33 *Central Crevice*

Action

The same as for Shangliao BL-31.

Comments

Same as for BL-31, with the only difference that this point has more of an influence on the Bladder.

XIALIAO BL-34 *Lower Crevice*

Action

Same as for Zhongliao BL-33.

Comments

Same as for BL-33.

CHENGFU BL-36 *Receiving Support*

Comments

This point is mostly used as a local point for lower backache with pain radiating down the back of the leg (sciatica).

YINMEN BL-37 *Huge Gate*

Comments

This is also frequently used as a local point for pain radiating down the back of the leg. It is particularly effective if it is gently heated with a moxa stick.

WEIYANG BL-39 *Supporting Yang*

Nature

Lower-Sea point for the Lower Burner.

Action

Opens the Water passages in the Lower Burner
Stimulates the transformation and excretion of fluids in the Lower Burner
Benefits the Bladder.

Comments

This is an important point to stimulate the transformation and excretion of fluids in the Lower Burner. It ensures that the Water passages of the Lower Burner are unobstructed so that dirty fluids can be excreted properly. It is therefore used in all Excess patterns of the Lower Burner characterized by the accumulation of fluids in the form of Dampness or oedema: this could manifest with urinary retention, burning on urination, difficult urination, oedema of the ankles, incontinence of urine or enuresis.

In particular, when the Lower Burner is in Excess, i.e. its Water passages obstructed (manifested with retention of urine), this point should be reduced so as to open the Water passages and stimulate the excretion of fluids. If the Lower Burner is Deficient, i.e. the Water passages are in a relaxed state and fluids are not contained (manifested with incontinence of urine or enuresis), this point should be tonified so as to strengthen Qi in the Lower Burner and "tighten" the Water passages so that fluids can be contained.

WEIZHONG BL-40 *Supporting Middle*

Nature

Sea Point
Earth point.

Action

Clears Heat
Resolves Dampness
Relaxes the sinews
Removes obstructions from the channel
Cools Blood
Eliminates stasis of Blood
Clears Summer-Heat.

Comments

This is a point with a very wide range of action. Firstly, it can clear Heat and resolve Dampness from the Bladder, and it can therefore be used for the symptom of burning during urination.

It relaxes the sinews and removes obstructions from the Bladder channel and is very much used for lower backache. It can be used for any kind of lower backache, whether chronic or acute and of the Excess or Deficiency type. However, it is best used in acute rather than chronic and Excess rather than Deficient type of lower backache. In fact, in very weak patients with pronounced Deficient and Cold symptoms, this point should not be used as it tends to have a reducing effect and it also cools Blood. In these cases, it can be replaced by Kunlun BL-60.

Finally, as far as the location of the backache is concerned, it is best used when the ache is either bilateral or unilateral, but not on the midline (i.e. on the spine itself).

This point also cools Blood and it is frequently used in skin diseases characterized by Heat in the Blood. It also moves Blood and is used mostly for pains in the lower legs from stasis of Blood.

Finally, it clears Summer-Heat and is used in acute attacks of Heat in summertime causing fever, delirium and a red skin rash.

POHU BL-42 *Door of the Corporeal Soul*

Nature

This is the point on the outer Bladder line corresponding to Feishu BL-13, the Back Transporting point for the Lungs.

Action

Stimulates the descending of Lung-Qi
Regulates Qi
Clears Heat
Stops cough and asthma
Subdues rebellious Qi.

Comments

This point has two main actions, on a physical and psychological level. On a physical level, it can be used to regulate and send Lung-Qi downwards in the treatment of cough and asthma.

It is also frequently used for Painful Obstruction Syndrome of the upper back and shoulders and is frequently tender on pressure. Needling this point can greatly relieve pain and stiffness of the upper back or scapula area.

On a psychological level, it is related to the Corporeal Soul ("*Po*") which is the mental-spiritual aspect residing in the Lungs (see page 86). It is therefore used for emotional problems related to the Lungs, particularly sadness, grief and worry. It has a very soothing effect on the spirit and it nourishes Qi when this is dispersed by a prolonged period of sadness or grief.

GAOHUANGSHU (or GAOHUANG) BL-43 *Vitals*

Nature

This is the point on the outer Bladder line

corresponding to BL-14, the Back Transporting point for the Pericardium.

Action

Tonifies Qi
Strengthens Deficiency
Nourishes Essence
Nourishes Lung-Yin
Invigorates the Mind
Stops cough and calms asthma.

Comments

This is an intriguing point. It has a very old history and is mentioned in one of the earliest references to acupuncture.[3] Its name is very difficult to translate. The two combined characters "*Gaohuang*" indicate the space between the heart and diaphragm. This is supposed to be the location of all chronic and nearly incurable diseases. Hence the use of this point in very chronic diseases with great debility.

This point tonifies the Qi of the whole body and is used when the person is very debilitated after a chronic illness. In these cases, it is usually treated with direct moxibustion with moxa cones.

It nourishes Essence, and can be used for Kidney deficiency manifesting with nocturnal emissions, low sexual energy or poor memory.

It nourishes Lung-Yin and is used to tonify the Lungs and promote the Yin after a chronic lung disease which has injured the Yin and left the person with a chronic dry cough and debility. In this case it is needled only and moxa is not used.

Finally, it invigorates the Mind, by promoting the Essence function of nourishing the brain. It therefore stimulates memory and lifts the spirit, especially after a long-standing disease.

SHENTANG BL-44 *Mind Hall*

Nature

This point is on the outer Bladder line in correspondence with Xinshu BL-15, the Back Transporting point for the Heart.

Action

Calms the Mind.

Comments

This point is mostly used for emotional and psychological problems related to the Heart. It is best used in conjunction with BL-15, for anxiety, insomnia and depression.

HUNMEN BL-47 *Door of the Ethereal Soul*

Nature

This point is on the outer Bladder line in correspondence with Ganshu BL-18, the Back Transporting point for the Liver.

Action

Regulates Liver-Qi
Roots the Ethereal Soul.

Comments

This point is used for emotional problems related to the Liver, such as depression, frustration and resentment over a long period of time.

In my experience, when used in conjunction with Ganshu LIV-8, it has a profound influence on a person's capacity of planning his or her life by rooting and steadying the Ethereal Soul. It can help a person find a sense of direction and purpose in life. This point will also help to lift mental depression associated with such difficulties.

Because it roots the Ethereal Soul, it can be used for a vague feeling of fear occurring at night in persons suffering from severe deficiency of Yin.

On a physical level, it can be combined with Ganshu BL-18 to eliminate stagnation of Liver-Qi.

YISHE BL-49 *Thought Shelter*

Nature

This point is on the outer Bladder line in

correspondence with Pishu BL-20, the Back Transporting point for the Spleen.

Action

Tonifies the Spleen
Stimulates memory and concentration.

Comments

This point tonifies the mental aspect of the Spleen, i.e. memory, concentration and capacity for study.

It can also be used for obsessive thoughts which are often related to a Spleen deficiency and are like the pathological correspondent of this organ's mental activity of memorization and concentration.

HUANGMEN BL-51 *Vitals Door*

Nature

This point is on the outer Bladder line in correspondence with BL-22, the Back Transporting point for the Triple Burner.

Action

Regulates the Triple Burner
Ensures the smooth spread of the Triple Burner Qi to the heart region.

Comments

This is another intriguing point, and in order to understand its functions, we have to recollect one of the Triple Burner functions. As was mentioned in the chapter on the functions of the Yang organs (see page 118), one of the Triple Burner's functions is that of being the "ambassador" or the "avenue" through which the Original Qi comes out of the Kidneys and spreads to the Internal Organs and the twelve channels. The Triple Burner also ensures the smooth flow of Qi in the region between the Heart and diaphragm, i.e. the "*Gaohuang*" region as mentioned in connection with point Gaohuangshu BL-43. Hence the name of this point: "*Huang*" indicates the "*Gaohuang*" region, i.e. below the heart and above the diaphragm, and "*men*" indicates "*door*" to describe the Triple Burner's function as an entrance or outlet for Qi in this region.

This point's name should be seen in conjunction with that of point "*Baohuang*" BL-53, two points below along the outer Bladder line in correspondence with Pangguangshu BL-28, the Back Transporting point for the Bladder. The "Acupuncture Textbook by Hui Yuan" says that the Triple Burner penetrates upwards to the "*Gaohuang*" region, and downwards to the "*Baohuang*" region, i.e. the uterus and bladder.[4] Thus this point regulates the movement of the Triple Burner upwards to the diaphragm region, whilst the point "*Baohuang*" BL-53 regulates the movement of the Triple Burner downwards to the uterus, genitals and urinary system.

In fact, the "Illustrated Classic of Acupuncture points as found on the Bronze Model" says that this point is indicated for a feeling of tightness below the heart and diseases of the breast in women.[5] It is interesting that this point which is in correspondence with Sanjiaoshu BL-22, the Back Transporting point for the Lower Burner, is not indicated for diseases of the Lower Burner, but for those of the Upper Burner.

ZHISHI BL-52 *Will Power Room*

Nature

This point is on the outer Bladder line in correspondence with Shenshu BL-23, the Back Transporting point for the Kidneys.

Action

Tonifies the Kidneys
Strengthens the back
Reinforces the will power.

Comments

This point is outside Shenshu BL-23, the Back Transporting point for the Kidneys. Similarly to Shenshu BL-23, it has a tonifying effect on the Kidneys and, combined with it, reinforces its effect.

It can be used in chronic lower backache especially if the point is tender on pressure, as it strengthens the back by tonifying the Kidneys.

Finally, this point strengthens will power and determination which are the mental-spiritual phenomena pertaining to the Kidneys. It is a very useful point in the treatment of certain types of depression, when the person is disoriented and lacks the will power and mental strength to make an effort to get better. Needling this point with reinforcing method, especially if combined with BL-23, will stimulate the will power and lift the spirit.

BAOHUANG BL-53 *Bladder Vitals*

Action

Opens the Water passages in the Lower Burner
Stimulates the transformation and excretion of fluids.

Comments

This point has a similar action to Sanjiaoshu BL-22, in so far as it stimulates the transformation and excretion of dirty fluids in the Lower Burner. It is mostly used for urinary problems such as retention of urine, difficult urination and burning urination.

The name of this point should be seen in conjunction with Huangmen BL-51, in so far as BL-51 controls the spread of Qi in the Upper Burner, and BL-53 controls the spread of Qi in the Lower Burner.

ZHIBIAN BL-54 *Lowermost Edge*

Comments

This point is not remarkable for its energetic action, but it is a very important local point for the treatment of lower backache radiating to buttocks and legs. It must always be checked for tenderness when treating ache extending to the buttocks and the back of the legs (along the Bladder channel). If it is tender, it should be needled with a long needle (i.e. at least 2 in.) and a good needling sensation obtained, preferably to radiate downwards some way towards the leg. If the needling sensation radiates all the way down to the foot, it may not be necessary to use any other point. If the buttock and leg ache is due to obstruction by Cold and Damp, moxibustion with a moxa stick is very effective and should always be used in conjunction with needling.

CHENGSHAN BL-57 *Supporting Mountain*

Action

Relaxes the sinews
Invigorates Blood
Clears Heat
Removes obstructions from the channel.

Comments

This point is used as a distal point for the treatment of lower backache and sciatica, with similar effect and range of action as Weizhong BL-40. It is also frequently used as an empirical distal point for the treatment of haemorrhoids.

It also invigorates Blood and can be used for menstrual pain or blood in the stools caused by stasis of Blood.

As a local point it relaxes the muscles and tendons of the lower leg and is therefore used in cramps of the gastrocnemius.

FEIYANG BL-58 *Flying Up*

Nature

Connecting point.

Action

Removes obstructions from the channel
Strengthens the Kidneys.

Comments

This point is used as a distal point in the treatment of lower backache and sciatica. A particular function of this point is to treat sciatica when the pain is somewhat in between the Bladder and Gall-Bladder channel in the leg.

It is also an empirical distal point for the treatment of haemorrhoids.

FUYANG BL-59 *Instep Yang*

Nature

Point of the Yang Heel Vessel
Accumulation point of the Yang Heel Vessel.

Action

Removes obstructions from the channel
Invigorates the Yang Heel Vessel
Strengthens the back.

Comments

This is a frequently used distal point in the treatment of lower back ache, particularly in chronic cases with weakness of the leg and back. This point strengthens the muscles and makes movement of the leg easier.

The Yang Heel Vessel corresponds to movement and agility and this point is its accumulation point, hence its effect in stimulating movement of the leg and back. It is effective only for unilateral backache.

KUNLUN BL-60 *Kunlun (Mountains)*

Nature

River point
Fire point.

Action

Expels Wind
Removes obstructions from the channel
Relaxes the sinews
Clears Heat
Invigorates Blood
Strengthens the back.

Comments

This point has a wide range of action. Firstly, it is very much used as a distal point in the treatment of backache. It differs from Weizhong BL-40, in so far as it is better for chronic rather than acute backache, and better for backache of Deficiency rather than Excess type.

Furthermore, its sphere of influence extends to the shoulders, neck and occiput (unlike BL-40), and is therefore much used for Painful Obstruction Syndrome of the shoulder, neck and head. This is also due to its effect in eliminating Wind (exterior or interior) which normally attacks the top part of the body.

Owing to its sphere of action being on the occiput and head, it is very much used as a distal point for headaches deriving from Kidney deficiency, particularly deficiency of Kidney-Yang.

BL-60 is also effective to clear internal Heat from the Bladder, hence its use for burning urination.

It also moves Blood and can be used for menstrual problems deriving from stasis of Blood, such as painful periods with dark-clotted blood.

Its name is probably due to the fact that the Kunlun mountains in Sichuan are where the source of the Yangtze river is. The Bladder channel is the longest channel of the body (just like the Yangtze river is the longest in China), and the point is near the prominence of the external malleolus which could be compared to the Kunlun mountains.

SHENMAI BL-62 *Ninth Channel*

Nature

Opening and beginning point of the Yang Heel Vessel.

Action

Removes obstructions from the channel
Benefits the eyes
Relaxes sinews
Opens the Yang Heel Vessel
Clears the mind
Eliminates interior Wind.

Comments

This point's action is mostly due to its being the opening and beginning point of the Yang Heel Vessel. This vessel controls movement and agility, and this point can be used in chronic backache in a similar way to Fuyang BL-59.

Shenmai BL-62 also relaxes the tendons and muscles of the outer leg, and is used when the muscles of the outer leg are tense, and those of the inner aspect of the leg are relaxed.

The Yang Heel Vessel flows up to the eye and meets the Yin Heel Vessel at Jingming BL-1. The Yang Heel Vessel brings Yang energy and the Yin Heel Vessel brings Yin energy to the eyes. The "Spiritual Axis" in chapter 17 says: *"The Yin Heel Vessel branches off from the Kidney channel [at Rangu KI-2], it travels upwards ... reaching the inner canthus of the eye. Here it meets the Yang Heel Vessel. When the Yin and Yang Heel Vessels are harmonized, the eyes will be moistened. When the energy of the Yin Heel Vessel is deficient, the eyes will not be able to close"*.[6]

As was mentioned before, BL-62 can be used in combination with Zhaohai KI-6 for the treatment of insomnia, in which case, BL-62 is reduced and KI-6 reinforced.

Besides its effect on the eye, BL-62 influences the spine and brain and eliminates interior Wind, and is therefore used in the treatment of epilepsy, but only if the attacks occur mostly in the daytime (if the attacks occur at night, KI-6 would be used).

The *"Shen"* character in the point's name indicates the 9th Earthly Branch, which is the time corresponding to the Bladder, hence the translation as "Ninth channel".

JINMEN BL-63 *Golden Door*

Nature

Accumulation point
Beginning point of Yang Linking Vessel.

Action

Clears Heat
Stops pain.

Comments

Like all Accumulation points, this point is used in acute cases to stop pain. It is frequently used in acute Bladder patterns to clear Heat and stop pain, for such symptoms as frequent and burning urination.

JINGGU BL-64 *Capital Bone*

Nature

Source point.

Action

Clears Heat
Eliminates Wind
Calms the Mind
Clears the brain
Strengthens the back.

Comments

This point clears Heat from the Bladder and is therefore used for burning pain on urination.

It eliminates interior Wind and is used in the treatment of epilepsy.

It strengthens the back and is frequently used to treat chronic lower backache.

SHUGU BL-65 *Binding Bone*

Nature

Stream point
Wood point
Sedation point.

Action

Removes obstructions from the channel
Clears Heat
Eliminates Wind.

Comments

This point can be used as a distal point for any problems along the Bladder channel, particularly if affecting the head. It is therefore used for Painful Obstruction Syndrome of the neck, for which it is particularly useful.

It clears Heat from the Bladder and can be used in acute cystitis.

It eliminates interior Wind and is used for epilepsy. It also eliminates exterior Wind and is frequently used in the beginning stages of an attack of Wind-Cold (Greater Yang stage) with pronounced headache and stiff neck.

TONGGU BL-66 *Passing Valley*

Nature

Spring point
Water point.

Action

Clears Heat
Removes obstructions from the channel
Eliminates Wind.

Comments

Like all Spring points, this point clears Heat and is particularly useful to clear Bladder-Heat in acute cases of cystitis as it is more dynamic and powerful than other Bladder points in its clearing Heat action.

Since it clears Heat and eliminates Wind, it is frequently used for the beginning stages of attacks of Wind-Heat (Defensive-Qi Level) with fever, headache and stiff neck.

ZHIYIN BL-67 *Reaching Yin*

Nature

Well point
Metal point
Tonification point.

Action

Eliminates Wind
Removes obstructions from the channel
Invigorates Blood
Clears the eye.

Comments

As a Well point, it eliminates Wind (both interior and exterior) and is frequently used for headache from exterior or interior Wind.

Being the end point of the channel, it can be used to affect the opposite end, and it is therefore used to clear the eyes, for such symptoms as blurred vision or pain in the eye (usually from Wind).

It is used empirically for malposition of the fetus. This is normally done in the 8th month of pregnancy, burning 5 moxa cones on each side, once a day for ten days.

KIDNEY CHANNEL

肾经

CHANNEL PATHWAY

The Kidney channel starts under the 5th toe and runs to the sole of the foot (at Yongquan KI-1). Running under the navicular bone and behind the medial malleolus, it ascends the medial side of the leg up to the inner aspect of the thigh. It then goes towards the sacrum (at Changqiang Du-1), it ascends along the lumbar spine and enters the kidney and urinary bladder. It then goes forwards to enter the liver, pass through the diaphragm and enter the lung. From here it ascends to the throat and terminates at the root of the tongue.

From the lung, a branch joins the heart and flows to the chest to connect with the Pericardium channel (Fig. 86).

CONNECTING CHANNEL PATHWAY

The Kidney Connecting channel starts at Dazhong KI-4 from where a branch connects with the Bladder channel. A branch runs along the main Kidney channel to the perineum and ascends through the lumbar spine (Fig. 86A).

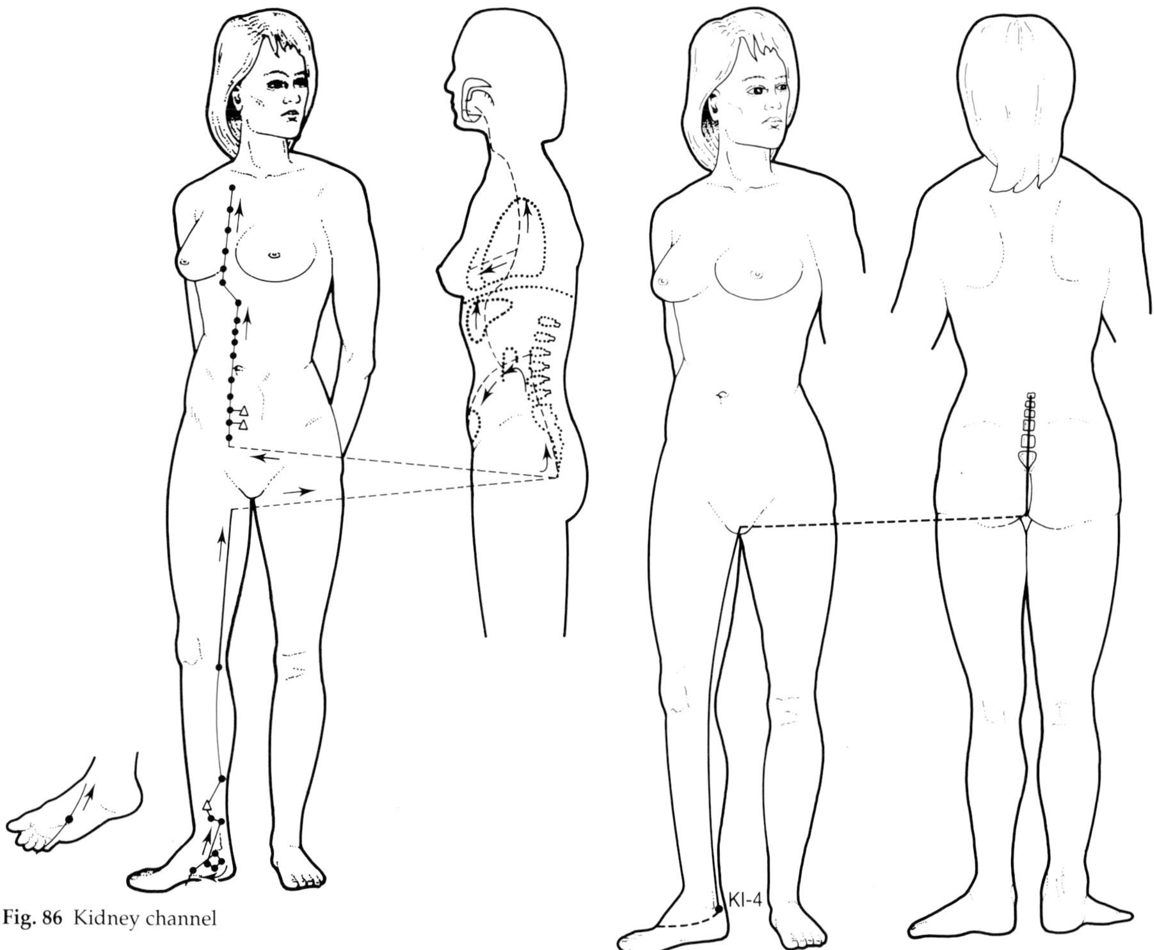

Fig. 86 Kidney channel

Fig. 86A Kidney Connecting channel

YONGQUAN KI-1 *Bubbling Spring*

Nature

Well point
Wood point
Sedation point.

Action

Tonifies Yin
Clears Heat
Subdues Wind
Subdues Empty-Heat
Calms the Mind
Restores consciousness
Clears the brain.

Comments

This point has a marked reducing effect on the body's Qi and is used in Excess patterns.

Firstly, it tonifies Yin and especially reduces Empty-Heat deriving from Yin deficiency.

It also clears Full-Heat and subdues Wind, hence its use for epilepsy and to promote resuscitation. It can be used in acute situations when the person is unconscious, to restore consciousness and clear the brain.

It has a very strong calming effect on the Mind, and is used in severe anxiety or mental illness such as hypomania.

Being on the sole of the foot, it has a strong sinking action, i.e. it eliminates pathogenic factors (such as Wind or Empty-Heat) from the head and it brings down rebellious ascending Qi (particularly Liver-Yang or Liver-Wind).

Since it tonifies Yin and subdues Empty-Heat, it is frequently used for the pattern of Yin deficiency with Empty-Heat in the Heart (Heart and Kidney not harmonized).

RANGU KI-2 *Blazing Valley*

Nature

Spring point
Fire point
Beginning point of Yin Heel Vessel.

Action

Clears Empty-Heat
Invigorates the Yin Heel Vessel
Cools Blood.

Comments

This is the main point to clear Empty-Heat from the Kidneys. It is very much used in such symptoms as red cheekbones, feeling of heat in the head in the evening, mental restlessness, thirst without desire to drink and dry throat and mouth at night. It can be combined with Yuji LU-10 to clear Empty-Heat from the Lungs, or with Yinxi HE-6 to clear Empty-Heat from the Heart.

Being the Spring point, it is a very dynamic point and more used in Excess patterns.

Being the beginning point of the Yin Heel Vessel, it can be used to strengthen this vessel in order to nourish Yin.

TAIXI KI-3 *Greater Stream*

Nature

Stream and Source point
Earth point.

Action

Tonifies the Kidneys
Benefits Essence
Strengthens the lower back and knees
Regulates the uterus.

Comments

This is an extremely important point used to tonify the Kidneys in any deficiency pattern of Kidney-Yin or Kidney-Yang. Being the Source point, it is in contact with the Original Qi of the Kidney channel, and since the Kidneys are the foundation of all the Qi of the body and the seat of the Original Qi, this point goes straight to the core of the Original Qi. As the Kidneys also store Essence, this point can tonify the Essence, the bones and Marrow.

Essence nourishes the uterus and this point can regulate the function of the uterus, and is therefore used in such symptoms as irregular periods, amenorrhoea and excessive bleeding.

Finally, the Kidneys rule the lower back and KI-3 can be used to treat any type of chronic ache of the lower back.

DAZHONG KI-4 *Big Bell*

Nature

Connecting point.

Action

Strengthens the back
Lifts the spirit.

Comments

Being the Connecting point, this point connects with the Bladder channel and is therefore very useful to treat chronic backache from Kidney deficiency.

It also has a marked effect on the Mind and can be used to "lift" the spirit when the person is exhausted and depressed from a chronic Kidney deficiency.

SHUIQUAN KI-5 *Water Spring*

Nature

Accumulation point.

Action

Benefits urination
Promotes circulation of Blood
Stops abdominal pain
Regulates the uterus.

Comments

Being the Accumulation point, KI-5 can be used in acute conditions to stop pain, and is therefore used in acute cystitis or urethritis.

It also stops abdominal pain around the umbilicus and it regulates Blood in the uterus. In particular, it is used for amenorrhoea from Kidney deficiency.

ZHAOHAI KI-6 *Shining Sea*

Nature

Opening point of Yin Heel Vessel.

Action

Nourishes Yin
Benefits the eyes
Calms the Mind
Invigorates the Yin Heel Vessel
Cools the Blood
Benefits the throat
Promotes the function of the uterus
Opens the chest.

Comments

This is a major point with many different functions. First of all, it is the best point on the Kidney channel to nourish Kidney-Yin and is widely used in Yin deficiency. It is also very useful to nourish fluids and moisten dryness, for such symptoms as dry throat and dry eyes.

As was mentioned before, the Yin Heel Vessel carries Yin energy to the eyes to nourish and moisten them, so this point can stimulate the Qi of the Yin Heel Vessel to flow up to the eyes. It is a very important point to use in all chronic eye diseases, particularly in old people with deficiency of Yin.

By nourishing Yin, KI-6 also calms the Mind, in cases of anxiety and restlessness deriving from Yin deficiency. Furthermore, it is used to treat insomnia, as its use brings Yin energy to the eyes and makes them close at night.

By tonifying the Yin and promoting fluids, KI-6 also cools the Blood and is therefore used for skin diseases characterized by Heat in the Blood.

By carrying Yin energy upwards, it moistens and benefits the throat, and is an important point to use for chronic dryness or soreness of the throat deriving from Yin deficiency.

KI-6 also influences the uterus and can be used for amenorrhoea from Kidney deficiency and prolapse of the uterus.

Finally, combined with Neiguan P-6, it opens the chest and moves Qi in the chest, so that it can be used for chest pain.

FULIU KI-7 *Returning Current*

Nature

River point
Metal point
Tonification point.

Action

Tonifies the Kidneys
Resolves Damp
Eliminates oedema
Strengthens the lower back
Regulates sweating.

Comments

This point can tonify the Kidneys in a similar way to KI-3, the only difference being that KI-7 is better to tonify Kidney-Yang.

KI-7 is an important point to resolve Damp in the Lower Burner and to eliminate oedema in the legs.

It can either promote or stop sweating: it is frequently used in combination with Hegu L.I.-4 to cause sweating in attacks of exterior Wind-Cold, and with Yinxi HE-6 to stop sweating from Kidney-Yin deficiency. In the former case the point would be reduced, while in the latter case it would be reinforced.

JIAOXIN KI-8 *Meeting the Spleen channel*

Nature

Accumulation point of the Yin Heel Vessel.

Action

Removes obstructions from the channel
Stops abdominal pain
Removes masses
Regulates menstruation.

Comments

Being the accumulation point of the Yin Heel Vessel, this point can invigorate this vessel and is particularly good to eliminate obstructions along the vessel and dissolve abdominal "masses". These "masses" are due to stagnation of Qi or stasis of Blood and are found in women. The Yin Heel Vessel can move Qi, eliminate Yin excesses and dissolve masses. This point is therefore important for abdominal pain deriving from obstruction and stagnation in the Yin Heel Vessel.

It is also important to regulate menstruation, particularly for menstrual problems deriving from stasis of Blood.

ZHUBIN KI-9 *Guest Building*

Nature

Accumulation point of Yin Linking Vessel.

Action

Calms the Mind
Tonifies Kidney-Yin
Opens the chest
Regulates the Yin Linking Vessel.

Comments

This is an excellent point to calm the Mind in cases of deep anxiety and mental restlessness deriving from Kidney-Yin deficiency. It has a profound calming effect and tonifies Kidney-Yin at the same time.

It also relaxes any tension or feeling of oppression felt in the chest, often with palpitations. Because it tonifies Kidney-Yin, calms the Mind and treats palpitations, this point is particularly indicated in the pattern of "Heart and Kidneys not harmonized".

YINGU KI-10 *Yin Valley*

Nature

Sea point
Water point.

Action

Expels Dampness from the Lower Burner
Tonifies Kidney-Yin.

Comments

This point has two main uses. First of all, in common with the other two Yin Sea points around the knee Yinlingquan SP-9 and Ququan LIV-8, it resolves Dampness from the Lower Burner, and is therefore used for urinary symptoms such as difficulty, pain, and frequency of urination.

Secondly, this point can also be used to nourish Kidney-Yin, but is not as effective from this point of view as Zhaohai KI-6 or Zhubin KI-9.

QIXUE KI-13 *Qi Hole*

Nature

Point of the Penetrating Vessel.

Action

Tonifies the Kidneys and Essence
Removes obstructions from the channel.

Comments

This point has a dual function, one to tonify and one to reduce. First of all, it can be used as a powerful tonification of the Kidneys and the Kidney-Essence (it is also level with Guanyuan Ren-4 which tonifies the Kidneys and Essence). This is due also to its being a point of the Penetrating Vessel which circulates the Kidney-Essence.

On the other hand, the Penetrating Vessel is also responsible for circulation of Qi and Blood in the abdomen and for removing masses and obstructions in abdomen and chest. This point can therefore be used for Excess patterns characterized by abdominal fullness and "masses".

HUANGSHU KI-16 *Vitals Transporting Point*

Nature

Point of the Penetrating Vessel.

Action

Removes obstructions from the channel
Tonifies the Kidneys
Benefits the Heart.

Comments

This point is related to "*Gaohuang*", i.e. the space between the heart and the diaphragm. The Kidney energy goes through this point to connect upwards with the diaphragm and the Heart, hence the name of this point.

This means that this point can be used to tonify the Kidneys, and, at the same time, tonify the Heart and calm the Mind. It is therefore useful when Kidney-Yin is deficient and fails to nourish the Heart.

SHENFENG KI-23 *Mind Seal*

LINGXU KI-24 *Spirit Burial-Ground*

SHENCANG KI-25 *Mind Storage*

Action

Tonify the Kidneys
Calm the Mind.

Comments

These three points can be considered together as they have similar functions. Their names also all relate to "Spirit" or "Mind" and the Heart. These three points are close to the heart, and they can all calm the Mind. They are therefore used to calm anxiety and mental restlessness deriving from Kidney deficiency.

In addition, Shencang KI-25 is an important local point to use for asthma due to Kidney not receiving Qi.

SHUFU KI-27 *Transporting point Mansion*

Action

Stimulates the Kidney function of reception of Qi
Subdues rebellious Qi
Stops cough
Calms asthma
Resolves Phlegm.

Comments

This is an important local point for the treatment of asthma from Kidney deficiency. By stimulating the Kidney to receive and hold Qi down, it will subdue ascending Qi and therefore stop cough and allay asthma.

NOTES

1 This combination of points was first mentiond in the "Gatherings of Eminent Acupuncturists" (*Zhen Jiu Ju Ying* 针灸聚英) by Gao Wu, AD 1529.
2 Spiritual Axis, p 73.
3 The name "*Gaohuang*" is mentioned in the *Zuo Chuan*, historical annals from the Spring and Autumn Period (770-476 BC). This is also the first historical mention of acupuncture. The annals report that a certain prince of Jin was severely ill and a famous doctor was sent for. The text then reports the conversation of two demons inside the prince's body deciding what would be the best place to hide in order to escape the doctor's subtle diagnostic skills. They decide to hide in the region of *Gaohuang* between the heart and diaphragm so that no

therapeutic method, whether acupuncture or herbs, could possibly reach them. Ever since then, the name Gaohuang indicates a chronic disease which is very difficult to cure. A complete account of this reference can be found in Needham J-Lu G D 1980 Celestial Lancets. Cambridge University Press, Cambridge, p 78.

4 Jiao Hui Yuan, Acupuncture Textbook by Hui Yuan (*Hui Yuan Zhen Jiu Xue* 会元针灸学). In: An explanation of the meaning of acupuncture points names, p 167.

5 The Illustrated Classic of Acupuncture Points as Found on the Bronze Model. In: An Explanation of the Meaning of Acupuncture Points names, p 167.

6 Spiritual Axis, p 50.

44 Pericardium and Triple Burner Channels

心包经三焦经

PERICARDIUM CHANNEL

心包经

MAIN CHANNEL PATHWAY

The Pericardium channel originates from the chest and enters the pericardium. It then descends through the diaphragm to the abdomen to communicate with the upper, middle and lower Burner.

A branch from the centre of the chest emerges laterally from the nipple to run along the superficial channel to the axilla and down the medial aspect of the arm to end at the medial side of the middle finger.

A branch from Laogong P-8 links with the Triple Burner channel at the point Guanchong T.B.-1 (Fig. 87).

CONNECTING CHANNEL PATHWAY

The Connecting channel starts from the point Neiguan P-6 and flows up to the chest to the pericardium and heart (Fig. 87A).

TIANCHI P-1 *Heavenly Pond*

Nature

Meeting point of Terminal Yin (Pericardium and Liver).

Comments

This point can be used as a local point for distension and pain of the breast caused by stagnation of Liver-Qi. However, it is hardly ever used for this purpose as it would be very inconvenient to needle in women especially when the breasts are tender and distended.

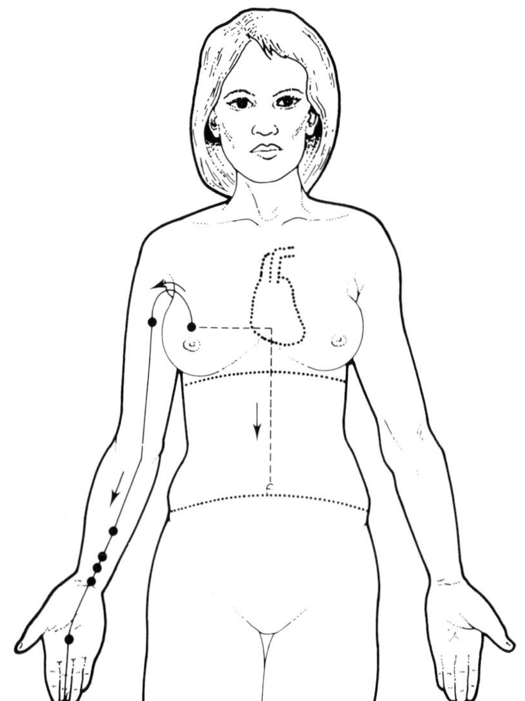

Fig. 87 Pericardium channel

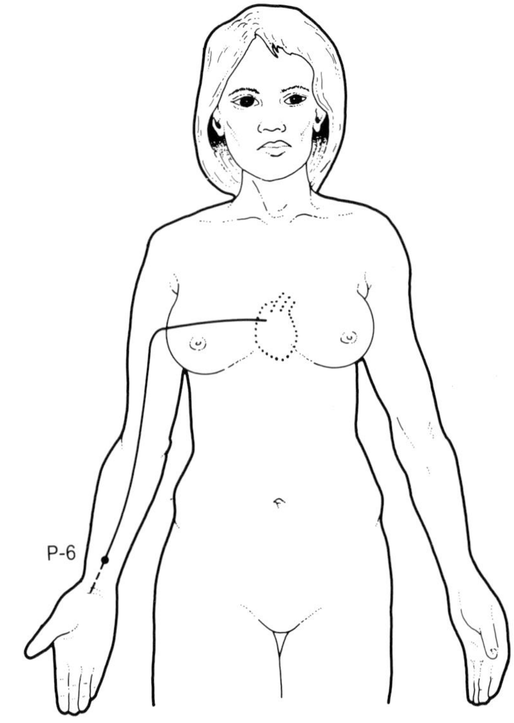

Fig. 87A Pericardium Connecting channel

QUZE P-3 *Marsh on Bend*

Nature

Sea point
Water point.

Action

Pacifies the Stomach
Clears Heat
Cools Blood
Expels Fire-Poison
Opens the orifices
Stops convulsions
Moves Blood and dispels stasis
Calms the Mind.

Comments

This point clears Heat at the Qi level (of the 4-Level Pattern Identification) and is used for acute sun-stroke and Heat in the Intestines. It also clears Heat and cools Blood at the Blood Level and is used for the late stages of febrile diseases with skin eruptions and convulsions.

It stimulates the descending of Stomach-Qi and is used to subdue rebellious Stomach-Qi which manifests with nausea and vomiting.

It clears Heat in the Pericardium during febrile diseases which can cause coma. It also opens the Heart orifices, thus promoting resuscitation.

Besides cooling Blood, it also moves Blood and removes stasis. It is therefore useful in chronic conditions of Blood Heat, when the Heat over a long period of time congeals the Blood and causes stasis. For example, this happens when Blood Heat causes excessive menstrual bleeding. Over a long period of time, the Heat concentrates the Blood and makes it stagnate, giving rise to uterine fibroids.

Finally, P-3 can also be used to calm the Mind, when there is severe anxiety caused by Heart-Fire.

XIMEN P-4 *Cleft Door*

Nature

Accumulation point.

Action

Removes obstructions from the channel
Stops pain
Calms the Heart
Opens the chest
Regulates Blood
Cools the Blood
Strengthens the Mind.

Comments

This is an important point of the Pericardium channel and being the Accumulation point, it is used in acute conditions particularly to stop pain.

P-4 has a special action in calming the Heart and regulating its rhythm, so it is the point of choice to use for arrhythmia and palpitations, particularly in acute cases.

It also regulates the Blood and removes Blood stasis, especially in the chest, so that it is a very important point to use for chest-pain due to stasis of Heart-Blood.

It also cools Blood and can be used for skin diseases caused by Blood Heat.

Finally, P-4 strengthens the Mind in cases of Heart deficiency which may give rise to fears and lack of mental strength.

JIANSHI P-5 *Intermediary*

Nature

River point
Metal point.
Meeting of the three Yin channels of the arm.

Action

Resolves Phlegm in the Heart
Regulates Heart-Qi
Opens the chest
Regulates the Stomach
Clears Heat.

Comments

This is a very important point to resolve Phlegm obstructing the Heart orifices. This is the non-substantial Phlegm obstructing the Heart and "misting" the mental faculties resulting in delirium, aphasia and coma. In acute cases, this happens at the Blood level (of the 4-Level Pattern Identification) of febrile diseases.

In chronic cases, Phlegm obstructing the Heart can cause mental illness, such as manic depression, with periods of deep depression alternating with periods of manic behaviour with incessant talking, uncontrolled activity and reckless behaviour.

In other cases, the same pathology of Phlegm obstructing the Heart can cause epilepsy, with the person losing consciousness during the epileptic fit and foaming heavily from the mouth (which is indicative of Phlegm).

This point regulates Heart-Qi and is used to dispel stagnation of Qi in the chest: it is therefore effective for discomfort of the chest due to stagnation of Qi.

It also has an effect on the Stomach, mostly in subduing rebellious Stomach-Qi which is the cause of nausea and vomiting.

It clears Heart-Fire and can be used for insomnia, tongue ulcers, bitter taste, dry mouth and mental agitation.

Finally, it is an empirical point for malaria.

NEIGUAN P-6 *Inner Gate*

Nature

Connecting point
Opening point of the Yin Linking Vessel.

Action

Opens the chest
Regulates Heart Qi and Blood
Regulates and clears the Triple Burner
Calms the Mind
Regulates the Terminal Yin
Harmonizes the Stomach.

Comments

This is one of the fundamental points of acupuncture with a great number of different functions.

It has a specific action on the chest, and can therefore be used for any chest problems. More specifically it moves Qi and Blood in the chest and is the point of choice for discomfort or pain of the chest due to stagnation of Qi or Blood.

It has a powerful calming action on the Mind and can be used in anxiety caused by any of the Heart patterns.

It also calms the Mind by its indirect action on the Liver (to which the Pericardium is related within the Terminal Yin). It can therefore be used for irritability due to stagnation of Liver-Qi, particularly if combined with anxiety from a Heart pattern.

It is particularly effective in women and is most useful to calm the Mind in women suffering from pre-menstrual depression and irritability. It also promotes sleep.

In addition to its action on the Heart and Liver, it is a major point to affect the Stomach, particularly the upper and middle part of the Stomach. It subdues rebellious Stomach-Qi and is the point of choice to treat nausea and vomiting. It can also be used in most Stomach patterns characterized by epigastric pain, acid regurgitation, hiccup and belching.

As it is the Connecting point of the Pericardium channel, it connects with the Triple Burner channel and is effective in treating neck ache on the occiput, especially in women. Women often suffer from neck ache after a hysterectomy and this point is very effective in treating it.

Finally, owing to its relationship with the Liver and its action of moving Blood, this point indirectly connects with the Blood of the uterus, and can be used to regulate irregular or painful periods.

DALING P-7 *Great Hill*

Nature

Source and Stream point
Earth point
Sedation point.

Action

Calms the Mind
Clears Heat.

Comments

This point's most important function is that of calming the Mind. In this respect, it has all the same functions as Shenmen HE-7. As a matter of fact, historically, Daling P-7 was used as the Source point of the Heart channel. The first chapter of the "Spiritual Axis" lists P-7 as the Source point of the Heart.[1]

In my experience, P-7 is more effective in women and HE-7 more effective in men to calm the Mind. P-7 is also better to deal with the emotional consequences of the breaking-up of relationships.

P-7 also clears Heart-Fire and is particularly important to use when Heart-Fire causes mental problems such as great anxiety and mental restlessness or even manic behaviour.

It is useful to compare and contrast the actions of Shenmen HE-7 and Daling P-7:

SHENMEN HE-7	*DALING P-7*
Both can nourish Heart-Blood and calm the Mind	
More for Deficiency patterns	More for Excess patterns
Not for Warm diseases	Important for Warm diseases, Heat in Pericardium (Nutritive-Qi level)
Gentle action in calming Mind	Better for severe anxiety and mania
Does not open Heart orifices	Opens Heart orifices
Better for men	Better for women
	Especially indicated for emotional upsets deriving from the breaking of relationships

LAOGONG P-8 *Labour Palace*

Nature

Spring point
Fire point.

Action

Clears Heart-Fire
Calms the Mind.

Comments

This is the most effective point on the Pericardium channel to clear Heart-Fire. Being the Spring point, it is a particularly dynamic point to clear Heat. In particular, it has a specific effect in clearing tongue ulcers deriving from Heart-Fire.

It can be used to clear Heart-Fire in chronic situations with mental symptoms, or in acute situations in febrile diseases at the Nutritive Qi level, characterized by Heat in the Pericardium, with high fever and delirium.

ZHONGCHONG P-9 *Centre Rush*

Nature

Well point
Wood point
Tonification point.

Action

Clears Heat
Restores consciousness
Expels Wind.

Comments

This point is mostly used to clear Heat either in chronic conditions with mental symptoms, or in acute cases of exterior Heat at the Qi or Nutritive Qi level.

It also expels interior Wind and restores consciousness and is used in acute Wind-stroke, together with all the other Well points of the hands.

The following is a comparison between Quze P-3, Ximen P-4, Jianshi P-5, Neiguan P-6 and Daling P-7. They can all calm the Mind:

P-3 clears Heat and cools Blood. Its functions of regulating the Intestines and cooling Blood are important.

P-4 regulates the Pericardium and stops pain in acute conditions. Its use in acute conditions with pain is the most important one.

P-5 resolves Phlegm from the Heart, for symptoms of Phlegm misting the Heart.

P-6 opens the chest, calms the Mind and regulates Liver-Qi. Its most important aspects are those of relieving oppression of the chest associated with a Heart pattern, calming anxiety particularly in women and indirectly moving Liver-Qi and its resulting emotional tightness.

P-7 calms the Mind, particularly for emotional problems deriving from difficult relationships. More often used for women than men.

TRIPLE BURNER CHANNEL
三焦经

MAIN CHANNEL PATHWAY

The Triple Burner channel starts at the tip of the ring finger. Running between the 4th and 5th metacarpal bones, it flows to the wrist and up the lateral aspect of the arm between the radius and ulna. It then reaches the shoulder joint and the supraclavicular fossa from where it goes down to the chest to connect with the pericardium. It then descends through the diaphragm to the abdomen to join the middle and lower Burners.

From the chest, a branch goes up to the supraclavicular fossa from where it ascends to the neck and the region behind the ear. It then turns downwards to the cheek and terminates in the infra-orbital region.

From behind the ear, a branch enters the ear, re-emerges in front of the ear and links with the Gall-Bladder channel (Fig. 88).

CONNECTING CHANNEL PATHWAY

The Connecting channel starts at Waiguan T.B.-5 and flows up the arm along the main channel to the shoulder and chest where it links with the Pericardium channel (Fig. 88A).

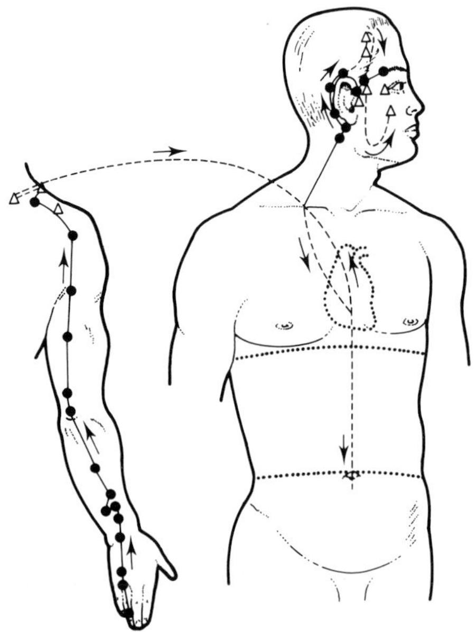

Fig. 88 Triple Burner channel

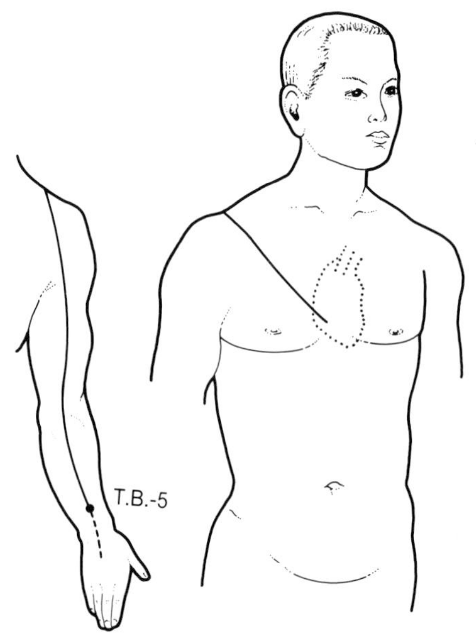

Fig. 88A Triple Burner Connecting channel

GUANCHONG T.B.-1 *Gate Rush*

Nature

Well point
Metal point.

Action

Clears Heat
Expels Wind
Invigorates Blood
Restores consciousness
Stops convulsions.

Comments

This point is used mostly in exterior patterns of invasion of exterior Wind-Heat causing fever, sore throat or earache. The Triple Burner channel is particularly indicated if there is fever and earache.

This point can be used for both the Greater Yang and the Lesser Yang stage of the 6-Stage Pattern Identification.

Being a Well point, it is used to restore consciousness in the acute stage of Wind-stroke.

Finally, it can also be used as a distal point to clear the channel for the treatment of painful and stiff shoulder joint. In this case, it is often bled.

YEMEN T.B.-2 *Fluid Door*

Nature

Spring point
Water point.

Action

Clears Heat
Expels Wind
Benefits the ear
Removes obstructions from the channel.

Comments

Some of the actions of this point in relation to invasions of exterior Wind-Heat are the same as those of Guanchong T.B.-1. In particular, Yemen T.B.-2 has a pronounced action on the ear and is used in cases of earache due to infection of the middle ear (which could accompany invasions of exterior Wind-Heat). It is also effective in treating tinnitus.

It clears interior Heat from the Triple Burner and Gall-Bladder channel especially in relation to the ear, such as in ear infections or tinnitus and deafness from Liver-Fire.

This point is also widely used for Painful Obstruction Syndrome of the fingers.

ZHONGZHU T.B.-3 *Middle Islet*

Nature

Stream point
Wood point
Tonification point.

Action

Clears Heat
Expels Wind
Benefits the ear
Removes obstructions from the channel
Regulates Qi
Lifts the Mind.

Comments

Some of the actions of this point are basically the same as those of Yemen T.B.-2. Zhongzhu T.B.-3, however, is more widely used as it has some additional functions.

It regulates Qi and indirectly affects the Liver, so that it can be used to remove stagnation of Liver-Qi manifesting with hypochondriac pain and mood swings. On a psychological level, it moves Qi and lifts depression deriving from stagnation of Liver-Qi, particularly in combination with Baihui Du-20. It is extremely effective in lifting the Mind when a person is depressed.

YANGCHI T.B.-4 *Yang Pond*

Nature

Source point.

Action

Relaxes sinews
Removes obstructions from the channel
Clears Heat
Regulates the Stomach
Promotes fluids transformation
Benefits Original Qi
Tonifies Penetrating and Directing Vessels.

Comments

This point has many different functions. Firstly, it relaxes sinews and removes obstructions from the channel, which means that it can be used to treat Painful Obstruction Syndrome of the arm and shoulder. It is also very effective for headaches of the occiput deriving from exterior invasion of Wind.

It regulates the function of the Stomach and tonifies the Stomach, especially in conjunction with Chongyang ST-42. The combination of these two points is very effective in tonifying Stomach and Spleen and giving energy if the person is very tired.

The Triple Burner, and particularly the Lower Burner, is in charge of the transformation of fluids, and this point can stimulate this function whenever fluids are not being transformed properly and Dampness accumulates in the Lower Burner. T.B.-4 is particularly effective in this connection combined with Jinggu BL-64: the combination of these two points stimulates the transformation and excretion of fluids in the Lower Burner very effectively.

As explained in chapter 38 dealing with the functions of the Source points, these points are in relation with the Original Qi. In particular, according to the "Classic of Difficulties", Original Qi arises between the Kidneys and spreads to the Internal Organs via the Triple Burner, so that the Triple Burner is like the "ambassador" or "intermediary" for the Original Qi.[2] This point is therefore not just a Source point, but the Source point of the Triple Burner which is the intermediary for the Original Qi. T.B.-4 can thus be used to tonify Original Qi in all chronic diseases when the Kidneys have become deficient and the person's energy is greatly weakened.

Because of its connection with Original Qi, this point is also connected with the Penetrating and Directing Vessels and can be used to regulate their Qi and Blood. It is therefore used in irregular or painful periods and amenorrhoea.

WAIGUAN T.B.-5 *Outer Gate*

Nature

Connecting point
Opening point of the Yang Linking Vessel.

Action

Expels Wind-Heat
Releases the Exterior
Removes obstruction from the channel
Benefits the ear
Subdues Liver-Yang.

Comments

This is a major point to release the Exterior and expel Wind-Heat. It must nearly always be used to expel Wind-Heat when there are such symptoms as fever, sore throat, slight sweating, aversion to cold and a Floating-Rapid pulse. It can be used for the Greater-Yang Stage of the 6 Stages (Wind-Heat type), or the Defensive-Qi Level of the 4 Levels.

In addition, it is the main point to regulate the Lesser Yang, when the pathogenic factor is half in the Exterior and half in the Interior, with such symptoms as alternation of chills and fever, irritability, hypochondriac pain, bitter taste, blurred vision and a Wiry pulse. According to some sources, this point can actually expel all six pathogenic factors, i.e. Wind, Heat, Cold, Dampness, Dryness and Fire.[3]

This point is also a major point for the treatment of Painful Obstruction Syndrome of the arm, shoulder and neck and is, indeed, a general point for Painful Obstruction Syndrome from Wind.

T.B.-5 benefits the ear and can be used whenever there is an ear infection from an invasion of exterior Wind-Heat or tinnitus and deafness from Liver-Fire or Liver-Yang rising.

Finally, T.B.-5 indirectly subdues Liver-Yang rising (because of the Triple Burner connection with the Gall Bladder within the Lesser Yang), and is very much used as a distal point to treat migraine headaches on the temples from rising of Liver-Yang.

ZHIGOU T.B.-6 *Branching Ditch*

Nature

River point
Fire point.

Action

Regulates Qi
Removes obstructions from the channel
Removes obstruction from the Large Intestine
Clears Heat
Expels Wind.

Comments

This point regulates Qi in the three Burners and removes stagnation of Liver-Qi, especially when combined with Yanglingquan G.B.-34. Its area of action is on the flanks.

It clears Heat and can be used at the Qi level of invasions of Heat when there is constipation and abdominal pain.

It expels Wind-Heat in the Blood affecting the skin and is widely used in skin diseases from Wind characterized by red rashes and hives that come and go or move quickly, such as in urticaria. In this case, it is combined with Fengshi G.B.-31.

Because of its action in expelling Wind-Heat, it is a major point for the treatment of herpes zoster when combined with G.B.-31, especially if the skin eruptions are on the flanks.

HUIZONG T.B.-7 *Converging Channels*

Nature

Accumulation point.

Action

Removes obstructions from the channel
Benefits the eyes and ears
Stops pain.

Comments

Like all Accumulation points, this point can be used in acute Excess patterns to stop pain. Its areas of action are the ears, temples and eyebrows. It is also effective for muscle ache in the arms in post-viral fatigue syndrome.

SANYANGLUO T.B.-8 *Connecting Three Yang*

Nature

Meeting point of the three Yang channels of the arm.

Action

Clears Heat
Removes obstructions from the channel.

Comments

This point is mostly used for Painful Obstruction Syndrome of the arm, neck, shoulders and occiput. It is particularly effective when the area of pain involves more than one channel on the Yang surface of arm and shoulders. It relaxes the sinews and relieves pain and stiffness.

TIANJING T.B.-10 *Heavenly Well*

Nature

Sea point
Earth point
Sedation point.

Action

Relaxes tendons
Resolves Dampness and Phlegm
Dispels "masses"
Clears Heat
Dispels stagnation
Regulates Nutritive and Defensive Qi.

Comments

First of all, this point is used in the treatment of Painful Obstruction Syndrome along the course of the channel. It relaxes the tendons and will stop pain and relieve stiffness particularly of the elbow.

It resolves Dampness and Phlegm and is used particularly for external invasions of Damp-Heat manifesting with such symptoms as swelling of glands and tonsils.

It dispels "masses", which is another aspect of its action in resolving Dampness, and is used to treat lymph-glands swelling.

It can be used in invasions of exterior Wind-Cold with prevalence of Wind to regulate Nutritive and Defensive Qi, stop sweating and release the Exterior.

Finally, it can be used in a similar way to Zhongzhu T.B.-3 to relieve stagnation of Liver-Qi and allay depression and mood swings.

NAOHUI T.B.-13 *Shoulder Convergence*

Nature

Point of the Yang Linking Vessel.

Comments

This is used as a local point for pain in the upper arm, and should always be tested for tenderness.

JIANLIAO T.B.-14 *Shoulder crevice*

Comments

This is an important local point for pain and arthritis of the shoulder joint, and should also always be tested for tenderness when choosing between this point and Jianyu L.I.-15.

TIANLIAO T.B.-15 *Heavenly Crevice*

Nature

Point of the Yang Linking Vessel.

Comments

This is an important local point for pain in the shoulder and should always be tested for tenderness. It is nearly always tender in cases of pain and stiffness of the shoulders and it gives very good results when needled with moxa.

YIFENG T.B.-17 *Wind Screen*

Nature

Meeting point of Triple Burner and Gall Bladder.

Action

Expels Wind
Benefits the ears.

Comments

This is a major local point for ear problems. It can be used in all ear problems of exterior or interior origin. It is used in ear infections from exterior Wind-Heat, or for deafness and tinnitus from rising of Liver-Yang or Liver-Fire.

As it expels Wind from the face, it is also used in other problems caused by exterior Wind, such as trigeminal neuralgia and facial paralysis. According to some doctors, needling this point fairly deeply (at least an inch) and obtaining a good needling sensation is an effective treatment for facial paralysis. In such disease it should always be needled if there is tenderness on pressure on the mastoid area.

ERMEN T.B.-21 *Ear Door*

Comments

This is only used as a local point for ear problems (mostly tinnitus and deafness) especially if deriving from rising of Liver-Yang.

SIZHUKONG T.B.-23 *Silk Bamboo Hole*

Action

Expels Wind
Brightens the eyes
Stops pain.

Comments

This point is used as a local point for eye problems and particularly headache around the outer corner of the eyebrow, especially if due to rising of Liver-Yang.

It is also used as a local point in facial paralysis, if there is inability to raise the outer corner of the eyebrow.

NOTES

1 Spiritual Axis, p 3.
2 Classic of Difficulties, p 144.
3 Tai Yi Shen Acupuncture, p 46.

45 Gall-Bladder and Liver Channels

胆经肝经

GALL-BLADDER CHANNEL

胆经

MAIN CHANNEL PATHWAY

The Gall-Bladder channel starts at the outer canthus of the eye. It ascends the forehead and curves downwards to the region behind the ear (at Fengchi G.B.-20). From here it runs down the neck to the supraclavicular fossa.

A branch from the region behind the ear enters the ear. Another branch from the outer canthus meets the Triple Burner channel in the infra-orbital region. It then descends to the neck and the supraclavicular fossa where it meets the main branch. From here, it descends to the chest and, passing through the diaphragm, it enters the liver and gall-bladder. It then runs down the hypochondriac region and the lateral side of the abdomen to reach the point Huantiao G.B.-30.

The main portion of the channel from the supraclavicular fossa goes to the axilla and the lateral side of the chest to the ribs and hip where it meets the previous branch. It then descends along the lateral aspect of the thigh and leg to end at the lateral side of the 4th toe.

From Zulinqi G.B.-41, a branch goes to Dadun LIV-1 (Fig. 89).

CONNECTING CHANNEL PATHWAY

The Connecting channel starts at Guangming G.B.-37 and connects with the Liver channel. Another branch proceeds downwards and scatters over the dorsum of the foot (Fig. 89A).

TONGZILIAO G.B.-1 *Pupil Crevice*

Nature

Meeting point of Small Intestine, Gall Bladder and Triple Burner.

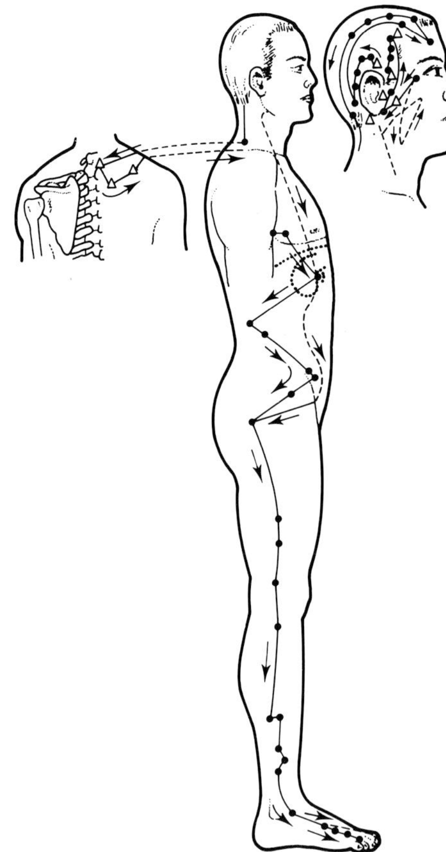

Fig. 89 Gall-Bladder channel.

Action
Expels Wind-Heat
Clears Fire
Brightens the eyes.

Comments

This is a widely used local point for problems of the eyes.

It expels Wind-Heat and is used for conjunctivitis from an exterior attack of Wind-Heat.

It clears Fire and is therefore used as a local point for eye problems caused by Liver-Fire, such as red, dry and painful eyes which may occur with iritis, keratitis or conjunctivitis.

It is also widely used as a local point for migraine headaches around the temple and outer corner of the eye due to rising of Liver-Fire or Liver-Yang.

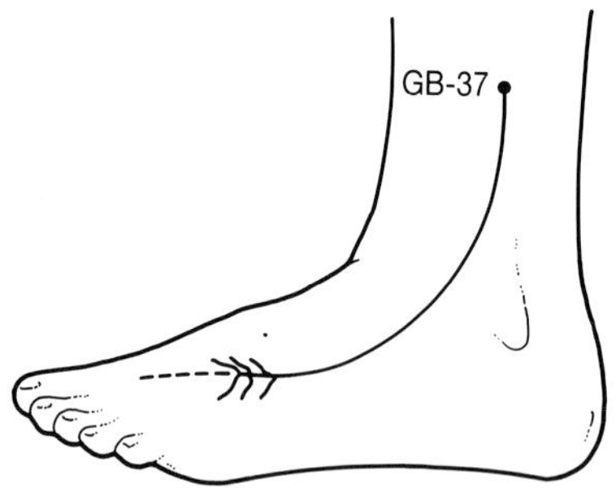

Fig. 89A Gall-Bladder Connecting channel

TINGHUI G.B.-2 *Hearing Convergence*

Action

Removes obstructions from the channel
Benefits the ears
Expels exterior Wind.

Comments

This is an important local point for ear problems. It is very much used as a local point for tinnitus and deafness caused by rising of Liver-Yang or Liver-Fire.

As it expels exterior Wind, in particular Wind-Heat, it is also an important local point for the treatment of otitis media from exterior Wind-Heat.

XUANLU G.B.-5 *Hanging Skull*

Comments

This point is used for disturbance of movement (such as convulsions and spasticity) and speech.[1]

XUANLI G.B.-6 *Deviation from Hanging Skull*

Nature

Meeting point of Gall Bladder, Triple Burner and Stomach.

Action

Removes obstructions from the channel
Benefits the ear.

Comments

This is an important local point for the treatment of migraine headaches on the side of the head due to rising of Liver-Yang, Liver-Fire or Liver-Wind. It should be needled horizontally (i.e. at 15 degree angle) towards the back of the head.

It can also be used for ear problems with pain extending to the side of the head, along the Gall-Bladder channel.

This point is also used in psychiatric practice for disturbance of will power, lack of motivation and speech difficulties.[2]

The name of this point is due to its vicinity to "Hanging Skull" G.B.-5.

SHUAIGU G.B.-8 *Leading Valley*

Nature

Meeting point of Gall-Bladder and Bladder.

Action

Removes obstruction from the channel
Benefits the ears.

Comments

This is widely used as a local point for ear problems from rising of Liver-Yang, such as tinnitus and deafness, and also for migraine headaches of the same origin.

TIANCHONG G.B.-9 *Penetrating Heaven*

Action

Removes obstructions from the channel
Subdues rising Qi
Eliminates interior Wind
Calms spasms
Calms the Mind.

Comments

This is a very important local point of the Gall-Bladder channel. First of all, it is very much used as a local point for migraine headaches on the side of the head from rising of Liver-Yang, Liver-Fire or Liver-Wind. This point helps to subdue the rising of rebellious Qi and conduct it downwards.

Another important function of this point is that of eliminating interior Wind and its manifestations, especially convulsions, epilepsy or contraction of muscles.

Finally, Tianchong G.B.-9 has a powerful mental effect, and is used to calm the Mind. In serious mental disorders such as hypomania, it is an important adjuvant to the treatment with distal points.

It is also used for disturbance of movement (such as ataxia) and speech originating from a central nervous system disease. When used in this way it is combined with Xuanlu G.B.-5, Quchi L.I.-11 and Yanglingquan G.B.-34.[3]

WANGU G.B.-12 *Whole Bone*

Nature

Meeting point of Gall-Bladder and Bladder.

Action

Eliminates Wind
Calms spasms
Subdues rising Qi
Calms the Mind.

Comments

This point can be used as a local point both to expel exterior Wind (such as in otitis media) and to subdue interior Wind (such as in epilepsy).

It is also a local point for migraine headaches along the Gall-Bladder channel on the posterior side of the head deriving from rising of Liver-Yang or Liver-Wind.

Finally, it is frequently used for insomnia from rising of Liver-Yang or Liver-Fire combined with Ganshu BL-18 and Danshu BL-19.

BENSHEN G.B.-13 *Mind Root*

Nature

Point of the Yang Linking Vessel.

Action

Calms the Mind
Eliminates Wind
Gathers Essence to the head
Clears the brain.

Comments

This is a very important point for mental and emotional problems. It is very much used in psychiatric practice for schizophrenia and split personality combined with Tongli HE-5 and Yangfu G.B.-38.[4] It is also indicated when the person has persistent and unreasonable feelings of jealousy and suspicion.

Apart from these mental traits, it has a powerful effect in calming the Mind and relieving anxiety deriving from constant worry and fixed thoughts. Its effect is enhanced if it is combined with Shenting Du-24.

Its deep mental and emotional effect is also due to its action of gathering Essence to the head. The Kidney-Essence is the root of our Pre-Heaven Qi and is the foundation for our mental and emotional life. A strong Essence is the fundamental prerequisite for a clear mind and a happy emotional life. When combined with other points to nourish Essence (such as Guangyuan Ren-4), G.B.-13 attracts Essence towards the head with the effect of calming the Mind and strengthening will power.

G.B.-13 also eliminates internal Wind and is effective for Wind-stroke and epilepsy.

YANGBAI G.B.-14 *Yang White*

Nature

Point of the Yang Linking Vessel.

Action

Eliminates exterior Wind
Subdues rising Qi.

Comments

This is an important and frequently used point to eliminate exterior Wind, especially in the treatment of facial paralysis. When treating facial paralysis, the choice of local points is made according to the area of paralysis, and this is determined by asking the patient to perform certain actions with the facial muscles. If the patient cannot form ridges on the forehead by raising the eyebrows; this point should be used on the affected side. It is needled horizontally downwards.

Yangbai G.B.-14 is also an important local point for unilateral frontal headaches on the Gall-Bladder channel.

LINQI G.B.-15 *Falling Tears*

Nature

Point of the Yang Linking Vessel
Meeting point of Gall-Bladder and Bladder.

Action

Regulates the Mind
Balances the emotions.

Comments

This point has a deep effect on the emotional life and is particularly indicated to balance the moods when the person oscillates between periods of low spirits and periods of elation.

CHENGLING G.B.-18 *Spirit Receiver*

Nature

Point of the Yang Linking Vessel.

Action

Calms the Mind
Clears the brain.

Comments

This point has a deep effect on mental problems such as obsessional thoughts and dementia.

FENGCHI G.B.-20 *Wind Pond*

Nature

Point of the Yang Linking Vessel.

Action

Eliminates Wind (interior and exterior)
Subdues Liver-Yang
Brightens the eyes
Benefits the ears
Clears Heat
Clears the brain.

Comments

This is a major point with many different actions. Firstly, it eliminates both interior and exterior Wind. It is very much used to eliminate exterior Wind-Cold or Wind-Heat, particularly if the headache and stiff neck that are normally caused by exterior Wind are very pronounced. It is combined with Lieque LU-7 to eliminate Wind-Cold, and Hegu L.I.-4 and Waiguan T.B.-5 to eliminate Wind-Heat.

It eliminates interior Wind and is used for such symptoms as dizziness and vertigo. It is the point to use for dizziness and vertigo from internal Wind or from rising of Liver-Yang or Liver-Fire. In all these cases, it is needled with reducing method.

It subdues Liver-Yang or Liver-Fire and is therefore used for occipital headaches deriving from rising of Liver-Yang.

It is a major point for eye problems, particularly if associated with a Liver disharmony. It can be used for blurred vision, cataract, iritis and optic nerve atrophy. It is particularly indicated for eye problems deriving from Liver-Fire, in which case it is needled with reducing method. However, it can also be used with reinforcing method to improve vision and clear the eyes when these are not nourished by deficient Liver-Blood.

It also has an effect on the ears, and can be used for tinnitus and deafness deriving from the rising of Liver-Yang.

Used with reinforcing method, it tonifies Marrow and nourishes the brain, so that it can be used for deficiency of the Sea of Marrow, with such symptoms as poor memory, dizziness and vertigo.

JIANJING G.B.-21 *Shoulder Well*

Nature

Meeting point of Gall-Bladder and Triple Burner
Point of the Yang Linking Vessel.

Action

Relaxes sinews
Promotes lactation
Promotes delivery.

Comments

This point has three main functions. Firstly, it is used as a local point for the treatment of Painful Obstruction Syndrome of the shoulders and neck. It relaxes the tendons and relieves stiffness, and is nearly always tender on pressure.

Secondly, it is an empirical point to promote lactation in nursing mothers.

Thirdly, it is an empirical point to use for many problems of childbirth such as retention of placenta, post-partum haemorrhage or threatened miscarriage.

RIYUE G.B.-24 *Sun and Moon*

Nature

Front Collecting point of the Gall Bladder.

Action

Resolves Damp-Heat
Promotes the function of the Gall-Bladder and Liver.

Comments

This is an important point to resolve Damp-Heat affecting the Gall-Bladder and Liver manifesting with such symptoms and signs as jaundice, hypochondriac pain, a feeling of heaviness, nausea and a sticky yellow tongue coating. In severe cases, it gives rise to the formation of gall stones. To resolve Damp-Heat this point is often combined with Yanglingquan G.B.-34 and Quchi L.I.-11.

It also promotes the free flow of Liver-Qi and is commonly used in the treatment of hypochondriac pain and distension.

JINGMEN G.B.-25 *Capital Door*

Nature

Front Collecting point of the Kidney.

Comments

Although this is the Front Collecting point for the Kidney, it is used more for diagnosis than treatment of Kidney problems.

DAIMAI G.B.-26 *Girdle Vessel*

Nature

Beginning point of the Girdle Vessel.

Action

Regulates the uterus
Resolves Damp-Heat
Regulates the Girdle Vessel.

Comments

This is an important point for gynaecological problems. It regulates the uterus and menstruation and can be used for irregular periods and dysmenorrhoea. It acts on the uterus and menstruation by regulating the Girdle Vessel which harmonizes the Liver and Gall-Bladder.

The Girdle Vessel encircles the leg channels and its dysfunction can lead to impaired circulation in these channels and to the formation of Damp-Heat in the Lower Burner. This point can therefore be used to treat chronic vaginal discharges and vaginal prolapse.

JULIAO G.B.-29 *Squatting Crevice*

Nature

Point of the Yang Heel Vessel.

Action

Removes obstructions from the channel.

Comments

This point is mostly used as a local point for Painful Obstruction Syndrome of the hip. It is often tender on pressure and is very effective in combination with Huantiao G.B.-30.

HUANTIAO G.B.-30 *Jumping Circle*

Nature

Meeting point of Gall-Bladder and Bladder.

Action

Removes obstructions from the channel
Tonifies Qi and Blood
Resolves Damp-Heat.

Comments

This is an important point with different functions extending beyond its obvious use as a local point for the hip joint. It is, of course, an important point for Painful Obstruction Syndrome of the hip and should always be needled in these cases at least two inches deep.

It is also an important point in the treatment of Atrophy Syndrome and sequelae of Wind-stroke: the use of Huantiao G.B.-30 can stimulate the circulation of Qi and Blood to the whole leg and strengthen the sinews.

It is also widely used in the treatment of sciatica with pain extending down the lateral side of the leg. In these cases, G.B.-30 should be needled trying to obtain the radiation of the needling sensation all the way down to the foot. If this is so, then no other point need be used. If the needling sensation extends only part of the way down the leg, other points may be used as a kind of "shuttle", such as Fengshi G.B.-31 or Yanglingquan G.B.-34, depending on how far the needling sensation from G.B.-30 has reached.

Apart from the above, this point also has a general tonifying effect on Qi and Blood of the whole body. This effect is almost as strong as that of Zusanli ST-36.

Finally, G.B.-30 also resolves Damp-Heat in the Lower Burner and can be used to affect the anus or genitals, depending on the direction of the needle. By resolving Damp-Heat, G.B.-30 can be used to treat such symptoms as itchy anus or groin, vaginal discharge and urethritis.

FENGSHI G.B.-31 *Wind Market*

Action

Expels Wind
Relaxes sinews
Strengthens the bones
Relieves itching.

Comments

This is an important point for the treatment of skin diseases due to Wind-Heat moving in the Blood. These would be manifested with the sudden appearance of red rashes which move from place to place, such as in urticaria. It is also used to expel Wind-Heat in herpes zoster, usually combined with Zhigou T.B.-6.

Apart from this, it is widely used for the treatment of Atrophy Syndrome and sequelae of Wind-stroke to relax the sinews and invigorate the circulation of Qi and Blood to the legs.

XIYANGGUAN G.B.-33 *Knee Yang gate*

Comments

This is mostly used as a local point for Painful Obstruction Syndrome of the knee, especially when there is great stiffness and the pain is on the lateral side of the knee. It is particularly indicated for problems of the ligaments and tendons of the knee, as the Liver and Gall-Bladder control sinews.

YANGLINGQUAN G.B.-34 *Yang Hill Spring*

Nature

Sea point
Earth point
Gathering point for sinews.

Action

Promotes the smooth flow of Liver-Qi
Resolves Damp-Heat
Removes obstruction from the channel
Relaxes the sinews
Subdues rebellious Qi.

Comments

This is one of the major points of the body. First of all, it is an extremely important point to promote the smooth flow of Liver-Qi. It is used whenever there is stagnation of Liver-Qi, especially in the hypochondriac area. When combined with other points, it can also affect stagnation of Liver-Qi in other areas, such as the epigastrium (combined with Zhongwan Ren-12) or the lower abdomen (combined with Qihai Ren-6).

By regulating Liver-Qi, it helps to make Stomach-Qi descend and can be used for such symptoms of ascending Stomach-Qi as nausea and vomiting.

It resolves Damp-Heat in Liver and Gall-Bladder, usually combined with Riyue G.B.-24.

It is an important point to relax tendons whenever there are contractions of the muscles, cramps or spasms.

It is also an important point in the treatment of Painful Obstruction Syndrome, Atrophy Syndrome and sequelae of Wind-stroke to invigorate the circulation of Qi and Blood in the legs and relax the tendons.

YANGJIAO G.B.-35 *Yang Crossing*

Nature

Crossing point of the three Yang channels of the leg
Accumulation point of the Yang Linking Vessel.

Action

Relaxes sinews
Removes obstructions from the channel
Stops pain.

Comments

This point is mostly used in acute pain along the Gall-Bladder channel with stiffness and cramp of the leg muscles.

WAIQIU G.B.-36 *Outer Mound*

Nature

Accumulation point of the Gall-Bladder channel.

Action

Removes obstruction from the channel
Stops pain.

Comments

Being the Accumulation point, G.B.-36 is used in all painful conditions of the channel or organ.

GUANGMING G.B.-37 *Brightness*

Nature

Connecting point.

Action

Brightens the eyes
Expels Wind
Clears Heat
Conducts Fire downwards.

Comments

The most important function of this point is that of benefiting the eyes, improving eyesight and eliminating "floaters" in the eyes.

It is particularly effective for eye problems due to Liver-Fire as it conducts Fire downwards.

YANGFU G.B.-38 *Yang Aid*

Nature

River point
Fire point
Sedation point.

Action

Subdues Liver-Yang
Clears Heat
Resolves Damp-Heat.

Comments

This point can be used to clear Liver-Fire and to subdue Liver-Yang. In this connection, it is an important distal point for chronic migraine headaches from rising of Liver-Yang or Liver-Fire.

XUANZHONG G.B.-39 *Hanging Bell*

Nature

Gathering point for Marrow.

Action

Benefits Essence
Nourishes Marrow
Eliminates Wind.

Comments

The most important function of this point is that of nourishing the Kidney-Essence and Marrow. It is used for chronic interior Wind with deficiency of Kidney Yin, especially in old people. The regular use of this point in old people helps to prevent Wind-stroke.

Apart from this, it is an important point to remove obstructions from the Lesser Yang channels from the lateral side of the neck, especially when the neck is very stiff and the person cannot turn the neck from side to side.

QIUXU G.B.-40 *Mound Ruins*

Nature

Source point.

Action

Promotes the smooth flow of Liver-Qi.

Comments

This point can be used to promote the smooth flow of Liver-Qi whenever Liver-Qi is stagnant, causing hypochondriac pain and distension and sighing.

In my experience, this point can be used to strengthen the Gall-Bladder mental aspect, i.e. the strength of character which allows one to take difficult decisions.

ZULINQI G.B.-41 (Foot) *Falling Tears*

Nature

Stream point
Wood point
Opening point of the Girdle Vessel.

Action

Resolves Damp-Heat
Promotes the smooth flow of Liver-Qi
Regulates the Girdle Vessel.

Comments

This point is important to resolve Damp-Heat in the genital region, with such symptoms as chronic vaginal discharge, cystitis and urethritis.

It promotes the smooth flow of Liver-Qi and is effective in treating headaches from stagnation of Liver-Qi or Liver-Fire.

It has an influence in Painful Obstruction Syndrome from Dampness, particularly of the knee and hip.

XIAXI G.B.-43 *Stream Insertion*

Nature

Spring point
Water point
Tonification point.

Action

Subdues Liver-Yang
Benefits the ears
Resolves Damp-Heat.

Comments

This point is effective in treating temporal headaches from rising of Liver-Yang. It is frequently used as a distal point for migraine headaches affecting the Gall-Bladder channel on the temples.

It is also effective for ear problems such as tinnitus from Liver-Yang rising or otitis media from exterior Damp-Heat.

ZUQIAOYIN G.B.-44 (Foot) *Orifice Yin*

Nature

Well point
Metal point.

Action

Subdues Liver-Yang
Benefits the eyes
Calms the Mind.

Comments

This point is used for migraine headaches around the eyes from rising of Liver-Yang. It has an influence on the eyes, and is used for red and painful eyes from the flaring up of Liver-Fire.

It also calms the Mind, in cases of insomnia and agitation deriving from Liver-Fire.

It will be useful to compare the action of the main Gall-Bladder points together with two of the Triple Burner points, as there is some overlap

Table 25 Comparison of Yanglingquan G.B.-34, Qiuxu G.B.-40, Zulinqi G.B.-41, Xiaxi G.B.-43, Zuqiaoyin G.B.-44, Zhigou T.B.-6. and Waiguan T.B.-5.

Point	Action	Area Affected
G.B.-34	Promotes the smooth flow of Liver-Qi	Hypochondrium
G.B.-40	Promotes the mental strength related to a strong Gall Bladder	Ears, temples, head
G.B.-41	Resolves Damp-Heat	Genital area and breast
G.B.-43	Subdues Liver-Yang	Temples and ears
G.B.-44	Calms the Mind	Eyes
T.B.-6	Moves Liver-Qi	Flanks
T.B.-5	Expels Wind-Heat	Temples, ears

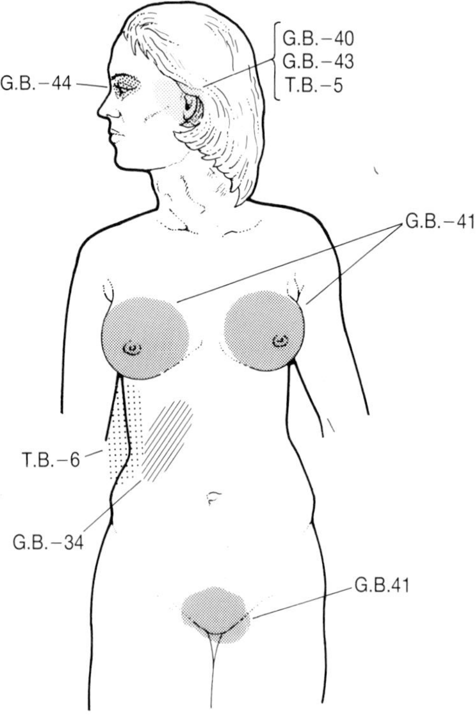

Fig. 90 Areas affected by Gall-Bladder and Triple Burner points

in the area influenced by these two channels (see Table 25 and Fig. 90).

LIVER CHANNEL

肝经

MAIN CHANNEL PATHWAY

The Liver channel starts on the big toe and runs upwards on the dorsum of the foot and medial malleolus and then up the medial aspect of the leg. It then reaches the genital region, curves around the genitalia and goes up to the lower abdomen. Proceeding further up, it curves around the stomach and enters the liver and gall-bladder. It then continues to ascend, passes through the diaphragm and branches out in the hypochondriac and costal region. From here, it ascends to the throat and reaches the eye. Running further upwards it goes to the top of the head to meet the Governing Vessel (Fig. 91).

CONNECTING CHANNEL PATHWAY

The Liver Connecting channel starts at Ligou LIV-5 and connects with the Gall-Bladder channel. Another branch flows upwards on the medial aspect of the leg and thigh to the genitals (Fig. 91A).

DADUN LIV-1 *Big Thick*

Nature

Well point
Wood point.

Action

Regulates menstruation
Resolves Damp-Heat
Promotes the smooth flow of Liver-Qi
Restores consciousness.

Comments

This point has a marked action on the Lower

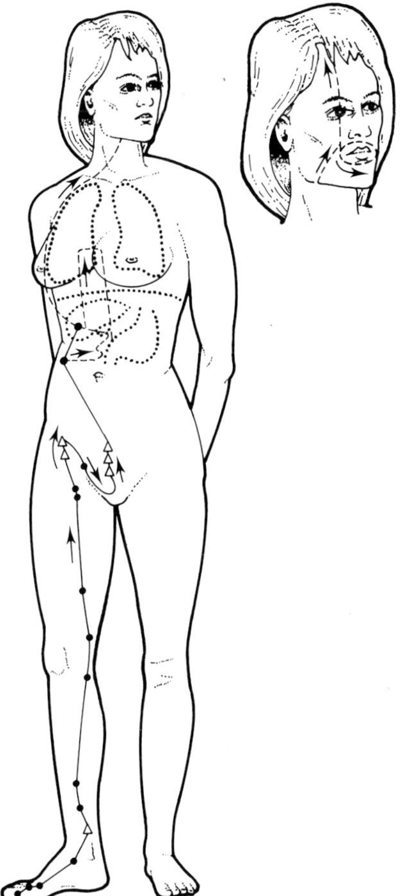

Fig. 91 Liver channel

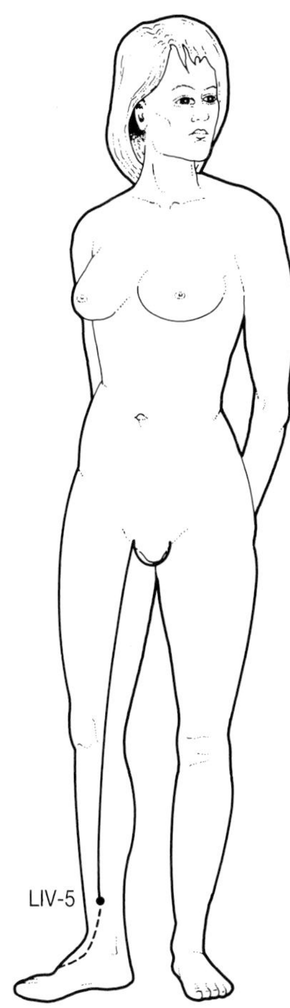

Fig. 91A Liver Connecting channel

Burner. First of all, it stops uterine bleeding from Heat in the Blood (it would not be indicated in uterine bleeding from Qi deficiency).

It resolves Damp-Heat in the Lower Burner and benefits urination so that it can be used for such symptoms as difficult urination, retention of urine, enlarged scrotum, itchy scrotum, vaginal discharge or pruritus vulvae. All these are symptoms of Damp-Heat in the urinary and genital area.

It also promotes the smooth flow of Liver-Qi in the same area, so that it can be used for pain on urination with distension of the hypogastrium due to stagnant Liver-Qi in the hypogastrium.

Finally, it restores consciousness (as many Well points do) and is used in the acute stage of Wind-stroke.

XINGJIAN LIV-2 *Temporary In-between*

Nature

Spring point
Fire point
Sedation point.

Action

Clears Liver-Fire
Subdues Liver-Yang
Cools Blood
Subdues interior Wind.

Comments

This is the point to clear Liver-Fire. It is a point

which is only used to sedate the Liver in Excess patterns, mostly to clear Liver-Fire, but also to subdue Liver-Yang and Liver-Wind.

Since it clears Liver-Fire, it is used for bitter taste, thirst, a red face, headaches, dream-disturbed sleep, scanty-dark urine, constipation, red eyes, a Red tongue with thick yellow coating and a Rapid-Wiry pulse. Since it subdues Liver-Yang, it is widely used to treat migraine headaches from rising Liver-Yang.

As it expels interior Wind, it is used for epilepsy and children's convulsions.

It is also the main point to clear Liver-Fire when this causes cough. The "Simple Questions" in chapter 38 says: "Each of the 5 Yin and 6 Yang organs can cause cough ... cough caused by the Liver is accompanied by pain below the ribs; in severe cases the person is unable to turn the body and has a sensation of swelling and fullness below the ribs".[5] In these cases, Liver-Fire "insults" the Lungs and obstructs the chest causing cough and breathlessness. This is frequently accompanied by Phlegm which combines with the Fire of the Liver to ascend to the chest.

TAICHONG LIV-3 *Bigger Rushing*

Nature

Source point
Stream point
Earth point.

Action

Subdues Liver-Yang
Expels interior Wind
Promotes the smooth flow of Liver-Qi
Calms the Mind
Calms spasms.

Comments

This is a major point. It is an extremely important point of the Liver channel used mostly to sedate the Liver in Excess patterns.

Its main action is that of subduing Liver-Yang, and is very frequently used in migraine headaches from rising of Liver-Yang. It is somewhat gentler than Xingjian LIV-2.

It expels interior Wind and it has a specific action in calming spasms, contraction and cramps of the muscles. Combined with Hegu L.I.-4, it expels Wind from the face, and is used for such symptoms as facial paralysis and tic.

It has a profound calming effect on the mind, and is effective in calming very tense people who are prone to short temper or experience feelings of deep frustration and repressed anger. However, its calming action is not limited to its action on feelings of anger which are typical of a Liver disharmony, as it is also effective in general nervous tension from stress. Its calming action is enhanced when combined with Hegu L.I.-4 : the combination of these four points is called the "Four Gates" (see p. 377).

Needled with reducing method and followed by moxibustion, it can expel Cold from the Liver channel, and treat genital swelling and orchitis in men, or chronic white vaginal discharge in women.

Finally, LIV-3 can also be needled with reinforcing method to nourish Liver-Blood. However, this is a secondary use for it, as this point is used far more often in Excess patterns of the Liver.

It is useful to compare the nature and action of Xingjian LIV-2 and Taichong LIV-3:

LIV-2	*LIV-3*
1 Specific to clear Liver-Fire	Not so much for Liver-Fire, more to subdue Liver-Yang
2 No strong mental effect	Strong mental calming effect
3 Used only to sedate	Can be used to nourish Liver-Blood
4 No specific effect on spasms	Specific effect on spasms
5 Quite a harsh point	Gentler point
6 Mostly to subdue rising Qi	To subdue rising Qi but also to promote the smooth flow of Qi when it stagnates "horizontally" (for example in epigastrium or hypochondrium)
7 Area affected is mostly head, secondarily genitals	Areas affected are head, epigastrium, hypochondrium, abdomen

ZHONGFENG LIV-4 *Middle Seal*

Nature

River point
Metal point.

Action

Promotes the smooth flow of Liver-Qi in the Lower Burner.

Comments

This point is mostly used to promote the smooth flow of Liver-Qi in the Lower Burner and more specifically in the genital and urinary region. It is thus used for urinary symptoms with a feeling of distension in the hypogastrium deriving from stagnation of Liver-Qi.

LIGOU LIV-5 *Gourd Ditch*

Nature

Connecting point.

Action

Promotes the smooth flow of Liver-Qi
Resolves Damp-Heat.

Comments

This point also has a specific affinity for the genital and urinary area. The Liver Connecting channel departs from this point and flows up the inner aspect of the thigh to encircle the genitals. This point can therefore be used for any urinary symptom deriving from stagnation of Liver-Qi, such as distension of the hypogastrium, distension and pain before urination and retention of urine.

It resolves Damp-Heat in this area and is therefore used for vaginal discharge or cloudy urine.

Besides influencing the genital area, this point also affects the throat and is used for stagnation of Liver-Qi in the throat causing the typical sensation of lump in the throat and of being unable to swallow. This sensation is related to emotional tension and it comes and goes according to the emotional state. It is called "plum-stone" sensation in Chinese Medicine, as the person feels as if he or she had an obstruction in the throat.

ZHONGDU LIV-6 *Middle Capital*

Nature

Accumulation point.

Action

Removes obstructions from the channel
Promotes the smooth flow of Liver-Qi
Stops pain.

Comments

This point also has an affinity with the genital and urinary area and has a similar action to Zhongfeng LIV-4 and Ligou LIV-5, the only difference being that it is the Accumulation point and is therefore useful in Excess patterns and acute cases to stop pain. For example, it is a very useful point for acute urinary pain (such as in cystitis) deriving from Damp-Heat and stagnation of Liver-Qi.

XIGUAN LIV-7 *Knee Gate*

Comments

This is used as a local point for Painful Obstruction Syndrome of the knee, particularly if from Wind and when the pain is on the inner aspect of the knee.

QUQUAN LIV-8 *Spring and Bend*

Nature

Sea point
Water point
Tonification point.

Action

Benefits the Bladder
Resolves Dampness from the Lower Burner
Relaxes the sinews
Nourishes Liver-Blood.

Comments

This point's main function is to eliminate Dampness obstructing the Lower Burner for such symptoms as urinary retention, cloudy urine, burning urination, vaginal discharge, pruritus vulvae. It is effective for both Damp-Heat and Damp-Cold.

Used with reinforcing method, it can also nourish Liver-Blood.

ZHANGMEN LIV-13 *Chapter Gate*

Nature

Front Collecting point of the Spleen
Gathering point for the 5 Yin organs.

Action

Promotes the smooth flow of Liver-Qi
Relieves retention of food
Benefits the Stomach and Spleen.

Comments

This point is very much used whenever Liver-Qi stagnates and invades the Stomach and Spleen, preventing Spleen-Qi from ascending (resulting in loose stools and abdominal distension) and Stomach-Qi from descending (resulting in retention of food, belching and fullness in the epigastrium). The use of this point will promote the smooth flow of Liver-Qi and eliminate stagnation, as well as strengthen the Spleen. It is therefore the main point to use whenever Liver and Spleen are not harmonized.

Needled with reinforcing method, this point can also be used to tonify Stomach and Spleen. If moxa is used in addition, it can tonify and warm the Spleen in deficiency of Spleen-Yang.[6]

QIMEN LIV-14 *Cyclic Gate*

Nature

Front Collecting point of the Liver
Point of the Yin Linking Vessel
Meeting point of Spleen and Liver.

Action

Promotes the smooth flow of Liver-Qi
Benefits the Stomach
Cools Blood.

Comments

This point has a similar function to that of Zhangmen LIV-13, the main difference being that this point affects mostly the Stomach, whilst LIV-13 affects more the Spleen.

This point is frequently used whenever Liver-Qi stagnates and invades the Stomach causing

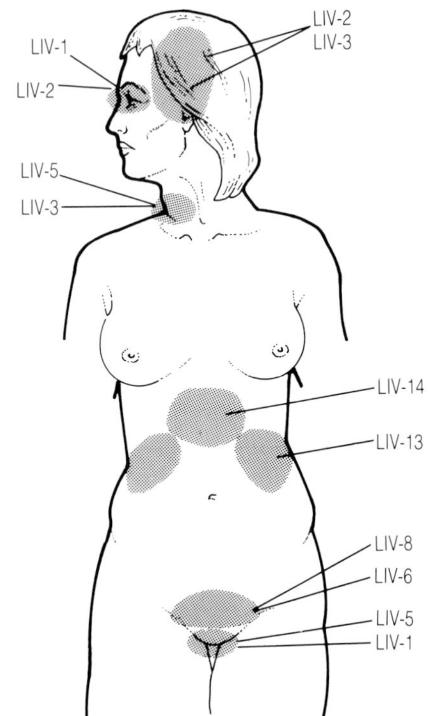

Fig. 92 Areas affected by Liver points.

belching, nausea, vomiting and hypochondriac distension and pain. It harmonizes Liver and Stomach Qi.

LIV-14 has also the effect of cooling Blood as the Liver stores Blood and using its Front Collecting point can eliminate Heat from the Blood.

Figure 92 illustrates the different areas influenced by various Liver-channel points in treatment.

NOTES

1 Dr Zhang Ming Jiu, personal communication, Nanjing 1982.
2 Dr Zhang Ming Jiu, personal communication, Nanjing 1982.
3 Dr Zhang Ming Jiu, personal communication, Nanjing 1982.
4 Dr Zhang Ming Jiu, personal communication, Nanjing 1982.
5 Simple Questions, p 215.
6 Clinical Application of Frequently Used Acupuncture Points, p 742.

Directing Vessel Points 46

任脉

MAIN CHANNEL PATHWAY

The Directing Vessel originates from the uterus (or deep in the lower abdomen in men) and emerges at the perineum. It runs anteriorly to the pubic region and all the way up to the throat along the midline of the body. From the throat it ascends to curve around the lips and up to the eyes to meet the Stomach channel at the point Chengqi ST-1 (Fig. 93).

CONNECTING CHANNEL PATHWAY

This channel starts at the tip of the xyphoid process from the point Jiuwei Ren-15 and spreads over the abdomen (Fig. 93A).

HUIYIN REN-1 *Meeting of Yin*

Nature

Beginning point of Directing, Penetrating and Governing Vessels
Connecting point of the Directing Vessel.

Action

Nourishes Yin
Promotes resuscitation
Resolves Damp-Heat
Benefits Essence.

Comments

This point nourishes Yin and benefits the Kidney-Essence: it is used for incontinence, enuresis and nocturnal emissions deriving from Yin deficiency.

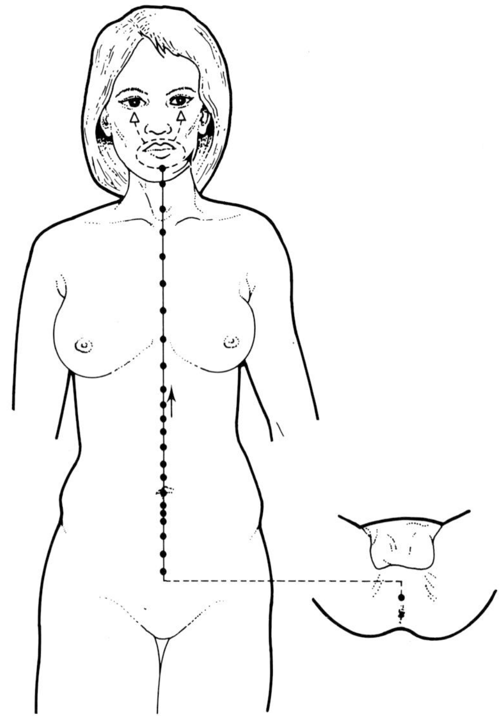

Fig. 93 Directing vessel

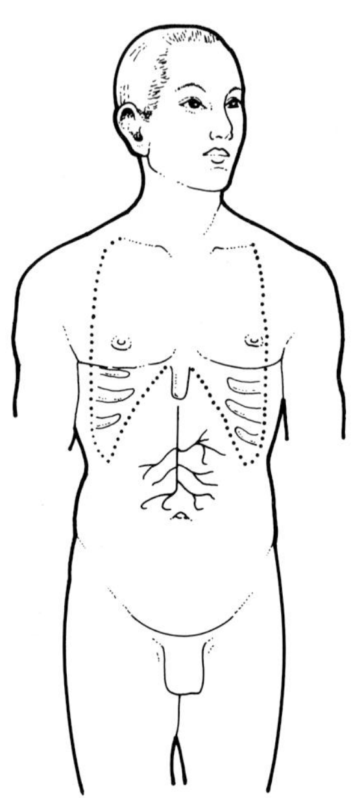

Fig. 93A Directing-Vessel Connecting channel

It resolves Damp-Heat in the genital area and can be used for vaginal discharge, pruritis vulvae or itching of scrotum.

It is an empirical point to promote resuscitation after drowning.

ZHONGJI REN-3 *Middle Extremity*

Nature

Front Collecting point of the Bladder
Meeting point of Directing Vessel, Spleen, Liver, Kidneys.

Action

Resolves Damp-Heat
Promotes the Bladder function of Qi transformation
Clears Heat.

Comments

This is a very important point for genito-urinary problems. It is the main point to affect the Bladder and its function of Qi transformation. It can therefore be used for any urinary problem, particularly acute ones. It is more frequently used with reducing method in Excess patterns. However, it can also be used with reinforcing method to strengthen the Bladder.

This point is specific to resolve Damp-Heat from the Bladder and is used for such symptoms as pain and burning on urination and interrupted flow of urine.

It clears Heat from the Bladder and is usually combined with some distal points for such symptoms as fever, burning on urination and blood in the urine. To treat these problems, it is often combined with Sanyinjiao SP-6, Yinlingquan SP-9 or Ligou LIV-5, depending on the presenting pattern.

GUANYUAN REN-4 *Gate to the Original Qi*

Nature

Front Collecting point of the Small Intestine

Meeting point of Directing Vessel, Spleen, Liver, Kidneys.

Action

Nourishes Blood and Yin
Strengthens Yang
Regulates the uterus
Benefits Original Qi
Tonifies the Kidneys
Calms the Mind
Roots the Ethereal Soul.

Comments

This is an extremely important point. It is one of the most powerful points to tonify Qi and Blood and strengthen the body and mind.

First of all, it can be used to tonify Blood and Yin in any pattern of deficiency of Blood and/or Yin.

Besides this, it also strengthens the Yang, when used with direct moxibustion and can be used in this way to rescue the Yang in the acute stages of Wind-stroke due to collapse of Yang. It can therefore be used in any pattern from deficiency of Yang, particularly Kidney-Yang.

Since it nourishes Blood, it has an effect on the uterus and menstruation, so that it is used for amenorrhoea or scanty periods.

It tonifies the Kidneys and Original Qi and is a very powerful point to strengthen the general level of energy and the Kidneys. It is thus an important point to treat chronic diseases or those patients with poor constitution or emaciation.

Ren-4 point can calm the Mind by nourishing Blood and Yin. It can strengthen the Lower Burner in persons who are very anxious, especially if such anxiety derives from Yin deficiency. This point tonifies the Qi of the Lower Burner, thus rooting Qi downwards and subduing the rising of Qi to the head, which happens in severe anxiety. In this way it has a powerful calming effect.

Finally, Ren-4 can root the Ethereal Soul and can be used for a vague feeling of fear at night which is said to be due to the floating of the Ethereal Soul.

It is useful to compare the action of Zhongji Ren-3 and Guanyuan Ren-4:

REN-3	*REN-4*
Affects the Bladder	Affects the Uterus
Mostly to reduce Excess	Mostly to tonify Deficiency
No general tonic effect	General tonic effect
No effect on the Mind	Powerful calming effect on the Mind
No effect on Original Qi	Tonifies Original Qi
Resolves Dampness	No effect to resolve Dampness
Clears Heat	Can tonify Yang

SHIMEN REN-5 *Stone Door*

Nature

Front Collecting point of the Triple Burner.

Action

Strengthens Original Qi
Promotes the transformation and excretion of fluids in the Lower Burner
Opens the Water passages.

Comments

In order to understand the function of this point, one must recall the role of the Triple Burner in relation to Original Qi. As was discussed in chapters 3 and 13, Original Qi arises from between the Kidneys and spreads to the 5 Yin and 6 Yang organs via the intermediary of the Triple Burner. This point is the Front Collecting point of the Triple Burner and rouses the Original Qi to circulate to all the organs and channels. It can therefore be used to tonify Original Qi in persons with Kidney deficiency and a poor constitution.

Besides this function, this point stimulates the Triple Burner (and specifically the Lower Burner) to transform and excrete fluids, and ensures that the Water passages of the Lower Burner are open. Its use is therefore indicated for oedema of the abdomen, urinary retention, difficult urination, diarrhoea or vaginal discharge.

QIHAI REN-6 *Sea of Qi*

Action

Tonifies Qi and Yang
Regulates Qi
Tonifies Original Qi
Resolves Dampness.

Comments

This is a major point of the body. First of all, it has a powerful tonifying effect on Qi and Yang, especially if used with direct moxibustion. It can be used for extreme physical and mental exhaustion and depression.

Besides tonifying Qi, this point also regulates Qi and dispels stagnant Qi. It can therefore be used for lower abdominal pain deriving from stagnation of Qi. Combined with Yanglingquan G.B.-34, it moves stagnant Qi in the lower abdomen and relieves pain and distension in this area.

Ren-6 tonifies Original Qi and Kidney-Yang, especially if used with direct moxibustion and can therefore be used for such symptoms as chilliness, loose stools, profuse pale urination, physical weakness, mental depression, lack of will power and a feeling that "everything is an effort".

Finally, by tonifying Qi in the lower abdomen, Ren-6 promotes the transformation of Dampness in the Lower Burner in all its manifestations, such as in urinary difficulty, vaginal discharges or loose stools with mucus.

It will be useful to compare the actions of Qihai Ren-6 with those of Guanyuan Ren-4:

REN-4	*REN-6*
Nourishes Blood and Yin	Tonifies Qi and Blood
No effect in moving Qi	Moves Qi and dispels stagnation
Affects Uterus	Affects Intestines
Tonifies the Kidneys	Tonifies the Spleen

YINJIAO REN-7 *Yin Crossing*

Action

Nourishes Yin
Regulates the uterus
Point of the Penetrating Vessel.

Comments

This point's main function is to nourish Yin and Blood and regulate the uterus. It is used in women's menstrual problems, particularly amenorrhoea, scanty periods or infertility.

It is frequently used in women during the menopause to nourish Blood and Yin.

SHENQUE REN-8 *Mind Palace*

Action

Rescues Yang
Strengthens the Spleen
Tonifies Original Qi.

Comments

This point's main function is to strongly tonify Yang. It is used to rescue Yang in the acute stage of Wind-stroke of the flaccid type characterized by collapse of Yang.

In other situations it can be used for severe deficiency of Yang with internal Cold and extreme weakness. This point is used with indirect moxibustion after filling the navel with salt.

It also strengthens Spleen-Yang and is particularly used for chronic diarrhoea from Spleen-Yang deficiency.

SHUIFEN REN-9 *Water Separation*

Action

Promotes the transformation of fluids
Controls the Water passages.

Comments

This is a very important point to promote the transportation, transformation and excretion of fluids in all parts of the body. It is used whenever there is Dampness, Phlegm or oedema. In particular, it is used for ascites (abdominal oedema).

XIAWAN REN-10 *Lower Epigastrium*

Nature

Meeting of Directing Vessel and Spleen.

Action

Promotes the descending of Stomach-Qi
Relieves stagnation of food
Tonifies the Spleen.

Comments

This is a useful point that combines a tonifying action on the Spleen and Stomach with a moving action in relation to Stomach-Qi. In particular, it promotes the descending of Stomach-Qi and is therefore useful for retention of food in the Stomach with such symptoms as abdominal distension, feeling of fullness after eating and sour regurgitation.

It also promotes the passage of food from the Stomach to the Intestines and removes obstructions.

This is one of three points that are in control of the three parts of the epigastrium. If one divides the epigastric area in three equal parts, Shangwan Ren-13 controls the upper part, Zhongwan Ren-12 the middle part, and Xiawan Ren-10 the lower part. From a Western anatomical point of view one can say that Ren-13 controls the *fundus* (upper part) of the stomach and oesophagus, Ren-12 the *body* (middle part) of the stomach, and Ren-10 the *pylorus* (lower part) of the stomach and the duodenum (Fig. 94).

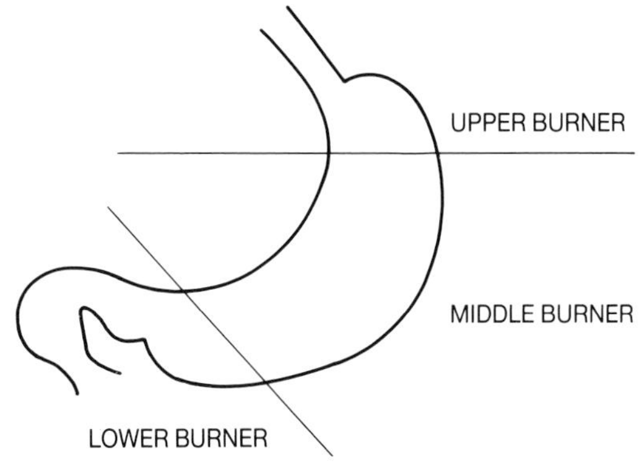

Fig. 94 Three divisions of the Stomach

Each of these three points can be used to affect the relevant part of the stomach with their related disorders. Thus Ren-10 is effective in stimulating the descending of Stomach-Qi, i.e. in promoting the movement of food down the pylorus and duodenum. Ren-12 affects the stomach digestion itself, and Ren-13 affects the oesophagus and stops hiccup, nausea and belching by subduing rebellious Stomach-Qi.

JIANLI REN-11 *Building Mile*

Action

Promotes the rotting and ripening of the Stomach
Stimulates the descending of Stomach-Qi.

Comments

This point is widely used for Stomach problems to promote digestion and stimulate the descending of Stomach-Qi. It is therefore used for a feeling of fullness and distension in the epigastrium, nausea, vomiting and epigastric pain. It is better for Excess patterns.

ZHONGWAN REN-12 *Middle of Epigastrium*

Nature

Front Collecting point of the Stomach
Gathering point for the Yang Organs
Front Collecting point of the Middle Burner.

Action

Tonifies Stomach and Spleen
Resolves Dampness
Regulates Stomach-Qi.

Comments

This is a major point for any Stomach problem. Although it can be used for practically any digestive system condition, it is best for Deficiency patterns (as opposed to Jianli Ren-11 and Shangwan Ren-13, which are better for Excess patterns).

Firstly, it tonifies Stomach and Spleen Qi,

especially if combined with Zusanli ST-36. It has a gentle action and is not a strong tonifying point. It can be used in any Deficiency pattern of Stomach and Spleen, with such symptoms and signs as lack of appetite, tiredness and dull epigastric pain relieved by eating.

It is the best point to use, particularly with moxa, for Empty-Cold patterns of the Stomach and Spleen. This could be used directly on the point with moxa cones, or the point can be heated with a moxa stick, or a "moxa box" can be applied on the area around the point. The moxa box is a wooden box without bottom with a metal griddle about 1/3 of the way down from the upper edge. Loose moxa is placed on the metal griddle and lit and a loose lid is placed over the box. This method of moxibustion is excellent for Empty-Cold conditions of Stomach and Spleen (Fig. 95).

Another important use of Ren-12 is to resolve Dampness. It does so by tonifying the Spleen function of transportation and transformation of fluids. It is very widely used in any pattern involving Dampness in any part of the body.

Finally, it also subdues rebellious Stomach-Qi (i.e. Stomach-Qi ascending instead of descending), but it is not as effective as Shangwan Ren-13 for this function.

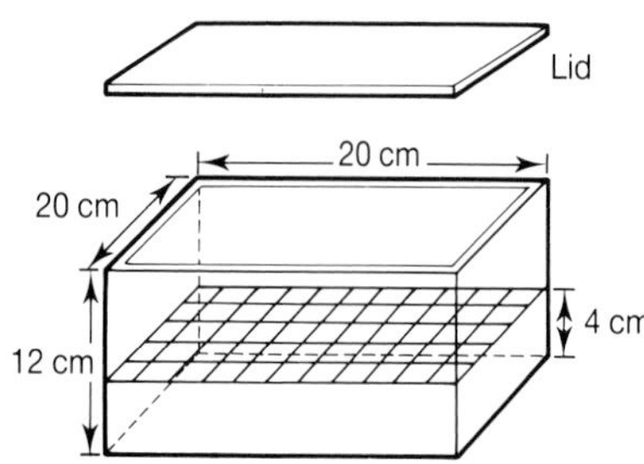

Fig. 95 Moxa box

SHANGWAN REN-13 *Upper Epigastrium*

Action

Subdues rebellious Stomach-Qi.

Comments

This is the best point to subdue rebellious Stomach-Qi, i.e. Stomach-Qi ascending, causing such symptoms as hiccup, belching, nausea, vomiting and a feeling of fullness in the upper epigastrium.

It is used mostly in Excess patterns of the Stomach.

JUQUE REN-14 *Great Palace*

Nature

Front Collecting point of the Heart.

Action

Subdues rebellious Stomach-Qi
Calms the Mind
Clears the Heart.

Comments

This point acts on the Stomach and on the Heart. It subdues rebellious Stomach-Qi in the same way as Shangwan Ren-13, and it is ideally indicated for digestive problems with rebellious Stomach-Qi of an emotional origin, as it treats both Stomach and Heart.

It clears Heart-Fire and calms the Mind and is frequently used for the pattern of Phlegm-Heat misting the Heart and leading to mental symptoms.

JIUWEI REN-15 *Dove Tail*

Nature

Connecting point of the Directing Vessel
Source point of the 5 Yin organs.

Action

Calms the Mind
Benefits Original Qi.

Comments

This is a very important and powerful point to calm the Mind. According to chapter 1 of the "Spiritual Axis", it is the source point of all the

Yin organs, which means that it affects the Original Qi of all Yin organs.[1]

This point nourishes all Yin organs and it calms the Mind particularly in Deficiency of Yin. It has a very powerful calming action in severe anxiety, worry, emotional upsets, fears or obsessions.

The Connecting channel of the Directing Vessel starts at this point which controls it. From this point, the Connecting Vessel branches out in numerous small branches fanning out over the abdomen. When the Connecting Vessel is empty there is itching of the abdomen, when it is in Excess there is pain of the abdomen. Ren-15 can be used for Empty or Full conditions of the Connecting channel.

This point is located at the tip of the xyphoid process which is commonly known as "dove-tail" in China, hence the name of the point.

SHANZHONG (OR TANZHONG) REN-17
Middle of Chest

Nature

Front Collecting point of the Pericardium
Front Collecting point of the Upper Burner
Gathering point for Qi
Point of the Sea of Qi.

Action

Tonifies Qi
Regulates Qi
Dispels fullness from the chest
Clears the Lungs
Resolves Phlegm
Benefits the diaphragm and the breasts.

Comments

This is a very important point to tonify Qi: it is both the Gathering point for Qi and a point of the Sea of Qi. It tonifies the Qi of the chest, which is related to Heart and Lungs.

Thus this point is used to tonify Qi, but only in relation to Lung-Qi and its action in dispersing and descending Qi. If the deficiency of Qi is due to weakness of the Stomach or Spleen, this point alone would not be enough to tonify Qi, but other points would have to be used, such as Zusanli ST-36, Zhongwan Ren-12 and Qihai Ren-6.

Besides tonifying Qi it also regulates Qi and dispels stagnation of Qi in the chest. It is therefore used in any condition of stagnation of Qi in the chest, with such symptoms as a feeling of constriction or tightness of the chest, breathlessness and pain in the chest.

Ren-17 dispels fullness from the chest and helps breathing. It is therefore used for breathlessness from any origin, whether it is from Lung-Qi or Heart-Qi deficiency or from obstruction of the chest by Phlegm.

This point also stimulates the Lung descending function and is thus used in chronic cough. It also resolves Phlegm from the Lungs, and is therefore used for chronic bronchitis.

Finally, it benefits the diaphragm and can be used to treat hiatus hernia. It also affects the breasts and can be used to treat insufficient lactation from deficiency of Qi and Blood.

TIANTU REN-22 *Heaven Projection*

Nature

Point of the Yin Linking Vessel.

Action

Stimulates the descending of Lung-Qi
Resolves Phlegm
Clears Heat
Stops cough
Benefits the throat
Soothes asthma.

Comments

This point stimulates the descending of Lung-Qi and is widely used in both acute and chronic cough and asthma.

It resolves Phlegm in the throat and lungs and promotes the expelling of sputum. It is used in acute situations such as acute bronchitis with profuse sputum, or chronic retention of Phlegm in the throat.

It clears Lung-Heat and is used in acute invasions of Wind-Heat in the Lungs both at the exterior or interior stage, with a sore throat.

LIANQUAN REN-23 *Corner Spring*

Nature

Point of Yin Linking Vessel.

Action

Dispels interior Wind
Promotes speech
Clears Fire
Resolves Phlegm
Subdues rebellious Qi.

Comments

This point is mostly used for aphasia or slurred speech following Wind-stroke. It affects the tongue directly and can be used in conjunction with Tongli HE-5 for speech difficulties or aphasia.

It is also used for local throat problems such as nodules on the vocal cords.

CHENGJIANG Ren-24 *Saliva Receiver*

Action

Expels exterior Wind.

Comments

This point is mostly used as a local point for exterior Wind invading the face and causing facial paralysis. It is used for paralysis of the mouth.

NOTES

1 Spiritual Axis, p 3.

Governing Vessel Points 47

督脉

MAIN CHANNEL PATHWAY

The Governing Vessel originates from the uterus (or deep inside the lower abdomen in men) and goes to the perineum where it emerges. It then ascends on the midline all the way up the back and neck to Fengfu Du-16 from where it enters the brain. It then ascends to the vertex and down the front of the face to the upper lip (Fig. 96).

CONNECTING CHANNEL PATHWAY

After separating from the point Changjiang Du-1, the Connecting channel flows upwards along both sides of the spine to the occiput from where it scatters over the top of the head. At the scapulae, a branch joins the Bladder channel and the upper spine (Fig. 96A).

CHANGQIANG DU-1 *Long Strength*

Nature

Connecting point of the Governing Vessel.

Action

Regulates Governing and Directing Vessels
Resolves Damp-Heat
Calms the Mind.

Comments

This is the beginning and Connecting point of the Governing Vessel. Being the Connecting point, it connects with the Directing Vessel. It can therefore be used to eliminate obstructions from both the Directing and the Governing Vessel.

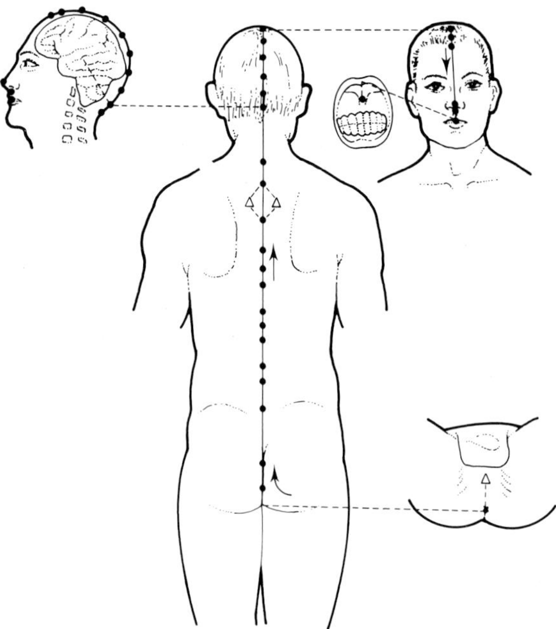

Fig. 96 Governing Vessel

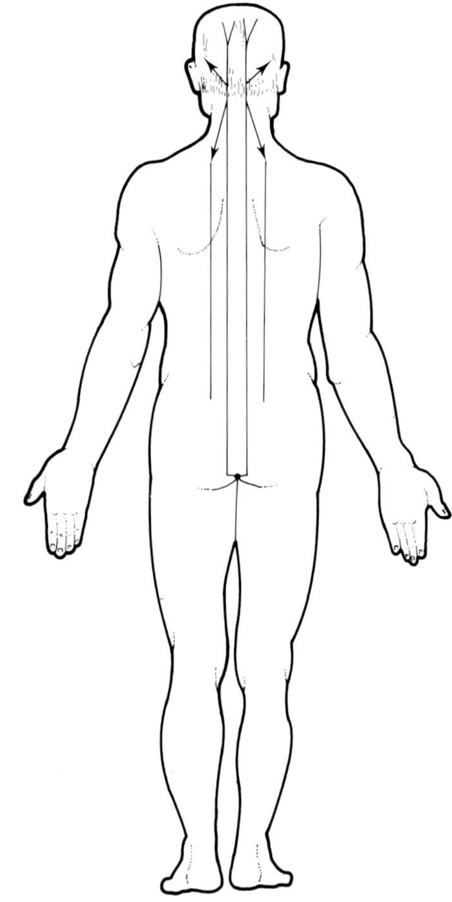

Fig. 96A Governing-Vessel connecting channel

It is very much used as a local point for prolapse of the anus. It also resolves Damp-Heat in the anus and is therefore used for haemorrhoids.

Being at the lowermost end of the Governing Vessel, Du-1 can be used to affect the top part, i.e. the brain. It is therefore used to calm the Mind in mental diseases characterized by agitation and hypomania.

YAOSHU DU-2 *Transporting Point of Lower Back*

Action

Extinguishes interior Wind
Calms spasms and convulsions
Strengthens the lower back.

Comments

This is an important point to eliminate interior Wind and its manifestations, particularly spasms and convulsions. For this reason, this is a major point to use to treat epilepsy. When used for epilepsy, it should be needled obliquely upwards, trying to obtain the needling sensation to travel upwards as far as possible.

Besides this, it can be used as a local point in chronic sacral backache from Kidney-Yang deficiency.

YAOYANGGUAN DU-3 *Lumbar Yang Gate*

Action

Strengthens the lower back
Tonifies Yang
Strengthens the legs.

Comments

This point is very frequently used as a local

point in lower back ache, particularly if due to Kidney-Yang deficiency. It is also especially indicated when the backache radiates to the legs.

Besides strengthening the lower back by tonifying Kidney-Yang, it also strengthens the legs, and is an important point to use for weakness of the legs in Atrophy Syndrome.

MINGMEN DU-4 *Gate of Life*

Action

Tonifies Kidney-Yang
Nourishes Original Qi
Warms the Gate of Vitality
Expels Cold
Strengthens the lower back
Benefits Essence.

Comments

This is the most powerful point to strengthen Kidney-Yang and all the Yang energies in general, especially if used with moxa. It tonifies and warms the Fire of the Gate of Vitality. It is therefore used for Kidney-Yang deficiency with such symptoms as chilliness, abundant-clear urination, tiredness, lack of vitality, depression, weak knees and legs, a Pale tongue and a Deep-Weak pulse. If this point is used with moxa, caution must be exercised, as it is a very warming point. One must therefore make sure not only that there is indeed a deficiency of Kidney-Yang, but also that there is internal Cold. A person may suffer from deficiency of Kidney-Yang, but also have some internal Heat somewhere else in the body (e.g. Damp-Heat in the Intestines). In such a case, this point would not be indicated as it would aggravate the Heat.

Original Qi is related to the Pre-Heaven Qi and to the person's constitution and basic vitality. This point strengthens Original Qi and is therefore indicated for chronic weakness on a physical and mental level.

It also benefits the Yang aspect of the Kidney-Essence and is indicated in all sexual disorders due to weakness of Essence, such as impotence, premature ejaculation or nocturnal emissions.

Du-4 is very effective in strengthening the lower back and knees and is indicated in chronic lower back ache deriving from deficiency of Kidney-Yang.

Finally, Du-4 is specific to eliminate interior Cold deriving from Yang deficiency. This could be in the Spleen, manifesting with chronic diarrhoea, in the Bladder, manifesting with profuse-clear urination, incontinence or enuresis, in the Intestines, manifesting with abdominal pain, or in the Uterus, manifesting with dysmenorrhoea or infertility.

JINSUO DU-8 *Tendon Spasm*

Action

Relaxes the sinews
Eliminates interior Wind.

Comments

As the name clearly implies, this point eliminates interior Wind and its manifestations. i.e. convulsions, muscle spasms, tremor or epilepsy.

ZHIYANG DU-9 *Reaching Yang*

Action

Regulates Liver and Gall Bladder
Moves Qi
Opens the chest and diaphragm
Resolves Damp-Heat

Comments

This point is related to the Liver and Gall-Bladder and promotes the smooth flow of Liver-Qi. It is used for hypochondriac pain and distension.

It moves Qi in general and is used for stagnation of Qi in the Middle Burner.

It affects the chest and diaphragm and resolves stagnation of Qi in these areas which give rise to a feeling of distension or oppression, hiccup and sighing.

Finally, it resolves Damp-Heat in the Gall-Bladder and Liver and is indicated for jaundice.

SHENDAO DU-11 *Mind Way*

Action

Regulates the Heart
Calms the Mind.

Comments

This point is on the same level as Xinshu BL-15 the Back Transporting point of the Heart, and its action mostly extends to the Heart. It clears Heart-Fire and calms the Mind, and is usually indicated for Excess patterns of the Heart.

SHENZHU DU-12 *Body Pillar*

Action

Eliminates interior Wind
Calms spasms
Tonifies Lung-Qi
Strengthens the body.

Comments

This point has two distinct functions according to whether it is reduced or reinforced. When used with reducing method it eliminates interior Wind and calms spasms, convulsions and tremors. It is also used for epilepsy.

When used with reinforcing method, it tonifies Lung-Qi (it is at the same level as the Back Transporting point of the Lungs Feishu BL-13) and generally strengthens the body. It is used to tonify the Lungs and to strengthen the body after a debilitating chronic illness.

TAODAO DU-13 *Kiln Way*

Nature

Meeting of Governing Vessel and Bladder.

Action

Clears Heat
Releases the Exterior
Regulates the Lesser Yang.

Comments

This point is mostly used to release the Exterior and clear Wind-Heat. It is used in the beginning stages of an attack of Wind-Heat.

In particular, it is effective to eliminate Heat at the Lesser Yang stage of the 6-Stage Pattern Identification, the cardinal sign of which is the alternation of chills and fever.

DAZHUI DU-14 *Big Vertebra*

Nature

Meeting point of Governing Vessel, Bladder, Gall Bladder and Stomach.

Action

Clears Heat
Releases the Exterior
Expels Wind
Regulates Nutritive and Defensive Qi
Clears the mind
Tonifies Yang.

Comments

This point can have opposite effects according to the needling method used. When used with a reducing method it releases the Exterior and is used in exterior attacks of Wind-Heat: this point will release the Exterior and eliminate Wind-Heat. It also regulates Nutritive and Defensive Qi when the person has been attacked by exterior Wind and is sweating.

It also clears interior Heat, and can be used in virtually any pattern of interior Heat.

If used with reinforcing method and, in particular, with direct moxa, it tonifies the Yang and can be used in any interior pattern of Yang deficiency. In particular, it tonifies Heart-Yang. Since it is also the meeting point of all the Yang channels which transport clear Yang upwards to the head, this point can also clear the mind and stimulate the brain.

YAMEN DU-15 *Gate to Dumbness*

Nature

Point of the Yang Linking Vessel.

Action

Clears the mind
Stimulates speech.

Comments

This point's main action is that of stimulating speech. It is used to promote the faculty of speech in children with speech difficulties or adults after a Wind-stroke.

Used with reinforcing method, it also nourishes the brain and clears the mind.

Many extraordinary claims were made during the Cultural Revolution in China regarding the effect of this point in treating deaf-mute children. Chinese doctors are now admitting that most of these claims were exaggerated if not outright false.

FENGFU DU-16 *Wind Palace*

Nature

Point of the Yang Linking Vessel
Point of the Sea of Marrow.

Action

Eliminates Wind
Clears the mind
Benefits the brain.

Comments

This point eliminates both exterior and interior Wind. It can therefore be used for exterior attacks of Wind-Cold or Wind-Heat, as well as for patterns of interior Wind, such as in Wind-stroke, epilepsy or severe giddiness.

It is a point of the Sea of Marrow. Marrow fills up the brain, and this point can clear the mind and stimulate the brain.

NAOHU DU-17 *Brain Window*

Nature

Meeting point of Governing Vessel and Bladder.

Action

Eliminates Wind
Benefits the brain
Clears the mind.

Comments

This point is used mostly to subdue interior Wind affecting the brain. It is therefore indicated for epilepsy, Wind-stroke and severe giddiness.

HOUDING DU-19 *Posterior Vertex*

Action

Calms the Mind.

Comments

This point has a powerful calming effect on the Mind and is very often used in severe anxiety, especially in combination with Jiuwei Ren-15.

BAIHUI DU-20 *Hundred Meetings*

Nature

Meeting point of all the Yang channels
Point of the Sea of Marrow.

Action

Clears the mind
Lifts the spirit
Tonifies Yang
Strengthens the ascending function of the Spleen
Eliminates interior Wind
Promotes resuscitation.

Comments

This is a meeting point of all the Yang channels

which carry clear Yang to the head: it therefore has a powerful effect in stimulating the ascending of Yang and clearing of the mind. It also has a good effect in lifting the spirits when the person is depressed.

When used with direct moxa, it tonifies Yang and strengthens the ascending function of the Spleen, and is therefore used for prolapse of the internal organs, such as stomach, uterus, bladder, anus or vagina.

When using this point with moxa to raise the Yang, caution must be exercised to make sure that there are no Heat symptoms at all. Also, this point should not be stimulated with moxa if the person suffers from high blood pressure.

When used with reducing method, it eliminates interior Wind, and can be used for giddiness.

Finally, it promotes resuscitation when the person is unconscious, especially combined with Renzhong Du-26 and Neiguan P-6.

SHANGXING DU-23 *Upper Star*

Action

Opens the nose.

Comments

This point is mostly used for chronic nose disorders such as allergic rhinitis or sinusitis, to open the nose and resolve Phlegm.

SHENTING DU-24 *Mind Courtyard*

Nature

Meeting point of Governing Vessel and Stomach.

Action

Calms the Mind.

Comments

This is a very important and powerful point to calm the Mind. It is frequently combined with Benshen G.B.-13 for severe anxiety and fears.

It is also used in psychiatric practice for schizophrenia and split thoughts.

RENZHONG DU-26 *Middle of Person*

Action

Promotes resuscitation
Benefits the lumbar spine.

Comments

This point is used to promote resuscitation when the person is unconscious.

An empirical use of this point is as a distal point for acute sprain of the lower back, but only when the pain is on the spine itself. In these cases it is usually reduced, while the patient is standing and gently bending backwards and forwards.

Extra Points 48

经外奇穴

YINTANG *Seal Hall*

Location

On the midline of the body in between the eyebrows.

Action

Eliminates Wind
Stops convulsions
Calms the Mind.

Comments

This point eliminates interior Wind and its manifestations particularly convulsions. It is therefore used at the late stages of children's febrile diseases.
More commonly in everyday practice, Yintang is used to calm the Mind and allay anxiety.

TAIYANG *Greater Yang*

Location

In a depression 1 *cun* posterior to the midpoint between the lateral end of the eyebrow and the outer canthus.

Action

Eliminates Wind
Clears Fire.

Comments

This point is very frequently used as a local point for headaches due to rising of Liver-Yang or Liver-Fire.

It can also be used for eye problems due to Heat, either exterior as in Wind-Heat or interior as in Liver-Fire.

BAXIE *Eight Pathogenic Factors*

Location

On the dorsum of the hand, on the webs between the five fingers of both hands.

Action

Relax the sinews
Expel Wind-Damp
Invigorate Blood.

Comments

These points are very frequently used for Painful Obstruction Syndrome of the hand and fingers. They eliminate Wind and Damp and relax the tendons.

They also move Blood in the hand and fingers and are therefore used for chronic Atrophy Syndrome of the hands.

BAFENG *Eight Winds*

Location

On the dorsum of the foot, on the webs between the five toes, proximal to the margins of the webs.

Action

Same as Baxie.

Comments

These points are used in a similar way to Baxie for Painful Obstruction Syndrome of the feet.

ZIGONG *Palace of Child*

Location

On the lower abdomen, 3 *cun* lateral to Zhongji Ren-3.

Action

Tonifies and warms Original Qi
Regulates menstruation
Calms the fetus.

Comments

This point is used to tonify the Kidneys and regulate menstruation. It is expecially indicated for menorrhagia, metrorrhagia and infertility in women.

YUYAO *Fish spine*

Location

In the middle of the eyebrow.

Action

Clears Heat
Removes obstructions from the channel
Brightens the eye.

Comments

This point is used mostly for eye disorders, such as blurred vision or floaters, particularly deriving from Liver-Blood deficiency.

SIFENG *Four cracks*

Location

On the palmar surface, in the transverse creases of the proximal interphalangeal joints of the four fingers (excluding the thumb).

Action

Expel Wind

Resolve Dampness
Promote digestion.

Comments

These points are mostly used in young children to promote digestion. The points should be needled and then a yellow fluid extracted from them. However, they are effective also if there is no yellow fluid coming out.

SHIXUAN *Ten declarations*

Location

On the tips of the ten fingers, about 0.1 *cun* distal to the nails.

Action

Clear Heat
Subdue interior Wind
Open the orifices.

Comments

These points are used in acute situations when the person is unconscious in cases of Wind-stroke.

XIYAN *Knee eyes*

Location

Two points in the depressions medial and lateral to the patellar ligaments. The lateral Xiyan is identical to Dubi ST-35.

Action

Expel Wind-Damp
Benefit the knees.

Comments

These are important local points for Painful Obstruction Syndrome of the knees, especially when the pain is in the front of the knee or deep inside the joint.

The needle should be inserted obliquely slightly upwards and medially towards the centre of the joint to a depth of at least 0.25 *cun*.

These points give particularly good results if moxa is burned on the needles.

JINGGONG *Palace of Essence*

Location

On the back, 0.5 *cun* lateral to the point Zhishi BL-52.

Action

Tonifies the Kidney-Essence.

Comments

This point is used to tonify the Kidney and specifically, the Kidney-Essence.

HUATUOJIAJI *Hua Tuo Back-filling points*

Location

A group of points on both sides of the spine 0.5 *cun* from the midline in correspondence of the intervertebral spaces from the 1st thoracic to the 5th lumbar vertebra.

Action

It varies according to the location of each point.

Comments

These points are named after the famous doctor *Hua Tuo* who lived during the Han dynasty. It is thought that he used these points as Back Transporting points.

The action of these points is similar to that of the corresponding Back Transporting points. However, they are not often used in this way as the Back Transporting points would be more effective. They are, however, frequently used as local points for backache and are particularly useful to actually correct deviations of vertebrae.

SISHENCONG *Four Mind Hearing*

Location

A group of four points at the vertex, one *cun* from Baihui Du-20 in a cross formation.

Action

Subdue interior Wind.

Comments

These points are mostly used as local points for the treatment of epilepsy.

DINGCHUAN *Stopping asthma*

Location

This point is 0.5 *cun* lateral to Dazhui Du-14.

Action

Expels exterior Wind
Calms asthma.

Comments

This point is mostly used to calm an acute attack of asthma.

SHIQIZHUIXIA *Below the 17th vertebra*

Location

This point is located on the midline of the back below the tip of the 5th lumbar vertebra.

Action

Removes obstructions from the channel
Benefits the back.

Comments

This point is excellent as a local point for the treatment of lower back ache whether the ache is on the midline or bilateral. It is only used if the ache is quite low down on the sacrum or just above it.

JIANNEILING *Inner shoulder mound*

Location

Midway between the end of the anterior axillary fold and Jianyu L.I.-15.

Action

Removes obstructions from the channel
Expels Dampness and Cold.

Comments

This is an extremely useful local point for the treatment of shoulder pain or frozen shoulder. It is only selected if the pain radiates towards the anterior aspect of the shoulder.

DANNANGXUE *Gall-Bladder point*

Location

This point is situated about one *cun* below Yanglingquan G.B.-34. Its location is not fixed as the needle is inserted in the area below G.B.-34 wherever it is tender on pressure.

Action

Resolves Damp-Heat from the Gall-Bladder.

Comments

This point is frequently used (if it is tender on pressure) to expel Damp-Heat from the Gall-Bladder in cholecystitis or cholelithiasis.

LANWEIXUE *Appendix point*

Location

On the Stomach channel in between Zusanli ST-36 and Shangjuxu ST-37, on the right leg only. The location of this point is also variable and it is wherever it is tender on pressure between ST-36 and ST-37.

Action

Stops abdominal pain
Resolves Damp-Heat.

Comments

This point is basically only used in an acute attack of appendicitis to stop pain. It is also a useful diagnostic aid in the diagnosis of appendicitis (including the chronic kind) if it is tender on pressure.

Appendix 1 Identification of Patterns According to the Six Stages[1]

GREATER YANG STAGE

GENERAL CLINICAL MANIFESTATIONS

Fever, aversion to cold, stiff neck, headache, aches in the body and Floating pulse.

ATTACK OF WIND

Fever, aversion to wind, stiff neck, aches in the body, sweating and Floating-Slow pulse.

ATTACK OF COLD

Fever, aversion to cold, stiff neck, headache, severe pains in the body, no sweating, shortness of breath and Floating-Tight pulse.

BRIGHT YANG STAGE

GENERAL CLINICAL MANIFESTATIONS

High fever, profuse sweating, aversion to heat, thirst and Overflowing pulse.

BRIGHT-YANG CHANNEL PATTERN

High fever, profuse sweating, aversion to heat, thirst with a desire to drink cold water, red face, restlessness, Red tongue with a yellow coating and Overflowing-Rapid pulse.

BRIGHT-YANG ORGAN PATTERN

High fever which is worse in the afternoon, profuse sweating, constipation, thirst with a desire to drink cold water, fullness and pain in the abdomen which becomes worse on pressure, restlessness and irritability, in severe cases delirium, Red tongue with a dry, yellow or black coating and Deep-Full pulse.

LESSER YANG STAGE

Alternation of chills and fever, fullness of the costal and hypochondriac regions, lack of appetite, irritability, dry throat, nausea, bitter taste, blurred vision, white-slippery tongue coating on one side only and Wiry pulse.

GREATER YIN STAGE

Abdominal fullness, vomiting, no appetite, diarrhoea, absence of thirst, Pale tongue and Deep-Slow pulse.

LESSER YIN STAGE

LESSER YIN COLD PATTERN

Chills, aversion to cold, listlessness, lethargy, cold limbs, diarrhoea, no thirst or desire to drink warm fluids, abundant-pale urine, Pale tongue and Deep-Fine pulse.

LESSER YIN HEAT PATTERN

Fever, irritability, insomnia, dry mouth and throat, scanty-dark urine, Red tongue without coating and Fine-Rapid pulse.

TERMINAL YIN

Thirst, feeling of energy rising to the chest, pain and feeling of heat in the chest, feeling of hunger with no desire to eat, cold limbs, diarrhoea and vomiting.

NOTES

1 For a more detailed discussion of these subjects please see: Maciocia G. 1987 Tongue Diagnosis in Chinese Medicine, Eastland Press, Seattle, p 131-146.

Appendix 2 Identification of Patterns According to the Four Levels

DEFENSIVE-QI LEVEL

Fever, aversion to cold, headache, slight sweating, runny nose with yellow discharge, slight thirst, sore throat, red and swollen tonsils, Red sides or tip of the tongue, Floating-Rapid pulse.

QI LEVEL

High fever, aversion to heat, cough with expectoration of thin-yellow sputum, asthma, thirst, Red tongue with thick-yellow coating, Slippery-Rapid pulse.

NUTRITIVE-QI LEVEL

Fever at night, dry mouth with no desire to drink, insomnia, mental restlessness, aphasia, spots on skin, in severe cases coma, Deep-Red tongue, Fine-Rapid pulse.

BLOOD LEVEL

High fever, skin eruptions, vomiting of blood, epistaxis, blood in stools, blood in urine, manic behaviour, in severe cases convulsions, Deep-Red tongue without coating, Wiry-Rapid pulse.

Appendix 3 Identification of Patterns According to the Three Burners

UPPER BURNER

WIND-HEAT INVADING THE LUNGS

The clinical manifestations of this pattern are the same as the Defensive Qi Level of the 4 Level patterns.

HEAT IN THE LUNGS

Fever, sweating, cough, asthma, thirst, stuffiness and pain in the chest, Red tongue with yellow tongue coating and Rapid pulse (this pattern corresponds to a Qi-Level pattern from the point of view of 4-Level Pattern Identification).

HEAT IN THE PERICARDIUM

Fever, burning sensation in the epigastrium, cold limbs, delirium, aphasia, stiff tongue, Deep-Red tongue without coating, Fine-Rapid pulse (this pattern corresponds to a Nutritive Qi-Level pattern from the points of view of 4-Level Pattern Identification).

MIDDLE BURNER

HEAT IN THE BRIGHT YANG

The clinical manifestations are the same as in the Bright Yang Organ pattern of the 6-Stage patterns.

DAMP-HEAT INVADING THE SPLEEN

Aversion to cold, slight fever which is worse in the afternoon, feeling of heaviness of head or of the whole body, fullness of the chest and epigastrium, nausea, vomiting, white-sticky tongue coating, Soft and Slow pulse.

LOWER BURNER

Low-grade fever in the afternoon, hot palms and soles, dry mouth, lassitude, deafness, in severe cases convulsions, Deep-Red tongue without coating, Fine-Rapid pulse.

Glossary of Chinese terms

General

丹田	*Dan Tian*	Field of Elixir
寸	*Cun*	*Cun* (acupuncture unit of measurement)

Symptoms

本	*Ben*	Root
鼻渊	*Bi Yuan*	'Nose pool' (sinusitis)
标	*Biao*	Manifestation
喘	*Chuan*	Breathlessness
积	*Ji*	Blood masses
结	*Jie*	Accumulation (or nodules)
聚	*Ju*	Qi masses
厥	*Jue*	Breakdown
口疮	*Kou Chuang*	Mouth ulcers
里急	*Li Ji*	Internal urgency (or tension of lining)
满	*Man*	Feeling of fullness
闷	*Men*	Feeling of oppression
逆经	*Ni Jing*	Reverse period
痞	*Pi*	Feeling of stuffiness
热毒	*Re Du*	Toxic Heat
实	*Shi*	Full, Fullness, Excess
胎气上逆	*Tai Qi Shang Ni*	Fetus's Qi rebelling upwards
脱	*Tuo*	Collapse
哮	*Xiao*	Wheezing
心烦	*Xin Fan*	Mental restlessness
虚	*Xu*	Empty, Emptiness, Deficiency
胀	*Zhang*	Feeling of distension

Disease-symptoms

崩漏	*Beng Lou*	Flooding and Trickling
闭经	*Bi Jing*	No Periods

痹证 *Bi Zheng*	Painful Obstruction Syndrome
膏淋 *Gao Lin*	Sticky Painful-Urination Syndrome
经间期出血 *Jing Jian Qi Chu Xue*	Bleeding between Periods
经期延长 *Jing Qi Yan Chang*	Long Periods
厥证 *Jue Zheng*	Breakdown Syndrome
劳淋 *Lao Lin*	Fatigue Painful-Urination Syndrome
淋证 *Lin Zheng*	Painful-Urination Syndrome
气淋 *Qi Lin*	Qi Painful-Urination Syndrome
热淋 *Re Lin*	Heat Painful-Urination Syndrome
石淋 *Shi Lin*	Stone Painful-Urination Syndrome
痿证 *Wei Zheng*	Atrophy Syndrome
温病 *Wen Bing*	Warm disease
虚劳 *Xu Lao*	Exhaustion
血淋 *Xue Lin*	Blood Painful-Urination Syndrome
月经过多 *Yue Jing Guo Duo*	Heavy Periods
月经过少 *Yue Jing Guo Shao*	Scanty Periods
月经后期 *Yue Jing Hou Qi*	Late Periods
月经先后无定期 *Yue Jing Xian Hou Wu Ding Qi*	Irregular Periods
月经先期 *Yue Jing Xian Qi*	Early Periods
中风 *Zhong Feng*	Wind-stroke
子淋 *Zi Lin*	Painful-Urination Syndrome of Pregnancy
子悬 *Zi Xuan*	Feeling of Suffocation in Pregnancy
子音 *Zi Yin*	Aphonia of Pregnancy
子晕 *Zi Yun*	Dizziness of Pregnancy
子肿 *Zi Zhong*	Oedema of Pregnancy

Vital substances

后天之气 *Hou Tian Zhi Qi*	Post-Natal Qi
魂 *Hun*	Ethereal Soul
精 *Jing*	Essence
君火 *Jun Huo*	Emperor Fire
命门 *Ming Men*	Gate of Life
命门火 *Ming Men Huo*	Fire of the Gate of Life
魄 *Po*	Corporeal Soul
神 *Shen*	Mind or Spirit
天癸 *Tian Gui*	Heavenly *Gui*
卫气 *Wei Qi*	Defensive Qi
先天之气 *Xian Tian Zhi Qi*	Pre-Natal Qi
相火 *Xiang Huo*	Minister Fire
意 *Yi*	Intellect
营气 *Ying Qi*	Nutritive Qi
原气 *Yuan Qi*	Original Qi
真气 *Zhen Qi*	True Qi
正气 *Zheng Qi*	Upright Qi
志 *Zhi*	Will-Power
中气 *Zhong Qi*	Central Qi
宗气 *Zong Qi*	Gathering Qi (of the chest)

Emotions

悲	*Bei*	Sadness
惊	*Jing*	Shock
恐	*Kong*	Fear
怒	*Nu*	Anger
思	*Si*	Pensiveness
喜	*Xi*	Joy
忧	*You*	Worry

Channels and points

胞络	*Bao Luo*	Uterus Channel
胞脉	*Bao Mai*	Uterus Vessel
别脉	*Bie Mai*	Divergent channels
冲脉	*Chong Mai*	Penetrating Vessel
腠理	*Cou Li*	Space between skin and muscles
带脉	*Dai Mai*	Girdle Vessel
督脉	*Du Mai*	Governing Vessel
会穴	*Hui Xue*	Gathering point
厥阴	*Jue Yin*	Terminal Yin
络脉（穴）	*Luo Mai (Xue)*	Connecting (point or channel)
幕穴	*Mu Xue*	Front-Collecting points
任脉	*Ren Mai*	Directing Vessel
少阳	*Shao Yang*	Lesser Yang
少阴	*Shao Yin*	Lesser Yin
（背）俞穴	*(Bei) Shu Xue*	Back-Transporting points
太阳	*Tai Yang*	Greater Yang
太阴	*Tai Yin*	Greater Yin
五输穴	*Wu Shu Xue*	Five Transporting points
郗穴	*Xi Xue*	Accumulation point
阳明	*Yang Ming*	Bright Yang
阳跷脉	*Yang Qiao Mai*	Yang Heel Vessel
阳维脉	*Yang Wei Mai*	Yang Linking Vessel
阴跷脉	*Yin Qiao Mai*	Yin Heel Vessel
阴维脉	*Yin Wei Mai*	Yin Linking Vessel
原穴	*Yuan Xue*	Source point

Pulse positions

尺	*Chi*	Rear (pulse position)
寸	*Cun*	Front (pulse position)
关	*Guan*	Middle (pulse position)

Pulse qualities

长	*Chang*	Long
沉	*Chen*	Deep
迟	*Chi*	Slow
促	*Cu*	Hasty

大 *Da*	Big
代 *Dai*	Irregular or Intermittent
动 *Dong*	Moving
短 *Duan*	Short
浮 *Fu*	Floating
伏 *Fu*	Hidden
革 *Ge*	Leather
洪 *Hong*	Overflowing
滑 *Hua*	Slippery
缓 *Huan*	Slowed-Down
急 *Ji*	Hurried
结 *Jie*	Knotted
紧 *Jin*	Tight
芤 *Kou*	Hollow
劳 *Lao*	Firm
濡 *Ru*	Weak-Floating
软 *Ruan*	Weak-Floating
弱 *Ruo*	Weak
散 *San*	Scattered
涩 *Se*	Choppy
实 *Shi*	Full
数 *Shu*	Rapid
微 *Wei*	Minute
细 *Xi*	Fine
弦 *Xian*	Wiry
虚 *Xu*	Empty

Methods of treatment

安胎 *An Tai*	Calm the Fetus
补 *Bu*	Tonify (or reinforce as a needle technique)
攻瘀 *Gong Yu*	Dispel stasis (of Blood)
固 *Gu*	Consolidate
固脱 *Gu Tuo*	Consolidate Collapse
化湿 *Hua Shi*	Resolve Dampness
化痰 *Hua Tan*	Resolve Phlegm
化瘀 *Hua Yu*	Eliminate stasis (of Blood)
缓急 *Huan Ji*	Moderate urgency
活血 *Huo Xue*	Invigorate Blood
解表 *Jie (Biao)*	Release (the Exterior)
解郁 *Jie Yu*	Eliminate stagnation (of Qi)
理气 *Li Qi*	Move Qi
利湿 *Li Shi*	Resolve Dampness
利水 *Li Shui*	Transform Water
平肝 *Ping Gan*	Calm the Liver
破血 *Po Xue*	Break-up Blood
清热 *Qing (Re)*	Clear Heat
祛风 *Qu (Feng)*	Expel (external Wind)
祛瘀 *Qu Yu*	Eliminate stasis (of Blood)

散寒 *San Han*	Scatter Cold
散结 *San Jie*	Dissipate accumulation, or dissipate nodules
生新 *Sheng Xin*	Promote healing of tissues
疏肝 *Shu (Gan)*	Pacify (the Liver)
调和营卫 *Tiao He Ying Wei*	Harmonize Nutritive and Defensive Qi
调经 *Tiao Jing*	Regulate the period
通络 *Tong Luo*	Remove obstructions from the Connecting channels
通窍 *Tong Qiao*	Open the orifices
通乳 *Tong Ru*	Remove obstructions from the breast's Connecting channels
温经 *Wen Jing*	Warm the menses
熄风 *Xi Feng*	Extinguish Wind (internal)
泻 *Xie*	Reduce (as a needle technique)
泄 *Xie*	Clear (Heat)
泻 *Xie*	Drain (Fire)
泻下 *Xie Xia*	Move downwards
辛开苦降 *Xin Kai Ku Jiang*	Use pungent herbs to open and bitter ones to make Qi descend
宣肺 *Xuan Fei*	Restore the diffusing of Lung-Qi
养血 *Yang (Xue)*	Nourish (Blood)

Pathogenic factors

风寒 *Feng Han*	Wind-Cold
风热 *Feng Re*	Wind-Heat
寒 *Han*	Cold
火 *Huo*	Fire
热 *Re*	Heat
热毒 *Re Du*	Toxic Heat
湿 *Shi*	Dampness
暑 *Shu*	Summer-Heat
痰 *Tan*	Phlegm
痰饮 *Tan Yin*	Phlegm-Fluids
燥 *Zao*	Dryness

Bibliography

ANCIENT CLASSICS

1 1979 The Yellow Emperor's Classic of Internal Medicine-Simple Questions (*Huang Ti Nei Jing Su Wen* 黄帝内经素问). People's Health Publishing House, Beijing, first published c. 100 BC.
2 1981 Spiritual Axis (*Ling Shu Jing* 灵枢经). People's Health Publishing House, Beijing, first published c. 100 BC.
3 Nanjing College of Traditional Chinese Medicine 1979 A Revised Explanation of the Classic of Difficulties (*Nan Jing Jiao Shi* 难经校释). People's Health Publishing House, Beijing, first published c. AD 100.
4 Hua Tuo 1985 The Classic of the Secret Transmission (*Zhong Cang Jing* 中藏经). Jiangsu Scientific Publishing House, first published c. AD 198.
5 Nanjing College of Traditional Chinese Medicine, Shang Han Lun Research Group 1980 Discussion on Cold-induced Diseases (*Shang Han Lun* 伤寒论) by Zhang Zhong Jing, Shanghai Scientific Publishing House, Shanghai, first published c. AD 220.
6 1981 Discussion of Prescriptions of the Golden Chest (*Jin Gui Yao Lue Fang Lun* 金匮要略方论). Zhejiang Scientific Publishing House, Zhejiang, first published c. AD 220.
7 Yang Ji Zhou 1980 Compendium of Acupuncture (*Zhen Jiu Da Cheng* 针灸大成). People's Health Publishing House, Beijing, first published in 1601.
8 Zhang Jie Bin (also called Zhang Jing Yue) 1982 Classic of Categories (*Lei Jing* 类经). People's Health Publishing House, Beijing, first published in 1624.
9 Zhang Jing Yue 1986 Complete Book of Jing Yue (*Jing Yue Quan Shu* 景岳全书). Shangai Scientific Publishing House, Shanghai, first published 1634.
10 Tang Zong Hai 1979 Discussion on Blood (*Xue Zheng Lun* 血证论). People's Health Publishing House, first published 1884.

MODERN TEXTS

1 Gu He Dao 1979 History of Chinese Medicine (*Zhong Guo Yi Xue Shi Lue* 中国医学史略). Shanxi People's Publishing House, Taiyuan.
2 1981 Syndromes and Treatment of the Internal Organs (*Zang Fu Zheng Zhi* 脏腑证治). Tianjin Scientific Publishing House, Tianjin.Scientific Publishing House, Tianjin.
3 1980 Concise Dictionary of Chinese Medicine (*Jian Ming Zhong Yi Ci Dian* 简明中医辞典). People's Health Publishing House, Beijing.
4 1983 Selected Historical Theories of Chinese Medicine (*Zhong Yi Li Dai Yi Lun Xuan* 中医历代医论选). Shandong Scientific Publishing House, Jinan.
5 1978 Fundamentals of Chinese Medicine (*Zhong Yi Ji Chu Xue* 中医基础学) Shandong Scientific Publishing House, Jinan.
6 1979 Patterns and Treatment of Kidney Diseases (*Shen Yu Shen Bing de Zheng Zhi* 肾与肾病的证治). Hebei People's Publishing House, Hebei.
7 Guangdong College of Traditional Chinese Medicine 1964 A Study of Diagnosis in Chinese Medicine (*Zhong Yi Zhen Duan Xue* 中医诊断学). Shanghai Scientific Publishing House, Shanghai.
8 Nanjing College of Traditional Chinese Medicine 1978 A Study of Warm Diseases (*Wen Bing Xue* 温病学). Shanghai Scientific Publishing House, Shanghai.
9 Li Wen Chuan, He Bao Yi 1987 Practical Acupuncture (*Shi Yong Zhen Jiu Xue* 实用针灸学). People's Health Publishing House, Beijing.
10 Zhai Ming Yi 1979 Clinical Chinese Medicine (*Zhong Yi Lin Chuang Ji Chu* 中医临床基础). Henan Publishing House, Henan.
11 Li Shi Zhen 1985 Clinical Application of Frequently Used Acupuncture Points (*Chang Yong Shu Xue Lin Chuang Fa Hui* 常用腧穴临床发挥). People's Health Publishing House, Beijing.
12 Shan Yu Dang 1984 Selection of Acupuncture Point Combinations from the Discussion on Cold-induced Diseases (*Shang Han Lun Zhen Jiu Pei Xue Xuan Zhu* 伤寒论针灸配穴选注). People's Health Publishing House, Beijing.
13 Ji Jie Yin 1984 Clinical Records of Tai Yi Shen Acupuncture (*Tai Yi Shen Zhen Jiu Lin Zheng Lu* 太乙神针灸临证录). Shanxi Province Scientific Publishing House, Shanxi.

14 Zhang Cheng Xing, and Qi Jin 1984 An Explanation of the Meaning of Acupunture Point Names (*Jing Xue Shi Yi Hui Jie* 经穴释义汇解) Shanghai Translations Publishing Company, Shanghai.
15 Zhang Shan Chen 1982 Essential Collection of Acupuncture Points from the ABC of Acupuncture (*Zhen Jiu Jia Yi Jing Shu Xue Zhong Ji* 针灸甲乙经腧穴重辑). Shandong Scientific Publishing House, Shandong.
16 Beijing College of Traditional Chinese Medicine 1980 Practical Chinese Medicine (*Shi Yong Zhong Yi Xue* 实用中医学). Beijing Publishing House, Beijing.
17 Anwei College of Traditional Chinese Medicine 1979 Clinical Manual of Chinese (*Zhong Yi Lin Chuang Shou Li* 中医临床手册). Anwei Scientific Publishing House, Anwei.
18 Zhang Yuan Ji 1985 Meng He Medical Collection of Four Doctors (*Meng He Si Jia Yi Ti* 孟河四家医集). Jiangsu Province Scientific Publishing House, Nanjing.
19 Zhang Shan You 1980 An Explanation of Passages Concerning Acupuncture from the Yellow Emperor's Classic of Internal Medicine (*Nei Jing Zhen Jiu Lei Fang Yu Shi* 内经针灸类方语释). Shandong Scientific Publishing House, Shandong.
20 Anwei College of Traditional Chinese Medicine and Shanghai College of Traditional Chinese Medicine 1987 **Dictionary of Acupunture (*Zhen Jiu Xue Ci Dian*** 针灸学辞典). Shanghai Scientific Publishing House, Shanghai.
21 Xu Ben Ren 1986 Clinical Acupuncture (*Lin Chuang Zhen Jiu Xue* 临床针灸学). Liaoning Scientific Publishing House, Liaoning.

Index